Development of the Gastrointestinal Tract

Development of the Gastrointestinal Tract

Ian R. Sanderson, MD, FRCPCH
Professor of Paediatric Gastroenterology
St. Bartholomew's and the Royal London School
of Medicine and Dentistry
Queen Mary and Westfield College
University of London
Honorary Consultant Paediatric Gastroenterologist
Royal Hospitals Trust
London, United Kingdom

W. Allan Walker, MD
Conrad Taff Professor of Nutrition and Pediatrics
Harvard Medical School
Director, Developmental Gastroenterology Laboratory
Massachusetts General Hospital
Chief, Combined Program in Pediatric Gastroenterology and Nutrition
Children's Hospital and Massachusetts General Hospital
Boston, Massachusetts

2000
B.C. *Decker* Inc.
Hamilton • London • Saint Louis

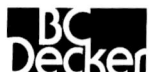

B.C. Decker Inc.
4 Hughson Street South
P.O. Box 620, L.C.D. 1
Hamilton, Ontario L8N 3K7
Tel: 905-522-7017; 1-800-568-7281
Fax: 905-522-7839
E-mail: info@bcdecker.com
Website: http://www.bcdecker.com

© 1999 Ian R. Sanderson, W. Allan Walker *Development of the Gastrointestinal Tract*

All rights reserved. No part of this publication may be reproduced, stored in a retrieval system, or transmitted, in any form or by any means, electronic, mechanical, photocopying, recording, or otherwise, without prior written permission from the publisher.

99 00 01 02 03 / EB / 6 5 4 3 2 1

Cover illustration by Gino Maulucci; adapted with permission from Glen Reid's The Forgut in Moore KL. *The Developing Human: Clinically Oriented Embryology. 6th ed.* Philadelphia W.B. Saunders; 1998.

ISBN 1–55009–081–X
Printed in Canada

Sales and Distribution

United States
B.C. Decker Inc.
P.O. Box 785
Lewiston, NY U.S.A. 14092-0785
Tel: 905-522-7017/1-800-568-7281
Fax: 905-522-7839
e-mail: info@bcdecker.com

Canada
B.C. Decker Inc.
4 Hughson Street South
P.O. Box 620, L.C.D. 1
Hamilton, Ontario L8N 3K7
Tel: 905-522-7017/1-800-568-7281
Fax: 905-522-7839
e-mail: info@bcdecker.com
website: http://www.bcdecker.com

Japan
Igaku-Shoin Ltd.
Foreign Publications Department
3-24-17 Hongo, Bunkyo-ku,
Tokyo 113-8719, Japan
Tel: 3 3817 5676
Fax: 3 3815 6776
e-mail: fmbook@ba2.so-net.or.jp

U.K., Europe, Scandinavia, Middle East
Blackwell Science Ltd.
Osney Mead
Oxford OX2 0EL
United Kingdom
Tel: 44-1865-206206
Fax: 44-1865-721205
e-mail: info@blackwell-science.com

Australia
Blackwell Science Asia Pty, Ltd.
54 University Street
Carlton, Victoria 3053
Australia
Tel: 03 9347 0300
Fax: 03 9349 3016
e-mail: info@blacksci.asia.com.au

South Korea
Seoul Medical Scientific Books Co.
C.P.O. Box 9794
Seoul 100-697
Seoul, Korea
Tel: 82-2925-5800
Fax: 82-2927-7283

South America
Ernesto Reichmann, Distribuidora de Livros Ltda.
Rua Coronel Marques
335-Tatuape, 03440-000
Sao Paulo-SP-Brazil
Tel/Fax: 011-218-2122

Foreign Rights
John Scott & Co.
International Publishers' Agency
P.O. Box 878
Kimberton, PA 19442
Tel: 610-827-1640
Fax: 610-827-1671

Notice: The authors and publisher have made every effort to ensure that the patient care recommended herein, including choice of drugs and drug dosages, is in accord with the accepted standard and practice at the time of publication. However, since research and regulation constantly change clinical standards, the reader is urged to check the product information sheet included in the package of each drug, which includes recommended doses, warnings, and contraindications. This is particularly important with new or infrequently used drugs.

Contributors

Ingegerd Adlerberth, MD, PhD
Department of Clinical Immunology
Göteborg University
Göteborg, Sweden

Yuriko Adkins, BS
Graduate Student, Department of Nutrition
University of California
Davis, California

John A. Barnard, MD
Associate Professor of Pediatrics
Vanderbilt University School of Medicine
Vanderbilt Children's Hospital
Nashville, Tennessee

Kenneth W. Beagley, PhD
Discipline of Immunology and Microbiology
The University of Newcastle
Callaghan, New South Wales, Australia

Charles L. Bevins, MD, PhD
Departments of Immunology,
Gastroenterology and Colo-rectal Surgery
Lerner Research Institute
The Cleveland Clinic Foundation
Cleveland, Ohio

W. Michael Bisset, MD, FRCPCH
Honorary Senior Lecturer
University of Aberdeen
Consultant Paediatric Gastroenterologist
Royal Aberdeen Children's Hospital
Aberdeen, United Kingdom

Randal K. Buddington, PhD
Professor in Biological Sciences
Mississippi State University
College of Veterinary Medicine
Mississippi State, Mississippi

David Calnek, PhD
Research Associate
Division of Pulmonary/Critical Care Medicine
Indiana University Medical Center
Indianapolis, Indiana

James E. Casanova, PhD
Assistant Professor of Pediatrics
Harvard Medical School
Combined Program in Pediatric Gastroenterology
  and Nutrition
Massachusetts General Hospital
Boston, Massachusetts

Elmer S. David, MD
Assistant Professor in Pediatrics
UMDNJ-New Jersey Medical School
Attending Neonatologist, The University Hospital
St. Michael's Medical Center
Newark, New Jersey

Ronaldo P. Ferraris, PhD
Associate Professor in Pharmacology and Physiology
UMDNJ-New Jersey Medical School
Department of Nutritional Sciences
Rutgers University
Newark, New Jersey

Jean-Noel Freund, PhD
INSERM U381
Strasbourg, France

Margit Hamosh, PhD
Professor of Pediatrics
Georgetown University Medical Center
Washington, DC

Paul Hamosh, PhD
Professor of Physiology and Biophysics
Georgetown University Medical Center
Washington, DC

Lars Åke Hanson, MD, PhD
Physician-in-Chief
Professor of Clinical Immunology
University of Göteborg
Göteborg, Sweden

Duncan Howie, PhD
Department of Paediatric Gastroenterology
St. Bartholomew's and the Royal London School
  of Medicine and Dentistry
London, United Kingdom

Michèle Kedinger, PhD
INSERM U381
Strasbourg, France

Jean-Francois Launay, PhD
INSERM U381
Strasbourg, France

Bo Lönnerdal, PhD
Professor of Nutrition and Internal Medicine
University of California
Davis, California

Thomas T. MacDonald, PhD, FRCPath
Professor of Mucosal Immunology
Department of Paediatric Gastroenterology
St. Bartholomew's and the Royal London School
  of Medicine and Dentistry
London, United Kingdom

Peter J. Milla, MSc, MBBS, FRCPCH
Professor of Paediatric Gastroenterology and Nutrition
University College London
Great Ormond Street Hospital for Sick Children
London, United Kingdom

Alan N. Mayer, MD, PhD
Instructor of Pediatrics
Harvard Medical School
Research Associate in Pediatric Gastroenterology
Combined Program in Pediatric Gastroenterology
 and Nutrition
Children's Hospital and Massachusetts General Hospital
Boston, Massachusetts

Dipa Natarajan, PhD
Postdoctoral Research Fellow
Division of Developmental Neurobiology
Medical Research Council
National Institute for Medical Research
London, United Kingdom

Andre J. Ouellette, PhD
Professor of Pathology and Microbiology
 and Molecular Genetics
College of Medicine
University of California
Irvine, California

Vassilis Pachnis, MD, PhD
Division of Developmental Neurobiology
Medical Research Council
National Institute for Medical Research
London, United Kingdom

D. Brent Polk, MD
Associate Professor of Pediatrics
Vanderbilt University School of Medicine
Vanderbilt Children's Hospital
Nashville, Tennessee

Andrea Quaroni, PhD
Professor of Physiology
Cornell University
Ithaca, New York

Alistair J. Ramsay, PhD
John Curtin School of Medical Research
Australian National University
Canberra, Australia

Drucilla J. Roberts, MD
Assistant Professor of Pathology
Harvard Medical School
Assistant Pathologist, Massachusetts General Hospital
Boston, Massachusetts

Ian R. Sanderson, MD, FRCPCH
Professor of Paediatric Gastroenterology
St. Bartholomew's and the Royal London School
 of Medicine and Dentistry
Queen Mary and Westfield College
University of London
Honorary Consultant Paediatric Gastroenterologist
Royal Hospitals Trust
London, United Kingdom

Tor C. Savidge, PhD
Assistant Professor of Pediatrics
Harvard Medical School
Developmental Gastroenterology Laboratory
Combined Program in Pediatric Gastroenterology
 and Nutrition
Massachusetts General Hospital
Boston, Massachusetts

Uzma Shah, MD
Instructor in Pediatrics,
Harvard Medical School
Research Associate, Developmental Gastroenterology
 Laboratory
Combined Program in Pediatric Gastroeneterology
 and Nutrition
Massachusetts General Hospital
Boston, Massachusetts

Patricia Simon-Assmann, PhD
INSERM U381
Strasbourg, France

Peter G. Traber, MD
Professor and Chair, Department of Medicine
University of Pennsylvania
Philadelphia, Pennsylvania

W. Allan Walker, MD
Conrad Taff Professor of Nutrition and Pediatrics
Harvard Medical School
Director, Developmental Gastroenterology Laboratory
Massachusetts General Hospital
Chief, Combined Program in Pediatric Gastroenterology
 and Nutrition
Children's Hospital and Massachusetts General Hospital
Boston, Massachusetts

Daniel A. Wiginton, PhD
Associate Professor, Department of Pediatrics
University of Cincinnati
Cincinnati, Ohio

Jean M. Wilson, PhD
Associate Professor
Department of Cell Biology and Anatomy
College of Medicine, University of Arizona
Tucson, Arizona

David L. Wingate, DM, FRCP
Professor of Gastrointestinal Science
Director, Gastrointestinal Research Unit
St. Bartholomew's and the Royal London Medical School
Consultant Gastroenterologist, Royal London Hospital
London, United Kingdom

Agnes E. Wold, MD, PhD
Department of Clinical Immunology, Göteborg University
Laboratory of Clinical Immunology, Sahlgren's University
Göteborg, Sweden

Preface

The evolution of multiorgan animals resulted from the specialization of certain cells acting as an epithelium dividing the outside world from the interior of the animal. This epithelium protected the animal from external harmful agents. Part of the epithelium, however, maintained the ability to absorb nutrients and to dominate the microenvironment close to its surface. The formation of the absorptive epithelium into a tube, its "outside world" now being a lumen, is the key to the ability of the epithelium to control its surroundings. The central importance of this evolutionary step is demonstrated by the presence of the gastrointestinal tract in all the species in the animal kingdom excepting sponges, jelly fish, and sea anemones. It predated the development of the spinal cord or neuronal cells by hundreds of millions of years.

During ontogeny, a simple fertilized egg must divide into cells that, to some extent, recapitulate this evolutionary success. In the human, the basic structure of the gut is formed soon after the beginning of organogenesis. Differentiation of cells into epithelial cells and their maturation for extrauterine life then ensues, followed by the changes necessary for extrauterine life and, finally, those changes necessary for adaptation to weaning and a normal adult diet.

The gastrointestinal tract contains a wide variety of cell types. These include epithelial cells, nerve cells, muscle cells, stromal cells, and immune cells. In addition, the fully functioning intestine surrounds a complex milieu of nutrients, growth factors, and bacteria. A study of the development of the gastrointestinal tract requires a coordinated study of many different disciplines, each examining a particular aspect. This textbook includes chapters representing each of these important areas. Each article describes one facet of the intestinal tract. The authors have not only reviewed their own field but also have related them to gastrointestinal development generally. The editors hope that publishing the current knowledge of the development of the gastrointestinal tract will result in new areas of study, which may eventually enhance the treatment of gastrointestinal disease. Intestinal failure in children results from a number of disorders that include the decreased absorptive capacity of the epithelial cell, the loss of motility and peristalsis, and the dysfunction of the intestinal tract as a whole. A better understanding of the genetic development of the gut provides us with a clearer insight into inherited diseases leading to severe disruption in the functioning of the gut and may provide the basis for future approaches to therapy. Replacement of epithelial cells with stem cell transplants or smooth muscle and/or neuronal cells presents therapeutic options that are currently a "pipe dream." Yet, it is our hope that understanding the development of the gastrointestinal tract will eventually enable researchers to realize these difficult goals.

Development of the Gastrointestinal Tract is relevant to developmental biologists, pediatric gastroenterologists, and gastroenterologists with an interest in gastrointestinal development. Each chapter author has emphasized three considerations. First, the mechanisms (both in terms of cell biology and molecular biology) of their field have been described and areas of further research have been suggested. Second, the information has been made relevant to an understanding of recognized disorders of gastrointestinal development that are encountered by pediatric gastroenterologists. Third, each author has been careful to include some background of their field.

We wish to thank our many authors for sharing their special expertise. By developing a specific format for the textbook and selecting the most appropriate authors in their fields, we have provided the most comprehensive and up-to-date text on the development of the gastrointestinal tract currently available.

We would like to thank Suzzette McCarron for her organizational talents and Jacqui Jenkins for her help in securing close communications between Boston and London.

The editors are also grateful to Brian Decker and to the staff of B.C. Decker Inc. for their help and support in developing and publishing this book.

Ian R. Sanderson, MD, FRCPCH
W. Allan Walker, MD
August 1999

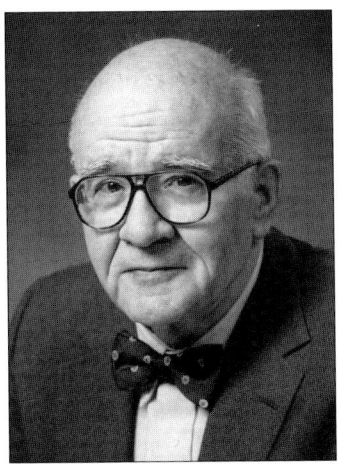

This book is dedicated to **Otakar Koldovsky, MD, PhD,** who died on April 5, 1998. Dr. Koldovsky's primary research interest was the development of the gastrointestinal tract; he published over 200 peer-reviewed articles and book chapters. In 1969, he wrote a single-author textbook titled *Development of the Functions of the Small Intestine in Mammals and Man*. In addition, he was responsible for the training of many students and young scientists.

Dr. Koldovsky was born in Prague, Czechoslovakia, the son of an ophthalmologist. He received his medical training at Charles University, Prague, and received a doctoral degree at the Institute of Physiology, Czechoslovak Academy of Sciences. It was in Czechoslovakia that his investigation of the development of the gastrointestinal tract began. In 1968, Dr. Koldovsky emigrated to the United States and took a Research Associate's position at Stanford University. He later moved to Philadelphia, where he remained for 11 years, and served as a faculty member at the University of Pennsylvania. At these institutions, he studied the biochemical and anatomic changes that occur during the ontogeny of the gastrointestinal tract, including the role of specific hormones such as steroids and thyroxin. In 1980, he moved to Tucson, Arizona, to become Professor at the University of Arizona College of Medicine. His recent research focused on breast milk composition, especially the effect of milk-borne growth factors on the development of the gastrointestinal tract.

Dr. Koldovsky was the recipient of many awards and honors, including the American Academy of Pediatrics Nutrition Award and the Harry Shwachman Award in Pediatric Gastroenterology and Nutrition. He will be greatly missed both as a scientist and as a human being.

Contents

1. Embryology of the Gastrointestinal Tract ...1
   Drucilla J. Roberts, MD

2. Gene Regulation: The Key to Intestinal Development ...13
   Daniel A. Wiginton, PhD

3. Hormones and Growth Factors in Intestinal Development ...37
   D. Brent Polk, MD, John A. Barnard, MD

4. Role of Cytokeratins in Epithelial Cell Development ...57
   Andrea Quaroni, PhD, David Calnek, PhD

5. Development of Endocytosis in the Intestinal Epithelium ...71
   Jean M. Wilson, PhD, James E. Casanova, PhD

6. Cell Interactions through the Basement Membrane in Intestinal Development and Differentiation ...83
   Michèle Kedinger, PhD, Jean-Noel Freund, PhD, Jean-Francois Launay, PhD, Patricia Simon-Assmann, PhD

7. Development of Brushborder Enzyme Activity ...103
   Peter G. Traber, MD

8. Ontogeny of Nutrient Transporters ...123
   Ronaldo P. Ferraris, PhD, Randal K. Buddington, PhD, Elmer S. David, MD

9. Development of Innate Immunity in the Small Intestine ...147
   Andre J. Ouellette, PhD, Charles L. Bevins, MD, PhD

10. Ontogeny of T Lymphocytes within the Human Intestine ...165
    Duncan Howie, PhD, Thomas T. MacDonald, PhD, FRCPath

11. Development of B Lymphocytes within the Mucosal Immune System ...175
    Alistair J. Ramsay, PhD, Kenneth W. Beagley, PhD

12. Development of the Enteric Nervous System ...197
    Dipa Natarajan, PhD, Vassilis Pachnis, MD, PhD

13. Gastrointestinal Motor Activity in the Fetus and Newborn ...211
    W. Michael Bisset, MD, FRCPCH, David L. Wingate, DM, FRCP, Peter J. Milla, MSc, MBBS, FRCPCH

14. Developmental Changes in Breast Milk Protein Composition during Lactation ...227
    Bo Lönnerdal, PhD, Yuriko Adkins, BS

15. Role of the Intestinal Lumen in the Ontogeny of the Gastrointestinal Tract 245
    Uzma Shah, MD, Ian R. Sanderson, MD, FRCPCH

16. Development of Digestive Enzyme Secretion 261
    Margit Hamosh, PhD, Paul Hamosh, MD

17. Ontogeny of the Intestinal Flora 279
    Ingegerd Adlerberth, MB, PhD, Lars Åke Hanson, MD, PhD, Agnes E. Wold, MD, PhD

18. Genetic Models of Gastrointestinal Development 293
    Alan N. Mayer, MD, PhD, W. Allan Walker, MD

19. Ectopic Transplantation Techniques for Evaluating Gastrointestinal Development 307
    Tor C. Savidge, PhD

Index 319

CHAPTER 1

Embryology of the Gastrointestinal Tract

Drucilla J. Roberts, MD

The gastrointestinal (GI) system is an early evolutionary innovation. The primitive tubular organism developed a tube within a tube, thus providing the ability to store and digest nutrients. The use of an internalized digestive system released the organism from developmental constraints on body size, and facilitated its ability to evolve other differentiated structures and systems. The GI system is also one of the first to polarize the embryo by forming an entry and exit to this system. This produced a patterned body plan, with an anterior and posterior (AP) axis (also known as the cranial-caudal axis).

The luminal part of the vertebrate GI system, the gut, is critical not only in its function as a digestive organ; embryologically, the gut endoderm is an essential collaborator in the formation of the heart[1–5] and in providing the anlage and signals to form the many gut-derived organs, including the thyroid, lungs, liver, and pancreas. Gut derivatives are formed by epithelial-mesenchymal (EM) interactions directing budding morphogenesis along the dorsal-ventral (DV) axis of the gut. In addition to the AP and DV axes, the gut has a coronal (cross-sectional) axis, in which there are differences in epithelial morphology and cytodifferentiation (the crypt-to-villus [CV] axis). This axis continues its growth and development into adult life. The AP and DV axes of the gut tube (without derivatives) are more or less symmetrical about their axes but with folding of the gut into the body cavity and differentiation of the AP regions of the gut, a distinct asymmetry evolves between left and right sides. How the gut tube rotates and folds is a complex area to study but has recently been tackled, with some interesting results. The embryogenesis of the vertebrate gut tube and the molecular controls of its pattern in the AP, DV, and LR axes will be reviewed in this chapter (Figure 1–1).

EARLY FORMATION OF THE GUT TUBE

Gut epithelium is derived from the ectoderm and endoderm. The origin of the smooth muscle of the gut wall is lateral plate-derived splanchnic mesenchyme. Most of the gut is composed of definitive endoderm and splanchnic mesoderm in a tube-like arrangement. The epithelium in the most anterior region of the gut (the mouth) and the most posterior region (the anus) is derived from ectoderm. The rest of the epithelial lining of the gut is formed from the endoderm. This chapter will focus on gut development of the endodermal-derived regions.

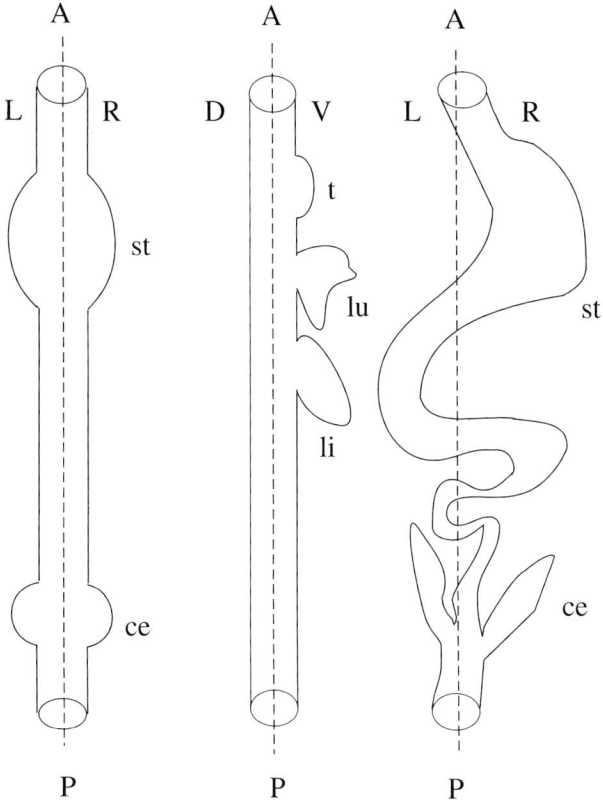

FIGURE 1–1A. Diagram of the axes of the gut. The anterior (A) and posterior (P) axes (*left*); dorsal (D) and ventral (V) axes (*middle*); and right (R) and left (L) axes (*right*) of the gut at approximately E4 in the chick. In humans and other bipedal vertebrates, the AP axis and the superior-inferior axis (or cranial-caudal axis) are the same.
st = stomach; t = thyroid; lu = lung; li = liver; ce = ceca.

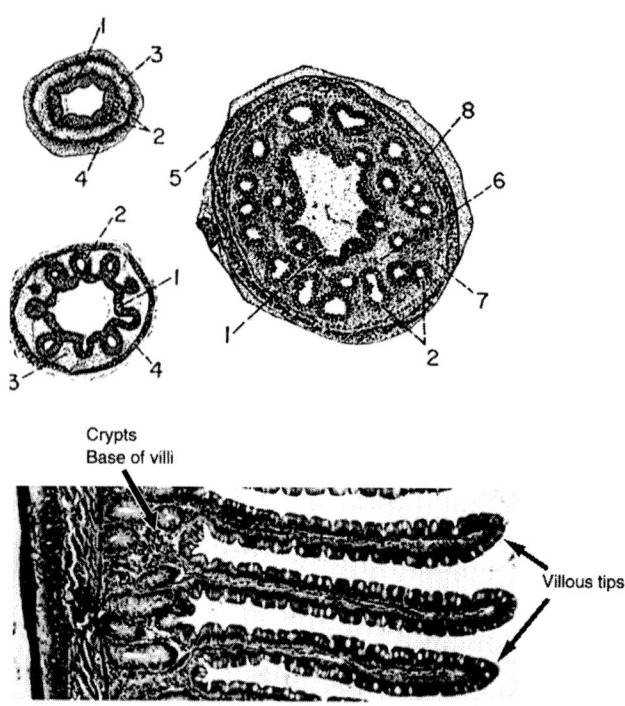
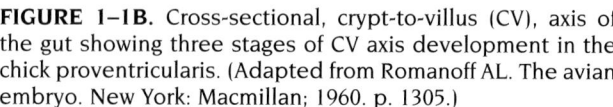

FIGURE 1–1B. Cross-sectional, crypt-to-villus (CV), axis of the gut showing three stages of CV axis development in the chick proventricularis. (Adapted from Romanoff AL. The avian embryo. New York: Macmillan; 1960. p. 1305.)

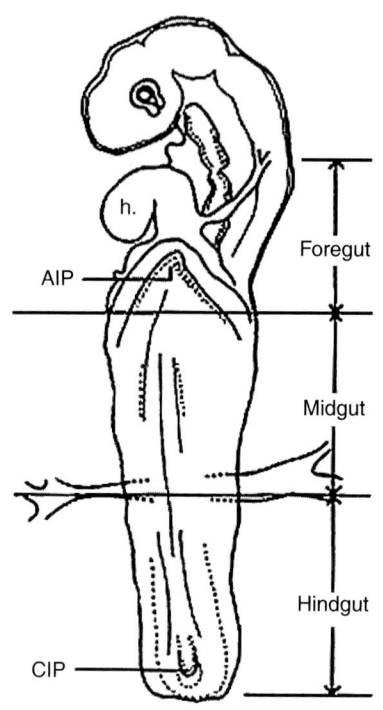

FIGURE 1–2. Diagram of AIP and CIP in the chick at approximately embryonic day 2 (E2). (Adapted from Romanoff AL. The avian embryo. New York: Macmillan; 1960. p. 1305.)

The embryogenesis of the gut is remarkably similar in all animals and nearly identical among vertebrates. Early gut-tube development is choreographed in synchrony with the turning and folding movements of the embryo during gastrulation. The blastula forms a three-dimensional polarized embryo by a complex series of movements that result in the internalization of organs, including the gut. Critical in early gut formation is the invagination of the primitive endoderm and the subsequent growth and differentiation of the subjacent splanchnic mesenchyme. The initial events include a sequence of two invaginations, starting with one at the anterior end of the embryo, forming the anterior intestinal portal (AIP), and followed temporally closely by a posterior invagination forming the caudal intestinal portal (CIP) (Figure 1–2). How these two invaginations occur is poorly understood. The AIP was thought to form as a passive response to the rapid growth of the central nervous system at the cranial end of the embryo (head-fold stage), forcing a folding ventrally and a pushing-in of the ventral endoderm.[6] But, as acranial-anencephalic embryos form the AIP quite normally and certain genetic mutations affect only the AIP formation and have normal cranial development,[7,8] the invagination is probably an active endoderm-specific function.[9] Subsequently, the splanchnic mesoderm closely associated with the endoderm undergoes smooth muscle differentiation as it forms a tube around the endoderm. This tube grows as an open cylinder, closing anteriorly during posterior elongation.

Shortly after the AIP is formed and has begun to elongate, the CIP forms at the posterior end of the embryo. The endoderm at the caudal end of the embryo invaginates ventrally and the subjacent mesenchymal mesoderm surrounds it, forming a tube similar to the formation of the AIP. Although this invagination mirrors that of the earlier AIP invagination, it is even more poorly understood. It has been suggested that the growth of the tail bud posteriorly may facilitate the CIP invagination.[6] Tailless mutants develop relatively normal guts so long as the endoderm is present,[10–14] suggesting that CIP formation (like AIP formation) is an active endoderm-specific function. The growth and elongation of the tubes formed from the AIP and CIP towards each other results in meeting and fusing, closing ventrally around the connection to the yolk sac-stalk in the middle of the embryo.

Initially, the gut tube is relatively straight and uniform in its gross morphology. Soon an AP pattern is formed with regionally distinct sections: fore-, mid-, and hindgut (Figure 1–3). One of the first gross morphologic regional distinctions is the rotation and distention in the posterior foregut at the start of the differentiation of the stomach. The liver diverticulum and the lung buds begin their development from specific ventral regions along the foregut at about this stage as well. Following this is elongation and looping of the midgut. A posterior gross morphologic distinction is the formation of short tubal structures at the midgut-hindgut boundary (appendix in mammals, ceca in birds). Many of these events occur before the ventral body wall closes, at limb-bud stages (by stage 23 in the chick;[15,16] Table 1–1). Therefore, in very early developmental stages, the three regions of the gut are formed: foregut from the AIP, hindgut

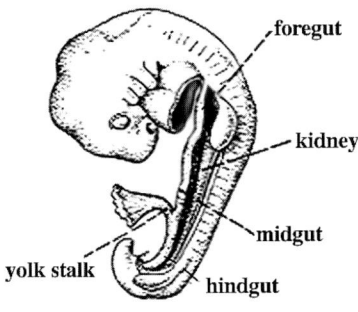
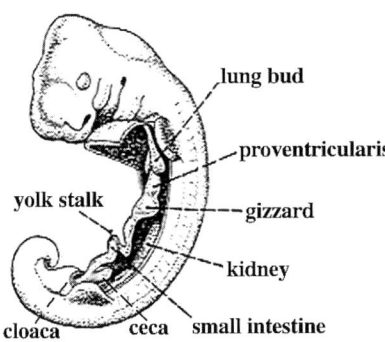

FIGURE 1–3. The AP regions of the chick gut. Approximately E3 (*top*) and E5 (*bottom*). (Adapted from Romanoff AL. The avian embryo. New York: Macmillan; 1960. p. 1305.)

TABLE 1–1
Stages of Chick Development

Somite #	Stage[15]	Embryonic Day
10	10	E1.4
19	13	E2
32	17	E3
40–44	21	E3–3.5
Nearly mature	44	E18
Newly hatched	46	E20–21

from the CIP, and midgut from both AIP and CIP. The mature gut pattern forms later by continued growth with characteristic rotations and organ-specific cellular differentiation in both the endoderm and mesoderm components (Table 1–2).

DIFFERENTIATION ALONG THE ANTERIOR-POSTERIOR AXIS: EPITHELIAL-MESENCHYMAL INTERACTIONS

The endoderm from the early gut-tube stages is essentially identical in its morphology along the length of the gut tube. There are no morphologic differences between the portions of tube formed by elongation of the AIP or by the CIP, and no distinctions in regions that will eventually form the AP portions of the gut: foregut, midgut, hindgut, and their adult phenotypes of esophagus-stomach, intestine, and colon. The primitive gut tube is lined by a single layer of a cuboidal-columnar endoderm-epithelium and encircled by a thin layer of splanchnic mesoderm. As the mesoderm grows and differentiates into smooth muscle, the gut tube alters its gross morphology, resulting in clear demarcations between the foregut, midgut, and hindgut. The epithelial morphology lags significantly in its regionally specific differentiation. In the chick, gross morphologic regional distinctions between the three primary AP subdivisions of the gut are evident by E3 to 5 but epithelial differences are not present until E14, and not clearly distinct until near hatching (E18 to 21) (Figure 1–4). In vertebrates, the gut epithelium continues to be plastic, often undergoing functional differentiation after birth, through weaning, before forming the adult phenotype.[17] The gut enjoys the remarkable ability of continued epithelial growth and differentiation throughout the life of the organism along the gut's CV axis (see Figure 1–4). It is this axis in which the regionalization of the gut is often described and distinguished, as morphologic and histologic differences are easily demonstrated (see Table 1–1 and Figure 1–4).

Throughout this remarkable process of gut development, the organ utilizes one of the most important phenomena of morphogenesis known in developmental biology: epithelial-mesenchymal (EM) interactions. It has been known for decades that the gut cannot develop normally without an interaction between the endoderm and mesoderm (see example,[18] and reviews[19–21]). When endodermal tissue is dissected from the primitive gut tube and cultured in isolation, tissue growth is achieved without differentiation. When the endoderm is cultured with its mesoderm, morphologic development is possible and gut-specific morphology can ensue.[19–21]

The direction of these EM-inductive events has been the focus of much work. While primitive foregut endoderm can differentiate to form gastric glands when cultured with prim-

TABLE 1–2
AP Regions of the Chick Gut

	Foregut (proventricularis)	Midgut	Hindgut-Cloaca
Histochemical		Neutral mucins[84]	Acid mucins[84,85] Sulfonomucins[84] Sialomucins[84]
Immunohistochemical	Pepsinogen[28,29,86,87] Gastrin-Releasing Peptide[88] Somatostatin[88] Avian Pancreatic peptide[88]	Brush border antigen[89] Sucrase[89] Motilin[88] Secretin[88]	
Molecular	Pepsinogen[28,29,86,87] HNF3B[63,64]	cNKX2.3&cNKX2.5[90] PDX-1[74,75,91–93] WNT5A[49] Lumican[49]	cNKX2.3&cNKX2.5[90] K-ATPase[94] HNF3Y[63,64]

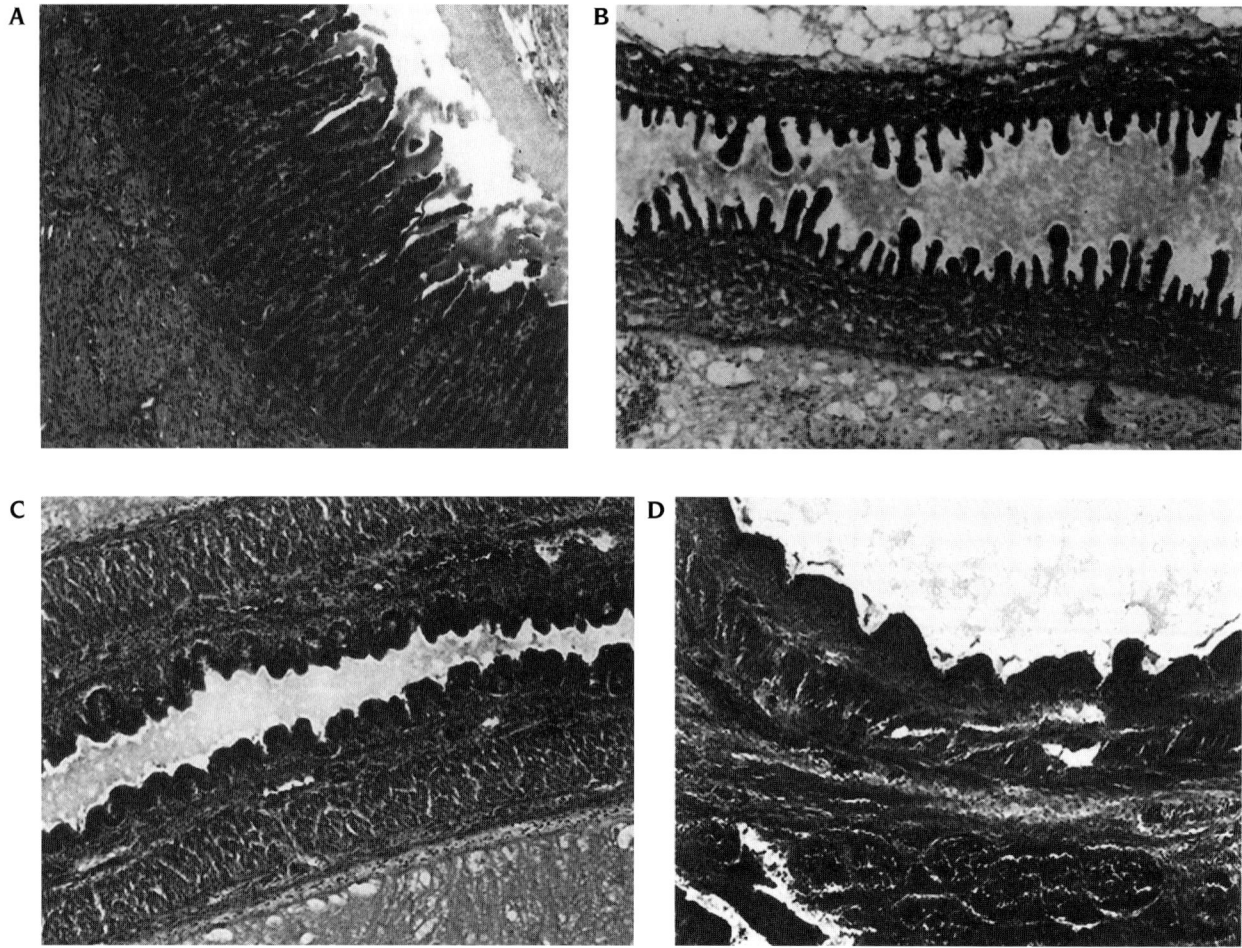

FIGURE 1–4. Histology of E18 chick gut regions; 5μ sections of paraffin-embedded, formalin-fixed E18 chick gut regions. A, Gizzard; B, small intestine; C, large intestine; D, cloaca.

itive foregut mesoderm, this result can also be obtained when the same endoderm is cultured with skin fibroblasts.[19,22] Is this a testament of the determined nature of the primitive stomach endoderm, or is this endoderm inducing the skin fibroblasts to become smooth muscle, in turn permitting stomach epithelial differentiation? Probably both answers are partly true. There is a developmental window after which the primitive gut endoderm, although still morphologically undifferentiated, is committed and develops into its regionally specified epithelium when cultured with a variety of tissues, including the vitelline membrane.[23] However, the same primitive endoderm cultured with non-gut-derived mesoderm (e.g., skin fibroblasts) in turn stimulates smooth muscle development, as assayed by histology and by induction of visceral mesodermal proteins: e.g., tenascin[24] and smooth-muscle actin.[22] Therefore, the endoderm is capable of inducting gut-specific (smooth muscle) differentiation of nonsplanchnic mesoderm (e.g., that derived from somitic mesoderm). Whether this transformed mesodermal tissue can subsequently induce precommitment-stage primitive endoderm is unknown. Many studies have demonstrated that when using undifferentiated (precommitment stage) gut endoderm cocultured with regionalized gut mesoderm, the endoderm will develop towards the epithelial fate of the mesoderm's region.[19,20,25,26] This demonstrates an inductive capability of the gut mesoderm.

In a simple model of gut development, the primitive endoderm first induces ventral invagination and then gut-specific differentiation of the splanchnic mesoderm. Later, the gut mesoderm induces epithelial-specific differentiation of its overlying endoderm. This simple model does not account for some epithelial autonomous function present in specific AP gut regions. The development of epithelial morphological differentiation may be independent (in some regions) of epithelial cytodifferentiation. The chick gut includes a two-part stomach, with the upper stomach (proventricularis) functioning in acid digestion and the lower stomach (gizzard) as a grinding-muscular organ. Small-intestinal epithelium has a microscopic morphology distinct from proventricular (see Figure 1–4). The epithelium is composed of a mucosa and submucosa forming villous projections into the lumen of the small intestine. The small-intestinal epithelium expresses enzymes distinct from the proventricularis. When presumptive small-intestinal endoderm is cultured with the proventricular mesoderm, the epithelium develops with a glandular (proventricular) morphology but the epithelial cells do not express pepsinogen.[27-29] This is true even when very early (15 to 20 somite stage, E2, approximately stage 13) endoderm is used.[30] In the converse experiment, the proventricular endoderm differentiates to small intestine in both morphology and cytodifferentiation, including formation of villi and expression of sucrase, a small-intestinal marker.[30]

The mesenchymal influence on endoderm patterning involves primarily specification of morphology that may not include cytodifferentiation. The difference between the ability of the midgut and foregut endoderm to undergo heterologous differentiation may be an endogenous characteristic of the small-intestinal endoderm, as it is evident in chicks (as described above) and rodents.[31] It may be that, unlike the foregut and hindgut endoderm, the midgut endoderm is self-determined, at least as far as some aspects of cytodifferentiation are concerned.

MOLECULAR CONTROLS OF ANTERIOR-POSTERIOR PATTERN FORMATION IN THE GUT

Since the AP pattern of the vertebrate gut has a positional relationship to the AP body plan (basically, the foregut is in the thorax, the midgut in the abdomen, and the hindgut in the pelvis), do the genes known to pattern the body plan also play a role in gut pattern? The HOX genes, vertebrate homologues of *Drosophila* HOM genes, are known to be regulators of the body plan in many organisms. The HOX genes probably emerged via quadruplication of an ancestral homeobox gene cluster in the vertebrate lineage. Four homologous complexes, HOXA, HOXB, HOXC, and HOXD, exist, each on different chromosomes. Homeodomain-sequence homologues have led to classification of HOX genes into subfamilies, each containing 2 to 4 related paralogous genes.[32] Genes within a cluster are expressed with spatial and temporal colinearity. The 3' genes are expressed in earlier and in more anterior domains, and the 5' genes are expressed later and in more posterior domains (see review[33]). The HOX genes are key regulators of AP pattern in the limb bud, axial tissues, and the hindbrain (see review[34,35]). In each of these tissues, the HOX genes are expressed in overlapping anteroposterior domains that correlate with structural boundaries.

The analysis of HOX gene expression and function in visceral pattern formation is a recent area of investigation. Visceral homeosis has been described in the uterus of murine HOXA-10 null mutants[36] and the vas deferens of HOXA-11 mutants.[37] Visceral anomalies have been described in the athymic and hypothyroid phenotype of HOXA-3 null mutants.[38] As discussed below, there are experimental data supporting a role for the HOX genes in gut patterning and development.

Several HOX genes are expressed in the vertebrate gut, including the HOXD genes in the ABD-B class.[39-41] 5' HOXD gene expression has been described in the mesoderm of the posterior midgut and hindgut. HOX gene expression in the chick hindgut has demonstrated that the ABD-B-like HOX genes of the A and D cluster have regionally restricted expression boundaries demarcating morphologic landmarks of the mid- and hindgut (Figure 1–5).[42,43] In general, the genes are expressed in a nested pattern, with sharp expression limits anteriorly, and overlapping expression at the most posterior hindgut region (Figure 1–5), reminiscent of the expression pattern of the ABD-B-like HOXD genes in the posterior region of the limb bud.[44,45] The expression patterns suggest that the restricted boundaries of expression of the ABD-B-like HOX genes demarcate the regions that will form the cloaca, large intestine, ceca, midceca at the midgut-hindgut border, and the posterior portion of the midgut (Figure 1–6). Moreover, these molecular events presage regional distinctions. Expression of all HOX genes could be detected by stage 14, well before the hindgut lumen is closed (stage 28) or cytodifferentiation of the hindgut mesoderm or epithelium at stages 29 to 31.[16]

Although all the genes analyzed are expressed in the mesoderm, with the 3' paralogues expressed more anteriorly than the 5', the 13th HOX paralogue gene is unique in its additional endodermal expression. Both HOXA-13 and HOXD-13 are expressed in the most posterior mesoderm of the gut, the chick cloaca (the common gut and urogenital orifice) and the murine anus; they are also both expressed in the endoderm of the hindgut.[42,46]

The 13th paralogue has been shown to play a role in chick and murine hindgut development. In mice, homozygous null mutants for HOXD-13 have a rectal phenotype demonstrable by gross morphology and histologic section of the region.[47] The loss of both the functional alleles resulted in anal-rectal prolapse due to maldevelopment of the anal sphincter. Microscopically, the anal sphincter muscle is disorganized and thin. Murine HOXA-13 null homozygotes are embryologically lethal.[48] Compound-mutant mice carrying null alleles of both HOXA-13 and HOXD-13 also show anomalies in both the epithelium of the rectum and the muscle of the anal sphincter.[46] Since these HOX genes are expressed in both tissue layers, with these studies it is impossible to determine whether the phenotype is the result of a specific function that is tissue type autonomous or nonautonomous.

We have used viral misexpression in the chick embryo to further elucidate the roles of HOXD-13 in the epithelial-mesenchymal interactions that guide the regionalization of the hindgut.[49] We have shown that misexpression of HOXD-13 into the embryonic chick midgut mesoderm results in induction of a hindgut morphology in the midgut epithelium. Therefore, mesodermal expression of HOX genes can function in the EM interaction-directing epithelial pattern. We have shown that the expression pattern of the other ABD-B-like HOX genes are not altered, nor are other factors regionally expressed in this area (e.g., WNT5A and lumican).[49] Clearly, other factors are in this pathway and are yet to be discovered.

Although the discovery of downstream targets of the HOX genes has proved elusive, an activator of the ABD-B-like HOX genes has been identified. Sonic hedgehog (Sonic), a vertebrate homologue of *Drosophila*'s hedgehog (hh), has been shown to be an upstream activator of HOXD genes in the vertebrate limb.[50] Sonic is a signaling molecule implicated in mediating pattern in several regions of the embryo, including the limb bud,[50] somite,[51,52] and neural tube.[53-55] Sonic is expressed in the endoderm of the gut and its derivatives[42,56,57] and is an excellent candidate for an early endodermally derived inductive signal in gut morphogenesis as its earliest endodermal expression is restricted to the endoderm of the AIP and CIP.[42]

Sonic is not the signal that initiates the invagination of the AIP or CIP as murine null mutants for Sonic develop a gut[58] although foregut abnormalities are present. The esophagus is malformed, with an enlarged lumen with disorganized or absent subjacent mesoderm (C. Chiang, personal communication). This finding suggests that the endodermally derived signal from Sonic is involved with mesodermal development, recruitment, or another aspect of foregut patterning. Indeed, Sonic must act as an EM signal from the endoderm to the mesoderm, since its receptor is present only in the gut mesoderm,[59] and ectopic expression or overexpression of Sonic results in a massive overproliferation of gut-specific mesoderm.[49]

One of the roles of Sonic's endodermal signal might be to induce HOX gene expression, analogous to its role in the limb bud.[50] At stages in which Sonic is expressed in the CIP endoderm of the chick (approximately stage 13), the ABD-B-like HOX genes are expressed in a nested mesodermal clus-

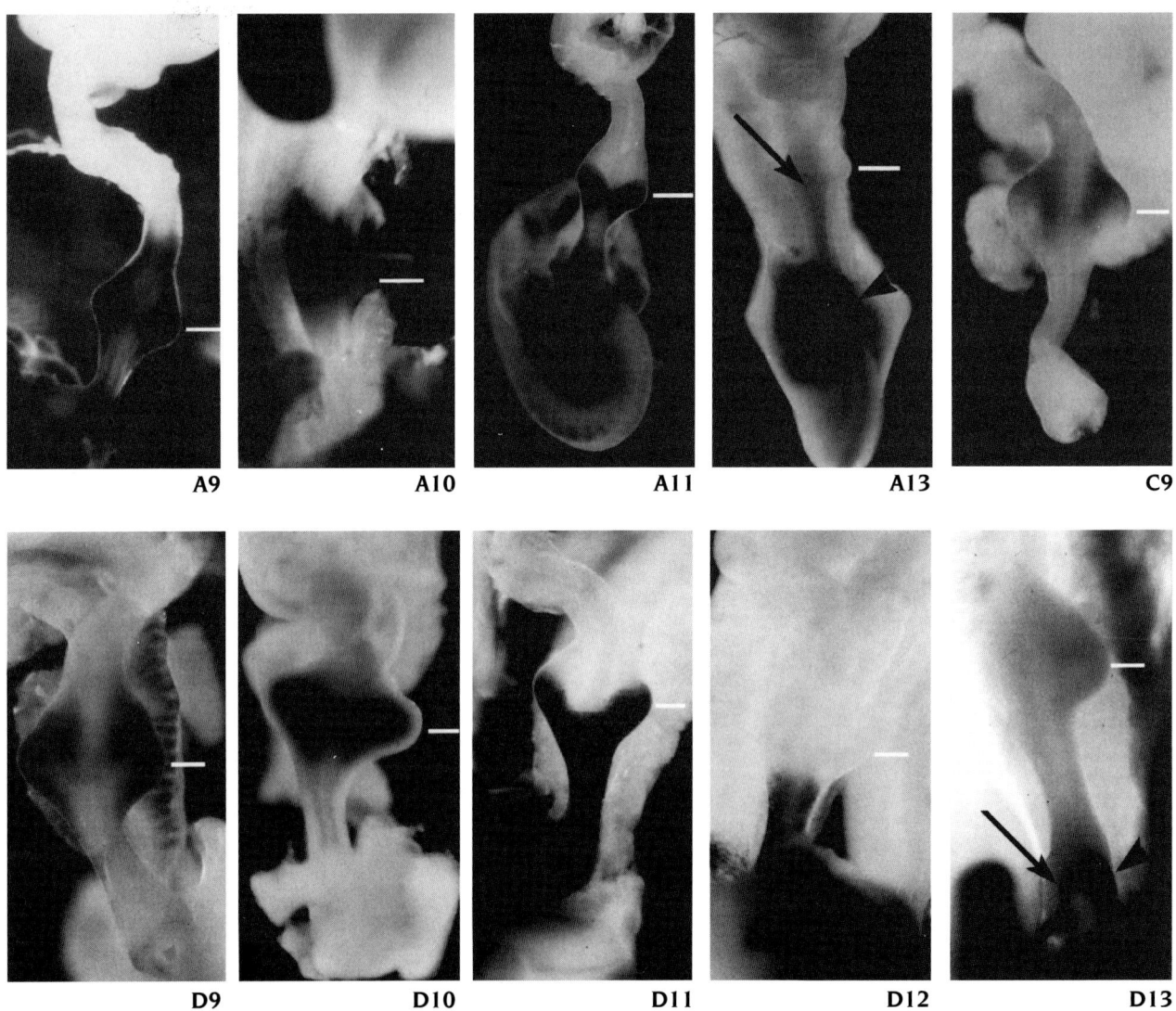

FIGURE 1–5. Expression of ABD-B-like HOX genes in the posterior chick gut at approximately E4. Expression of the 5' members of the HOX genes in stage 26 to 28 chick hindgut is studied by whole mount in situ hybridization. Paralogues are aligned. There is no paralogue of HOXD-12 in the HOXA cluster. Paralogues without detectable hindgut expression (HOXB-9, HOXC-10, HOXC-11) are not shown. HOXC-12 and HOXC-13 were not studied. Expression limits in the visceral mesoderm can be seen around the midgut and hindgut boundary of the ceca and the posterior limit of the hindgut, the cloaca. The ceca in each panel are highlighted by thin white lines. In general, paralogues of different clusters exhibit anterior expression borders in the hindgut similar to those in other embryonic tissues. HOXD-9 in the gut is an exception to this rule as it is expressed in a domain seemingly identical to HOXA-10 and HOXD-10 at this stage. The functional significance of this deviation from the paralogue expression "rule" is unclear. Expression of HOXA-13 and HOXD-13 is also found in the endoderm. (*Long arrow* indicates endodermal expression; *arrowhead* denotes mesodermal expression. The anterior extent of HOXD-13's endodermal expression is not evident in this photograph.) (With permission from Roberts DJ, Johnson RL, Burke AC, et al. *Sonic hedgehog* is an endodermal signal inducing BMP-4 and H*ox* genes during induction and regionalization of the chick hindgut. Development 1995;121:3163–74.)

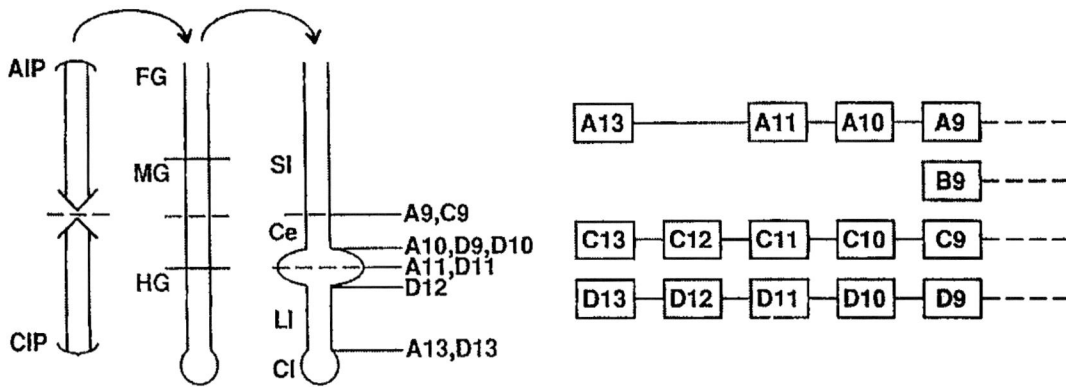

FIGURE 1–6. Diagram describing the apparent demarcation of gut regions by expression limits of the ABD-B-like HOX genes in the chick gut. Diagrammatic representation of vertebrate gut morphogenesis with the AIP and CIP growing and elongating (*large arrows*) towards the umbilicus (*dashed horizontal line*). The regionalization of the lumenal gut forms foregut, midgut, and hindgut, derived from the invaginations of the AIP (foregut and midgut) and CIP (midgut and hindgut). Cytodifferentiation of these regions forms the small intestine from the midgut; the ceca from both the midgut (anteriorly) and the hindgut (posteriorly); and, the large intestine and part of the cloaca from the hindgut. The regionally restricted pattern of expression of the ABD-B-like HOX genes demarcates morphologic distinctions in the midgut and hindgut visceral mesoderm, diagrammatically shown with anterior limits of expression noted. (Exception is HOXC-9; posterior limit of expression shown.) The genes expressed in the vertebrate abdominal region are from the 5' end of each cluster, related evolutionarily to the *Drosophila* gene ABD-B. The cognate genes (paralogues) of the ABD-B-like genes of the four HOX complexes are diagrammed with the most posteriorly expressed (5') genes aligned on the left.
AIP = anterior intestinal portal; Ce = ceca; CIP = caudal intestinal portal; Cl = cloaca; FG = foregut; MG = midgut; HG = hindgut; LI = large intestine; SI = small intestine.
(With permission from Roberts DJ, Johnson RL, Burke AC, et al. Sonic hedgehog is an endodermal signal inducing BMP-4 and Hox genes during induction and regionalization of the chick hindgut. Development 1995;121:3163–74.)

ter around the Sonic-expressing CIP endoderm,[42] in a manner reminiscent of Sonic in the developing limb bud.[50] In fact, just as virally mediated Sonic misexpression in the limb bud induces ectopic expression of the ABD-B-like HOX-genes,[50,60] misexpression of Sonic in stage 10 presumptive midgut region of the embryo induces expression of HOXD-11 and HOXD-13 in the subjacent splanchnic mesoderm.[42]

In each organ in which the endoderm-derived tissue expresses Sonic, there is closely associated mesenchymal mesoderm that expresses a homologue of *Drosophila*'s dpp.[42,56,57] There are two vertebrate homologues of dpp: BMP2 and BMP4. In the primitive hindgut, at the earliest time in which Sonic expression can be detected in the CIP region (even before invagination is apparent), BMP4 is expressed in the subjacent mesenchymal mesoderm.[42] In misexpression studies, Sonic ectopically induces BMP4 in the splanchnic mesoderm of the developing gut.[42,49]

A model has been proposed in which the endodermal role of Sonic at the CIP is to induce BMP4 expression in the splanchnic mesoderm, which then forms the smooth muscle of the gut, and to induce the expression of the ABD-B-like HOX genes in the mesoderm, to regionalize that portion of the gut formed by the elongation of the CIP (posterior midgut and hindgut).[42] This may be the signal to polarize the gut mesoderm along its AP axis, as a posterior signal has been proposed to be dominant.[61]

One of the many mysteries that remain in the initial events of gut formation is that although Sonic and BMP4 are expressed at both ends of the developing gut (the AIP and CIP), clearly different patterns emerge. The nested pattern of the ABD-B-like HOX genes at the CIP are not activated at the AIP. Are other proteins acting at these two critical poles of gut formation that confer differential tissue competency? Candidates for this aspect of patterning in the gut include those with differential AP expression before either Sonic is expressed or the HOX genes are expressed at the AIP or CIP. Candidate upstream activators of Sonic include vertebrate homologues of the FKH gene class, first identified in *Drosophila*. FKH encodes a novel transcription factor required for fore- and hindgut development in *Drosophila*. There are at least six vertebrate FKH homologues[62] that share homology with the DNA-binding domain. HNF-3α, β, and γ were originally identified for their importance in hepatic development. All are expressed in the murine gut endoderm, with slightly different expression patterns along the AP axis of the gut.[63,64] Detailed spatial-temporal expression patterns of the three have not been published, but HNF-3β is expressed in Hensen's node at the site of the origin of the definitive endoderm[63] and might be responsible for the induction of the early gut endoderm.[65] In the mouse, HNF-3β is expressed at both the AIP and CIP.[63,65,66] It has been suggested that HNF-3β regulates the production of Sonic in the notochord and floorplate[53,54,63] and interacts with Sonic at the node.[67] Similarly, HNF-3β expression may lead to transcription of Sonic within the AIP endoderm. We found HNF-3β expression limited to the chick AIP before expression of Sonic (Figure 1–7), with no expression at the CIP in stages studied. This difference in AP expression is consistent with a role for HNF-3β as an activator of Sonic at the AIP or may play a role in AP regionalization of Sonic's signal. Per-

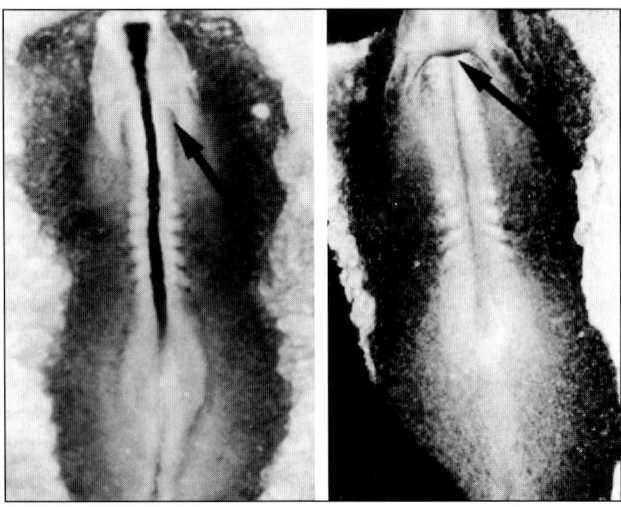

FIGURE 1-7. Whole-mount in situ hybridization pattern of HNF-3β and Sonic in the chick embryo at stage 7. Arrow points to AIP. Sonic expression on the *left*; HNF-3β on the *right*.

haps one of the other HNF-3 genes plays a similar regulatory role at the chick CIP.

Although the description of the molecular control of AP morphogenesis of the gut is just beginning to be explored, significant insight into the embryogenesis of gut formation has emerged. With the advantages of murine transgenics and chick misexpression systems as well as classic experimental embryologic techniques, the field will be active and productive in the coming years.

DORSAL-VENTRAL PATTERNING IN THE GUT

Although the studies described above just begin to decipher the AP regionalization of the gut, DV regionalization is at an even earlier stage of understanding. The molecular controls of gut-DV pattern have focused on the foregut derivatives: particularly the thyroid, lung, liver, and pancreas. All these organs start as ventral buds off the foregut except the pancreas, which in most vertebrates has both ventral and dorsal buds.

Ventral specification of the foregut is required for organogenesis of the thyroid and lung and involves a different class of homeobox-containing transcription factors, the NKX2 class, which are related to *Drosophila* NK2.[68] One of these genes, NKX2.1, is restricted in its gut expression to the ventral region of the foregut endoderm at the point where the thyroid and lungs will bud.[69,70] The null transgenic mouse phenotype shows agenesis of the thyroid and lung parenchyma.[71,72] Although the thyroid rudiment is formed, it never bifurcates or develops a gland.[72] Ventralization of the trachea from the esophagus, the first step in lung organogenesis, does not occur. The anterior foregut shows an uncompartmentalized single lumen that has a phenotype of a compound trachea and esophagus with rings of tracheal-like cartilage (although abnormal in number). The bronchi emerge bilaterally from this malformed luminal.[72] This is reminiscent of a human malformation of the trachea-esophagus in rare forms of congenital tracheoesophageal fistula.[73] It appears that NKX2.1 is required in an apparently inductive signaling pathway that is required for the ventralization of the foregut.

In pancreatic development, two buds off the posterior end of the foregut develop: one ventral and one dorsal. These buds eventually fuse. The ventral bud forms the dominant pancreatic duct as well as the bile ducts. Studies have shown that PDX1, another homeobox-containing transcription factor, is required in this pathway.[74,75] PDX1 is expressed in the endoderm of the foregut at the regions where both the ventral and dorsal buds will form.[74,76,77] Its expression is excluded from the lateral endoderm.[77] The reciprocal expression pattern is present for Sonic at the prepancreatic bud stage. Sonic is expressed in the endoderm in the regions lateral to the PDX1-expressing endoderm and is excluded from expression in the DV endoderm at this level.[77] (It remains to be elucidated whether PDX1 inhibits Sonic expression.) In PDX1 null mutant mice, the ventral bud forms but fails to grow, and the dorsal bud grows and becomes lobulated but arrests and never forms a functioning pancreas.[74,76] The pancreatic endoderm never fully differentiates but the mesoderm develops, apparently normally.[74,76] These findings implied that the PDX1 endodermal signal is required for normal pancreatic epithelial development but not for pancreatic-specific mesodermal development (at least dorsally[74,76]).

Complete pancreatic development of both mesoderm and endoderm tissues involves DV patterning of the foregut, with polarizing DV expression pattern of both PDX1 and Sonic. Evidence of this was elegantly shown when transgenic mice were designed such that the wild-type lateral Sonic expression was abrogated.[77] By using the PDX1 promoter, Sonic was expressed circumferentially in the endoderm of the pancreatic region. There was no difference in the wild-type expression of PDX1. The results of the experiment were very interesting, in that the position of the buds formed correctly and the epithelium showed pancreatic differentiation (expressing both exocrine and endocrine pancreatic-specific proteins) but the phenotype of the mesoderm was small intestinal (midgut). In fact, the mesoderm was entirely smooth muscle and showed peristalsis, as does wild-type small intestine. It appears that expression of Sonic in the gut endoderm induces gut-specific smooth muscle differentiation in its subjacent mesoderm (supporting the Sonic-BMP4-smooth muscle pathway described above). In addition, these studies show that the prepancreatic endoderm requires a positive signal, in which PDX1 plays a key role, to differentiate along a pancreatic endodermal fate.

There remain many questions about the molecular control of DV patterning in the gut. One paramount question concerns the "ground state" of the gut. Is a stimulatory signal required for ventralization, or is an inhibitory signal necessary? Is the ground state dorsal or ventral? The fact that nearly all the derivatives of the foregut are ventral can support either theory.

Experimental data suggest that a positive signal is needed to ventralize the mesoderm.[7-9,78] If you consider that smooth muscle (derived from splanchnic mesoderm) is ventral mesoderm, then Sonic is a candidate factor for ventralizing the mesoderm (via BMP4[42]). When the mesoderm is adjacent to Sonic-expressing endoderm, the mesoderm will develop gut-like smooth muscle. Where endodermal Sonic is not expressed, the mesoderm reverts to its "ground state" of dorsalized (non-gut-like) mesoderm (as in the pancreas). Rare gut duplications occur in humans, termed enteric cysts, which are always dorsal structures.[73] This may be a sequela of the normal anatomic proximity of the endoderm and pregut mesoderm to the notochord (a Sonic-expressing tissue). As the mesoderm infiltrates the region between the endoderm and the notochord, the endoderm separates from the notochord and becomes encased by the mesoderm, which carries Sonic's receptor complex, including Ptc. Sonic protein will be expressed from both the endoderm and the notochord. Therefore, this mesoderm, at the most dorsal region of the gut tube, sees the highest concentration of Sonic protein. As the mesoderm receives high concentration of Sonic, if abnormal separation of the endoderm from the notochord or aberrant endodermal budding occurs dorsally, then we would predict that the mesoderm should never develop into duplicated structures phenocopying gut derivatives, but rather gut-like mesoderm (smooth muscle). Morphologically, these cysts apparently always phenocopy the AP gut region in which they are present, at least in the mesoderm. The epithelium may not obey the dorsal ground state theory. Often these cysts contain heterotopic epithelial differentiation (usually of stomach and/or pancreatic epithelium), even though their mesoderm is always gut-like.

Another endodermal factor has been implicated in ventralization of the foregut. GATA-4, a transcription factor expressed in the ventral foregut endoderm and mesoderm, is necessary for normal ventral development of both the heart and foregut.[7,8] Null mutants fail to develop the AIP and therefore have abnormal heart and foregut morphogenesis. This phenotype can be rescued when GATA-4 is provided by GATA-4-expressing cells of endodermal origin only in a chimeric mouse.[9] The endodermal function of GATA-4 is likely to ensure normal AIP and, therefore, foregut development. These findings suggest that one key role of the anterior endoderm is as provider of a ventralizing factor required for AIP formation.

Although the above experimental and observational data suggest that an inductive signal is required for ventralization (therefore a dorsal ground state), other experimental data suggest that an inhibitory signal is present in the dorsal mesoderm that inhibits ventralization of the endoderm (a ventral ground state).[79] Hepatic development requires ventralized foregut endoderm in an EM interaction with cardiac mesoderm. Culture work has shown that nonforegut endoderm can be induced to develop as hepatic when cultured with cardiac mesoderm. An elegant experiment, in which early markers for endodermal hepatic differentiation were assayed from cocultures of ventral endoderm, cardiac mesoderm, and dorsal mesoderm from the posterior regions of the gut, found that the endoderm failed to undergo hepatic differentiation. When the dorsal mesoderm was removed from the coculture, the endoderm differentiated as hepatic, suggesting that a dorsal-mesodermal inhibitory signal prevents ventral specification. Therefore, many signaling sources may be present to ventralize the gut, including a dorsal inhibitory signal from the mesoderm (unknown), and a ventral stimulatory signal from the endoderm (e.g., GATA-4, PDX1, NKX2.1, Sonic). The DV-axis determination will be an exciting area to study, as conflicting data and theories presently remain unexplained.

DIFFERENTIATION OF THE GUT IN THE LEFT-RIGHT AXIS

Vertebrates demonstrate a general symmetry between the left and right sides of the embryo and adult, yet consistent asymmetry exists in this axis in the viscera (situs). This asymmetry is evidenced by a left-sided heart, spleen, and stomach, and a right-sided liver and gallbladder. Additionally, the paired lungs exhibit differences between left and right lobes. Looping of the gut is critical in the development of asymmetry in many aspects of visceral placement. The controls of left-right (LR) asymmetry are very poorly understood, yet many candidate factors have been proposed and studied.[80] Although generally the left-right asymmetry of the viscera appears controlled as a unit such that the heart and gut develop together their combined asymmetry (e.g., the heart and stomach are usually left sided), the molecular controls of the asymmetry may include independent controls for the GI system and heart.[81]

In the chick, asymmetrically expressed factors at the earliest stages of embryogenesis (at nodal stages of development) seem to control the LR fate of the heart and looping of the gut. When the asymmetrical expression of these factors is erased by misexpression such that bilateral expression is experimentally produced, randomization of the situs results.[67] A signaling pathway, in which Sonic again is a key player, exists such that when Sonic (which is normally expressed only on the left side of Hensen's node) is expressed bilaterally, randomization of the heart looping and gut looping occurs.[67,81] The two events apparently occur independently, such that the heart may have its normal left-sidedness, yet the stomach will develop right-sided (a heterotaxic phenomenon). Evidence of naturally occuring independent situs events is present in humans with isolated dextrocardia or malrotation of the gut.

This area of study is in the early stages of understanding, and we are sure to see rapid growth of our knowledge of the molecular controls of situs of the gut in the near future.

CONCLUSION

In humans, malformations of the GI tract are quite common. For example, duodenal atresia has an incidence of 1 in 3000 births.[82] Many, if not most, of these gut structural anomalies are sporadic, with an etiology that generally remains unexplained. The summary of the research findings in the molecular controls of gut development discussed in this chapter provide an opportunity to hypothesize and study the molecular etiology of, for example, anal agenesis, tracheoesophageal fistula, malrotation, annular pancreas, extralobar pulmonary sequestrations, and dorsal enteric cysts.

Although historically much work has been done using classic surgical embryologic techniques to attempt to explain the controls of gut development, the advent of molecular techniques to study visceral morphogenesis is a relatively new area of research. Much would be gained by more insight into the molecular controls of the axes of gut development, with particular focus on EM interactions, which are known to be critical in all areas of gut and gut-derivative formation. Despite the data summarized in this chapter that implicate the HOX genes in regulating the AP development of the gut, it remains unknown how they function in this role. The HOX genes are nuclear transcription factors that must activate genes that encode secretory proteins, which then, via EM interactions, induce AP-epithelial fate. Downstream targets of the HOX genes have proved elusive to identify to date. This is a critical area of investigation, which should receive aggressive attention in the near future.

It would seem a distinct advantage to integrate data and theories with naturally occurring developmental phenomena in the gut: a collaboration between anatomists, clinicians, and molecular developmental biologists. Despite recent advances in the understanding of the controls of pattern formation, especially along the AP axis of the gut, initial events in gut embryogenesis (such as AIP and CIP formation) and the control of the development along the DV axis are still obscure. With this area of investigation gaining interest, we will be sure to see a vibrant competition, with exciting discoveries over the next decade.

REFERENCES

1. Jacobson AG, Sater AK. Features of embryonic induction. Development 1988;104:341–59.
2. Sugi Y, Lough J. Anterior endoderm is a specific effector of terminal cardiac myocyte differentiation of cells from the embryonic heart forming region. Dev Dyn 1994;200:155–62.
3. Lough J, Barron M, Brogley M, et al. Combined BMP-2 and FGF-4, but neither factor alone, induces cardiogenesis in non-precardiac embryonic mesoderm. Dev Biol 1996;178:198–202.
4. Nascone N, Mercola M. An inductive role for the endoderm in *Xenopus* cardiogenesis. Development 1995;121:515–23.
5. Sugi Y, Markwald RR. Formation and early morphogenesis of endocardial endothelial precursor cells and the role of endoderm. Dev Biol 1996;175:66–83.
6. Gruenwald P. Normal and abnormal detachment of body and gut from the blastoderm in the chick embryo, with remarks on the early development of the allantois. J Morphol 1941;69:83–125.
7. Kuo CT, Morrisey EE, Anadappa R, et al. GATA4 transcription factor is required for ventral morphogenesis and heart tube formation. Genes Dev 1997;11:1048–60.
8. Molkentin JD, Lin Q, Duncan SA, Olson EN. Requirement of the transcription factor GATA4 for heart tube formation and ventral morphogenesis. Genes Dev 1997;11:1061–72.
9. Narita N, Bielinska M, Wilson DB. Wild-type endoderm abrogates the ventral developmental defects associated with GATA-4 deficiency in the mouse. Dev Biol 1997;189:270–4.
10. Rashbass P, Wilson V, Rosen B, Beddington RSP. Alterations in gene expression during mesoderm formation and axial patterning in Brachyury (T) embryos. Int J Dev Biol 1994;38:35–44.
11. Takada S, Stark KL, Shea MJ, et al. Wnt-3a regulates somite and tailbud formation in the mouse embryo genes. Dev Genes 1994;8:174–89.
12. Schier AF, Neuhauss SC, Helde KA, et al. The one-eyed pinhead gene functions in mesoderm and endoderm formation in zebrafish and interacts with no tail. Development 1997;124:327–42.
13. Schulte-Merker S, van Eeden FJ, Halpern ME, et al. no tail (ntl) is the zebrafish homologue of the mouse T (Brachyury). Development 1994;120:843–52.
14. Greco TL, Takada S, Newhouse MM, et al. Analysis of the vestigial tail mutation demonstrates that Wnt-3a gene dosage regulates mouse axial development. Genes Dev 1996;10:313–24.
15. Hamburger V, Hamilton HL. A series of normal stages in the development of the chick embryo. J Morphol 1951;88:49–92.
16. Romanoff AL. The avian embryo. New York: Macmillan; 1960. p. 1305.
17. Rings EHHM, Krasinski SD, Van Beers EH, et al. Restriction of lactase gene expression along the proximal-to-distal axis of rat small intestine occurs during postnatal development. Gastroenterology 1994;106:1223–32.
18. Le Douarin N. Etude experimentale de l'organeogenese du tube digestif et du foie chez l'embryon de poulet. Bull Biol France, Belg 1964;98:533–676.
19. Haffen K, Lacroix B, Kedinger M, Simon-Assman PM. Inductive properties of fibroblastic cell cultures derived from rat intestinal mucosa on epithelial differentiation. Differentiation 1983;23:226–33.
20. Haffen K, Kedinger M, Simon-Assman P. Mesenchyme-dependent differentiation of epithelial progenitor cells in the gut. J Pediatr Gastroenterol Nutr 1987;6:14–23.
21. Yasugi S. Role of epithelial-mesenchymal interactions in differentiation of epithelium of vertebrate digestive organs. Dev Growth Differ 1993;35:1–9.
22. Kedinger M, Simon-Assman PM, Bouziges F, et al. Smooth muscle actin expression during rat gut development and induction in fetal skin fibroblastic cells associated with intestinal embryonic epithelium. Differentiation 1990;43:87–97.
23. Sumiya M. Differentiation of the digestive tract epithelium of the chick embryo cultured in vitro enveloped in a fragment of vitelline membrane in the absence of mesenchyme. Roux's Archiv 1976;197:1–17.
24. Aufderheide E, Ekblom P. Tenascin during gut development: appearance in the mesenchyme, shift in molecular forms, and dependence on epithelial-mesenchymal interactions. J Cell Biol 1988;107:2341–9.
25. Kedinger M, Simon-Assman PM, Lacroix B, et al. Fetal gut mesenchyme induces differentiation of cultured intestinal endodermal and crypt cells. Dev Biol 1986;113:474–83.
26. Kedinger M, Simon-Assman P, Bouziges F, Haffen K. Epithelial-mesenchymal interactions in intestinal epithelial differentiation. Scand J Gastroenterol 1988;23:62–9.
27. Yasugi S. Differentiation of allantoic endoderm implanted into the presumptive digestive area in avian embryos. A study with organ-specific antigens. J Embryol Exp Morph 1984;80:137–53.
28. Yasugi S, Matsushita S, Mizuno T. Gland formation induced in the allantoic and small-intestinal endoderm by the proventricular mesenchyme is not coupled with pepsinogen expression. Differentiation 1985;30:47–52.
29. Hayashi K, Yasugi S, Mizuno T. Pepsinogen gene transcription induced in heterologous epithelial-mesenchymal recombinations of chicken endoderms and glandular stomach mesenchyme. Development 1988;103:725–31.
30. Yasugi S, Takeda H, Fukuda K. Early determination of developmental fate in presumptive intestinal endoderm of the chicken embryo. Dev Growth Differ 1991;33:235–41.
31. Duluc I, Freund J-N, Leberquier C, Kedinger M. Fetal endoderm primarily holds the temporal and positional information required for mammalian intestinal development. J Cell Biol 1994;126:211–21.

32. Scott MP. A rational nomenclature for vertebrate homeobox (HOX) genes. Nucleic Acids Res 1993;21:1687–8.
33. Dolle P, Izpisua-Belmonte JC, Brown J, et al. Hox genes and the morphogenesis of the vertebrate limb. Prog Clin Biol Res 1993;383A:11–20.
34. McGinnis W, Krumlauf R. Homeobox genes and axial patterning. Cell 1992;68:283–302.
35. Krumlauf R. Hox genes in vertebrate development. Cell 1994;78:191–201.
36. Benson GV, Lim H, Paria BC, et al. Mechanisms of reduced fertility in *Hoxa-10* mutant mice: uterine homeosis and loss of maternal *Hoxa-10* expression. Development 1996;122:2687–96.
37. Hsieh-Li HM, Witte DP, Weinstein M, et al. *Hoxa-11* structure, extensive antisense transcription, and function in male and female fertility. Development 1995;121:1373–85.
38. Manley NR, Capecchi MR. The role of *Hoxa-3* in mouse thymus and thyroid development. Development 1995;121:1989–2003.
39. Dolle P, Izpisua-Belmonte JC, Brown JM, et al. HOX-4 genes and the morphogenesis of mammalian genitalia. Genes Dev 1991;5:1767–7.
40. Izpisua-Belmonte JC, Falkenstein H, Dolle P, et al. Murine genes related to the *Drosophila AbdB* homeotic genes are sequentially expressed during development of the posterior part of the body. EMBO J 1991;10:2279–89.
41. Dolle P, Dierich A, LeMeur M, et al. Disruption of the *Hoxd13* gene induces localized heterchrony leading to mice with neotenic limbs. Cell 1993;75:431–41.
42. Roberts DJ, Johnson RL, Burke AC, et al. *Sonic Hedgehog* is an endodermal signal inducing *BMP-4* and *Hox* genes during induction and regionalization of the chick hindgut. Development 1995;121:3163–74.
43. Yokouchi Y, Sakiyama J, Kuroiwa A. Coordinated expression of *Abd-B* subfamily genes of the *HoxA* cluster in the developing digestive tract of the chick embryo. Dev Biol 1995;169:76–89.
44. Tabin CJ. Why we have (only) five fingers per hand: hox genes and the evolution of paired limbs [review]. Development 1992;116:289–96.
45. Nelson CE, Morgan BA, Burke AC, et al. Analysis of *Hox* gene expression in the chick limb bud. Development 1996;122:1449–66.
46. Warot X, Fromental-Ramain C, Fraulob V, et al. Gene dosage-dependent effects of the *Hoxa-13* and *Hoxd-13* mutations on morphogenesis of the terminal parts of the digestive and urogenital tracts. Development 1997;124:4781–91.
47. Kondo T, Dolle P, Zakany J, Duboule D. Function of Posterior *HoxD* genes in the morphogenesis of the anal sphincter. Development 1996;122:2651–9.
48. Fromental-Ramain C, Warot X, Lakkaraju S, et al. Specific and redundant functions of the paralogous *Hoxa-9* and *Hoxd-9* genes in forelimb and axial skeleton patterning. Development 1996;122:461–72.
49. Roberts DJ, Smith DM, Goff DJ, Tabin CJ. Epithelial-mesenchymal signaling during the regionalization of the chick gut. Development 1998;125:2791–874.
50. Riddle RD, Johnson RL, Laufer E, Tabin C. Sonic hedgehog mediates the polarizing activity of the ZPA. Cell 1993;75:1401–16.
51. Johnson RL, Laufer E, Riddle RD, Tabin C. Ectopic expression of *Sonic hedgehog* alters dorsal-ventral patterning of somites. Cell 1994;79:1165–73.
52. Fan CM, Tessier-Lavigne M. Patterning of mammalian somites by surface ectoderm and notochord: evidence for sclerotome induction by a hedgehog homolog. Cell 1994;79:1175–86.
53. Echelard Y, Epstein DJ, St-Jacques B, et al. Sonic hedgehog, a member of a family of putative secreted signaling molecules, is implicated in the regulation of CNS polarity. Cell 1993;75:1417–30.
54. Krauss S, Concordet J-P, Ingham PW. A functionally conserved homolog of the *Drosophila* segment polarity gene *hh* is expressed in tissues with polarizing activity in zebrafish. Cell 1993;75:1431–44.
55. Roelink H, Augsburger A, Heemskerk J, et al. Floor plate and motor neuron induction by *vhh-1*, a vertebrate homolog of *hedgehog* expressed by the notochord. Cell 1994;76:761–75.
56. Bitgood MJ, McMahon AP. Hedgehog and Bmp genes are coexpressed at many diverse sites of cell-cell interaction in the mouse embryo. Dev Biol 1995;172:126–38.
57. Marigo V, Roberts DJ, Lee SMK, et al. Cloning, expression, and chromosomal location of *SHH* and *IHH*: two human homologues of the *Drosophila* segment polarity gene *hedgehog*. Genomics 1995;28:44–51.
58. Chiang C, Litingtung Y, Lee E, et al. Cyclopia and defective axial patterning in mice lacking *Sonic hedgehog* gene function. Nature 1996; 383:407–13.
59. Marigo V, Scott MP, Johnson RL, et al. Conservation in *hedgehog* signaling: induction of a chicken patched homolog by Sonic hedgehog in the developing limb. Development 1996;122:1225–33.
60. Laufer E, Nelson CE, Johnson RL, et al. *Sonic hedgehog* and *Fgf-4* act through a signaling cascade and feedback loop to integrate growth and patterning of the developing limb bud. Cell 1994;79:993–1003.
61. Slack JMW, Isaacs HV, Johnson GE, et al. Specification of the body plan during Xenopus gastrulation: dorsoventral and anteroposterior patterning of the mesoderm. Development 1992;Suppl:143–9.
62. Kaestner KH, Lee K-H, Schlondorff J, et al. Six members of the mouse forkhead gene family are developmentally regulated. Proc Natl Acad Sci U S A 1993;90:7628–31.
63. Monaghan AP, Kaestner KH, Grau E, Schutz G. Postimplantation expression patterns indicate a role for the mouse *forkhead/HNF-3α*, β, γ genes in determination of the definitive endoderm, chordamEsoderm and neuroectoderm. Development 1993;119:567–78.
64. Sasaki H, Hogan BLM. Differential expression of multiple fork head related genes during gastrulation and axial pattern formation in the mouse embryo. Development 1993;118:47–59.
65. Ang S-L, Wierda A, Wong D, et al. The formation and maintenance of the definitive endoderm lineage in the mouse: involvement of HNF3/*forkhead* proteins. Development 1993;119:1301–5.
66. Sasaki H, Hogan BLM. *HNF-3β* as a regulator of floor plate development. Cell 1994;76:103–15.
67. Levin M, Johnson RL, Stern CD, et al. A molecular pathway determining left-right asymmetry in chick embryogenesis. Cell 1995;82:803–14.
68. Kim Y, Nirenberg M. Drosophila NK-homeobox genes. Proc Natl Acad Sci USA 1989;86:7716–20.
69. Lazzaro D, Price M, De Felice M, Di Lauro R. The transcription factor TTF-1 is expressed at the onset of thyroid and lung morphogenesis and in restricted regions of the foetal brain. Development 1991;113:1093–104.
70. Mizuno K, Gonzalez FJ, Kimura S. Thyroid-specific enhancer-binding protein (T/EBP): cDNA cloning, functional characterization, and structural identity with thyroid transcription factor TTF-1. Mol Cell Biol 1991;11:4927–33.
71. Kimura S, Hara Y, Pineau T, et al. The T/ebp null mouse: thyroid-specific enhancer-binding protein is essential for the organogen-

esis of the thryoid, lung, ventral forebrain, and pituitary. Genes Dev 1996;10:60–9.
72. Minoo P, Hamdam H, Bu D, et al. TTF-1 regulates lung epithelial morphogenesis. Dev Biol 1995;172:694–8.
73. Skandalakis JE, Gray SW, editors. Embryology for surgeons. The embryologic basis for the treatment of congenital anomalies. 2nd ed. Baltimore: Williams & Wilkins; 1994. p. 1101.
74. Offield MF, Jetton TL, Labosky PA, et al. PDX-1 is required for pancreatic outgrowth and differentiation of the rostral duodenom. Development 1996;122:983–95.
75. Ohlsson H, Karlsson K, Edlund T. IPF1, a homeodomain-containing transactivator of the insulin gene. EMBO J 1993;12:4251–9.
76. Ahlgren U, Jonsson J, Edlund H. The morphogenesis of the pancreatic mesenchyme is uncoupled from that of the pancreatic epithelium. Development; 1996;122:1409–16.
77. Apelqvist A, Ahlgren U, Edlund H. Sonic hedgehog directs specialised mesoderm differentiation in the intestine and pancreas. Curr Biol 1997;7:801–4.
78. Graff JM, Thies RS, Song JJ, et al. Studies with a Xenopus BMP receptor suggest that ventral mesoderm-inducing signals override dorsal signals in vivo. Cell 1994;79:169–79.
79. Gualdi R, Bossard P, Zheng M, et al. Hepatic specification of the gut endoderm in vitro: cell signaling and transcriptional control. Genes Devel 1996;10:1670–82.
80. Levin M. Left-right asymmetry in vertebrate embryogenesis. Bioessays 1997;19:287–96.
81. Levin M, Pagan S, Roberts DJ, et al. Left/right patterning signals and the independent regulation of different aspects of situs in the chick embryo. Dev Biol 1997;189:57–67.
82. Dillon PW, Cilley RE. Newborn surgical emergencies: gastrointestinal anomalies, abdominal wall defects. Pediatr Clin North Am 1993;40:1289–314.
83. Chuong C, editor. Molecular basis of epithelial appendage morphogenesis. Georgetown (TX): Landes Bioscience; 1998.
84. Whitehead R, editor. Gastrointestinal and oesophageal pathology. New York: Churchill Livingstone; 1989.
85. Suprasert A, Fujioka T, Yamada K. The histochemistry of glycoconjugates in the colonic epithelium of the chicken. Histochemistry 1987;86:491–7.
86. Takiguchi K, Yasugi S, Mizuno T. Gizzard epithelium of chick embryos can express embryonic pepsinogen antigen, a marker protein of proventriculus. Roux's Arch Dev Biol 1986;195:475–83.
87. Hayashi K, Agata K, Mochii M, et al. Molecular cloning and the nucleotide sequence of cDNA for embryonic chicken pepsinogen: phylogenetic relationship with prochymosin. J Biochem 1988;103:290–6.
88. Andrew A, Rawdon BB. Can a non-gut mesenchyme support differentiation of gut endocrine cells? Anat Embryol 1992;185:509–16.
89. Matsushita S. Appearance of brush-border antigens and sucrase in the allantoic endoderm cultured in recombination with digestive-tract mesenchymes. Roux's Arch Dev Biol 1984;193:211–8.
90. Buchberger A, Pabst O, Brand T, et al. Chick NKx2.3 represents a novel family member of vertebrate homologues to the *Drosophila* homeobox gene tinman: differential expression of cNKx2.3 and cNKx2.5 during heart and gut development. Mech Dev 1996;56:151–63.
91. Jonsson J, Carlsson L, Edlund T, Edlund H. Insulin-promoter-factor 1 is required for pancreas development in mice. Nature 1994;371:606–9.
92. Peshavaria M, Gamer L, Henderson E, et al. XlHbox 1, an endoderm-specific Xenopus homeodomain protein, is closely related to a mammalian insulin gene transcription factor. Mol Endocrinol 1994;8:806–16.
93. Guz Y, Montiminy MR, Stein R, et al. Expression of murine STF-1, a putative insulin gene transcription factor, in beta cells of pancreas, duodenal epithelium and pancreatic exocrine and endocrine progenitors during ontogeny. Development 1995;121:11–8.
94. Lee J, Rajendran VM, Mann AS, et al. Functional expression and segmental localization of rat colonic K-Adenosine Triphosphatase. J Clin Invest 1995;96:2002–8.

CHAPTER 2

Gene Regulation: The Key to Intestinal Development

Daniel A. Wiginton, PhD

GENOMIC REGULATORY SYSTEMS

In mammals and other higher eukaryotes, just as in all metazoans, the body is composed of cells that have differentiated and developed into tissues and organs with distinct structures and functions. In fact, any organism or species is defined by the structure and function of these tissues and organs. The master plan or blueprint for the development of each organism is genetically encoded within the nuclear DNA of each cell of that organism. This much is a fairly obvious extrapolation of our knowledge of the structure and function of DNA and of the fact that all cells within an organism can originate from a single cell derived from the union of DNA from two parental germ cells. Not so obvious are the mechanisms by which the genetic information in the cell's genomic DNA is accessed, interpreted, and used to produce the myriad distinct, differentiated cell types present in the tissue structures and organs of a particular organism. Studies to understand these mechanisms are a principal focus of modern developmental biology and are the key to understanding the development of any tissue or organ, such as those in the gastrointestinal tract.

The nature of any cell within a differentiated organism is defined by the pattern of specific gene products expressed from the large ensemble of genes within the cell's genomic DNA. Not all genes within the ensemble will express products within any particular cell type. Also, the level and timing of expression of a particular gene product may vary widely among cell types in which it is expressed. How are these complex patterns of cell-type-specific and tissue-specific gene expression established and regulated?

It appears that the regulatory programs governing these patterns of gene expression during development are "hardwired" into the genomic DNA.[1] These developmental regulatory programs are principally encoded in cis-regulatory genomic sequences, through which the expression of individual genes is controlled. While a particular cell or tissue may respond to changes in its internal or external environment by modifying patterns or levels of gene expression, in the end these changes are also moderated through the cis-regulatory sequences associated with the gene. While the structure and function of some gene products may be specifically modified after their expression, these modifications are carried out by factors whose expression is itself specifically controlled by other cis-regulatory sequences. Thus, the essence of understanding the cell differentiation and tissue formation that underlie development is an understanding of the nature and function of cis-regulatory genomic sequences.

Regulation through Control of Transcription Initiation

A general characteristic of cis-regulatory genomic DNA sequences is that they are recognized and bound in a sequence-specific manner by proteins that are generically termed specific transcription factors. Gene expression is thought to be controlled principally at the level of transcription, especially transcription initiation. The principal role of transcription factors bound at a gene's cis-regulatory sequences is to influence, directly or indirectly, the rate of transcription initiation. Deoxyribonucleic acid binding is not a prerequisite for a factor to function as a transcription factor. Some factors influence transcription through protein-protein interactions alone. Transcription in eukaryotic cells is carried out by several distinct RNA polymerases. Ribonucleic acid polymerase I transcribes ribosomal RNA (rRNA) from ribosomal DNA (rDNA) and accounts for most of the transcriptional activity within the cell. Ribonucleic acid polymerase II transcribes RNA from structural genes, and these RNAs are processed into mRNAs that encode the wide variety of proteins produced by the cell. Ribonucleic acid polymerase III transcribes small RNAs, such as the transfer RNAs (tRNAs). The rest of this chapter will be focused on factors that affect the transcriptional function of RNA polymerase II.

Eukaryotic RNA polymerase II, itself a multisubunit protein, does not initiate transcription alone, but as a larger complex with a number of other proteins, termed general or basal transcription factors.[2] These general transcription factors (GTFs) include TFIID, TFIIA, TFIIB, TFIIE, TFIIF, and TFIIH. A detailed description of the assembly, structure, and function of this general transcription complex (sometimes called the basal transcription or preinitiation complex) and its subunits is well beyond the scope of this chapter but a few general principles and relevant observations will be described.

The GTFs recruit RNA polymerase II to a region called the core promoter of the gene and assembly of the preinitiation complex at that site. In so doing they determine the site of transcription initiation and prepare the polymerase for that event. A key player in the formation of the preinitiation complex, TFIID has been found to be a complex of at least six to eight separate proteins. One of these, TATA binding protein (TBP) recognizes and binds a DNA sequence (the TATA box) found in many, but not all, core promoters. The remaining proteins in the TFIID complex are called TBP associated factors (TAFs). Transcription factors bound to some cis-regulatory DNA sequences in a gene have a regulatory influence on the transcription of that gene by directly or indirectly interacting with components of the preinitiation complex to affect the efficiency of the formation and stability of that complex.[3] These interactions can be with TBP, other GTFs (such as TFIIA or TFIIB), or TAFs (sometimes called coactivators or adapters). In some cases there may be simultaneous interactions with more than one component. Transcription factors bound at the distant sites of cis-regulatory DNA sequences can interact with the preinitiation complex by bending and/or looping out of the intervening DNA. Sequence-specific transcription factors that function as activators normally do so through a subdomain of the factor called the activator domain (discussed in more detail below). The transcription factors may act alone to use the activator domain to interact with factors in the preinitiation complex, or as a dimer or higher-order regulatory complex. Multiple proteins in a single regulatory complex or multiple proteins bound at separate distinct regulatory sites may make contacts with the preinitiation complex simultaneously. In summary, the major determinant of the level of transcription initiation (and subsequent transcription and gene product formation) of a gene in a cell is probably the identity and functional nature of the sequence-specific transcription factors bound on the cis-regulatory DNA sequences of that gene.

Organization of Cis-regulatory DNA Sequences

Historically, cis-regulatory DNA sequences for eukaryotic genes have been categorized into several distinct groups, such as promoter elements, enhancers, and silencers. These categories have been based on both functional and structural criteria. Promoter elements are normally found upstream of the core promoter and transcription start site. There are proximal promoter elements that are near the transcription start site and distal promoter elements that are farther upstream and can even be several kilobases from the start site. Transcription factors bound to promoter elements can have a positive or negative effect on transcription initiation (as activators or repressors). The function of factors bound to promoter elements can sometimes be highly dependent on physical constraints, such as the distance of the promoter element from the transcription start site. The classic definition of an enhancer is a DNA segment, often found a large distance upstream or downstream of the transcription start site, that can activate transcription in an orientation- and distance-independent manner. These enhancers are normally compact DNA segments of 200 to 300 bases containing multiple cis-regulatory DNA sequences. Enhancers may be intragenic or intergenic in nature. Enhancers have often been found to exert their functional influence on transcription in a tissue-specific or stage-specific manner. Silencer is a functional name for a DNA segment that has a negative impact on transcription initiation. Silencers may contain cis-regulatory DNA sequences that bind repressor factors. The functional distinction between certain promoter elements and enhancers or silencers can sometimes be quite blurred. Care should be taken to discern the meaning that is being implied by use of these terms in any discussion of gene regulation.

Regulatory Networks and Cascades

As described above, the expression of protein gene products, such as enzymes and structural proteins, is governed at the level of transcription by factors bound by the gene's cis-regulatory DNA sequences. Since these transcription factors themselves are proteins, their expression is also governed by other transcription factors bound at cis-regulatory DNA sequences associated with the genes that encode them. In an obvious extrapolation of this logic, there are cascades of gene regulation that control expression of the array of functional proteins present in a cell. Since multiple transcription factors are normally involved in regulation of a particular gene, and a particular type of transcription factor may be involved in the regulation of multiple genes, it is obvious that these cascades are only part of a complex, interconnected regulatory network. The complexity of this network is further increased by observations such as feedback loops of self-regulation, functional modification of transcription factors by enzymes such as kinases and phosphatases, the ability of different factors to bind to the same cis-regulatory element, and the ability of some factors to heterodimerize with a variety of partners. This complex network represents the circuitry of the hardwired pattern of development described earlier in this section. In order to understand development as a whole or development of any particular organ or tissue, we must understand this regulatory network and the factors and elements that compose it.

MODULARITY: A CRITICAL ASPECT OF EUKARYOTIC GENE REGULATION

The concept of modules is a consistent underlying theme in the regulation of eukaryotic genes.[1] A module is defined as a self-contained unit or item that is used in combination with other units to produce the function of the group as a whole. Modularity is observed at several different levels of eukaryotic gene regulation and is the basis for much of the

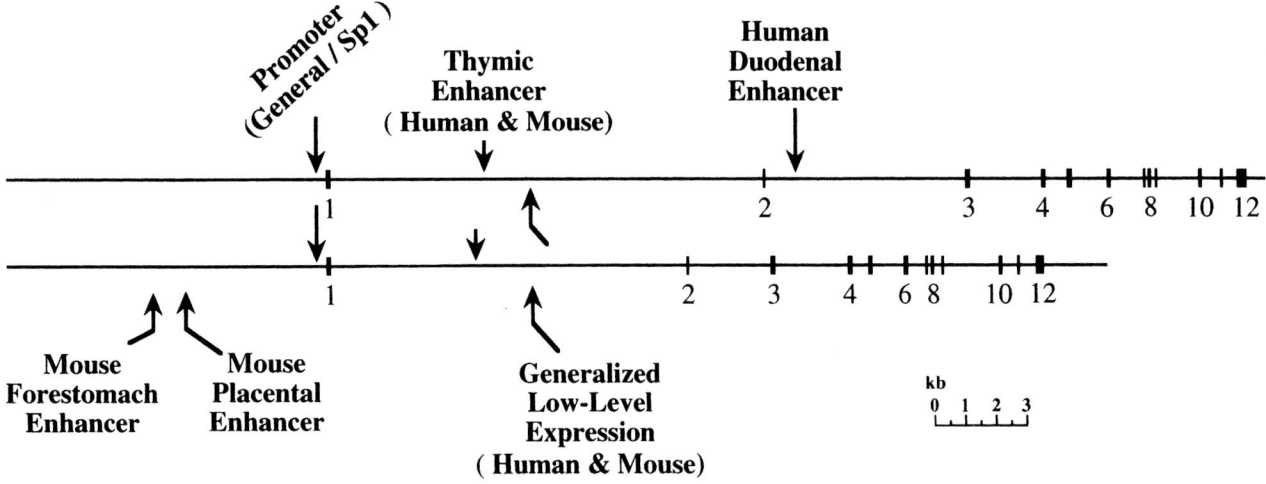

FIGURE 2–1. Modular regulation of adenosine deaminase. The human (top) and mouse (bottom) adenosine deaminase (ADA) genes are shown to scale in a linear, graphic representation. Exons are shown as solid vertical rectangles. Also shown are the approximate locations of various regulatory modules that govern the tissue-specific and generalized expression of these ADA genes.

subtle and sophisticated patterns of gene expression observed in higher organisms. If a gene is expressed in different tissues or in distinct domains or time frames during development, often distinct cis-regulatory modules carry out the different parts of the regulatory job. These modules can be a single cis-regulatory element but are usually modular themselves, comprising multiple distinct elements that are binding sites for different transcription factors. Finally, there is modularity at yet a third level since transcription factors that bind to the regulatory elements themselves often have modular protein structure. Distinct protein subdomains (or modules) carry out the protein's different functions, such as DNA binding, transactivation, and dimerization.

Different Modules for Different Jobs

As mentioned, when a gene is to be expressed (or repressed) in different circumstances during development or expressed in a tissue-specific pattern in the mature organism, different modules may control different aspects of the patterns of expression. These modules can be positive or negative, and many have been characterized as distinct enhancers or silencers although those terms often carry additional denotations. An experimental definition of a cis-regulatory module is a fragment of DNA containing multiple transcription-factor target sites that, when tested in a gene-transfer protocol, produces some subelement of the overall pattern of expression of the gene.[4] These modules are separate and distinct from the basal promoter but may interact with the preinitiation complex that assembles there, as described. Also, these modules are functionally separable from their natural promoters and should interact with at least some heterologous promoters. They also may interact with one another to supplement or modify functionality in gene regulation. It should also be noted that some genes that have a fairly straightforward pattern of expression, such as one that is ubiquitously expressed at a relatively uniform level or one that has a very limited pattern of tissue-specific expression, may be regulated by what could be considered a single regulatory module.

Modularity is an important characteristic of a number of complex cis-regulatory systems that have been characterized in Drosophila and sea urchin.[4] For example, in Drosophila, the Krüppel gene includes modules that control expression in certain regions of early- and later-stage blastoderm embryos, plus at least 10 distinct elements specifying expression in different developing tissue-structures and cellular precursors.[5] Modularity in cis-regulatory systems is by no means limited to lower organisms, and a number of examples have been found in mammals. One example, regulation of the genes for human and mouse adenosine deaminase (ADA), is described in Figure 2–1. Adenosine deaminase (an enzyme involved in purine salvage and degradation) is expressed ubiquitously in mice and humans but the levels of expression vary dramatically between various tissues. In addition to a proximal promoter module, which is driven principally by the transcription factor Sp1 and activates low-level expression in a non-tissue-specific manner, several modules that activate high-level expression in tissues have been identified.[6] These include thymus-specific and generalized enhancers identified in both the human and mouse genes,[7,8] placental and forestomach-specific enhancers identified in the mouse gene,[9] and an intestine-specific enhancer element identified in the human gene.[10]

Intramodular Complexity

Whether expression of a gene is governed by multiple regulatory modules or a single regulatory module, normally there is significant complexity within the individual modules themselves. They are usually composed of multiple DNA elements that bind separate factors since transcription factors almost never work alone. These elements represent the second level of modularity in the systems that regulate eukaryotic gene expression. The output that comes from any regulatory module is the product of all the bound factors working together, in conjunction with any factors that may be bound by protein-protein interactions without contacting DNA. A corollary to this statement is that the quality and quantity of output from a module depends on the nature and concentration of the factors available within a particular cell to bind the module's elements. In addition, sometimes impediments such as chromatin structure of the DNA must be overcome before the array of available factors can bind and interact. The structure of a number of complex modules has been reviewed recently.[1]

An Array of Elements and Factors

There are a number of aspects of the intramodular DNA elements and their binding factors that increase the complexity and functional flexibility of modules. Some of these will be listed here. (1) Individual factors may have a positive (activator) or negative (repressor) effect on module function. A particular factor's positive or negative character may vary, depending on the context of other factors present within the module. (2) Some factors' presentation and/or activity are directly affected in response to signal transduction systems. (3) Covalent modification, such as phosphorylation or dephosphorylation, may be required for factor binding and/or function. In some cases, the modification may be required for binding or, alternatively, the modification may occur only after binding. (4) Different transcription factors may bind the same or overlapping DNA elements. Many factors are members of transcription factor families that recognize and bind the same or similar DNA elements. This makes aspects such as relative concentration, avidity of binding, and surrounding environment (such as contiguous DNA sequence and bound factors adjacent to the element) critical in determining which factor binds to and functions from a particular element. (5) Direct physical contact with other proteins may be critical to a factor's ability to bind DNA or carry out its function. These interactions can occur before or after DNA binding. Some factors bind only as monomers while others bind only as dimers (or higher-order complexes). The factors that require dimerization may bind and function only as homodimers, only as heterodimers, or, in some instances, as either. The latter two instances lend a great deal of variety to the regulatory potential of a particular module since multiple heterodimer partners may be possible. Different dimers may form with different kinetics, may recognize different DNA elements, or may recognize the same element with different avidities. Some dimer pairs may result in an inability to bind DNA and/or loss of function compared to other dimer pairs, imparting a subtle negative regulatory capability to the system. (6) Some transcription factors are expressed ubiquitously, some in a tissue-restricted pattern, and some in a cell- or tissue-specific manner. The tissues and cell types in which a module functions at any given time are those in which the module elements are accessible and the specific combination of factors required for module function are present at appropriate levels.

Architecture of the Module

So far our discussion has focused principally on elements of regulatory modules that bind transcription factors that affect transcription initiation directly, either by themselves or in conjunction with other proteins. There are other types of elements that bind factors whose roles are architectural in nature.[3] We have already talked about the large preinitiation complex of general transcription factors and polymerase that forms on the core promoter. Similarly, stereospecific multiprotein complexes also form on DNA in some cis-regulatory modules, such as some enhancers. The role of certain factors within these regulatory complexes is obviously the modulation of transcription initiation through their transactivation domains, as described above. However, some proteins in the complex may bind DNA in a sequence-specific manner but function as architectural components.[3] A prototypical example of this is the LEF-1 binding site in the T-cell receptor α-enhancer. This site binds members of the LEF-1/TCF-1 transcription factor family that are known to severely bend DNA (~120°) upon binding.[11] LEF-1 has been shown to activate transcription in vitro only in a context-specific manner and only in conjunction with other transcription factors. The DNA bending is a critical step that allows factor interaction in the formation of a T-cell-specific enhancer complex of at least four DNA-bound transcription factors (Figure 2–2).[12] Interaction of proteins bound within the module are thus crucial, and relative positions and orientations of elements within the module are essential to proper complex formation and module function.

The Chromatin Obstacle

Another architectural role of some factors that bind DNA elements in regulatory modules is the modification of chromatin structure on the module's DNA. Chromatin is composed principally of nucleosome structures in which the DNA is packaged by wrapping it in a specific way around a core of histone proteins. Chromatin's nucleosomal structure has a

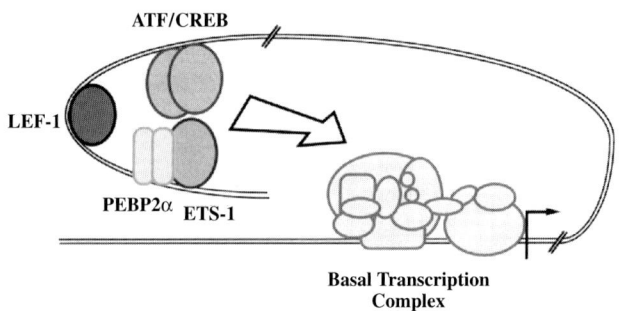

FIGURE 2–2. Model of T-cell receptor α-enhancer function. A regulatory complex is known to form on the T-cell receptor α-enhancer DNA segment in the thymocytes and T-cells in which it functions.[12] This is a model representation of that complex in which LEF-1 bends the DNA to allow interaction of the other bound factors during complex formation. The complex, once formed, is thought to interact indirectly or directly by DNA looping with the general transcription complex as it forms near the transcription start site.

generally repressive effect on transcriptional activation,[13] probably due in great part to limitation of access of transcription factors to their DNA binding site. One component of the gene activation process is the disruption of repressive chromatin structures.[14] Therefore, a role of one or more factors that bind in a particular regulatory module may be the modification, disruption, displacement, or realignment of nucleosomes along the module's DNA. These regions of modified or disrupted nucleosome structure are often seen as DNase I-hypersensitive sites associated with functional modules in the DNA of intact nuclei.[15] The mechanisms by which factors modify and disrupt nucleosome structure in the process of gene activation are just beginning to be worked out. It appears to be a multistep process in which the nucleosomes are initially modified and destabilized, allowing eventual access of all transcription factors necessary for module function.[14,16] Recent studies have shown that destabilization and stabilization of nucleosomes can occur by acetylation and deacetylation, respectively, of particular histones.[17] The histone acetylase and deacetylase activities are carried out by cofactor proteins associated with transcription factors known to bind elements in the regulatory modules studied.

Specialized Modules

A number of specialized modules have been identified that do not affect transcription directly but are known to have profound effects on the ability of associated genes to be transcribed. For purposes of our discussion, we will consider these modules to be cis-regulatory modules. Many, if not all, of these specialized modules are thought to exert their function by affecting the higher-order structures associated with genes, such as chromatin structure and formation of other regulatory complexes.[18] One such module, the locus control region (LCR), was first identified in association with the β-globin locus.[19] An LCR is experimentally defined as a DNA segment which in transgenic mice or stable transformation assays confers integration site-independent expression to a linked gene (independent of the chromatin environment at the site of insertion). This expression is often tissue-specific, and sometimes the level of expression is copy number-dependent (directly proportional to the number of gene copies introduced). Locus control regions normally have associated with them multiple binding sites for transcription factors.[20] In this and other ways, LCRs closely resemble enhancers. In fact, LCRs sometimes have enhancer activity associated with them. A clearer understanding of the similarities and differences between LCRs and enhancers awaits better knowledge of the mechanisms by which these two types of modules actually function.

Another type of specialized module affecting gene transcription, variously called insulator or boundary element, was originally identified as an element that could functionally isolate neighboring genes by blocking interactions between distal enhancers and inappropriate target promoters.[21] Recently, it has been proposed that their role might not be so restricted, and that they might also function as flexible regulatory elements that modulate promoter-enhancer interactions in complex genetic loci.[22] Experiments have shown that when one of these modules is artificially placed between an enhancer and its natural promoter target, it can block the promoter-enhancer interaction. Similar effects of insulators have been noted on the interaction of these enhancers with heterologous promoters. The mechanisms by which insulators and proteins associated with them exert their positional and polar effects are not well understood but establishment of chromatin domains and/or DNA loops have been proposed as part of the system.[23] Biochemical studies have identified segments of DNA called matrix-attachment regions (MARs) or scaffold-associated regions (SARs) that bind factors that can promote attachment to the nuclear matrix-scaffold.[24] Because of this attachment, they have been implicated in DNA looping and domain formation in vivo. The exact relationship between MARs and boundary elements-insulators is the subject of considerable debate. Matrix attachment regions have also been found in or flanking DNA segments that contain enhancers and have been implicated in the formation and/or function of the enhancer complex.[25]

As mentioned above, some modules have associated with them more than one functionality, such as enhancer-LCR or enhancer-MAR. In such cases, the distinct nature of the functions begins to blur, and their distinctness may be an arbitrary result of the nature of the experiments used to define them. One such case is the T-cell enhancer of the human ADA gene.[26] This enhancer has an LCR-like activity associated with it in transgenic mouse studies, and both the enhancer and LCR function in vivo are dependent on flanking segments called facilitators.[7] These facilitators are position- and orientation-dependent, and appear to be functionally different from insulators and, probably, MARs.[27] While the enhancer, LCR, and facilitator activities can be seen as distinct, in reality they function together as a single module to activate high-level ADA activity in thymocytes in vivo.

Transcription Factors are Modular

As alluded to, the third and last level of modularity in eukaryotic gene regulatory systems is within the transcription factors themselves.[28,29] Separate small subregions (or modules) of a transcription factor protein can account for the factor's ability to bind DNA, activate transcription, dimerize with other proteins, or other functions. As shown in Figure 2–3,[30–33] these subregions are linear stretches of contiguous amino acids that are on average from 50 to 100 residues long. Sometimes a particular function, such as DNA binding, requires more than one subregion but often these subregional modules function alone. This has been demonstrated repeatedly in experiments in which partial complementary DNA (cDNA) sequences for transcription factors are expressed either as truncated proteins (when expressed alone) or hybrid fusion proteins (when joined to and expressed with cDNA for another protein). The truncated or fusion protein is often able to maintain the function of the module(s) included, independent of the missing regions found normally in the native transcription factor.

DNA-Binding Domains: Transcription Factor Classification

One of the most significant observations to come from structural studies and amino acid sequence comparisons of tran-

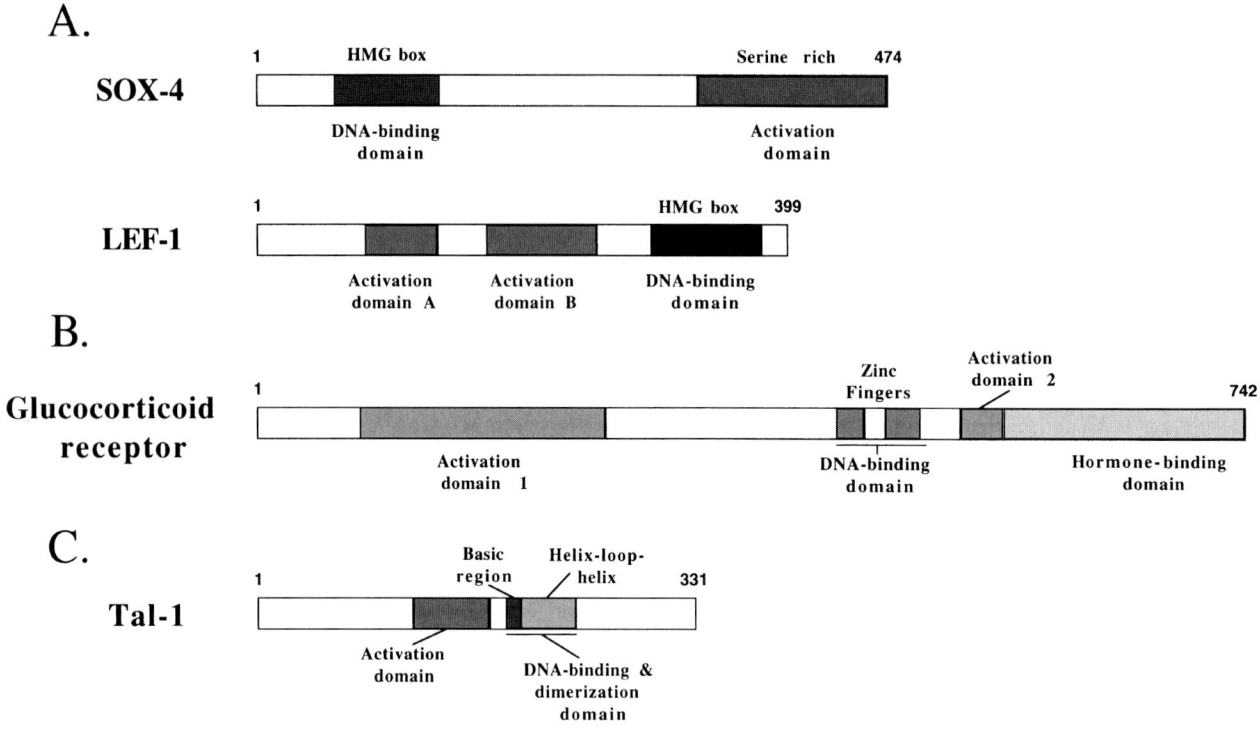

FIGURE 2–3. Modular subregions of several human transcription factors. Shown are linear schematic representations of members of three different classes of transcription factors: A, HMG domain factors, SOX-4 and LEF-1;[30,31] B, a zinc-finger factor glucocorticoid receptor;[32] and C, a bHLH family member, Tal-1.[33] SOX-4 and LEF-1 have very similar HMG DNA-binding domains but dramatically different activation domains.

scription factors is that they can be grouped into classes and families based on relatedness of structural motifs or modules. This classification has most often been done by comparison of the DNA recognition-binding modules of transcription factors. One such classification system, that of the TRANSFAC database at GBF Bioinformatics in Braunschweig, Germany, will be described here.[34] Most of the factors are listed as a member of one of four superclasses, each of which is subdivided into five to eight factor classes. Each class is further subdivided into families and subfamilies. The four superclasses are (1) basic domains, (2) zinc-coordinating DNA-binding domains, (3) helix-turn-helix, and (4) β-scaffold factors with minor groove contacts. The structural differences between these groups show that nature has solved the problem of DNA binding in a variety of different ways.

Among the eight classes in the basic domain superclass are the leucine zipper factors (bZIP), the helix-loop-helix factors (bHLH), helix-loop-helix/leucine-zipper factors (bHLH-ZIP), and NF-1-like factors. Many of the factors in this superclass have been shown to have roles in differentiation and development. In addition, they illustrate the important roles that heterodimer formation plays in gene regulation.[35] Factors in this superclass contact DNA through a highly basic domain. Most can dimerize, forming both homodimers and heterodimers, with the dimerization occurring through an adjacent domain, such as the leucine-zipper domain or helix-loop-helix domain. Deoxyribonucleic acid binding normally requires the dimerization while dimerization can occur in the absence of the basic DNA-binding domain. Among the seven families of factors within the bZIP class are AP-1 (and AP-1-like factors), the CREB family, and C/EBP-like factors. The bHLH factors include E2A-like ubiquitous factors, the myogenic transcription factor family (including MYOD, myogenin, and MYF-5), the Tal-Twist group, and six other families. The two principal families of bHLH-ZIP factors are ubiquitous factors (such as TFE3 and USF) and cell-cycle controlling factors (such as MYC and MAD-MAX).

The superclass of factors with zinc-coordinating, DNA-binding domains are principally composed of a variety of zinc-finger proteins. While protein zinc fingers have been shown to have other functions, a principal role of many is specific DNA binding. The zinc fingers are composed of a zinc ion coordinated and complexed by several amino acid residues (usually Cys or His), forming a finger-like protrusion. Most proteins have multiple fingers present that are involved in or influence DNA binding. The Cys4 zinc finger of nuclear receptor is a class that includes the steroid hormone receptor family (corticoid, progesterone, androgen, and estrogen receptors) and thyroid-hormone receptor-like factors (including thyroid hormone receptors, RAR receptors, Vitamin D receptor, and HNF-4). Another class, the diverse Cys4 zinc fingers class, contains the family of GATA factors. A number of ubiquitous factors (such as Sp1 and YY1), as well as developmental and cell cycle regulators (such as the EGR-KROX family and the Krüppel family) are found in the Cys2His2 zinc finger class. Other classes in this superclass are Cys6 cysteine-zinc cluster factors and zinc fingers of alternating composition.

There are a very large number of factors grouped in the helix-turn-helix superclass. Many of them fall within the homeodomain class. The homeodomain is a highly conserved region of about 60 amino acids that forms a stable, folded structure that is capable of binding DNA alone.[34] This class includes clustered and dispersed homeobox (HOX) genes that bind DNA through this homeodomain. Many are related to Abdominal B (ABDB), Antennapedia (ANTP), caudal (CAD), paired (PRD) and other homeobox genes in *Drosophila*. The factors CDX1 and CDX2 are members of the CAD subfamily. The HNF-1 group of factors are also part of the homeodomain family. Many homeodomain factors have domains with conserved sequence motifs that flank the homeodomain and modulate its DNA-binding specificity. These include the POU-domain family (such as PIT-1 and OCT factors) and LIM-domain family. Other classes within the helix-turn-helix superclass are the paired box factors (including the PAX family), fork head-winged helix factors (including the HNF-3 factors), heat shock factors, tryptophan cluster factors (such as MYB and the ETS family), and TEA domain factors.

The final superclass is a diverse group of factors that are called β-scaffold factors with minor groove contacts. Classes within this superclass include Rel homology region (RHR) factors, p53 factors, MADS box factors (including a number of regulators of differentiation and homeotic genes), β-barrel α-helix factors, TBP, and HMG factors (such as LEF-1 and TCF-1 mentioned above). There are also small but important groups of factors that fall into structural classes that are not related to any of the four major superclasses. These include the Runt (PEBP2 factors), STAT, and pocket domain (RB and CBP) classes. New transcription factors are being discovered at a rapid pace. Many fit into previously defined classes but it is likely that new classes and perhaps even superclasses remain to be discovered.

Other Modular Domains

In addition to the DNA-binding domains or modules, there are several other types of functional modules found in transcription factors. Some of these modules function alone and/or in conjunction with other modules. Dimerization domains or modules have been described above. The other major type of module found in transcription factors is the activation domain. Compared to DNA-binding and dimerization domains, whose roles are relatively straightforward, the functional roles and mechanisms of activation domains are not as easily understood. This is probably due to (1) great variability in the mechanisms by which activation is accomplished (i.e., with which components of the transcriptional apparatus does it interact?); (2) heterogeneity in the sequence of the activation domains themselves; and (3) the fact that transcriptional activation by a factor sometimes requires several distinct activation domains (or modules) within the factor working in concert. Nevertheless, several distinct types of activation domains have been identified. These types include acidic, glutamine-rich, and proline-rich domains.[3] As one would expect, distinct subtypes of these have been shown to exist. Interestingly, the individual predominant residues that give the activation domain its name may not be the most important, with more critical residues being dispersed among the predominant. These domains seem to have some conformational flexibility, with the conformation potentially being modulated both by partners within a dimer-regulatory complex and by the specific activation target.[3] This would provide a mechanism to achieve both specificity and flexibility.

GENE EXPRESSION IN THE INTESTINE

We have introduced in a general manner some of the current concepts and information about the mechanisms and factors involved in regulating gene transcription and the regulatory networks that underpin tissue development and cell differentiation. Now we will describe studies that have made application of this information and these principles in initial attempts to understand intestinal gene regulation and its role in orchestrating intestinal development and function. These studies can be grouped, primarily, into two broad categories. One category of studies examines the regulation of "end-product" genes that encode proteins and peptides that carry out specific jobs in the intestine, such as enzymes and structural proteins. The expression of these genes is the end product of the regulatory pathways and network. The complete array of such products expressed within a particular cell in the intestine defines, in large part, the nature and function of that cell. The other category of studies examines particular transcription factors and their role in the regulatory network within the intestine. These studies often seek to define the expression pattern of the factor, what target genes it regulates, and what factors regulate its expression. In this way, the place and role of an individual factor within the intestinal gene regulatory network and cascades can be defined. The eventual goal of both categories of study is that their results will merge into a pattern that will define the entire hardwired network of gene expression that governs intestinal development, maintenance, and function.

Organization of Mammalian Intestinal Epithelium

A number of the genes and factors that have been examined in intestinal gene regulation studies are expressed more broadly than just in intestine. However, many of the experimental studies have been designed to focus on the intestine-specific aspect of their regulation or function. Other studies have focused on genes whose expression is strictly limited to intestine. Often, intestine-specific studies of either type have further focused on or identified expression within one of the multiple tissue compartments within the intestine, such as the epithelium or muscularis. Perhaps the most widely studied of these has been the mammalian intestinal epithelium. Therefore, a brief review of the structure of that compartment in small intestine will be presented here.

The mammalian gastrointestinal epithelium has a complex but highly defined architecture. In small intestine, the primary components of this architecture are the crypt and villus (Figure 2–4). Committed stem cells in the crypt are the precursors of all four of the major specialized epithelial cell types. After cell division and initiation of differentiation, the immature cells begin an interesting bipolar migration. Enterocytes, goblet cells, and enteroendocrine cells migrate linearly in a band up along the villus, while Paneth cells migrate down into the crypt. The absorptive enterocytes represent 90 to 95% of the cells on the villus surface. The goblet cells produce mucus to protect the luminal surface, diverse enteroendocrine cells produce a variety of neuropeptides, and Paneth cells produce antibacterial peptides, digestive enzymes, and growth factors. The process of differentiation into each of these cell types involves activation of a specific program of gene expression characteristic of that epithelial cell type.

Intestinal Gene Regulation in the Epithelium along Three Axes

Changes in gene expression are observed within a particular epithelial cell type during differentiation and migration along the crypt-villus (CV) axis. In addition, there are large variations in gene expression along two other axes in the small intestine, the cephalocaudal or anterior and posterior (AP) axis from duodenum to ileum and the developmental time axis. Therefore, there are three separate but obviously interrelated axes on which intestinal gene expression can be evaluated (Figure 2–5). The network of regulatory factors and elements that specify and determine gene expression along these various axes is, in general, poorly understood.

During development there are changes in gene expression corresponding to both establishment of the intestinal architecture and to activation of genes at specific developmental times. The developmental timeframe and profile is obviously very different among different organisms. Even in mammalian systems there are important timing differences related to the length of gestation. Among mammalian systems, probably the best characterized developmental model is the mouse. In the mouse embryo, the primitive gut tube, comprised of endoderm surrounded by mesenchyme, is established around embryonic day 5 (E5). Morphogenesis of the gut epithelium occurs rather late in mouse development, from E15 through approximately postnatal day 21 (P21). The mouse gut endoderm undergoes rapid remodeling from E15 to E19 as a proximal-to-distal wave of cytodifferentiation converts it from a pseudostratified to a simple columnar epithelium. The intestinal-specific expression of certain end-product genes first occurs during this period. In the columnar epithelium, a monolayer covers nascent villi that are separated from one another by a polyclonal proliferative compartment known as the intervillus epithelium, the precursor of the intestinal crypt. Starting at E19, the crypts develop and the villi lengthen. A process of cell selection somehow occurs during crypt formation that converts them to monoclonal compartments by P14. As one might expect,

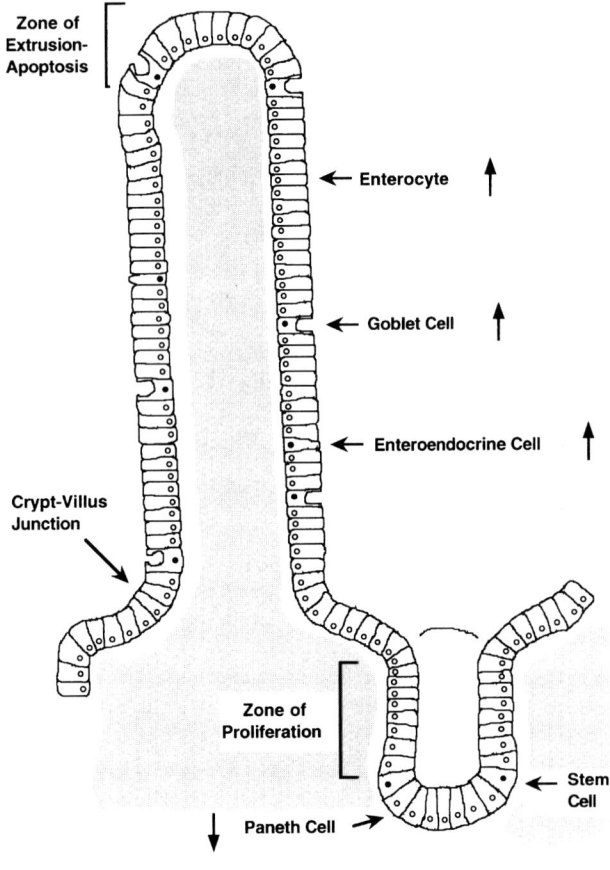

FIGURE 2–4. Crypt-villus structure of the mammalian small intestine. A simplified graphic representation of an intestinal villus and adjacent crypt of Lieberkühn is shown. Up and down arrows indicate the relative direction of migration for enterocytes, goblet cells, enteroendocrine cells, and Paneth cells.

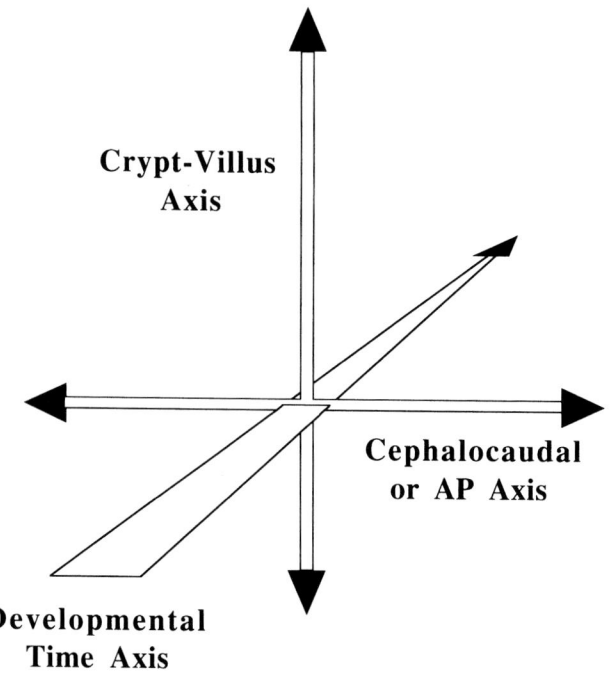

FIGURE 2–5. Three axes of development and cell differentiation in intestine.

there are changes in enzyme expression pattern along the gut that are associated with this developmental sequence of events. Days P14 to P21 are characterized by dramatic increases in crypt number as the result of crypt fission, and the final product is an adult epithelium in which well-formed villus structures are covered with columns of epithelial cells emanating from several adjacent crypts. During this time the suckling-weanling transition occurs, which is marked by a wave of cytodifferentiation and induction of gene expression from proximal to distal along the AP axis. In humans, most temporal changes during development of the intestine are observed relatively earlier, while in utero. Villi appear along the length of the human small intestine between 8 and 12 weeks of gestation, developing in a caudal wave from duodenum to ileum. Primitive crypts appear soon after. Late fetal intestine in humans has a CV morphology and enzyme expression pattern very similar to that in adult intestine. Once the adult pattern of gene expression is established along the AP axis in mice or humans, it is maintained despite a continuous and rapid turnover of epithelial cells throughout life.

Along this horizontal AP axis of the small intestine, in the duodenum, jejunum, and ileum, the epithelial cells show significant regional variation in metabolic capabilities and patterns of gene expression. As mentioned above, these regional differences are sustained throughout life despite the continuous, rapid renewal of the epithelium. A wide variety of studies have shown that outside factors such as diet, luminal contents, and hormones can modulate intestinal levels of certain proteins. However, a number of transplantation and isograft studies have clearly shown that the patterns of expression principally reflect an intrinsic program of development and differentiation in the epithelium. The molecular basis of this positional variation in differentiation programs is unclear, as is the actual source of the positional address. Perhaps the two most likely sources are the stem cell itself and mesenchyme-derived cells (such as fibroblasts) that are closely associated with the epithelium.

Along the CV axis there are many significant questions that remain unanswered as well. What are the stages, factors, and mechanisms involved in lineage allocation to the various cell types from the committed epithelial stem cells? What are the genetic mechanisms that drive the process of cellular differentiation once lineage allocation has occurred? Studies of the regulation of genes expressed in a cell type-specific manner in the epithelium are likely to lead to a better understanding of both processes, allocation and differentiation. Cellular differentiation appears to be tightly coupled to the cell migration that occurs subsequent to cell division. Proliferation ceases in the upper third of the crypt, and cell division does not occur once the cells migrate onto the villus. In enterocytes, emergence from the crypt onto the villus at the CV junction corresponds to a time at which expression of a wide variety of genes is first observed.[36] The timing suggests that this transcriptional induction of differentiated expression is intimately associated with cessation of proliferation. It is not clear whether this is generally true of gene expression in other differentiated villus cell types as well, although some evidence indicates that it is not.[36] Therefore, mechanisms behind the process of differentiation may vary with cell lineage.

Studies of Gene Regulation in the Epithelium

Significant efforts to understand gene regulation in intestinal cells began in the late 1980s, with transgenic mouse experiments examining expression and regulation of members of the fatty acid binding protein family carried out by Gordon and colleagues.[37,38] These studies have also produced many insights into the biology of intestinal epithelial cells, as reviewed above.[39] As in most of the genes whose intestinal regulation we will discuss below, the regulatory modules discovered and analyzed were located in the promoter regions, both proximal and distal to the transcription start sites.

Fatty Acid Binding Protein Genes

Two members of the fatty acid binding protein (FABP) family of proteins are found in abundance in the cytoplasm of epithelial cells in mammalian small intestine. These proteins were named intestinal (I-) FABP and liver (L-) FABP, based on their initial sites of isolation. Expression of I-FABP is confined to the gut, with a gradient of expression along the AP axis of the intestine. Highest levels of expression are observed in the distal jejunum, with graded decreases toward the duodenum and proximal colon, where lowest levels are observed. In addition, variation in expression is observed along the CV axis where expression first appears at the CV junction and persists to the villus tip. Expression of I-FABP is normally confined to cells of the enterocyte lineage. Transgenic mice were used to map cis-acting elements that control this complex pattern of expression for the I-FABP gene.[38-41] Early observations indicated that different, distinct mechanisms probably regulate I-FABP expression along the AP and CV axes.[38] Detailed transgenic studies showed that nucleotides −103 to +28 of the rat I-FABP gene were able to restrict transgene expression to the enterocytic lineage and establish an appropriate AP gradient, as well as correctly initiate transgene expression in late fetal life.[40] However, expression during development and differentiation, as well as along the AP gradient, was influenced by elements upstream of the −103 to +28 segment. Sequences in a −1178 to −278 segment were found to be involved in sustained expression in adulthood. The sequences between −277 and −185 repressed distal expression in ileum-colon and in crypt cells. An element was identified in this region (−263 to −244) that binds small intestinal nuclear proteins and functions to suppress expression in ileum-colon, in the crypt, and in Paneth cells.[42] The only specific factors identified, to date, that function in the −1178 to +28 I-FABP promoter segment were identified by studies in cell lines.[41] Two members of the Cys4 zinc finger-type nuclear receptor class of transcription factors, hepatic nuclear factor-4 (HNF-4) and apolipoprotein regulatory factor-1 (ARP-1), were found to interact with a conserved 14 bp element in the −103 to +28 promoter segment. Studies suggested that HNF-4 and ARP-1 function to activate expression through this element, and that this activation is affected by other elements/factors.

Similar transgenic studies have been carried out on L-FABP, whose synthesis is confined to liver and the gastrointestinal tract from stomach to colon in man and rat.[37,39,43] In the small intestine and liver, L-FABP expression is limited to villus enterocytes and hepatocytes respectively. Along the AP axis of the small intestine, highest L-FABP levels are found in proximal jejunum. Along the CV axis, expression is activated in the villus enterocytes as they emerge from the crypt in a manner similar to that described above for a number of proteins. Sequences from −4000 to +21 of the rat L-FABP gene were tested in transgenic animals.[37,39] Again, a small proximal promoter fragment (−132 to +21) was sufficient to establish and maintain a pattern of expression similar to that of the endogenous gene in villus enterocytes along the AP axis of the small intestine (as well as appropriate hepatocyte expression). However, the segment from −4000 to +21 did not contain sequences necessary to suppress precocious expression in crypt cells, with inappropriate regulation along the CV differentiation axis. This is further evidence that different sequences regulate regional- and differentiation-dependent patterns of expression. Several segments upstream of −132 were found to suppress expression in colon, cecum, and kidney, but no homology was obvious, with segments having similar activity in the I-FABP gene. Subsequent studies identified a heptad repeat sequence located between −186 and −133 that functions as a suppressor in several different cell types, including kidney cells.[44] This repeat sequence appears to bind novel regulatory factors. Thus, both the I-FABP and L-FABP genes are regulated by the functional interplay of multiple positive and negative regulatory modules, with some of the endogenous silencer or repressor modules probably lying outside the tested promoter fragments.

Sucrase-Isomaltase Gene

Perhaps the best understood intestinal regulatory system at the molecular level is that of the sucrase-isomaltase (SI) gene. Regulation studies of the human and mouse SI genes have been carried out in both cell culture and transgenic mouse systems by Traber and colleagues.[45–48] Sucrase-isomaltase is a brush-border disaccharidase whose expression in adults is confined to villus enterocytes of the small intestine, where transcriptional activation of the gene is once again first evident at the CV junction. Sucrase-isomaltase is expressed at significant levels throughout the small intestine, with highest levels in the proximal jejunum.[47] Studies with transgenic mice indicated that the −3424 to +54 fragment flanking the human SI gene was sufficient to direct transgene transcription solely to the intestine and to give an appropriate CV expression pattern.[47] However, the AP pattern was aberrant, with high expression in distal jejunum and ileum and little or no expression in duodenum and proximal jejunum. A larger (−8500 to +54) fragment of the mouse SI gene, however, gave a pattern of intestinal-specific transgene expression along the AP axis much more similar to that of the endogenous gene.[48] This might indicate the presence of a different regulatory module(s) within the additional 5 kb of sequence in the mouse fragment, although species differences were not ruled out. Both mouse and human fragments gave inappropriate ectopic expression in some colonic cells. In addition, inappropriate expression of the transgene was observed in small intestine in enteroendocrine, Paneth, and goblet cells.[48] It was postulated that negative elements or silencers were missing from the transgene fragments tested, resulting in the inappropriate or ectopic expression. Thus, again it would appear that multiple positive and negative modules are required to function together to give the intestinal-specific pattern of SI expression observed in vivo.

Transfection studies in cell culture[45] and transgenic mouse studies[49] have shown that short segments of 200 to 300 bp of the most proximal 5′-flanking promoter sequence from the human and mouse SI genes were sufficient to direct transcription specifically to intestinal epithelial cells. Footprinting with DNase I and gel-shift experiments were used to identify three segments within the −180 to −30 region (SIF-1,-2 and-3) that acted as positive-regulatory elements.[46] The SIF-2 and SIF-3 segments were found to be bound by factors that were ubiquitous and related. Subsequently these elements were found to bind two divergent members of the homeodomain family of transcription factors, hepatocyte nuclear factor 1α (HNF-1α) and HNF-1β, with different affinities.[50] HNF-1α was shown to activate transcription in cotransfection studies with the SI promoter. The SIF-1 element binds an intestine-specific factor, which has been identified as the caudal-related homeodomain factor CDX2.[51] Cotransfection studies showed that CDX2 can activate transcription of the SI promoter. Other studies have shown that CDX1 can also bind the SIF-1 element.[49] There is a proposed GATA-type binding site between SIF-1 and SIF-2. Preliminary results with a fourth segment (SIF-4) show that it can bind factors of the basic-leucine-zipper class.[36] Examination of the expression patterns of the CDX and HNF factors that are known to bind the proximal promoters of the SI genes indicate that they alone are not sufficient to explain the spatial and temporal patterns of SI expression. Among the many possibilities proposed are the combinatorial effects of all the bound factors (including other, as yet undefined, factors that bind in the SI proximal promoter), functional modification of the known factors by phosphorylation or other means, interaction of the known factors with proteins that do not bind DNA (such as coactivator or adapter molecules), role of regulatory modules outside the proximal promoter, and requirements for chromatin modulation.[49,52] Recent studies have indicated that factors other than CDX2 can bind the SIF-1 element, and the nature of these factors may change during postnatal development.[53]

Intestinal-Specific Regulation of Other Genes

In recent years, studies have begun on the regulation of a wide variety of other intestinally expressed genes. We will examine some of them here. Aminopeptidase N (APN) is a metallopeptidase found at high levels in the brushborder of intestinal enterocytes and at lower levels in liver and myeloid cells. The APN gene has two distinct promoters separated by several kb of DNA. The upstream promoter activates expression in myeloid cells while the downstream promoter is responsible for expression in intestine and liver. Functional binding sites for HNF-1 factors and for Sp1 have been identified in the porcine intestinal-liver promoter between −85 and −30.[54] An enhancer-like segment has been identified between the promoters that seems to be capable of activating either promoter.[55] This segment has potential binding sites for Ets factors, C/EBP factors, and Sp1.[55]

The disaccharidase enzyme lactase-phlorizin hydrolase (LPH) is a membrane-bound protein expressed in enterocytes. Most newborn mammals have high levels of LPH, which decline dramatically at about the time of weaning. This pattern of expression is almost diametrically opposed to that of the predominant adult disaccharidase, SI. A 1-kb segment of the proximal porcine LPH promoter was shown to direct postweaning decline and small intestinal-specific expression in transgenic mice.[56] Transfection studies, DNase I footprinting, and EMSA studies demonstrated that there are several distinct elements or modules in this region with positive and negative character,[57,58] and the most proximal of the positive elements was shown to bind CDX2.[58] It has also been proposed that post-transcriptional mechanisms may have a significant impact on levels of LPH observed in adults.[53]

The calbindin-D9k gene is expressed at high levels in rat duodenal epithelium, principally in differentiated enterocytes, as well as lung and uterus. The calbindin-D9k gene is transcriptionally regulated in intestine by 1,25-dihydroxyvitamin D3 through a receptor response element located in the rat promoter between −489 and −445.[59] Transgenic mouse studies determined that distinct promoter elements (or modules) were responsible for activating calbindin-D9k expression in various tissues, including a segment between −4400 and −1011 that was required for intestinal expression.[60] This region encompasses a previously observed intestinal-specific DNase I hypersensitive site (HS) at −3.5 kb. Transient transfection studies in intestinal (CaCo-2) and non-intestinal (HeLa) cells were used to define functional regions in the proximal promoter.[61] A minimal promoter fragment (−117 to +20) activated expression in both cell types, while addition of sequences out to −559 repressed expression in the HeLa cells but not the CaCo-2 cells. This region contains the only additional intestinal-specific HS observed. DNase I footprinting and EMSA experiments were used to evaluate factor binding in the proximal promoter region.[61] Apparent binding sites for CDX2, C/EBP α and β factors, HNF-1 factors, and HNF-4-COUP were identified between −270 and −10. Several other footprints that bind factors of unknown nature were observed between −800 and −300, including two that were duodenal-specific.

Guanylin, a 15-amino-acid peptide, is an endogenous ligand for the receptor guanylyl cyclase C. Both guanylin and the receptor are principally expressed in intestine, where they are involved in mediation of fluid and electrolyte secretion and balance. Initial regulatory studies have been carried out on the promoters of the mouse[62] and human[63] guanylin genes and the human guanylyl cyclase C gene.[64] Transfection studies have implicated HNF-1α in activation of expression of the mouse guanylin gene through a very proximal site in the promoter.[62]

Apolipoprotein B (APOB) is a major constituent of the plasma lipoproteins. In adult mammals, it is synthesized principally in two tissues, liver and intestine. The human APOB gene has a proximal promoter located in the first few hundred bp of 5′-flanking sequence that binds multiple factors and is comprised of both positive and negative elements.[65,66] Binding sites for HNF-4 and C/EBP factors were identified in the positive elements.[66,67] This promoter activates expression in both liver- and intestine-derived cultured cells but requires additional sequences, including flanking MAR sequences, to recapitulate tissue-specific expression in transgenic mice.[68,69] The additional required sequences appear to be different for liver and intestine, in that a liver-specific enhancer was identified in the second intron of the human APOB gene that does not activate expression in intestine.[68] Although a comparable enhancer module that activates intestinal expression of APOB in vivo has not been identified, a segment in the third intron was studied that represses transcription in intestinal CaCo-2 cells.[70] Interestingly, binding sites for members of the caudal family (such as CDX2) and for HNF-1 factors were identified within this apparent repressor module. An interaction between factors bound in the repressor and C/EBP factor(s) bound in the promoter was proposed as a requirement for repression.[70]

Carbonic anhydrase 1 (CA1), a member of a large family of mammalian carbonic anhydrase proteins with different tissue and subcellular localization, is expressed principally in colonic epithelium and erythroid cells, where it is abundant. Carbonic anhydrase 1 catalyzes reversible hydration of CO_2 and is important for cellular diffusion of CO_2, ion transport, and pH regulation. The CA1 gene is unusual in that it has two distinct promoters: one that functions in colon and one that is erythroid cell-specific.[71] DNase I hypersensitivity and EMSA studies were used to identify a CDX2 binding site within the colon-specific promoter.[72]

In addition to the gene regulatory systems described above, the promoters of a wide variety of other genes have been examined that have an intestinal component to their expression pattern. Transgenic mouse studies that have identified promoters or promoter segments that activate intestinal expression include, but are not limited to, studies of ileal lipid-binding protein, α-fetoprotein, ornithine transcarbamylase, carbamyl phosphate synthetase, pyruvate kinase, PEPCK, HMG-CoA synthetase, cholesteryl ester transfer protein, the P450 family member CYP1A1, and glutamine synthetase. Transfection studies in intestinal cell culture have been used to examine the intestinal promoter function of a wide variety of genes, including the genes encoding villin, alcohol dehydrogenase, apolipoprotein A-II, dipeptidyl-peptidase IV, the Na^+/H^+ exchanger NHE3, Factor B, and inducible nitric oxide synthetase.

Intestinal-Specific Enhancers

The studies in intestinal gene regulation that have been described almost exclusively examined regulatory modules and elements located in the proximal and distal promoter regions of the genes studied. Intestinal-specific regulatory modules have also been identified in other locations for a few genes. As mentioned above, and shown in Figure 2–1, one of the several regulatory modules identified that orchestrate the complex tissue-specific regulation of the human ADA gene is an intestinal-specific enhancer located 15 kb downstream of the transcription initiation site.[10] This enhancer activates high-level reporter gene expression in transgenic mice that is specific to the duodenal epithelium and was found to have associated with it several duodenal-

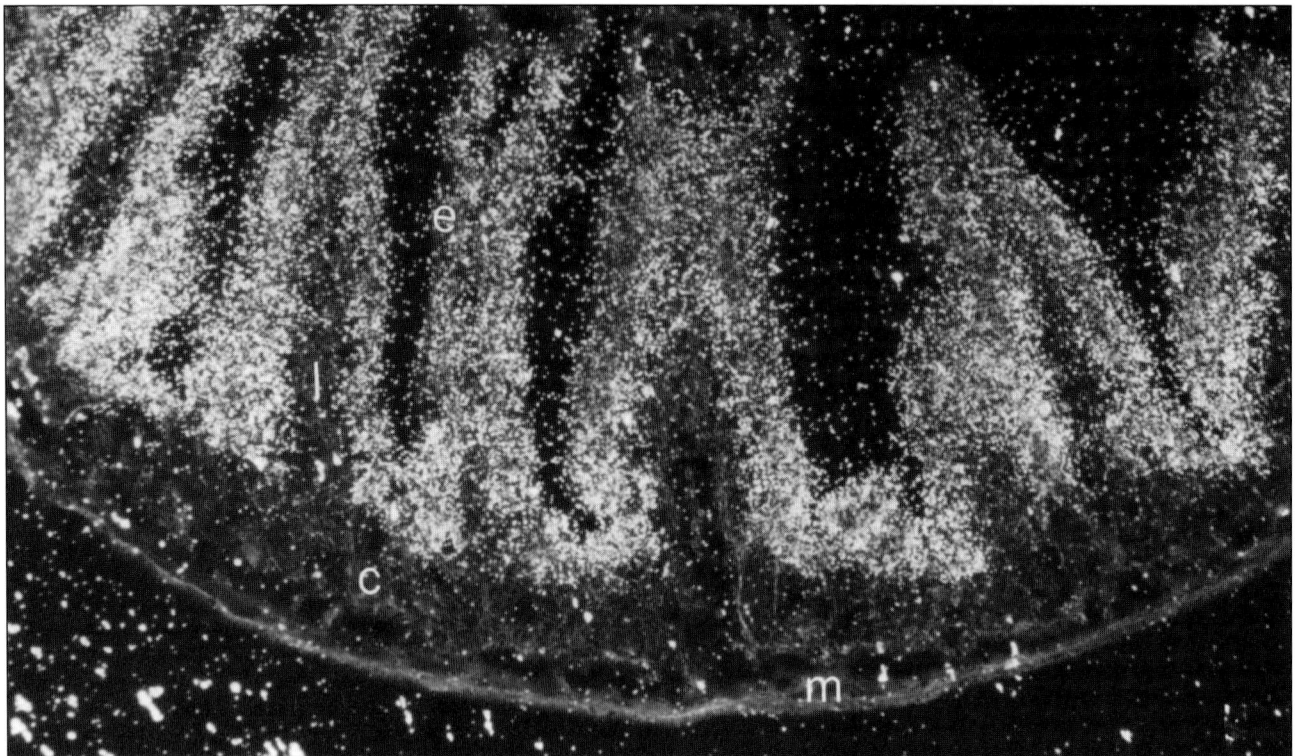

FIGURE 2–6. In situ hybridization to CAT mRNA in ADA-promoter-CAT-reporter transgenic mouse duodenum. A duodenum from a transgenic mouse expressing chloramphenicol acetyl transferase (CAT) was sectioned and hybridized to a radiolabelled CAT antisense probe. Original magnification ×100. The CAT-reporter gene expression was activated to high levels, specifically in duodenum, when a duodenal-specific enhancer segment from the human ADA gene was included in the transgene construction along with the ADA promoter and the CAT coding sequences.[10] Deposition of signal is seen in along the duodenal villi, over the villous epithelium (e), but absent from crypt (c), lamina propria (l), and intestinal muscular layer (m). This pattern of expression is identical to that observed for the endogenous murine ADA gene in duodenum.

specific HSs. The enhancer appears to be principally responsible for the pattern of endogenous ADA expression observed along the intestinal AP axis, where ADA is expressed at very high levels in duodenum and much lower levels in the more distal parts of the small and large intestine. In addition, the enhancer drives appropriate expression along the duodenal CV axis, where reporter-gene activation at the CV junction and expression in villus enterocytes closely resemble the pattern observed for endogenous ADA (Figure 2–6). Developmental activation of ADA transgene expression was precocious compared to endogenous mouse ADA expression, and may more closely resemble the developmental activation pattern of the human ADA gene.[10]

The apolipoprotein genes constitute a multigene family with strong similarities in structure, genomic structure, and functional domains. In humans, apolipoprotein A-I (APOA-I), apolipoprotein A-IV (APOA-IV), and apolipoprotein C-III (APOC-III) are expressed primarily in liver and intestine. These three genes are tandemly organized in a closely linked gene cluster of about 15 kb, with the APOC-III gene in the middle. The APOC-III gene is transcribed in the opposite orientation to that in which the other two genes are transcribed. Transgenic mice and cell culture transfection studies have been used to identify several positive and negative regulatory modules in this gene cluster. Transgenic mouse studies identified a 260-bp enhancer (−780 to −520) in the promoter of the human APOC-III gene that is capable of activating expression of the convergently transcribed APOA-I gene in intestine.[73,74] Transfection studies indicate that there are two separable cell-specific proximal promoters for APOA-I: one that functions in liver, and one in intestine.[75] The intestinal promoter contains an HNF-4 site (−214 to −192) that is required for enhancer-activated expression.[75] The APOA-IV proximal promoter (−380 to +10) also has been shown to function alone only at low levels in transfection studies using liver HepG2- and intestinal CaCo-2-cultured cells, and requires the enhancer located in the APOC-III promoter for higher-level activation.[76] Another functional HNF-4 binding site was identified within a DNase I footprint (−148 to −92) in the APOA-IV promoter. Other transfection studies have identified additional positive and negative segments lying between the APOC-III and APOA-IV promoters that are involved in regulating both these genes, and further demonstrated the importance of HNF-4 in regulating the expression of this gene cluster.[77]

As one can see in examining the studies on the apolipoprotein genes and the ADA gene, it is important to examine intronic and downstream intergenic sequences for the presence of regulatory modules, in addition to examining the promoter and 5′-flanking sequences. These regulatory modules can, moreover, sometimes be located long distances away. One additional example of an intronic enhancer is that found in the first intron of the rat aldolase B gene.[78] In transgenic mice this segment was found to be essential for expression in kidney, liver, and intestinal epithelium.

Gene Regulation in Goblet, Paneth, and Enteroendocrine Cells

Most of the studies in gene regulation described involved genes that are expressed in the intestine principally or exclusively in enterocytes. A number of studies have also been initiated examining regulation of genes whose intestinal expression is limited to one of the other epithelial cell types. Transgenic mouse studies demonstrated that nucleotides −6500 to +34 of the Paneth cell-specific cryptdin 2 gene could direct reporter gene expression specifically to the Paneth cell lineage in the crypt.[79] Intestinal trefoil factor (ITF) is a small peptide whose expression is localized primarily to goblet cells of the small and large intestine. Transient transfection studies with various segments of the rat ITF gene promoter indicated that the first 153 base pairs of proximal promoter were sufficient to drive goblet cell-specific expression.[80] Transient transfection studies have been carried out to analyze the extended promoter region of the human MUC2 gene, which expresses mucin principally in goblet cells.[81,82] Sequences were identified within the first several hundred bases of the promoter that activated expression in intestinal cell lines, including a potential Sp1 site.[82] More distal sequences exerted a negative effect on expression although it was not clear that the sequences examined were sufficient to produce the normal tissue-specific pattern observed for the gene.[81]

The intestinal regulation of genes that produce two different hormones, secretin and glucagon, in enteroendocrine cells has been examined. Secretin is produced in the rat by the enteroendocrine S cells in the small intestine and a subpopulation of developing pancreatic β-islet cells. Transgenic mouse studies showed that a promoter segment (−1600 to +34) of the rat secretin gene could direct expression to fetal islet cells and intestinal enteroendocrine cells in the proper distribution, with some ectopic expression in other tissues.[83] Transfection studies identified within this region an activator segment (−174 to −53) with two potential binding sites for Sp1 and a consensus E box binding site for bHLH factors.[84] Additional studies indicated that this site was functionally bound by the tissue-specific bHLH factor BETA2/NeuroD, heterodimerized with one of the ubiquitous bHLH factors, Pan1 or Pan2 (rodent homologues of E47 and E12).[85] Mice lacking BETA2 expression have been generated by gene-targeting methods.[86] Homozygous BETA2 null mice developed diabetes and died perinatally, with reduced beta cell numbers and defective islet development. In addition, secretin and cholecystokinin production was absent in the intestinal enteroendocrine cells.

The proglucagon gene is expressed in certain brain cells, intestinal enteroendocrine L cells, and pancreatic A cells. Transgenic mouse studies indicate that extended promoter segments of the rat proglucagon gene out to −2000 support expression in all three tissues, but segments out to −1300 support expression in brain and pancreas but not intestine.[87,88] This could indicate the existence of an intestinal-specific regulatory module. The homeobox transcription factor CDX2 has been shown to bind a proximal region of the rat proglucagon promoter called G1 (−94 to −37) that is important to activation of expression in both intestine and pancreas[89] and to activate expression through that promoter segment.[90] The regulatory studies on secretin and glucagon provide evidence of the developmental relationship between pancreas and intestine, and indicate the likelihood that the different enteroendocrine cell types have a common earlier epithelial progenitor.

The gene for neurotensin-neuromedin N (NT-N) is expressed principally in brain and enteroendocrine N cells in the distal small intestine. An N cell-like line, BON, was used for transfection studies to analyze the function of the NT-N gene proximal promoter. The proximal 216 bp of 5′-flanking sequence was identified as essential for NT-N expression in BON cells, and footprinting and EMSA experiments identified a number of putative factor-binding sites in this promoter region.[91] Further characterization of the systems described above and other similar gene regulatory systems in goblet, Paneth, and enteroendocrine cells should provide significant insight into the transcription factors and mechanisms that underlie cellular differentiation into all the various cell types along the epithelial CV axis.

Muscle-Specific Gene Regulation in the Intestine

So far, our discussion of gene regulation in the intestine has focused on expression within the epithelium of the intestine. Studies in other intestinal compartments have also been carried out, especially in the muscularis. The adult mammalian intestine normally contains two primary smooth muscle layers within the muscularis compartment, the muscularis mucosae and the muscularis propria. The muscularis mucosae lies between the lamina propria and the submucosa while the muscularis propria lies between the submucosa and the serosa. The muscularis propria is itself divided into two distinct layers, the circular smooth muscle layer and the longitudinal smooth muscle layer. The muscularis mucosae function is mucosal movement for mixing and absorption. The primary functions of the muscularis propria are motility, mixing, and sphincter formation. Development of these muscle layers occurs in a proximal-to-distal gradient along the AP axis, from amorphous mesenchyme positioned between a primitive epithelium on the luminal side and a primitive mesothelium on the serosal side.[92] This development from mesoderm requires a series of complex mutual interactions, both between the mesenchyme and developing epithelium (derived from the endoderm) and between the mesenchyme and developing enteric nervous system (derived from the ectoderm). It appears that normal intestinal smooth muscle development proceeds by the linear differentiation of distinct smooth muscle cell (SMC) phenotypes that result from the hierarchic expression of specific gene products.[92] The sequential smooth muscle phenotypes are undifferentiated mesenchyme cell, smooth muscle myoblast, immature smooth muscle myocyte, and mature smooth muscle myocyte. Intestinal smooth muscle development in the mouse involves at least three stages that correspond to inductive events that lead to initiation of differentiation in the circular layer of the muscularis propria, in the longitudinal layer of the muscularis propria, and in the muscularis mucosae. Many important questions about the developmental process and the gene expression and regulation that underlie it remain unanswered.

Skeletal, cardiac, and smooth muscle cells express many of the same muscle-specific genes during development and cell differentiation. Each cell type, however, also expresses a different set of muscle-specific genes, the products of which give each muscle cell type its unique properties. A significant part of the regulation of skeletal muscle genes is due to the combinatorial control of bHLH factors (MYOD, MYOGENIN, MYF5, and MRF4) and members of the MEF-2 (MADS-box) family.[93] It has been proposed that similar types of combinatorial systems may regulate gene expression in cardiac muscle cells and smooth muscle cells, as well as probably being involved in other regulatory pathways that are cell type specific.[92,93] Loss of function mutations of the single Drosophila MEF-2 gene (D-MEF2) resulted in embryos completely lacking skeletal, cardiac, and visceral muscle, evidence of critical involvement in differentiation of myocytes of all three lineages.[94] The bHLH factor nautilus functions in skeletal muscle cells in Drosophila but potential cofactors (bHLH or otherwise) for MEF-2 in the cardiac and visceral lineages have not been identified in Drosophila or other systems.[93,95] Studies in transgenic mice have shown that several regulatory modules are often required to direct the complete developmental pattern of expression of individual muscle-specific genes, even within a single muscle cell type.[95]

Detailed analysis of the modules, elements, and factors involved in transcriptional regulation of several genes expressed in intestinal SMCs has been initiated. The actin multigene family contains at least six distinct members, two of which are smooth muscle γ-actin (SMGA) and smooth muscle α-actin (SMAA). These isoactins are extremely highly conserved during evolution. Smooth muscle γ-actin expression is almost exclusively limited to SMCs with some expression in postmeiotic spermatocytes.[96] Smooth muscle γ-actin is the predominant actin in visceral SMCs and is also present in vascular and airway smooth muscle. Transgenic mouse studies have been carried out examining segments of the murine SMGA gene and promoter for regulatory function.[96] Various DNA fragments from a 13.7-kb segment, extending from 4.5 upstream of the transcription start site to the translation start codon in exon 2, were tested for their ability to activate expression of a CAT reporter transgene. Transgenes with the largest 13.7-kb fragment demonstrated high-level CAT expression that was limited to SMCs. Analysis of transgenes with truncations and deletions of this 13.7-kb region suggest a modular regulatory system. Both distal 5′ promoter sequences (−2.7 to −0.57 kb) and intron 1 sequences strongly enhance SMGA expression from the proximal promoter in vivo. This study also provides some evidence of differences in the regulatory segments required for expression in visceral smooth muscle versus airway and vascular smooth muscle.

The other smooth muscle isoactin, SMAA, is primarily restricted to SMCs in adults where it is widely expressed in all SMC types. However, during the early stages of embryogenesis, SMAA expression is also seen in cardiac and skeletal muscle. Transfection studies have been carried out with promoter segments from several SMAA genes, including those from mouse, human, rat, and chicken. These studies have identified a number of positive and negative regulatory segments that include several conserved CArG boxes and bHLH-type E box sequences.[97–100] Two conserved, proximal CArG boxes were shown to be part of serum response-type elements that were capable of binding serum response factor complexes in some cells.[98,99] Just upstream of these CArG boxes, a polypurine-polypyrimidine tract was identified that binds the TEA-class transcriptional activator, TEF-1, and two single-stranded DNA-binding factors, designated as VACssBF1 and VACssBF2.[100] It was proposed that VACssBF1 and VACssBF2 act as repressors to inhibit TEF-1 binding and activation. Most of the transfection studies carried out in SMCs were done in vascular SMCs, making it unclear about the role of the defined elements and factors in visceral/intestinal SMCs. However, in transgenic mouse studies, 1.1 kb of promoter sequence and 2.5 kb of first intron sequence from the mouse SMAA gene were able to drive expression of an attached insulin-like growth factor cDNA specifically in SMC-containing tissues, including intestine.[101]

The protein SM22α is expressed in cardiac, skeletal, and smooth muscle lineages during mouse embryogenesis and expressed exclusively in smooth muscle-containing tissues in the adult animal.[102] It is one of the earliest markers of differentiated SMCs. Transgenic mouse studies have been conducted examining segments of the mouse SM22α gene promoter and first intron for regulatory function. The largest segment tested extended from −2735 to +1093. None of the segments examined were sufficient to drive reporter-gene expression in visceral and venous SMCs, even though appropriate expression was observed in skeletal and cardiac cell lineages and arterial smooth muscle cells.[102] This suggests that separate regulatory mechanisms exist to control expression of SM22α in different SMC lineages and an additional regulatory module(s) lies outside the investigated region of the SM22α gene. An enhancer or enhancers of visceral and venous expression were postulated to exist.

Smooth muscle myosin heavy chain (SMHC) gene products are expressed exclusively in SMCs. Transfection analyses of various segments of the rabbit and rat SMHC promoter have been carried out in vascular SMCs.[103–105] Multiple positive and negative elements were defined, and putative CArG box, E box, and MEF-2 sites were identified.[103,104] Again, the significance of the transfection results and their relevance to visceral-intestinal SMC expression of SMHC are unclear. The carboxy terminus of the smooth muscle myosin light chain kinase (SMMLCK) is expressed as an independent protein, telokin, exclusively in smooth muscle cells.[106] Telokin is expressed from a promoter within the SMMLCK gene, which is SMC specific. A 2.4-kb fragment of the telokin promoter was found to recapitulate the telokin pattern of expression in transgenic mice while a smaller promoter segment of about 300 bp was found to contain all the elements necessary to control SMC-specific expression in transfection studies.[106] Within this smaller promoter, a functional CArG box-serum response element and potential E box- and MEF-2-type sites were identified.[107]

As one can see from the studies described, there are some common themes and factors involved in regulation of smooth muscle gene expression, many of which may overlap with those observed for other muscle types. However, it is already clear that distinct segments and modules are often involved in smooth muscle cell expression when a gene is expressed in multiple muscle types. It is likely that there will be significant mechanisms and factors that are unique to smooth muscle. This may especially be true in the inductive regulatory events that occur between both the developing epithelium and the developing enteric nervous system and smooth muscle as it develops from the mesenchyme. Progress in this area is occurring rapidly and should soon give us insight into the molecular bases of these events.

TRANSCRIPTION FACTORS INVOLVED IN INTESTINAL DEVELOPMENT AND GENE REGULATION

One of the basic premises of the concept of a regulatory network that specifies development of a tissue through gene regulation is that common transcription factors will be involved, regulating the expression of a number of genes. The review above of studies examining end-product gene regulation demonstrates that this is clearly the case. A number of factors, such as CDX2, HNF-4, the HNF-1 family, and the C/EBP family, have been directly implicated in regulating the intestinal expression of a number of genes. As mentioned, the second major category of studies (other than examination of end-product genes) being carried out in an attempt to understand intestinal regulatory network is examination of transcription factors central to the network. As mentioned earlier, these studies often seek to define the expression pattern of the factor, what target genes it regulates, and what factors regulate its expression, so that the place and role of the individual factors within the intestinal gene regulatory network and cascades can be defined. We will discuss here the factors that have been directly and indirectly implicated in this network.

Caudal-Related CDX Factors

The *Drosophila* gene caudal encodes one of the homeobox factors whose expression is involved in the complex process of body segmentation and global body patterning. A number of caudal homologues have been identified in various vertebrates, including the genes for CDX1 and CDX2 in mouse,[108,109] CDXA in chicken,[110] and CDX in rat.[111] It has been proposed that the mouse CDX genes and, by inference, their homologues in other vertebrate systems are an integral part of the regulatory network that orchestrates development and differentiation in intestinal epithelium and maintenance of gene expression in differentiated epithelial cells.[112] This proposal is based on a number of lines of evidence. As outlined above, CDX2 has been directly implicated in regulating the expression of at least six different genes in the intestinal epithelium. CDX2 and CDX1 in mice and humans and CDXA in chickens are expressed almost exclusively in the adult intestinal epithelium.[108,109,113,114] CDX1 and CDX2 in mice and CDX in rat show a gradient of expression,[109,111] increasing from proximal small intestine to colon, that has been proposed to have a role in positional gene expression along the intestinal AP axis.[115] In the developing mouse embryo, CDX2 and CDX1 are expressed at the time when gut endoderm transforms into a simple columnar epithelium with nascent villi.[108,115,116] In chicken, CDXA is expressed during gastrulation, where it exhibits a posterior localization along the primitive streak, suggesting that it may be involved in axial determination.[117] CDXA also appears to play a role in gut closure.[114] The main CDXA spatial distribution pattern during intestinal morphogenesis suggests that a tight linkage to the formation and differentiation of the epithelium exists.[114] Conditional expression of CDX2 in IEC-6 cells, an undifferentiated rat intestinal cell line, produced arrest of proliferation, followed by a period of growth resulting in multicellular structures containing a well-formed columnar layer of cells with many morphologic characteristics of intestinal epithelial cells.[112] Both enterocyte- and goblet-like cells were evident. Evidence of differentiation was shown by the demonstration that the cells were expressing SI, a marker of mature enterocytes.

Several additional studies have been carried out involving CDX1 and CDX2 that give insight into the functional roles of these factors. Homologous recombination has been used to functionally inactivate the mouse CDX1 and CDX2 genes.[118,119] In the CDX1 "knockout," viable fertile homozygous mice were obtained with anterior homeotic transformations of vertebrae, which were concomitant with posterior shifts in HOX gene expression domains in the somitic mesoderm.[118] A possible regulatory relationship, with CDX1 impacting expression of other HOX genes, was proposed. Possible effects on developing intestine were not described. In the CDX2 knockout, homozygous null mutants die between 3.5 and 5.5 days postcoitum.[119] The CDX2 heterozygote mutants survive, showing a variable phenotype with stunted growth and skeletal abnormalities. Interestingly, within the first 3 months of life, 90% of the CDX2 heterozygotes develop multiple adenomatous polyps, especially in the proximal colon. The neoplastic cells do not express CDX2 from the remaining functional gene, indicating that CDX2 mutation may be a primary event in some intestinal tumors.

Isolation and preliminary characterization of the murine CDX1 gene has been carried out.[120] Initial studies on the promoter indicate that there are several distinct positive and negative modules in the region from −1040 to +66, including a silencer element between −589 and −380. Molecular studies with CDX2 have shown that it can bind two well-defined elements in the HOXC8 enhancer and that it can activate heterologous promoters in a cell-line dependent manner.[121] The data suggest that either a coactivator protein or differential phosphorylation of the activation domain may be the mechanism for the intestinal cell line-specific function. Studies such as these will eventually lead to an understanding of the place and role of CDX1 and CDX2 in the intestinal gene regulatory network.

HNF-1 Gene Family

The hepatocyte nuclear factor 1 (HNF-1) family of factors have, as indicated in the sections above, been implicated in the regulation of a number of genes that are expressed in intestine. These factors were first identified, as the name indicates, in liver.[122] Subsequently they were found to be more widely expressed in tissues such as kidney, stomach, pancreas, and large and small intestine. These transcription factors contain a very divergent type DNA-binding homeodomain and bind as dimers.[122] In most of the cases in which HNF-1 factors have been implicated in the regulation of intestinal expression of genes (such as SI, APN, and calbindin-D9K), they have been implicated in concert with other factors binding distinct elements within the same module. In vertebrates, the two primary members of the HNF-1 family are the closely related HNF-1α and HNF-1β, which have closely related dimerization and DNA-binding domains but different activation domains.[123] These factors can homodimerize or heterodimerize with each other.[123] It has been proposed that the relative ratio of these factors is important in determining which dimers are formed and, therefore, the pattern and level of gene activation in tissues such as liver[123] and intestine.[36] In addition, it has been reported that different forms of both HNF-1α and HNF-1β can be generated by alternate mRNA processing and are differentially expressed in fetal and adult liver, kidney, and intestine.[124] The resulting isoforms have transactivation domains of different strengths or, in one case, no transactivation domain at all. These are all reported to have the ability to homodimerize or heterodimerize, further increasing the potential for regulatory capability and complexity.[124]

Mice lacking expression of HNF-1α have been generated by homologous recombination.[125] Mice homozygous for HNF-1α deficiency fail to thrive and die around weaning after a progressive wasting syndrome with severe liver enlargement, while heterozygotes are phenotypically indistinguishable from wild type. Absence of HNF-1α had variable effects on the hepatic expression of genes with known or proposed HNF-1-type binding sites. Most showed reduced expression of various extents, with phenylalanine hydroxylase (PAH) showing complete loss of expression.[125] Subsequent investigation demonstrated that HNF-1α inactivation impaired chromatin remodeling and demethylation necessary to expression of the PAH gene.[126] Effects of HNF-1α inactivation on intestinal gene expression were not reported.

HNF-4 Factors

Hepatocyte nuclear factor 4 (HNF-4) is a member of the "Cys4 zinc finger of nuclear receptor type" class transcription factor. As such, it is a member of the hormone receptor superfamily.[127] It is expressed principally in liver, kidney, and intestine, and normally binds DNA as a homodimer. HNF-4 factors have been extensively studied as regulators of liver- and kidney-specific gene expression. As mentioned above, it has been implicated in regulation of intestinal expression of several genes as well. HNF-4 is also involved in the regulation of the gene that encodes HNF-1α.[128] There is an HNF-4 binding site in the HNF-1α promoter that is required for promoter function, and cotransfection studies show that HNF-4 potently transactivates this promoter. Therefore, HNF-4 and HNF-1α form part of a regulatory cascade or transcriptional hierarchy in liver (and probably intestinal) gene expression and development.[128] Interestingly, a natural mutation that disrupts the HNF-4 binding site in the HNF-1α promoter has been identified as a cause of maturity-onset diabetes due to decreased HNF-1α expression.[129] It has been reported that HNF-1α negatively regulates its own expression and that of other HNF-4-dependent genes by a direct interaction with the activation domain of HNF-4.[130]

In situ hybridization studies in the developing mouse indicate that HNF-4 has a role in early stages of postimplantation development, as well as organogenesis.[131] Expression was found in the primary endoderm at day 4.5 and was restricted to columnar visceral endoderm cells of the yolk sac from day 5.5 to day 8.5. At day 8.5, HNF-4 mRNA was first detected in the liver diverticulum and the hindgut. At later times, expression was observed in developing kidney, pancreas, stomach, and intestine. Disruption of the HNF-4 gene was accomplished by homologous recombination, and homozygous loss of HNF-4 is embryonic lethal, with evidence of cell death as early as 6.5 days.[132]

Initial studies on the regulation of the gene that encodes HNF-4 have indicated that it is likely regulated by several distinct modules.[133,134] Multiple tissue-specific DNase I HSs were identified in a region of up to 22 kb upstream of the transcription start site in the mouse gene. A proximal promoter segment containing an HNF-1 site (between −98 and −68) had promoter function in transfection assays, but distal enhancer elements located at −5.5 kb and −6.5 kb were required for correct expression in transgenic animals.[134] These two enhancer modules mapped to two of the promoter DNase I HSs. Multiple isoforms of HNF-4 have been reported, and it has been postulated that the distinct isoforms may play different roles in various cell types, including differentiating enterocytes.[135]

C/EBP Gene Family

Members of the CCAAT-enhancer binding protein (C/EBP) family have been implicated in the regulation of several genes in the intestine. These factors have been widely studied as regulators of expression in hepatocytes and adipocytes but much less is known of their function in intestine. The C/EBP factors are members of the basic leucine zipper class of transcription factors. In vertebrates, there are multiple closely related members of this family that can form homodimers and heterodimers, including C/EBPα, C/EBPβ, and C/EBPδ, which are expressed in intestinal epithelial cells.[136,137] Transcripts for some of the family members can be translated into more than one protein, with the different products having different transcription activation potentials.[138] The factor C/EBPα has been characterized as part of a differentiation switch in adipocytes that promotes a cessation of cell growth and movement toward terminal differentiation.[139] A similar role has been proposed for this factor (and possibly related factors) in cells of the intestinal epithelium, based on its expression pattern in adult mice.[137] Patterns of C/EBP isoform expression were determined and correlated with intestinal marker gene expression and intestinal development in fetal rat.[140] It was determined that expression of all three isoforms, C/EBPα, C/EBPβ, and C/EBPδ, was detected at 17 days of gestation, which preceded villus formation and differentiation marker expression. A role for the C/EBP factors in fetal intestinal differentiation was implied. If the C/EBP factors are involved in cessation of cellular proliferation and initiation of differentiation, they are unlikely to act alone. Recently, a zinc-finger transcription factor named gut-enriched Krüppel-like factor (GKLF) was identified as a potential negative regulator of cell growth in tissues such as gut mucosa.[141] In colonic epithelium, where GKLF is expressed at highest levels, it is enriched in epithelial cells of the middle to upper crypt region, where cell growth ceases and terminal differentiation initiates. Cells transfected with a GKLF-expressing plasmid show an inhibition of DNA synthesis.[141]

PDX1

The homeodomain transcription factor PDX1 (also widely known as IPF1, STF-1, and IDX-1) is expressed almost exclusively in the pancreas and duodenum.[142] PDX1 function is critical to the development of both tissues. Disruption by homologous recombination of the mouse gene that encodes PDX1 results in failure of the pancreas to develop, disruption of the epithelium in the proximal duodenum, and absence of Brunner's glands.[143,144] The pancreatic buds do form in homozygous mutants but the buds show limited proliferation and outgrowth.[144] The proximal duodenum shows a local absence of normal columnar epithelium and villi.[144] A single base-pair deletion was recently identified in the human PDX1 gene that appears to be responsible for pancreatic agenesis in a patient who is homozygous for the mutation.[145] Early studies with the gene XLHBOX8, the *Xenopus* homologue of PDX1, suggested that it was involved in endodermal differentiation during pancreatic and duodenal development.[146] Studies of the expression pattern in mouse embryos during development support this idea.[144,147] The factor PDX1 has been shown to be an important part of the regulation of a number of genes in the pancreas, including insulin and somatostatin genes.[148] It is also likely to be involved in the regulation of genes in the intestinal epithelium, especially in the duodenum. Because of the likelihood of PDX1 being involved in the cascade of factors that regulate development of pancreas and duodenum, it is of interest to know what factors regulate PDX1 transcription. Studies with the promoter of the rat PDX1 gene identified two distinct regulatory modules within a segment that activates expression specifically in pancreas and duodenum of transgenic mice.[149] These are a proximal region that contains a binding site for the E-box binding factor USF at −104, and a distal enhancer-like region between −6.5 and −3 kb.[149] Within the latter module, two functional elements that bind BETA-2 and HNF-3β were identified and found to act in a synergistic manner.[150] Transfection and transgenic mouse studies with the mouse PDX1 promoter confirmed a role for HNF-3β in tissue-specific expression from a site at −2 kb.[151] HNF-3β will be discussed in more detail in the section below.

HNF-3-Fork Head Family of Factors

The HNF-3 factors are members of a large family of fork head-winged helix class transcription factors in the helix-turn-helix superclass of factors that bind DNA as a monomer.[152] The founding members of this family were identified at about the same time in *Drosophila* and in rat liver.[153,154] The gene fork head (FKH) was identified as a homeotic gene in *Drosophila* that was essential for proper formation of terminal structures in the embryo.[153] In situ localization studies showed that it was present at early stages, primarily in the developing anterior and posterior gut of the fly. Shortly after the identification of FKH in *Drosophila*, the family of hepatocyte nuclear factor-3 (HNF-3) genes were identified as FKH homologues in rat liver.[154] The original members of this family in rodents are HNF-3α, HNF-3β, and HNF-3γ.[152] Subsequently other groups, such as the FD family in *Drosophila*, the HFH family in rodents, the MF-1/MF-2 and FKH family in mouse, and the XFD family in *Xenopus* were identified.[152] A large number of studies have implicated various members of these FKH groups as transcription factors that are developmental and tissue-specific regulators of expression in a wide variety of tissues.[152] A number of these factors are known to be expressed in embryonic endodermal and gut precursor cells (FKH; FD1; HNF-3α, -3β, -3γ) in *Drosophila* and mouse and in adult intestine (HFH-2; HFH-6; HFH-11; HNF-3α, -3β, -3γ; FKH-6) in rat, human, and mouse.[152] Thus, it seemed likely that these factors, their homologues, and related factors have a role in intestinal gene regulation and intestinal development.

The patterns of expression of the murine HNF-3 factors have been examined during embryogenesis.[155] Mouse HNF-3α, HNF-3β, and HNF-3γ are activated sequentially during development of the definitive endoderm. HNF-3β is activated first and is expressed in the node at the anterior end of the primitive streak in all three germ layers. Next, HNF-3α is activated in the primitive endoderm in the region of the invaginating foregut. Finally, HNF-3γ is expressed upon hindgut differentiation. The different anterior boundaries of HNF-3α, HNF-3β, and HNF-3γ expression during development suggest they may function in definitive endoderm regionalization.[155,156] Homozygous deletion of HNF-3β in mice is embryonically lethal, apparently due to defects in the node and the absence of a neural tube.[157,158] Assessment of endodermal cells in these mutants indicates that HNF-3β is not necessary for initial specification of endodermal cells but may be necessary for further development.[159] The HNF-3 factors are known to be involved in regulating the expression of a number of genes in liver, lung, and pancreas. The strong structural similarities between the HNF-3 DNA binding domain and linker histone molecules, and the proven ability of HNF-3-like proteins to help organize nucleosome position indicate that part of their ability to activate genes in vivo might occur at the level of chromatin organization.[159] In situ hybridization studies in adult mouse intestine showed that HNF-3α is expressed at high levels in the crypts and in a decreasing gradient along the CV axis, while HNF-3β is principally restricted to the crypts.[160] Potential HNF-3 binding sites were identified in a number of intestinally-expressed genes.[160]

Experiments with the proximal promoters of the rat genes for HNF-3β and HNF-3α show that they contain functional HNF-3-type binding sites,[161,162] indicating the likelihood of auto- and/or cross-regulatory functions. An additional factor, HNF-6, was implicated in the regulation of the HNF-3β gene's promoter as well.[163] Potential binding sites for HNF-6 were also identified in several other genes expressed in liver and intestine, and HNF-6 binding activity was detected in an intestinal epithelial cell line, HT-29. Recently a 3'-enhancer segment was identified 16 kb downstream of the transcription start site for the mouse gene encoding HNF-3γ.[164] This enhancer, which was necessary and sufficient in transgenic mice to direct reporter-gene expression to liver, pancreas, stomach, and intestine, contains a binding site for HNF-1 factors. HNF-1β was proposed as the in vivo activator.

A human homologue of the HNF-3 factors, HFH-11, was recently identified and isolated from the colon carcinoma HT-29 cell line.[160] In 16-day mouse embryos, HFH-11 was expressed in mesenchymal and epithelial cells of the liver, lung, intestine, renal cortex, and urinary tract. In adults, however, expression was limited to epithelial cells in the intestinal crypts and cells in the testis, thymus, and colon. Experiments were carried out that indicate, that HFH-11 expression can be induced by proliferative signals in adult epithelial cells. Differentiation of CaCo-2 cells toward the enterocyte lineage resulted in decreased HFH-11 expression and reciprocal increases in HNF-3α and HNF-3β expression. These studies suggest that HFH-11 might regulate genes mediating the transition between proliferating intestinal epithelial cells and enterocyte differentiation that occurs after exiting the cell cycle.[160]

The gene for the winged helix, fork head factor FKH-6, is expressed in the mesenchyme of the gut, lung, head, and tongue of developing mouse embryos.[165] In the mesenchyme of the gastrointestinal tract, FKH-6 is expressed directly adjacent to the endoderm-derived epithelium.[166] Homozygous null mice for FKH-6 showed postnatal growth retardation, secondary to structural abnormalities of the stomach, duodenum, and jejunum.[166] Abnormal crypt structure and changes in villus length were observed, apparently as a consequence of a fourfold increase in the number of dividing epithelial cells and a marked expansion of the proliferative zone. Epithelial cell-lineage allocation or differentiation seemed to be affected to some extent. The expression pattern of a number of intestinal transcription factors was unaffected, including CDX-1, CDX-2, HNF-3α, HNF-3β, and HNF-3γ. The possible role of FKH-6 in activation or repression of mesenchymal growth or differentiation factors that act on the gut epithelium to control proliferation and differentiation was investigated.[166] Several candidates for such mesenchymal signal mediators, TGF-α, TGF-β1, TGF-β2, TGF-β3, neuregulin, and scatter factor-hepatocyte growth factor, were found to be unaffected. Several classes of secreted polypeptides that are expressed either in the mesenchyme or epithelium of the GI tract and have been implicated in cell-cell signaling were investigated. No changes were observed for either the WNT genes WNT2 and WNT5A or for the hedgehog homologous SHH and IHH. However, significant reductions in the expression of decapentaplegic homologues BMP2 and BMP4 were observed, indicating that they might be downstream targets, either direct or indirect, in a signaling cascade with FKH6.

GATA Factors

The GATA family of factors are members of the diverse Cys4 zinc-finger class of transcription factors that recognize a distinctive consensus DNA sequence of (A/T)GATA(A/G). The founding member of this family, GATA-1, was identified because of its role in development and gene regulation in erythroid and other hematopoietic systems. Recently, three members of this family, GATA-4, GATA-5, and GATA-6, have been identified that are expressed in vertebrates in the developing gut and adult epithelium of the stomach and intestine, as well as heart and other tissues.[167-172] These factors have been studied principally for their role in heart development and cardiac gene regulation. However, they are almost certainly involved in intestinal gene regulation and development of the intestinal epithelium as well. Targeted mutagenesis of the GATA-4 gene in mouse ES cells resulted in a specific block in visceral endoderm formation, under in vitro culture conditions.[173]

The nematode *Caenorhabditis elegans* is an excellent model system for studying the molecular mechanisms of cellular differentiation programs and lineage relationship. In *C. elegans,* the main body of the intestine consists of a tube of 20 cells that are derived from the E blastomere of the eight-cell embryo. Investigation of the regulatory network and factors involved in intestinal cell specification, and differentiation is an area of active research. Two intestine-specific genes, the gut esterase gene (GES-1) and the vitellogenin gene (VIT-2) have been shown to have GATA-like consensus elements in their promoters that are important for expression in intestine.[174,175] A 36-bp deletion encompassing the GATA sequences in the GES-1 promoter not only eliminated intestinal expression but activated expression in cells of the pharynx/tail that belong to a different cell lineage.[175] The results of mutation of the GATA sequences suggest that gut activation and pharynx/tail suppression are modulated by separate factors. Thus, these regulatory elements seem to be part of a module that acts as an enhancer in intestinal cells and a silencer in other related cell lineages. Several GATA factors have been identified in *C. elegans,* including the factors ELT-1 and ELT-2.[176,177]

Other Factors

As our understanding of the regulatory networks that govern intestinal development and intestinal gene regulation increases, new factors and families of factors will be implicated at an increasing pace. The NKX homeodomain proteins are members of a large and rapidly growing family of vertebrate transcription factors that have strong homology to the NK-2 genes (including tinman) in *Drosophila*.[178] Mutant flies lacking tinman function fail to develop heart and gut muscle progenitor cells, as well as some of the body wall muscles.[178] The initial emphasis in vertebrates has been to examine the role of family members in heart development. However, several NKX factors are known to be expressed in the developing gut and mature visceral organs.[179-181] The factor NKX2-3 is expressed in the gut mesoderm, among other locations, during pre- and postnatal development of the mouse, and a role in gut muscle layer development was proposed.[180]

Surveys have been carried out on adult intestinal expression of homeobox genes in mouse[109] and man.[182] Expression of up to 13 different genes from the A, B, C, and D groups of clustered homeobox (HOX) genes was observed. The relative levels of expression in various intestinal segments along the AP axis were quite variable for many of these genes. Little is known about the gene targets of these factors or their role in intestinal function and maintenance.

Nonmammalian Model Systems

As has been amply illustrated in the sections above, nonvertebrate model systems such as *Drosophila* and *C. elegans* have been absolutely critical to our present state of knowledge of vertebrate intestinal gene regulation and its role in intestinal development. This will undoubtedly continue to be the case, as a steady stream of "homologies and analogies" passes back and forth. At least two GATA factors, SRP and DGATAC, have been identified in the gut of developing *Drosophila* embryos.[183,184] Studies with these and related factors will give us information about the roles and targets of GATA factors in mammalian intestinal development. A homologue of the HNF-3-fork head family, called CE-FKH-1, has recently been cloned from *C. elegans*.[185] The CE-FKH-1 gene is expressed in the pharynx and intestine at the midproliferation stage. Studies with this factor will shed light on the role of HNF-3 factors in the endoderm of mammalian embryos. Similarly an HNF-3 homologue, axial, has been cloned from zebrafish and appears to encode the counterpart of HNF-3β.[186,187] The zebrafish gastrointestinal tract matures in a manner similar to that of higher vertebrates; therefore, it serves as another useful model that can be manipulated to increase our understanding of intestinal development in vertebrates. Nine mutations were produced and characterized in zebrafish that perturb development of organs in the gastrointestinal tract.[188] Seven mutations cause arrest of intestinal epithelial development after formation of the tube but before cell polarization is achieved. These perturb different regions of the intestine, with six preferentially affecting the foregut and one the hindgut. In the foregut mutation that affects the anterior intestine, the esophagus does not form, while in four others, the pancreas fails to develop. Detailed characterization of one or more of these mutations would be yet another source of light on the puzzle of genes that form the network that regulates intestinal development.

REFERENCES

1. Arnone MI, Davidson EH. The hardwiring of development: organization and function of genomic regulatory systems. Development 1997;124:1851–64.
2. Zawel L, Reinberg D. Common themes in assembly and function of eukaryotic transcription complexes. Annu Rev Biochem 1995;64:533–61.
3. Tjian R, Maniatis T. Transcriptional activation: a complex puzzle with few easy pieces. Cell 1994;77:5–8.
4. Kirchamer CV, Yuh C-H, Davidson EH. Modular cis-regulatory organization of developmentally expressed genes. Proc Natl Acad Sci U S A 1996;93:9322–8.
5. Hoch M, Schroder C, Seifert E, Jäckle H. cis-Acting control elements for Krüppel expression in the *Drosophila* embryo. EMBO J 1990;9:2587–95.
6. Blackburn MR, Kellems RE. Regulation and function of adenosine deaminase in mice. Prog Nucleic Acid Res Mol Biol 1996;55:195–226.
7. Aronow BJ, Silbiger RN, Dusing MR, et al. Functional analysis of the human adenosine deaminase gene thymic regulatory region and its ability to generate position-independent transgene expression. Mol Cell Biol 1992;12:4170–85.
8. Winston JH, Hong L, Datta SJ, Kellems RE. An intron 1 regulatory region from the murine adenosine deaminase gene can activate heterologous promoters for ubiquitous expression in transgenic mice. Somat Cell Mol Genet 1996;22:261–78.
9. Shi D, Winston JH, Blackburn MR, et al. Diverse genetic regulatory motifs required for murine adenosine deaminase gene expression in the placenta. J Biol Chem 1997;272:2334–41.
10. Dusing MR, Brickner AG, Thomas MB, Wiginton DA. Regulation of duodenal specific expression of the human adenosine deaminase gene. J Biol Chem 1997;272:26634–42.
11. Giese K, Cox J, Grosschedl R. The HMG domain of lymphoid enhancer factor 1 bends DNA and facilitates assembly of functional nucleoprotein structures. Cell 1992;69:185–95.
12. Giese K, Kingsley C, Kirshner JR, Grosschedl R. Assembly and function of a TCRα enhancer complex is dependent on LEF-1-induced DNA bending and multiple protein-protein interactions. Genes Dev 1995;9:995–1008.
13. Kornberg RD, Lorch Y. Irresistible force meets immovable object: transcription and the nucleosome. Cell 1991;67:833–6.
14. Wolffe AP. Transcription: in tune with the histones. Cell 1994;77:13–6.
15. Gross DS, Garrard WT. Nuclease hypersensitive sites in chromatin. Annu Rev Biochem 1988;57:159–97.
16. Jenuwein T, Forrester W, Grosschedl R. Role of enhancer sequences in regulating accessibility of DNA in nuclear chromatin. Cold Spring Harb Symp Quant Biol 1993;LVIII:97–103.
17. Wolffe AP. Sinful repression. Nature 1997;387:16–8.
18. Paranjape SM, Kamakaka RT, Kadonaga JT. Role of chromatin structure in the regulation of transcription by RNA polymerase II. Annu Rev Biochem 1994;63:265–97.
19. Grosveld F, van Assendelft GB, Greaves DR, Kolias G. Position-independent, high-level expression of the human β-globin gene in transgenic mice. Cell 1987;51:975–85.
20. Felsenfeld G. Chromatin as an essential part of the transcriptional mechanism. Nature 1992;355:219–24.
21. Kellum R, Schedl P. A position-effect assay for boundaries of higher order chromosomal domains. Cell 1991;64:941–50.
22. Cal H, Levine M. Modulation of enhancer-promoter interactions by insulators in the *Drosophila* embryo. Nature 1995;376:533–6.
23. Corces VG. Keeping enhancers under control. Nature 1995;376:462–3.
24. Laemmli UK, Kas E, Poljak L, Adachi Y. Scaffold-associated regions: cis-acting determinants of chromatin structural loops and functional domains. Curr Opin Genet Dev 1992;2:275–85.
25. Forrester W, van Genderen C, Jenuwein T, Grosschedl R. Dependence of enhancer-mediated transcription of the immunoglobulin μ gene on nuclear matrix attachment regions. Science 1994;265:1221–5.
26. Aronow B, Lattier D, Silbiger R, et al. Evidence for a complex regulatory array in the first intron of the human adenosine deaminase gene. Genes Dev 1989;3:1384–400.
27. Aronow BJ, Ebert CA, Valerius MT, et al. Dissecting a locus control region: facilitation of enhancer function by extended enhancer-flanking sequences. Mol Cell Biol 1995;15:1123–35.
28. Mitchell PJ, Tjian R. Transcriptional regulation in mammalian cells by sequence-specific DNA binding proteins. Science 1989;245:371–7.
29. Pabo CO, Sauer RT. Transcription factors: structural families and principles of DNA recognition. Annu Rev Biochem 1992;61:1053–95.

30. Carlsson P, Waterman ML, Jones KA. The hLEF/TCF-1α HMG protein contains a context-dependent transcriptional activation domain that induces the TCRα enhancer in T cells. Genes Dev 1993;7:2418–30.
31. van de Wetering M, Oosterwegel M, van Norren K, Clevers H. Sox-4, an Sry-like HMG box protein, is a transcriptional activator in lymphocytes. EMBO J 1993;12:3847–54.
32. Evans RM. The steroid and thyroid hormone receptor superfamily. Science 1988;240:889–95.
33. Hsu H-L, Cheng J-T, Chen Q, Baer R. Enhancer-binding activity of the tal-1 oncoprotein in association with the E47/E12 helix-loop-helix proteins. Mol Cell Biol 1991;11:3037–42.
34. Wingender E, Dietze P, Karas H, Knüppel R. TRANSFAC: a database on transcription factors and their DNA binding sites. Nucleic Acids Res 1996;24:238–41.
35. Vinson CR, Garcia KC. Molecular model for DNA recognition by the family of basic-helix-loop-helix-zipper proteins. New Biologist 1992;4:396–403.
36. Traber PG, Silberg DG. Intestine-specific gene transcription. Annu Rev Physiol 1996;58:275–97.
37. Sweetser DA, Birkenmeier EH, Hoppe PC, et al. Mechanisms underlying generation of gradients in gene expression within the intestine: an analysis using transgenic mice containing fatty acid binding protein-human growth hormone fusion genes. Genes Dev 1988;2:1318–32.
38. Sweetser DA, Hauft SM, Hoppe PC, et al. Transgenic mice containing intestinal fatty acid-binding protein-human growth hormone fusion genes exhibit correct regional and cell-specific expression of the reporter gene in their small intestine. Proc Natl Acad Sci U S A 1988;85:9611–5.
39. Gordon JI. Intestinal epithelial differentiation: new insights from chimeric and transgenic mice. J Cell Biol 1989;108:1187–94.
40. Cohn SM, Simon TC, Roth KA, et al. Use of transgenic mice to map cis-acting elements in the intestinal fatty acid binding protein gene (*Fabpi*) that control its cell lineage-specific and regional patterns of expression along the duodenal-colonic and crypt-villus axes of the gut epithelium. J Cell Biol 1992;119:27–44.
41. Rottman JN, Gordon JI. Comparison of the patterns of expression of the rat intestinal fatty acid binding protein/human growth hormone fusion genes in cultured intestinal epithelial cell lines and in the gut epithelium of transgenic mice. J Biol Chem 1993;268:11994–2002.
42. Simon TC, Roberts LJJ, Gordon JI. A 20-nucleotide element in the intestinal fatty acid binding protein gene modulates its cell lineage-specific, differentiation-dependent, and cephalocaudal patterns of expression in transgenic mice. Proc Natl Acad Sci U S A 1995;92:8685–9.
43. Simon TC, Roth KA, Gordon JI. Use of transgenic mice to map cis-acting elements in the liver fatty acid-binding protein gene (*Fabpl*) that regulate its cell lineage-specific, differentiation-dependent, and spatial patterns of expression in the gut epithelium and in the liver acinus. J Biol Chem 1993;268:18345–58.
44. Simon TC, Cho A, Tso P, Gordon JI. Suppressor and activator functions mediated by a repeated heptad sequence in the liver fatty acid-binding protein gene (*Fabpl*). J Biol Chem 1997;272:10652–63.
45. Wu GD, Wang W, Traber PG. Isolation and characterization of the human sucrase-isomaltase gene and demonstration of intestine-specific transcriptional elements. J Biol Chem 1992;267:7863–70.
46. Traber PG, Wu GD, Wang W. Novel DNA-binding proteins regulate intestine-specific transcription of the sucrase-isomaltase gene. Mol Cell Biol 1992;2:3614–27.
47. Markowitz AJ, Wu GD, Birkenmeier EH, Traber PG. The human sucrase-isomaltase gene directs complex patterns of gene expression in transgenic mice. Am J Physiol 1993;265:G526–39.
48. Markowitz AJ, Wu GD, Bader A, et al. Regulation of lineage-specific transcription of the sucrase-isomaltase gene in transgenic mice and cell lines. Am J Physiol 1995;269:G925–39.
49. Tung J, Markowitz AJ, Silberg DG, Traber PG. Developmental expression of SI is regulated in transgenic mice by an evolutionarily conserved promoter. Am J Physiol 1997;273:G83–92.
50. Wu GD, Chen L, Forslund K, Traber PG. Hepatocyte nuclear factor-1α (HNF-1α) and HNF-1β regulate transcription via two elements in an intestine-specific promoter. J Biol Chem 1994;269:17080–5.
51. Suh E, Chen L, Taylor J, Traber PG. A homeodomain protein related to caudal regulates intestine-specific gene transcription. Mol Cell Biol 1994;14:7340–51.
52. Traber PG. Epithelial cell growth and differentiation V. Transcriptional regulation, development, and neoplasia of the intestinal epithelium. Am J Physiol 1997;273:G979–81.
53. Hecht A, Torbey CF, Korsmo HA, Olsen WA. Regulation of sucrase and lactase in developing rats: role of nuclear factors that bind to two gene regulatory elements. Gastroenterology 1997;112:803–12.
54. Olsen J, Lausten L, Kärnström U, et al. Tissue-specific interactions between nuclear proteins and the aminopeptidase N promoter. J Biol Chem 1991;266:18089–96.
55. Olsen J, Kokholm K, Troelsen JT, Lausten L. An enhancer with cell-type dependent activity is located between the myeloid and epithelial aminopeptidase N (CD 13) promoters. Biochem J 1997;322:899–908.
56. Troelsen JT, Mehlum A, Olsen J, et al. 1 kb of the lactase-phlorizin hydrolase promoter directs post-weaning decline and small intestinal-specific expression in transgenic mice. FEBS Lett 1994;342:219–96.
57. Troelsen JT, Olsen J, Nóren O, Sjöström H. A novel intestinal trans-factor (NF-LPH1) interacts with the lactase-phlorizin hydrolase promoter and co-varies with the enzymatic activity. J Biol Chem 1992;267:20407–11.
58. Troelsen JT, Mitchelmore C, Spodsberg N, et al. Regulation of lactase-phlorizin hydrolase gene expression by the caudal-related homeodomain protein CDX-2. Biochem J 1997;322:833–8.
59. Darwish HM, DeLuca HF. Identification of a 1.25-dihydroxyvitamin D3-response element in the 5′-flanking region of the rat calbindin D-9k gene. Proc Natl Acad Sci USA 1992;89:603–7.
60. Romagnolo B, Cluzeaud F, Lambert M, et al. Tissue-specific and hormonal regulation of calbindin-D9K fusion genes in transgenic mice. J Biol Chem 1996;271:1820–6.
61. Lambert M, Colnot S, Suh E, et al. *cis*-Acting elements and transcription factors involved in the intestinal specific expression of the rat calbindin-D9k gene. Eur J Biochem 1996;236:778–88.
62. Hochman JA, Sciaky D, Whitaker TL, et al. Hepatocyte nuclear factor-1α regulates transcription of the guanylin gene. Am J Physiol 1997;273:G833–41.
63. Pardiol A, Magert HJ, Hill O, Forssmann WG. Functional analysis of the human guanylin gene promoter. Biochem Biophys Res Commun 1996;224:638–44.
64. Mann EA, Jump ML, Gianella RA. Cell line-specific transcriptional activation of the promoter of the human guanylyl cyclase C/heat-stable enterotoxin/receptor gene. Biochim Biophys Acta 1996;1305:7–10.
65. Kardassis D, Hadzopoulou-Cladaras M, Ramji DP, et al. Characterization of the promoter elements required for hepatic and intestinal transcription of the human apoB gene: definition of the DNA-binding site of a tissue-specific transcription factor. Mol Cell Biol 1990;10:253–9.

66. Carlsson P, Eriksson P, Bjursell G. Two nuclear proteins bind to the major positive element of the apolipoprotein B gene promoter. Gene 1990;94:295–301.
67. Metzger S, Halaas JL, Breslow JL, Sladek FM. Orphan receptor HNF-4 and bZip protein C/EBPα bind to overlapping regions of the apolipoprotein B gene promoter and synergistically activate transcription. J Biol Chem 1993;28:16831–8.
68. Brooks AR, Nagy BP, Taylor S, et al. Sequences containing the second-intron enhancer are essential for transcription of the human apolipoprotein B gene in the livers of transgenic mice. Mol Cell Biol 1994;14:2243–56.
69. Wang D-M, Taylor S, Levy-Wilson B. Evaluation of the function of the human apolipoprotein B gene nuclear matrix association regions in transgenic mice. J Lipid Res 1996; 37:2117–24.
70. Lee SY, Nagy BP, Brooks AR, et al. Members of the caudal family of homeodomain proteins repress transcription from the human apolipoprotein B promoter in intestinal cells. J Biol Chem 1996;271:707–18.
71. Sowden J, Leigh S, Talbot I, et al. Expression from the proximal promoter of the carbonic anhydrase 1 gene as a marker for differentiation in colon epithelia. Differentiation 1993;53:67–74.
72. Drummond F, Sowden J, Morrison K, Edwards YH. The *caudal*-type homeobox protein CDX-2 binds to the colon promoter of the carbonic anhydrase 1 gene. Eur J Biochem 1996; 236:670–81.
73. Walsh A, Azrolan N, Wang K, et al. Intestinal expression of the human apoA-I gene in transgenic mice is controlled by a DNA region 3′ to the gene in the promoter of the adjacent convergently transcribed apoC-III gene. J Lipid Res 1993; 34:617–23.
74. Bisaha JG, Simon TC, Gordon JI, Breslow JL. Characterization of an enhancer element in the human apolipoprotein C-III gene that regulates human apolipoprotein A-I gene expression in the intestinal epithelium. J Biol Chem 1995;270:19979–88.
75. Ginsburg GS, Ozer J, Karathanasis SK. Intestinal apolipoprotein AI gene transcription is regulated by multiple distinct DNA elements and is synergistically activated by the orphan nuclear receptor, hepatocyte nuclear factor 4. J Clin Invest 1995;9:528–38.
76. Ktistaki E, Lacorte J-M, Katrakili N, et al. Transcriptional regulation of the apolipoprotein A-IV gene involves synergism between a proximal orphan receptor response element and a distant enhancer located in the upstream promoter region of the apolipoprotein C-III gene. Nucleic Acids Res 1994;22:4689–96.
77. Vergnes L, Taniguchi T, Omori K, et al. The apolipoprotein A-I/C-III/A-IV gene cluster: ApoC-III and ApoA-IV expression is regulated by two common enhancers. Biochim Biophys Acta 1997;1348:299–310.
78. Sabourin JC, Kern AS, Gregori C, et al. An intronic enhancer essential for tissue-specific expression of the aldolase B transgenes. J Biol Chem 1996;271:3469–73.
79. Bry L, Falk P, Huttner K, et al. Paneth cell differentiation in the developing intestine of normal and transgenic mice. Proc Natl Acad Sci U S A 1994;91:10335–9.
80. Sands BE, Ogata H, Lynch-Devaney K, et al. Molecular cloning of the rat intestinal trefoil factor gene. J Biol Chem 1995;270:9353–61.
81. Velcich A, Palumbo L, Selleri L, et al. Organization and regulatory aspects of the human intestinal mucin gene (*MUC2*) locus. J Biol Chem 1997;272:7968–76.
82. Gum JR, Hicks JW, Kim YS. Identification and characterization of the *MUC2* (human intestinal mucin) gene 5′-flanking region: promoter activity in cultured cells. Biochem J 1997; 325:259–67.
83. Lopez MJ, Upchurch BH, Rindi G, Leiter AB. Studies in transgenic mice reveal potential relationships between secretin-producing cells and other endocrine cell types. J Biol Chem 1995;270:885–91.
84. Nishitani J, Rindi G, Lopez MJ, et al. Transcriptional regulation of secretin gene expression. J Clin Gastroenterol 1995; 21:S50–5.
85. Mutoh H, Fung BP, Naya FJ, et al. The basic helix-loop-helix transcription factor BETA2/NeuroD is expressed in mammalian enteroendocrine cells and activates secretin gene expression. Proc Natl Acad Sci U S A 1997;94:3560–4.
86. Naya FJ, Huang H-P, Qiu Y, et al. Diabetes, defective pancreatic morphogenesis, and abnormal enteroendocrine differentiation in BETA2/NeuroD-deficient mice. Genes Dev 1997;11: 2323–34.
87. Efrat S, Teitelman G, Anwar M, et al. Glucagon gene regulatory region directs oncoprotein expression to neurons and pancreatic alpha cells. Neuron 1988;1:605–13.
88. Lee YC, Asa SL, Drucker DJ. Glucagon gene 5′-flanking sequences direct expression of simian virus 40 large T antigen to the intestine producing carcinoma of the large bowel in transgenic mice. J Biol Chem 1992 May;267:10705–8.
89. Jin T, Drucker DJ. Activation of proglucagon gene transcription through a novel promoter element by the caudal-related homeodomain protein cdx-2/3. Mol Cell Biol 1996;16: 19–28.
90. Jin T, Trinh DKY, Wang F, Drucker DJ. The *caudal* homeobox protein cdx-2/3 activates endogenous proglucagon gene expression in InR1-G9 islet cells. Mol Endocrinol 1997; 11:203–9.
91. Evers BM, Wang X, Zhou Z, et al. Characterization of promoter elements required for cell-specific expression of the neurotensin/neuromedin N gene in a human endocrine cell line. Mol Cell Biol 1995;15:3870–81.
92. McHugh K. Molecular analysis of gastrointestinal smooth muscle development. J Pediatr Gastroenterol Nutr 1996; 23:379–94.
93. Molkentin JD, Olsen EN. Combinatorial control of muscle development by basic helix-loop-helix and MADS-box transcription factors. Proc Natl Acad Sci U S A 1996;93:9366–73.
94. Lilly B, Zhao B, Ranganayakulu G, et al. Requirement of MADS domain transcription factor D-MEF2 for muscle formation in *Drosophila*. Science 1995;267:688–93.
95. Firulli AB, Olson EN. Modular regulation of muscle gene transcription: a mechanism for muscle cell diversity. Trends Genet 1997;13:364–9.
96. Qian J, Kumar A, Szucsik JC, Lessard JL. Tissue and developmental specific expression of murine smooth muscle γ-actin fusion genes in transgenic mice. Dev Dyn 1996;207: 135–44.
97. Foster DN, Min B, Foster LK, et al. Positive and negative *cis*-acting regulatory elements mediate expression of the mouse vascular smooth muscle α-actin gene. J Biol Chem 1992; 27:11995–2003.
98. Shimizu RT, Blank RS, Jervis R, et al. The smooth muscle α-actin gene promoter is differentially regulated in smooth muscle versus non-smooth muscle cells. J Biol Chem 1995;270:7631–43.
99. Bushel P, Kim JH, Chang W, et al. Two serum response elements mediate transcriptional repression of human smooth muscle α-actin promoter in *ras*-transformed cells. Oncogene 1995;10:1361–70.
100. Sun S, Stoflet ES, Cogan JG, et al. Negative regulation of the vascular smooth muscle α-actin gene in fibroblasts and myoblasts: disruption of enhancer function by sequence-specific single-stranded-DNA-binding proteins. Mol Cell Biol 1995;15:2429–36.

101. Wang J, Niu W, Nikiforov Y, et al. Targeted overexpression of IGF-I evokes distinct patterns of organ remodeling in smooth muscle cell tissue beds of transgenic mice. J Clin Invest 1997; 100:1425–39.
102. Li L, Miano M, Mercer B, Olson EN. Expression of the SM22α promoter in transgenic mice provides evidence for distinct transcriptional regulatory programs in vascular and visceral smooth muscle cells. J Cell Biol 1996;132:849–59.
103. Katoh Y, Loukianov E, Kopras E, et al. Identification of functional promoter elements in the rabbit smooth muscle myosin heavy chain gene. J Biol Chem 1994;269:30538–45.
104. Madsen CS, Hershey JC, Hautmann MB, et al. Expression of the smooth muscle myosin heavy chain gene is regulated by a negative-acting GC-rich element located between two positive-acting serum response factor-binding elements. J Biol Chem 1997;272:6332–40.
105. White SL, Low RB. Identification of promoter elements involved in cell-specific regulation of rat smooth muscle myosin heavy chain gene regulation. J Biol Chem 1996; 271:15008–17.
106. Herring BP, Smith AF. Telokin expression is mediated by a smooth muscle cell-specific promoter. Am J Physiol 1996; 270:C1656–65.
107. Herring BP, Smith AF. Telokin expression in A10 smooth muscle cells requires serum response factor. Am J Physiol 1997;272:C1394–404.
108. Duprey P, Chowdhury K, Dressler GR, et al. A mouse gene homologous to the Drosophila gene caudal is expressed in epithelial cells from the embryonic intestine. Genes Dev 1988;2:1647–54.
109. James R, Kazenwadel J. Homeobox gene expression in the intestinal epithelium of adult mice. J Biol Chem 1991; 266:3246–51.
110. Frumkin A, Rangini Z, Ben-Yehuda A, et al. A chicken caudal homologue, Chox-cad, is expressed in the epiblast with posterior localization and in early endodermal lineage. Development 1991;112:207–19.
111. Freund J-N, Boukamel R, Benazzouz A. Gradient expression of Cdx along the rat intestine throughout postnatal development. FEBS Lett 1992;314:163–6.
112. Suh E, Traber PG. An intestine-specific homeobox gene regulates proliferation and differentiation. Mol Cell Biol 1996; 16:619–25.
113. Mallo G, Rechreche H, Frigerio J-M, et al. Molecular cloning, sequencing and expression of the mRNA encoding human Cdx1 and Cdx2 homeobox. Down-regulation of Cdx1 and Cdx2 mRNA expression during colorectal carcinogenesis. Int J Cancer 1997;74:35–44.
114. Frumkin A, Pillemer G, Haffner R, et al. A role for CdxA in gut closure and intestinal epithelia differentiation. Development 1994;120:253–63.
115. James R, Erler T, Kazenwadel J. Structure of the murine homeobox gene cdx-2. J Biol Chem 1994;269:15229–37.
116. Meyer BI, Gruss P. Mouse Cdx-1 expression during gastrulation. Development 1993;117:191–203.
117. Frumkin A, Haffner R, Shapira E, et al. The chicken CdxA homeobox gene and axial positioning during gastrulation. Development 1993;118:553–62.
118. Subramanian V, Meyer BI, Gruss P. Disruption of the murine homeobox gene Cdx1 affects axial skeletal identities by altering the mesodermal expression domains of Hox genes. Cell 1995;83:641–53.
119. Chawengsaksophak K, James R, Hammond VE, et al. Homeosis and intestinal tumours in Cdx2 mutant mice. Nature 1997;38:84–7.
120. Hu Y, Kazenwadel J, James R. Isolation and characterization of the murine homeobox gene Cdx-1. J Biol Chem 1993; 28:27214–25.
121. Taylor JK, Levy T, Suh ER, Traber PG. Activation of enhancer elements by the homeobox gene Cdx2 is cell line specific. Nucleic Acids Res 1997;25:2293–300.
122. Mendel DB, Crabtree GR. HNF-1, a member of a novel class of dimerizing homeodomain proteins. J Biol Chem 1991;266:677–80.
123. Mendel DB, Hansen LP, Graves MK, et al. HNF-1α and HNF-1β (vHNF-1) share dimerization and homeo domains, but not activation domains, and form heterodimers in vitro. Genes Dev 1991;5:1042–56.
124. Bach I, Yaniv M. More potent transcriptional activators or a transdominant inhibitor of the HNF1 homeodomain family are generated by alternative splicing. EMBO J 1993; 12:4229–42.
125. Pontoglio M, Barra J, Hadchouel M, et al. Hepatocyte nuclear factor 1α inactivation results in hepatic dysfunction, phenylketonuria, and renal Fanconi syndrome. Cell 1996; 84:575–85.
126. Pontoglio M, Faust DM, Doyen A, et al. Hepatocyte nuclear factor 1α gene inactivation impairs chromatin remodeling and demethylation of the phenylalanine hydroxylase gene. Mol Cell Biol 1997;17:4948–56.
127. Sladek FM, Zhong WM, Lai E, Darnell JE. Liver-enriched transcription factor HNF-4 is a novel member of the steroid hormone receptor superfamily. Genes Dev 1990;4:2353–65.
128. Kuo CJ, Conley PB, Chen L, et al. A transcriptional hierarchy involved in mammalian cell-type specification. Nature 1992;355:457–61.
129. Gragnoli C, Lindner T, Cockburn BN, et al. Maturity-onset diabetes of the young due to a mutation in the hepatocyte nuclear factor-4α binding site in the promoter of the hepatocyte nuclear factor-1α gene. Diabetes 1997;46:1648–51.
130. Ktistaki E, Taliadis I. Modulation of hepatic gene expression by hepatocyte nuclear factor 1. Science 1997;277:109–12.
131. Duncan SA, Manova K, Chen WS, et al. Expression of the transcription factor HNF-4 in the extraembryonic endoderm, gut, and nephrogenic tissue of the developing mouse embryo: HNF-4 is a marker for primary endoderm in the implanting blastocyst. Proc Natl Acad Sci U S A 1994;91: 7598–602.
132. Chen WS, Manova K, Weinstein DC, et al. Disruption of the HNF-4 gene, expressed in visceral endoderm, leads to cell death in embryonic ectoderm and impaired gastrulation of mouse embryos. Genes Dev 1994;8:2466–77.
133. Taraviras S, Monaghan AP, Schütz G, Kelsey G. Characterization of the mouse HNF-4 gene and its expression during mouse embryogenesis. Mech Dev 1994;48:67–79.
134. Zhong WM, Mirkovitch J, Darnell JE. Tissue-specific regulation of mouse hepatocyte nuclear factor 4 expression. Mol Cell Biol 1994;14:7276–84.
135. Suaud L, Joseph B, Formstecher P, Laine B. mRNA expression of HNF-4 isoforms and of HNF-1α/HNF-1β variants and differentiation of human cell lines that mimic highly specialized phenotypes of intestinal epithelium. Biochem Biophys Res Commun 1997;235:820–5.
136. Boudreau F, Blais S, Asselin C. Regulation of CCAAT/enhancer binding protein isoforms by serum and glucocorticoids in the rat intestinal epithelial crypt cell line IEC-6. Exp Cell Res 1996;222:1–9.
137. Chandrasekaran C, Gordon JI. Cell lineage-specific and differentiation-dependent patterns of CCAAT/enhancer binding protein α expression in the gut epithelium of normal and transgenic mice. Proc Natl Acad Sci U S A 1993;90:8871–5.
138. Ossipow V, Descombes P, Schibler U. CCAAT/enhancer-binding protein mRNA is translated into multiple proteins with different transcription activation potentials. Proc Natl Acad Sci U S A 1993;90:8219–23.

139. Umek R, Friedman AD, McKnight SL. CAAT/enhancer-binding protein: a component of a differentiation switch. Science 1991;251:288–92.
140. Montgomery RK, Rings EHHM, Thompson JF, et al. Increased C/EBP in fetal rat small intestine precedes initiation of differentiation marker mRNA synthesis. Am J Physiol 1997;272:G534–44.
141. Shields JM, Christy RJ, Yang VW. Identification and characterization of a gene encoding a gut-enriched Krüppel-like factor expressed during growth arrest. J Biol Chem 1996; 271:20009–17.
142. Miller C, McGehee RE, Habener JF. IDX-1: a new homeodomain transcription factor expressed in rat pancreatic islets and duodenum that transactivates the somatostatin gene. EMBO J 1994;13:1145–56.
143. Jonsson J, Carlsson L, Edlund T, Edlund H. Insulin-promoter-factor 1 is required for pancreatic development in mice. Nature 1994;371:606–9.
144. Offield MF, Jetton TL, Labosky PA, et al. PDX-1 is required for pancreatic outgrowth and differentiation of the rostral duodenum. Development 1996;122:983–95.
145. Stoffers DA, Zinkin NT, Stanojevic V, et al. Pancreatic agenesis attributable to a single nucleotide deletion in the human IPF1 gene coding sequence. Nat Genet 1997;15:106–10.
146. Wright CVE, Schnegelsberg P, De Robertis EM. XlHbox 8: a novel Xenopus homeo protein restricted to a narrow band of endoderm. Development 1988;104:787–94.
147. Guz Y, Montminy MR, Stein R, et al. Expression of murine STF-1, a putative insulin gene transcription factor, in β cells of pancreas, duodenal epithelium and pancreatic exocrine and endocrine progenitors during ontogeny. Development 1995; 121:11–8.
148. Sander M, German MS. The β cell transcription factors and development of the pancreas. J Mol Med 1997;75:327–40.
149. Sharma S, Leonard J, Lee S, et al. Pancreatic islet expression of the homeobox factor STF-1 relies on an E-box motif that binds USF. J Biol Chem 1996;271:2294–9.
150. Sharma S, Jhala US, Johnson T, et al. Hormonal regulation of an islet-specific enhancer in the pancreatic homeobox gene STF-1. Mol Cell Biol 1997;17:2598–604.
151. Wu K-L, Gannon M, Peshavaria M, et al. Hepatocyte nuclear factor 3β is involved in pancreatic β-cell-specific transcription of the pdx-1 gene. Mol Cell Biol 1997;17:6002–13.
152. Kaufmann E, Knöckel W. Five years on the wings of forkhead. Mech Dev 1996;57:3–20.
153. Weigel D, Jürgens G, Küttner F, et al. The homeotic gene fork head encodes a nuclear protein and is expressed in the terminal regions of the Drosophila embryo. Cell 1989; 57:645–58.
154. Lai E, Prezioso VR, Smith E, et al. HNF-3A, a hepatocyte-enriched transcription factor of novel structure is regulated transcriptionally. Genes Dev 1990;4:1427–36.
155. Monaghan AP, Kaestner KH, Grau E, Schütz G. Postimplantation expression patterns indicate a role for the mouse forkhead/ HNF-3α, β, and γ genes in determination of the definitive endoderm, chordamesoderm and neuroectoderm. Development 1993;119:567–78.
156. Ang SL, Wierda A, Wong D, et al. The formation and maintenance of the definitive endoderm lineage in the mouse: involvement of HNF-3/forkhead proteins. Development 1993;119:1302–15.
157. Ang SL, Roussant J. HNF-3β is essential for node and notochord formation in mouse development. Cell 1994;78: 561–74.
158. Weinstein DC, Ruiz i Altaba A, Chen WS, et al. The winged-helix transcription factor HNF-3β is required for notochord development in the mouse embryo. Cell 1994;78:575–88.
159. Zaret KS. Molecular genetics of early liver development. Annu Rev Physiol 1996;58:231–51.
160. Ye H, Kelly TF, Samadani U, et al. Hepatocyte nuclear factor 3/fork head homolog 11 expressed in proliferating epithelial and mesenchymal cells of embryonic and adult tissues. Mol Cell Biol 1997;17:1626–41.
161. Pani L, Quian XB, Clevidence D, Costa RH. The restricted promoter activity of the liver transcription factor hepatocyte nuclear factor 3β involves a cell-specific factor and positive autoactivation. Mol Cell Biol 1992;12:552–62.
162. Peterson RS, Clevidence DE, Ye H, Costa RH. Hepatocyte nuclear factor 3α promoter regulation involves recognition by cell specific factors, thyroid transcription factor-1, and autoactivation. Cell Growth Diff 1997;8:69–82.
163. Samadani U, Costa RH. The transcriptional activator hepatocyte nuclear factor 6 regulates liver gene expression. Mol Cell Biol 1996;16:6273–84.
164. Hiemisch H, Schütz G, Kaestner KH. Transcriptional regulation in endoderm development: characterization of an enhancer controlling Hnf3g expression by transgenesis and targeted mutagenesis. EMBO J 1997;16:3995–4006.
165. Kaestner KH, Bleckmann SC, Monaghan AP, et al. Clustered arrangement of winged helix genes fkh-6 and MFH-1: possible implications for mesoderm development. Development 1996;122:1751–8.
166. Kaestner KH, Silberg DG, Traber PG, Schütz G. The mesenchymal winged helix transcription factor Fkh6 is required for the control of gastrointestinal proliferation and differentiation. Genes Dev 1997;11:1583–95.
167. Arceci RJ, King AAJ, Simon MC, et al. Mouse GATA-4: a retinoic acid-inducible GATA-binding transcription factor expressed in endodermally derived tissues and heart. Mol Cell Biol 1993;13:2235–46.
168. Lavierriere AC, MacNeill C, Mueller C, et al. GATA-4/5/6, a subfamily of three transcription factors transcribed in developing heart and gut. J Biol Chem 1994;269:23177–84.
169. Jiang Y, Evans T. The Xenopus GATA-4/5/6 genes are associated with cardiac specification and can regulate cardiac-specific transcription during embryogenesis. Dev Biol 1996; 174:258–70.
170. Morrisey EE, Ip HS, Lu MM, Parmacek MS. GATA-6: a zinc finger transcription factor that is expressed in multiple cell lineages derived from lateral mesoderm. Dev Biol 1996;177: 309–22.
171. Morrisey EE, Ip HS, Tand Z, et al. GATA-5: a transcriptional activator expressed in a novel temporally and spatially-restricted pattern during embryonic development. Dev Biol 1997;183:21–36.
172. Huggon IC, Davies A, Gove C, et al. Molecular cloning of human GATA-6 DNA binding protein: high levels of expression in heart and gut. Biochim Biophys Acta 1997;1353: 98–102.
173. Soudais C, Bielinska M, Heikinheimo M, et al. Targeted mutagenesis of the transcription factor GATA-4 gene in mouse embryonic stem cells disrupts visceral endoderm differentiation in vitro. Development 1995;121:3877–88.
174. Mac Morris M, Broverman S, Greenspoon S, et al. Regulation of vitellogenin gene expression in transgenic Caenorhabditis elegans: short sequences required for activation of the vit-2 promoter. Mol Cell Biol 1992;12:1652–62.
175. Egan CR, Chung MA, Allen FL, et al. A gut-to-pharynx/tail switch in embryonic expression of the Caenorhabditis elegans ges-1 gene centers on two GATA sequences. Dev Biol 1995;170:397–419.
176. Spieth J, Shim YH, Lea K, et al. Elt-1, an embryonically expressed Caenorhabditis elegans: gene homologous to the GATA transcription factor family. Mol Cell Biol 1991;11:4651–9.

177. Hawkins MG, McGhee JD. *Elt-2*, a second GATA factor from the nematode *Caenorhabditis elegans*. J Biol Chem 1995; 270:14666–71.
178. Harvey RP. *NK-2* homeobox genes and heart development. Dev Biol 1996;178:203–16.
179. Buchberger A, Pabst O, Brand T, et al. Chick *NKx-2.3* represents a novel family member of vertebrate homologues to the *Drosophila* homeobox gene *tinman*: differential expression *cNKx-2.3* and *cNKx-2.5* during heart and gut development. Mech Dev 1996;56:151–63.
180. Pabst O, Schneider A, Brand T, Arnold HH. The mouse Nkx2-3 homeodomain gene is expressed in gut mesenchyme during pre- and postnatal mouse development. Dev Dyn 1997; 209:29–35.
181. Evans SM, Yan W, Murillo MP, et al. *Tinman*, a *Drosophila* homeobox gene required for heart and visceral mesoderm specification, may be represented by a family of genes in vertebrates: *XNkx-2.3*, a second vertebrate homologue of *tinman*. Development 1995;121:3889–99.
182. Walters JRF, Howard A, Rumble HEE, et al. Differences in expression of homeobox transcription factors in proximal and distal human small intestine. Gastroenterology 1997;113:472–7.
183. Lin W-H, Huang L-H, Yeh J-H, et al. Expression of a *Drosophila* GATA transcription factor in multiple tissues in the developing embryos. J Biol Chem 1995;270:25150–8.
184. Rehorn K-P, Thelen H, Michelson AM, Reuter R. A molecular aspect of hematopoiesis and endoderm development common to vertebrates and *Drosophila*. Development 1996;122: 4023–41.
185. Azzaria M, Goszczynski B, Chung MA, et al. A *forkhead/HNF-3* homolog expressed in the pharynx and intestine of the *Caenorhabditis elegans* embryo. Dev Biol 1996;178:289–303.
186. Strahle U, Blader P, Henrique D, Ingham PW. *Axial*, a zebrafish gene expressed along the developing body axis, shows altered expression in cyclops mutant embryos. Genes Dev 1993;7:1436–46.
187. Strahle U, Blader P, Ingham PW. Expression of *axial* and *sonic hedgehog* in wildtype and midline defective zebrafish embryos. Int J Dev Biol 1996;40:929–40.
188. Pack M, Solnicka-Krezel L, Malicki J, et al. Mutations affecting development of zebrafish digestive organs. Development 1996;123:321–8.

CHAPTER 3

Hormones and Growth Factors in Intestinal Development

D. Brent Polk, MD

John A. Barnard, MD

In this chapter, recent advances in the study of selected growth factors and hormones important in intestinal development are presented. At the cellular level several advances have been made in understanding of the mechanisms of signal transduction by the respective receptors. At the whole-animal level, on the other hand, selected disruption of growth factors, hormones or their receptors has added insight into potential roles for these factors in development as well as in intestinal cell biology. For an extensive compendium of additional factors with putative roles in intestinal development readers are referred to a recent publication on gut peptides.[1]

GLUCOCORTICOIDS

Overview

The effect of glucocorticoids on intestinal development has been extensively studied, perhaps more so than any other hormone or growth factor. In part, at least, the intense focus has been prompted by extensive characterization of the rat model of postnatal intestinal development, in which glucocorticoids appear to play a prominent role.[2] The current discussion will be restricted to studies of the rat model of development, with occasional reference to the limited information available in humans. The rat model is particularly valuable because at the time of birth the rat intestine is immature. During the first 3 postnatal weeks rapid and dramatic changes in intestinal structure and function occur in the context of an orderly, well-defined change in glucocorticoid metabolism. Precise definition of developmental changes in glucocorticoid secretion and glucocorticoid receptor expression has led to discovery of direct cause-and-effect relationships and correlations with a variety of intestinal developmental processes, as outlined below.

Structure and Biochemistry

The anterior pituitary adrenocorticotropic hormone, ACTH, stimulates biosynthesis of adrenal steroids, lipid-soluble hormones synthesized from a cholesterol nucleus by the adrenal cortex. There is a large number of adrenal cortex hormones, but the predominant circulating form in humans is cortisol (hydrocortisone), whereas the principal form in mice and rats is corticosterone.[3] The majority of circulating glucocorticoids are bound to corticosteroid-binding globulin (transcortin), a plasma protein synthesized in the liver. The reader is referred to standard biochemistry texts for further information on the biochemistry of adrenal steroid hormones and steroidogenesis.

Receptors

Glucocorticoid receptors belong to the steroid-thyroid hormone receptor superfamily, which includes the receptors for glucocorticoids, mineralocorticoids, vitamin D, thyroid hormones, retinoic acids, and steroid sex hormones such as estrogen. These receptors function as transcription factors. In general, it is thought that glucocorticoids and other steroids pass through the cell membrane and into the cytoplasm by simple diffusion. Within the cytoplasm, glucocorticoids bind the glucocorticoid receptor, and the receptor-ligand complex is translocated into the nucleus to directly participate in transcriptional regulation of target genes.

The glucocorticoid receptor has three major structural domains.[4,5] The ligand-binding domain is located at the C-terminus. The DNA-binding domain is located N-terminal to the ligand-binding domain, and its sequence is the most conserved region among all the steroid receptor superfamily sequences. The N-terminal sequence contains the transcriptional transactivation domain. There are three mechanisms by which the glucocorticoid receptor modifies expression of target genes: (1) recognition of a specific DNA consensus sequence (the glucocorticoid response element or GRE); (2) titration of other transcription factors independent of DNA binding; and (3) modification of chromatin structure allowing assembly and function of other transcriptional machinery.

Developmental phenomena in the intestine related to the action of glucocorticoids require the presence of functional, high-affinity glucocorticoid receptors. In rat small intestine, high-affinity receptors for [3H]-dexamethasone are present in cytosolic fractions of the jejunum throughout late fetal life and into adulthood.[6] The level of binding is somewhat greater during the first 2 postnatal weeks than in the post-weaning interval. All intestinal epithelial cells appear to bind [3H]-dexamethasone, but cell fractions isolated from the crypt epithelium bind approximately twofold more than villus tip cells.[7] In limited studies of tissue obtained from human embryos, prominent nuclear immunostaining was noted in the epithelium of the stomach and foregut.[8]

Disruption of gene expression by homologous recombination (gene targeting) may provide clues to the biologic function of glucocorticoids in intestinal development. The glucocorticoid receptor has been disrupted in mice but the majority of these mice die a few hours after birth from respiratory failure due to impaired development of alveoli and terminal bronchioles.[9] These mice also have adrenal abnormalities. Structural and functional abnormalities in the intestine have not been reported.

Biology

The postnatal development of serum glucocorticoid and corticosteroid-binding globulin levels was defined in seminal studies reported by Dr. Susan Henning in the 1970s.[2] Henning first reported that both free and total corticosterone concentrations in rats rose dramatically between postnatal days 12 and 14 and reached maximum concentrations at day 24. Nearly parallel observations were made for corticosteroid-binding globulin. In the same studies, the developmental changes in lactase and sucrase activity occurred 2 days following the surge in glucocorticoid levels. Subsequent studies more closely scrutinized the effect of glucocorticoids on development of disaccharidase activities. Many of these are discussed in more detail in Chapter 7. A focused discussion is provided in the current chapter.

Effect of Glucocorticoids on Sucrase and Lactase Development

In the rat, sucrase-isomaltase activity is not detectable until approximately postnatal day 16, about 48 hours after the developmental surge of corticosterone, implying a cause-and-effect relationship. Over 30 years ago, it was found that administration of hydrocortisone induces the precocious appearance of sucrase hydrolytic activity in the rat intestine, as early as postnatal day 9.[10] More recent analyses have determined that glucocorticoids precociously induce sucrase activity by early induction of sucrase mRNA expression.[11] Interestingly, however, there is only a brief window of time during which exogenous glucocorticoid is capable of inducing sucrase.

Sometime between postnatal days 16 and 18 in the rat, exogenous administration of dexamethasone no longer induces sucrase activity and mRNA above control levels, and this glucocorticoid independence persists into adulthood.[11] Surgical adrenalectomy performed prior to the normal corticosterone surge in rats offers an interesting insight into the requirement for endogenous glucocorticoids in sucrase development.[12] Adrenalectomy results in a 2-day *delay* in the developmental appearance of sucrase enzymatic activity and mRNA expression but by postnatal day 26 levels are equivalent in controls and adrenalectomized animals. Collectively these studies indicate that glucocorticoids are a covariable but are not absolutely required for development of sucrase activity.

The effects of glucocorticoids on lactase expression are less straightforward and precipitous than effects on sucrase. Lactase activity is highest at birth during the first 12 to 14 postnatal days.[13] Thereafter, levels slowly decline over the next 7 to 10 days. While adrenalectomy[12] delays the decline by several days, and administration of glucocorticoid at the time of maturational decline somewhat increases the rate of decline,[14] a true precocious decline in lactase activity earlier in postnatal life is not observed with glucocorticoid administration.

Of course the effects of glucocorticoids on development of intestinal disaccharidases do not occur in isolation. Complex interactions and, in some cases, synergy between components of the thyroid hormone axis and the glucocorticoid hormone axis have been described by several investigators.[14–17]

Effect of Glucocorticoids on Intestinal Bile Salt Transport

During the first 2 weeks of postnatal development of the rat intestine, bile salts are absorbed in the jejunum and ileum by passive (nonsaturable) diffusion.[18,19] Active (saturable), sodium-dependent cotransport by the ileal brushborder membrane is first detectable on postnatal day 17, a developmental pattern reminiscent of the development of sucrase activity (see above), suggesting a potential role for glucocorticoids in the development of ileal bile salt transport. Administration of daily pharmacologic doses of the glucocorticoid methylprednisolone (days 11, 12, and 13) to suckling rats results in the precocious appearance of sodium-dependent taurocholate transport on day 14.[20] In contrast, administration of corticosterone in physiologic doses does not appear to induce precocious development of active bile salt transport.[21]

The relatively recent molecular cloning of a sodium-dependent ileal bile salt transporter has permitted further examination of developmental phenomena related to bile salt transport.[22] While both the cotransporter mRNA and protein are induced by exogenous administration of corticosterone to adult rats,[23] the ontogenic pattern of mRNA and protein expression is somewhat unanticipated. Expression of both the ileal brushborder membrane transporter mRNA and protein follow a biphasic pattern, with increased levels detectable late in gestation followed by a pronounced reduction until late in weaning, when expression is markedly induced by a transcriptional mechanism.[22,24] Interestingly, these prominent ontogenic changes in intestinal bile salt transport occur while the renal transporter is constitutively expressed.[25] Additional study will be required to more completely delineate the role for glucocorticoid hormones in intestinal bile salt transport.

In humans, the intestinal absorption of bile salts has received limited attention. Accumulation of taurocholate into gut rings from human intestine occurred against a concentration gradient in infants beyond 8 months of age, implying a postnatal maturation of bile salt transport.[26] However, there is no definitive evidence in support of glucocorticoid-mediated effects on bile salt transport in humans.

Effect of Glucocorticoids on Other Intestinal Functions

A number of additional intestinal functions potentially relevant to development are influenced by glucocorticoids, although these are less well studied. These include regulation of cellular proliferation,[27] ion transport,[28,29] vitamin D metabolism,[30] and collagen synthesis.[31]

THYROID HORMONES

Overview

Thyroxine (T4) and triiodothyronine (T3) have been reviewed extensively as potential regulatory hormones for intestinal development.[2,32] One of the criteria suggested by Henning as necessary to establish a role for specific hormones in intestinal ontogeny is that physiologic administration of a hormone induces precocious maturation.[2] Whereas physiologic levels of locally-produced growth factors such as epidermal growth factor (EGF) and transforming growth factor α (TGFα) are not readily measurable, the levels of circulating hormones, such as T4, glucocorticoids, or insulin are more apparent. A study of physiologic levels of T4 clearly demonstrated that this hormone has no significant effect on post-natal ontogeny of the rat intestine.[17] Interestingly, the investigators clearly demonstrated synergistic effects on the maturation of various enzymes when T4 was administered concomitantly with dexamethasone. In spite of evidence that thyroid hormone does not play a significant role in later intestinal ontogeny, recent exciting findings in *Xenopus* have suggested a primary role for thyroid hormones during intestinal morphogenesis.[32]

Structure and Biochemistry

Thyroid hormones are produced in the thyroid follicular cells of the thyroid gland and secreted as either T4 or T3 in response to thyroid stimulating hormone. The primary active form is T3, and T4 must be converted to T3 to render biologic activity. For a detailed review of the regulation of thyroid hormone synthesis, secretion and transport, the reader is referred to a recent review by LoPresti and Singer.[33] Interestingly, the enzyme responsible for conversion of T4 to T3, iodothyronine deiodinase, is developmentally regulated in the amphibian intestine.[34] Also, the availability of T3 for receptor binding during intestinal development may be regulated by expression of a cytosolic thyroid hormone-binding protein.[35] In a study of steady-state organ distribution of T3 and T4 in adult male rats the greatest extrathyroidal pool (33%) was found in the intestine.[36]

Thyroid hormone receptors are nuclear-localized proteins expressed as two separate gene products, α and β, and

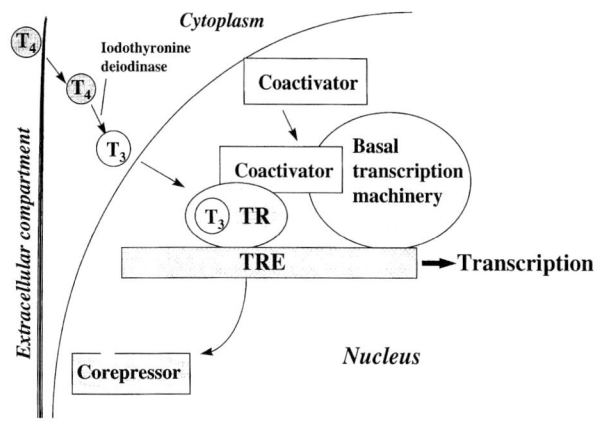

FIGURE 3-1. Thyroid hormone receptor binding and initiation of transcription.

belong to the nuclear receptor superfamily, which includes steroid and retinoid receptors. The receptors are bound to DNA thyroid response elements as dimers in a complex of proteins, including corepressor proteins, which block receptor transcription function. Ligation of thyroid hormone receptor by T3 displaces the repressor protein, permitting association with a coactivator protein and initiation of transcription (Figure 3–1).[37] Mutations in the ligand-binding domain of the thyroid hormone receptor gene cause resistance to thyroid hormone function.[38]

Receptors

Thyroid hormone receptors are expressed in the nucleus of intestinal epithelial cells. The predominant form expressed in the developing and adult rat intestine is the Trβ-1.[39] During intestinal development, a nonhormone binding thyroid receptor isoform, c-erbAα-2, is significantly downregulated between 5 and 25 days postnatal, at a time when the rat small intestinal expression of intestinal alkaline phosphatase is increasingly T3-responsive.[39]

Biologic Effect on Intestinal Development

The organism *Xenopus* has proven an excellent model for studying early intestinal growth and morphogenesis.[32] Organ cultures of larval intestine were shown to undergo transition to adult-type epithelium in the presence of T3, cortisol, and insulin.[40] Interestingly, T3 alone could induce the apoptotic changes of early morphogenesis but not the proliferation and differentiation of later ontogeny. By isolating larval and adult intestinal epithelial cells and fibroblasts, the same laboratory was able to demonstrate proliferation of fibroblasts and adult epithelial cells by T3.[41] However, T3-induced apoptosis of larval epithelial cells was inhibited by extracellular matrix. The signal transduction pathway regulating thyroid hormone-induced apoptosis in larval intestinal cells can be inhibited by cyclosporin A, but not tacrolimus (FK506); whereas both immunosuppressive drugs block T-cell apoptosis.[42] Identification of the target of cyclosporin A in this pathway may provide novel information about regulating apoptosis during intestinal morphogenesis.

The patterns of intestinal fatty acid-binding protein (IFABP) have been well-characterized in the developing mouse intestine.[43] The biphasic expression of IFABP in developing *Xenopus* intestine has been highly correlated with intestinal cell apoptosis.[44] Intestinal fatty acid-binding protein expression is normally downregulated over a 20-day period just prior to the onset of massive epithelial cell death during intestinal remodeling. This entire effect could be reproduced in just 3 days if tadpoles were treated with thyroid hormone prior to the normal reduction in IFABP.[44] Subsequently, a regional pattern of regulation for IFABP expression was uncovered by organ culture.[45] The proximal but not distal larval intestinal expression of IFABP was downregulated by thyroid hormone, suggesting that other endogenous factors may play regional regulatory roles in this process.

The maturational effect in early ontogeny is not restricted to the epithelium. In a series of epithelial and supporting matrix recombinations, induction of connective tissue differentiation required the presence of epithelium and T3.[46] This crosstalk between the epithelium, connective tissue, and T3 also altered immune cell development in the connective tissue; without epithelium and T3, there was a reduction in macrophage-like cells in the connective tissue. The potential importance of thyroid hormone regulation of intestinal immune function has been recently underscored by a report of mice lacking thyroid-stimulating hormone receptor expression with selective impairment of intestinal T-cell repertoire.[47]

As noted, thyroid hormones exert cellular effects primarily by regulating gene transcription through direct binding to two nuclear thyroid hormone receptors. Several potential target genes have been identified in intestinal epithelial cells with either direct or indirect transcriptional regulation by thyroid hormone receptor binding.[48–53] The expression of the matrix metalloproteinase gene, stromelysin-3, is upregulated in intestinal fibroblasts during thyroid hormone-induced morphogenesis in *Xenopus*.[48] This suggests a functional role for stromelysin-3 in the modification of extracellular matrix that is necessary for the accompanying massive cell death in this developmental process.

The Hedgehog family of secreted proteins are key regulatory molecules in establishing positional information and tissue patterning during development.[54] The *Xenopus* homolog of Hedgehog was isolated by subtractive hybridization screening analysis of thyroid hormone-induced expression in the metamorphosis of *Xenopus laevis* gastrointestinal tract.[49] Both normal thyroid hormone-dependent and precocious thyroid hormone-induced morphogenesis in the intestine were accompanied by upregulated expression of Hedgehog. Inhibitors of protein expression blocked thyroid hormone-induced expression in the intestine, suggesting Hedgehog is a direct thyroid hormone response gene.[49] Other transcriptional targets of thyroid hormone in the *Xenopus* intestine have been identified, including a novel collagenase, a plasma membrane immediate-early gene product, and a leucine zipper-containing transcription factor.[50–52]

There is convincing evidence that thyroid hormones play an integral role in regulating the expression, or function, of several transporters expressed on the intestinal epithelial cell.[55–59] The administration of T4 to adult rats inhibits Cl^--HCO_3^- anion exchange activity in the intestine, which appears to be via transcriptional regulation.[56] The apical membrane Na^+-H^+ exchanger NHE3 expression is upregulated by both glucocorticoids and T4 through cis-acting elements in the 5′-flanking promoter region.[57] Amiloride-sensitive Na^+ transport in the rat colon is regulated by T4, independent of glucocorticoids.[58] Expression of Na^+-K^+ATPase in the rat small intestine and the CaCo-2 cell line were shown to be responsive to thyroid hormone.[59] This appears to be regulated by the transcription of the beta-1 subunit of the Na^+-K^+ATPase pump.

Thyroid hormone regulation of the brushborder enzymes has been extensively reviewed elsewhere.[2,60] There now appears to be little evidence to suggest a major role for T3 or T4 in most brushborder enzymes studied, with the exception of intestinal alkaline phosphatase.[61,62] This upregulation appears to be at the transcriptional level in the villus cells but is not detected in crypt cells.[62] Similar findings were noted in studies with the conditionally differentiated HT29 colon cancer cell line.[62] Cotransfection of the T3 receptor with a reporter plasmid construct for the intestinal alkaline phosphatase (IAP) gene induced greater IAP reporter activity in differentiated, compared to undifferentiated, HT29 cells. The authors localized this thyroid hormone response cis-element to a 2.4 kb segment of the reporter gene.[62]

The strongest evidence for thyroid hormone as a regulatory molecule in early intestinal development comes from a recent description of disruption of expression of the T3Rα gene in a knockout mouse model that is a lethal mutation at about 5 weeks postnatal age.[63] The small intestine appeared to be particularly affected in this mouse line. The entire small intestine was described as smaller, softer, and more fragile than in wild-type mice. The overall diameter of jejunal and ileal sections was reduced two- to three-fold in the TR3α-/- mice with a decrease in both the number and size of the villi. The epithelial cell mass was decreased by approximately 65%. Goblet cell numbers were reduced 2.5-fold. A significant reduction in underlying circular and smooth muscle layers correlated with altered motility based on several functional assays. Interestingly, while there was a twofold reduction in total dipeptidase and disaccharidase activities neither cellular expression nor functional absorption appeared altered.

Taken together these findings demonstrate a clear role for thyroid hormones in early intestinal morphogenesis of amphibian and mammalian intestine and suggest a potential role in regulation of mucosal immunity and ion transport.

INSULIN AND INSULIN-LIKE GROWTH FACTORS

Overview

The insulin-like growth factor (IGF) ligand-receptor system includes the three structurally-related peptide ligands (insulin, IGF-I, and IGF-II) and two high-affinity, membrane-associated tyrosine kinase receptors (IGF type I and IGF type II receptors). The interaction between IGFs and their receptors is modulated by a family of IGF-binding proteins (IGFBP1–6). Collectively, these proteins function in a

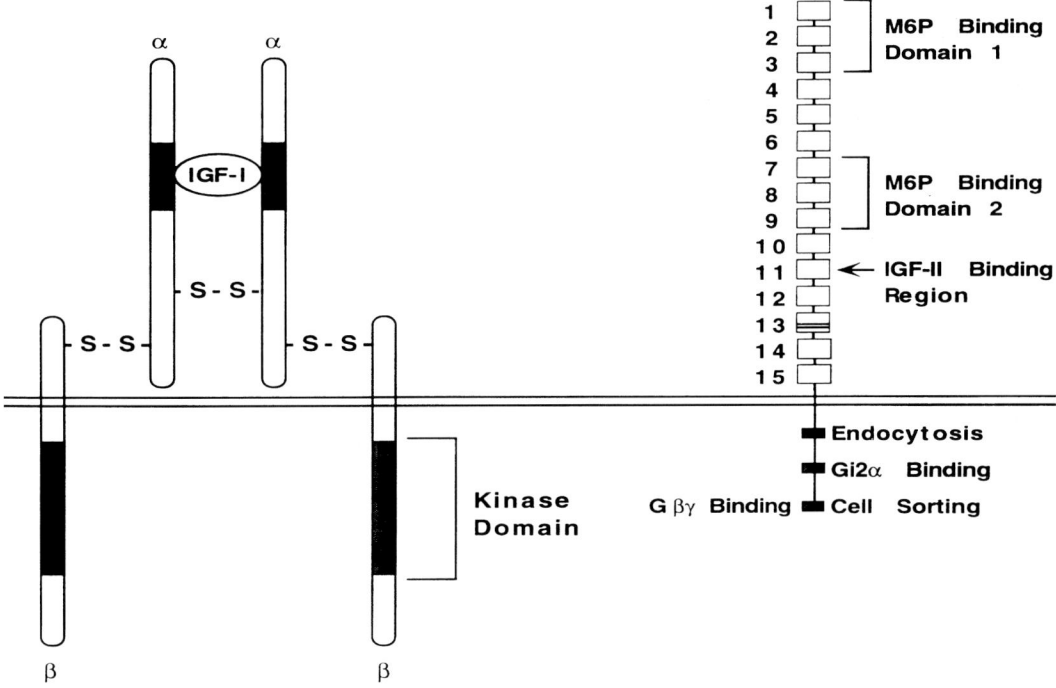

FIGURE 3–2. The IGF-I and IGF-II-mannose-6-phosphate receptors.

wide variety of cells and tissues to regulate a host of biologic functions related to cellular growth and differentiation. A great deal of information is known about the structure, function, and biology of the IGFs, and the reader is referred to a number of excellent, comprehensive reviews.[64–69]

Much remains to be learned about the role of the IGFs in gastrointestinal biology. In this section, the relevant biochemistry of IGFs will be reviewed, along with selected observations regarding the role of IGFs in gastrointestinal biology and development. A complete review of the biology of insulin is beyond the scope of this discussion, and its role in the gastrointestinal biology tract will be mentioned only in the context of IGF-I and IGF-II.

Insulin-Like Growth Factor Genes and Proteins

The human IGF-I gene is located on chromosome 12 and comprises 6 exons.[70] The genomic DNA sequence is large, spanning more than 80 kB. A complex pattern of alternate splicing occurs, the biologic significance of which is uncertain but that may reflect tissue-specific or developmentally-regulated functions. Insulin-like growth factor-I RNA sequences range from about 1.0 to 8.0 kB, and at least four precursor sequences are recognized for the IGF-I protein. The structure of these is highly conserved across evolution.[71] The aminoterminal precursor sequence is not characteristic for a typical signal peptide, and the carboxyterminal precursor sequence does not contain classic dibasic cleavage sites characteristic of other proteins. The most commonly recognized mature peptide sequence contains 70 amino acids. There is evidence that cellular secretion of IGF-I occurs prior to processing of the carboxyterminal precursor sequence.[72] The majority of circulating IGF-I is synthesized in the liver in response to pituitary growth hormone, and it appears that all the growth-stimulating activities of growth hormone can be mimicked by IGF-I. It is clear that growth hormone regulates IGF production in other tissues as well, including the gastrointestinal tract as described below.

The human IGF-II gene is located on chromosome 11. Insulin-like growth factor-I and IGF-II share approximately 70% identity and have a close structural homology with insulin. Like IGF-I, the IGF-II precursor is large, and a variety of splice variants have been described many of which are developmentally regulated and contain gut-specific promoters.[73] The IGF-II precursor contains an aminoterminal signal peptide. Like IGF-I, a pro-IGF-II-containing carboxyterminal precursor sequence is secreted from cells prior to processing to the mature 67 amino acid protein.[69] The biologic function of IGF-II is not clearly understood.

Insulin-Like Growth Factor Receptor Genes and Proteins

The IGF type I receptor gene is located on human chromosome 15 and is homologous to the insulin receptor gene.[74] The protein is synthesized as a single polypeptide chain that is cleaved by proteolysis at a tetrabasic amino acid site resulting in an alpha (α) and beta (β) subunit (Figure 3–2). Alpha and β subunits associate by disulfide bridging into a heterodimer (αβ heterodimer or half-receptor), and these heterodimers further associate by disulfide bridging to the mature heterotetrameric receptor, designated α2β2 receptor.

The α subunits are extracellular sequences and harbor the ligand-binding domain, whereas the β subunits are primarily intracellular sequences and contain the tyrosine kinase signaling domain.[66] This receptor assembly is closely analogous to the insulin receptor. The IGF type I receptor binds IGF-I and IGF II with high affinity (Kd in the nanomolar range) and binds insulin with a much lower affinity. Interestingly, hybrid receptors resulting from association of insulin receptor subunits and IGF type I receptor subunits have been described,[75] but the physiologic significance of these will require further study.

Most of the biologic activities of IGF-I and IGF-II are mediated by the IGF type I receptor. Insulin-like growth factor I binding results in tyrosine phosphorylation of a key 185 kD signaling protein termed the insulin receptor substrate 1 (IRS-1).[76] Insulin receptor substrate 1 contains a large number of potential phosphorylation sites and SH domains, permitting docking of a variety of intracellular signaling molecules, the end result of which is activation of a variety of signaling cascades including the Ras and phosphoinositide 3-kinase pathways. A number of immediate early genes associated with traverse through the G1 phase of the cell cycle, including c-fos, c-myc, and c-jun, are activated by stimulation of the IGF type I receptor.

The IGF type II receptor is a single, transmembrane polypeptide chain that binds IGF-II with high affinity and IGF-I with low affinity. The IGF type II receptor is identical to the mannose-6-phosphate receptor and has no structural homology with the insulin and IGF type I receptor. The IGF type II receptor contains 15 cysteine-laden, contiguous extracellular repeats and a short intracellular sequence without a recognizable signaling domain.[68] Recognition of mannose-6-phosphate residues by the IGF type II-mannose-6-phosphate receptor on proteins in the Golgi apparatus targets these proteins to the lysosome. There is clear evidence that the IGF type II receptor mediates binding and intracellular degradation of IGF-II, thus functioning as a scavenger receptor. There is much less evidence for activation of signaling pathways by the IGF type II receptor.[67]

Insulin-Like Growth Factor Binding Proteins

Six IGFBPs have been cloned and characterized to date. All six are structurally related, but the central portion of each is structurally unique. Additional information about the gene organization, protein structure, and molecular biology of IGFBPs can be found in the reviews referenced at the beginning of this section.

Insulin-like growth factor binding proteins are detectable in plasma and extracellular fluids and are expressed during development as well as during adult life. Postulated actions of IGFBPs include potentiation or inhibition of IGF activity, reservation of IGF in a biologically inaccessible pool, transport of IGFs in extracellular fluids, and activities that take place independent of IGF binding.[77] In part, these activities are possible because the affinity of IGF-I and IGF-II for their binding proteins is greater than their affinity for the IGF receptors. Both IGFs bind to all six binding proteins, albeit with some differences in affinity.

Insulin-Like Growth Factor Family Distribution in the Gastrointestinal Tract

A large number of studies have described the presence and distribution of IGFs and IGF receptors in the gastrointestinal tract in a variety of species, including humans,[73] rats,[72,78–83] rabbits,[84] and pigs.[85] It is clear that IGF-I, IGF-II, and the IGF type I receptor are expressed throughout the gastrointestinal tract; however, a concise portrayal of the distribution of these factors within gastrointestinal tissues is not possible. Interpretation of the available literature is complicated by the variety of species studied, the variety of technical and molecular approaches used to study the distribution of IGF family members and, in some instances, conflicting results. A thorough review of the studies published to date is nicely presented in the review by Lund.[71] A few general conclusions will be stated herein. First, sufficient analysis of the binding of [^{125}I]-IGF-I and II to cell membranes isolated from the intestinal epithelium has been done to conclude that receptors are localized on the epithelium of the native gastrointestinal tract and in cultured intestinal epithelial cells.[79,85–89] It is less apparent if there is a consistent differential distribution along the CV axis, a specific pattern of localization in the muscularis mucosae or if there is targeting to a specific epithelial membrane domain. A systemic approach using the latest immunolocalization and in situ hybridization techniques in a single species is sorely needed to address these important issues.

Changes in IGF-II and IGF type II receptor expression during rat development are quite prominent. Intestinal IGF-II RNA transcripts are readily detectable during late fetal gestation, but much less in adult rat samples.[83] Others have described a similar pattern, in which RNA transcripts decrease to adults levels by the eleventh postnatal day.[82] Insulin-like growth factor type II receptor levels also decrease during rat development,[90] suggesting that the IGF-II-IGF type II receptor axis may play an important role in intestinal development. A clear pattern of developmental expression of IGF-I-IGF type I receptor has not emerged. Fluctuations in expression are observed, and the degree of change is less apparent than that described for IGF-I.[83,85,91]

Biology of Insulin-Like Growth Factor Family in the Gastrointestinal Tract

Insulin-like growth factors have a wide variety of biologic activities, including effects on glucose, carbohydrate, and protein metabolism and pronounced effects relevant to the stimulation of cellular proliferation in a great number of cell types. The most prominent effect relevant to the gastrointestinal tract is the stimulation of intestinal epithelial proliferation. The effect of IGFs on intestinal epithelial differentiation appears minimal.

Three major lines of evidence support the potent mitogenic activities of IGFs on the intestinal epithelium. First, intestinal epithelial cells in culture proliferate in response to IGFs. Second, exogenous administration of IGF stimulates epithelial cell proliferation in the intestine. Last, transgenic mice with increased expression of IGF demonstrate increased growth of the gastrointestinal tract. Each of these lines of evidence will be examined separately below.

The paucity of nontransformed intestinal epithelial cell lines available for cell culture studies has limited the number of in vitro studies on the mitogenic properties of IGFs. Collectively the reported studies support a role for IGFs in stimulation of intestinal epithelial growth although the potency appears significantly less than that of EGF[89,92–94] When EGF is administered with IGF-I or insulin, a synergistic effect on intestinal epithelial proliferation is observed.[93,94]

The evidence for a proliferative effect of IGF on the intestine is much more substantially supported by in vivo analyses. Both enteral and parenteral routes of IGF administration have been studied. The biologic justification for investigation of enteral IGF administration on intestinal growth is supported by the occurrence of both IGF-I and IGF-II in human milk[95] and IGF-I in human gastrointestinal secretions.[96] At least a portion of enterally administered [^{125}I]-IGF-I and II can be recovered intact from gastrointestinal tissues of suckling rats, indicating that the peptide is stable in the milieu of the neonatal stomach and small intestine.[97] In support of this, addition of a "supraphysiologic" IGF-I dose to neonatal pigs from birth to 4 days of age increased certain indices of small intestinal growth, such as weight, DNA content, protein content, and villus height of the small intestine.[98] These effects were most prominent in the proximal small intestine. No effect was observed in the pancreas or stomach. Analogous observations occur in the jejunum and ileum of fetal sheep.[99] In the sheep model, the fetal esophagus is ligated in utero, thus depriving the distal intestinal tract from growth regulatory peptides in amniotic fluid. A 10-day infusion of IGF-I distal to the ligation results in increased parameters of small intestinal growth, indicating that IGF-I in amniotic fluid may play an important role in in utero growth of the sheep intestine.

Stimulation of intestinal growth also occurs following parenteral administration of IGF. Potten and co-workers found a modest stimulation of small intestinal crypt labeling index after brief treatment of mice with an intraperitoneal injection of IGF-I.[100] Similarly a 14-day parenteral treatment of adult rats with IGF-I increased crypt depth and villus height 30% over control values.[101] Again, the proximal small intestine was the most responsive region of the intestinal tract. These same investigators later found a shorter-term infusion (3 days) by osmotic minipump of LR^{3}IGF-I, an N-terminal extended analog of IGF-I with more potency than the parent peptide, stimulated parameters of proliferation in the small intestinal epithelium of adults rats.[102] Similar findings were observed in suckling and weanling rats in the small intestinal epithelium and in the muscularis.[103]

A variety of studies have examined the effect of parenteral IGF-I on intestinal growth under pathophysiologic conditions. For example, IGF-I enhances adaptive mucosal proliferation in the small intestine and colon of rats that have undergone a massive small intestinal resection.[104,105] Peterson and colleagues found that atrophy of the jejunal mucosa occurring in conjunction with total parenteral nutrition in rats was ameliorated by inclusion of IGF-I in the parenteral nutrition solution.[106] Atrophy of the rat small intestine occurring in conjunction with chronic liver disease or sepsis is also reduced by administration of IGF-I.[107,108]

The final experimental data supporting a proliferative effect of IGFs on the intestinal mucosa come from recent studies on the effect of IGF-I overexpression in transgenic mice. The background for these studies is interesting. It has previously been reported that transgenic mice overexpressing growth hormone have increased bowel length and mass but a normal intestinal crypt cell proliferation rate, suggesting that growth hormone increases survival of intestinal epithelial cells.[109] These mice, as expected, had increased levels of plasma IGF-I and increased IGF-I expression in the intestinal mucosa. The finding that IGF is a survival factor for the intestinal epithelium is interesting in light of observations that IGF-I inhibits apoptosis (programmed cell death) in a variety of cultured cell lines.[110] Matthews and colleagues subsequently generated transgenic mice overexpressing IGF-I under the metallothionein (MT) I promoter.[111] In these mice, circulating GH levels are undetectable because of negative feedback from overexpression of IGF-I, thus permitting a dissociation between the effects of GH and IGF-I. Ohneda and co-workers[112] used MT-IGF-I mice to determine the effect of IGF-I on intestinal proliferation. After exposure of the mice to zinc for 30 to 40 days to activate the promoter, these animals exhibited a significantly greater small intestinal length and mass, an increased villus height, crypt depth, and crypt cell mitotic index than their littermates. Indices of differentiation were not altered. Overexpression of IGF-II in a transgenic mouse either does[113] or does not[114] increase the mass of the gastrointestinal tract but detailed effects on the gastrointestinal tract were not reported in either case. Thus far no specific details of the development and function of the intestine in IGFBP overexpressing mice have been described.

Scattered additional observations relevant to the IGF system and intestinal biology have been reported. For example, it is well known that fasting leads to intestinal mucosal atrophy and reduced levels of serum IGF-I.[115] Refeeding stimulates intestinal epithelial cell proliferation. Several investigators[116,117] have made the intriguing observation that rat jejunal IGF-I mRNA levels decrease by at least half during fasting and return to control levels with refeeding. In parallel studies, Winesett and co-workers[116] found that IGFBP-3 mRNA levels decrease with fasting, but *do not* increase with refeeding, leading to speculation that the proliferative actions of IGF-I are thereby amplified. These observations emphasize the complex relationship between the IGFs and their binding proteins. Indeed, one can conceive an almost bewildering array of permutations in the interactions between these peptides and how they are regulated by other growth factors as well as physiologic and pathophysiologic states. Studies in cell culture have just begun to scratch the surface.[118,119]

Elimination of Insulin-Like Growth Factor Function by Gene Targeting

The technique of gene targeting (knockout) by homologous recombination has been used extensively to study the function of the IGF peptide and receptor family.[120] Interestingly, distinctive effects on development of the gastrointestinal system have not been found. A prominent effect is fetal growth retardation. For example, mice rendered IGF type I receptor-deficient had a birth weight approximately 45% of their normal littermates.[121] The animals were cyanotic at birth and died of respiratory failure within minutes. The lung structure of late-stage embryos was normal, indicating respiratory failure was not due to defective morphogenesis. Significant abnormalities were detected in several organ systems and included hypoplasia of skeletal muscle, central nervous system anomalies, skin and hair follicle abnormalities and delayed bone development. Insulin-like growth factor-I deficient mice were about 60% of normal birth weight. Depending on the genetic background, some mice died in the newborn period, similar to the IGF type I receptor animals, while some survived into adulthood. Placental development in both gene-targeted mice is normal.[122] Gene targeting of selected IGFBPs has been accomplished but no intestinal phenotype has been described.

EPIDERMAL GROWTH FACTOR RECEPTOR LIGANDS

Overview

The epidermal growth factor receptor is the prototypical member of a family of transmembrane proteins containing intrinsic cytoplasmic tyrosine kinase activity that is enhanced by ligation with any of at least nine different peptides, EGF, TGFα, heparin-binding (HB) EGF, amphiregulin (AR), betacellulin (BTC), cripto, heregulin (HR), and epiregulin. There are currently four members of the class I receptor subfamily, which includes ErbB1 (EGF receptor), ErbB2, ErbB3, and ErbB4.[123] The focus of this review will be on the EGF receptor and the two best-characterized ligands for this receptor family, EGF and TGFα. Epidermal growth factor was originally isolated by Cohen from the salivary secretions of mice based on the ability to stimulate proliferation and differentiation of the eyelid with epidermal thickening and keratinization, eruption of incisors, and inhibition of hair growth.[124] Significant progress has been made in understanding the molecular mechanisms of signal transduction of the ErbB family members from ligand binding to proliferative and nonproliferative cellular responses. Several lines of evidence have suggested a role for the EGF receptor in gastrointestinal development, though very little is known regarding expression or regulation of the other ErbB family members in either the developing or mature intestine.

Epidermal Growth Factor, Transforming Growth Factor α, and Epidermal Growth Factor Receptor Genes and Proteins

Epidermal growth factor is a 53-amino acid protein member of a family of peptides that include TGFα, AR, BTC, and HB-EGF and that share 11 invariant amino acid residues including six cysteines that form the three disulfide bonds defining the structure of the EGF family. Overall sequence homology between the members of this growth factor family is 20%; however, this is significantly enhanced if the invariant amino acids are weighted in the calculations.[125,126] The EGF receptor ligands are produced as glycosylated, membrane-anchored precursors ranging in size from 160 to 1207 amino acids, which are cleaved into soluble, mature proteins in a range from 6 to 17 kDa.[125]

In humans, the gene-encoding EGF is located on chromosome 4 while TGFα is located on chromosome 2.[127,128] The EGF gene is estimated to span 120 kilobases (kb), including 24 exons and 23 introns, with the mature EGF composed of exons 20 and 21.[129] The TGFα gene is composed of 6 exons, with the sequence for mature TGFα encoded by exons 3 and 4.[130] The human EGF receptor gene is located on chromosome 7 where it is estimated to cover 110 kb, including 26 exons encoding the receptor sequence.[131] The mature EGF receptor, of approximately 170 kDa, is expressed in most adult tissues except for the hematopoietic system.[125] It is expressed as a transmembrane protein composed of a glycosylated cysteine-rich extracellular ligand-binding domain and a cytoplasmic domain containing an intrinsic tyrosine kinase activity and five cytoplasmic tyrosines that are autophosphorylated and important in regulating receptor-protein interactions and signal transduction pathways from the receptor to various cellular compartments.[123,132] Epidermal growth factor receptor ligands, such as EGF or TGFα, bind to the extracellular domain of the receptor and induce dimerization or clustering of receptors, activating the receptor's intrinsic tyrosine kinase activity and initiating signal transduction pathways that may include transphosphorylation of other ErbB proteins.[133–135]

Distribution of Epidermal Growth Factor and Transforming Growth Factor α

The gastrointestinal distribution of EGF is more limited than that of TGFα. As noted above, EGF was initially isolated from salivary secretions and has also been detected in the pancreas and Brunner's glands of the duodenum.[136] Additionally, a novel ulcer-associated crypt-derived cell lineage has been described that secretes immunoreactive EGF into the intestinal lumen.[137,138] Both EGF and TGFα have been isolated in human fetal gut, with TGFα levels as much as 10 times those of EGF.[139] Gastric acid and proteases present in gastrointestinal secretions digest EGF to smaller, less active forms, an effect that can be inhibited by ingestion of food.[140,141] Enterally administered EGF has been detected throughout the body, though the content in gastrointestinal secretions may be regulated by postnatal age.[142–144] Epidermal growth factor has been shown to be the most active mitogen present in breast milk, with levels varying based on postnatal age in the rodent, but relatively constant in human milk.[145–147] Transforming growth factor α is also expressed in human milk but, interestingly, not in rat milk.[148,149] The predominant source of TGFα appears to be the epithelial cell with detection throughout the gastrointestinal tract including the stomach, pancreas, small intestine, and colon.[150–154] It has been suggested by several investigators that TGFα may be the relevant ligand for the intestinal EGF receptor in intact mucosa and that EGF may have a greater role in mucosal repair.[137,155,156]

Distribution of Epidermal Growth Factor Receptors

Epidermal growth factor receptors have been localized by binding analysis, mRNA, and protein immunodetection throughout the gastrointestinal tract.[157–162] Scheving demonstrated basolateral localization of the EGF receptor on the surface of the polarized intestinal cell, which has subsequently been substantiated by others.[158,163,164] The receptor expression appears to progressively increase from the crypt to the villus tip.[165,166] There is also evidence suggesting that intestinal expression and signal transduction of the EGF receptor are developmentally regulated, with the greatest expression during the weaning period in mice and rats.[167,168] However, it has also been suggested that the enhanced signal transduction during weaning is regulated by mucosal permeability.[164]

Biologic Effect on Intestinal Development

Numerous investigators have demonstrated enhanced intestinal cell proliferation by both EGF and TGFα in vivo and in cell culture.[100,169–173] The majority of in vivo studies have involved the systemic administration of pharmacologic doses of EGF or TGFα, including studies performed in human infants.[174] However, the most compelling evidence for a physiologic role of EGF receptor ligand regulation in enterocyte proliferation was shown by feeding neonatal rats pooled rat milk containing either antibody to EGF or normal rabbit serum. Intestinal DNA synthesis was decreased in the anti-EGF antibody-treated-milk-fed group while no effect was seen in the group fed milk treated with normal rabbit serum.[170] Enteral administration of physiologic concentrations of EGF have also shown increased DNA in the colon of suckling rats.[144] Organ cultures of human intestinal mucosa have provided conflicting results. In one study of fetal human jejunum, DNA synthesis was significantly decreased by EGF while higher concentrations of EGF employed in matched mucosal biopsies from adult duodenum showed an increased crypt cell production rate.[175,176] An in vivo model of proliferation using parenteral administration of nutrients to induce atrophy and decreased crypt cell proliferation showed that concomitant administration of EGF reversed the atrophic effects and enhanced cellular proliferation.[177]

The strongest evidence of a regulatory role for EGF receptor ligands in normal intestinal development is provided by studies of gene targeting to disrupt expression of the EGF receptor in mice. One of the three laboratories reporting EGF receptor null mice described animals demonstrating impaired intestinal development with shortened villi, a pseudostratified epithelium, and death associated with a necrotizing enterocolitis-like disorder.[178] A similar phenotype was not observed in the other EGF receptor null mouse lines;[179,180] however, the successful oocyte implantation and fetal development varied significantly between mouse strains, suggesting that genetic background may be important in regulating the relative importance of growth factor or receptor signaling systems in the mice.[178–180] Because of the complexity of studying a ubiquitously expressed protein like the EGF receptor in whole animal knockout studies, a clear picture of the importance of EGF receptor signal transduction in intestinal development will likely require specific disruption of intestinal expression only, perhaps by use of a dominant negative approach.[138,181,182]

Another in vivo model of gastrointestinal development has been the use of massive small bowel resection, which has shown EGF to enhance body weight and mucosal mass in a number of laboratories.[183–186] This effect is associated with an increase in expression of both EGF and its receptor.[183,187] Interestingly, small bowel resection in mice with defective EGF receptor signal transduction shows attenuated adaptation compared to heterozygous or wild-type controls.[188]

Administration of EGF has been shown to enhance the absorptive function of the gastrointestinal mucosa for glucose, amino acids, electrolytes, and calcium. The addition of EGF to the perfusate in a rabbit intestinal perfusion model enhanced the uptake of glucose, Na^+, and Cl^-.[189] It has been shown that EGF can immediately enhance the total absorptive surface area of the intestine in this model, suggesting reorganization of the actin cytoskeleton by a mechanism dependent on extracellular calcium.[190] Net calcium transport in suckling rats was enhanced by systemic EGF administration.[191] This effect may be partly explained by the ability of EGF to induce precocious expression of vitamin D-dependent calcium-binding proteins.[192] Intragastric administration of EGF increased the transport of sodium, glucose, and glycine in a similar rat model.[193] A caveat of these studies was the ability of intragastric feeding of formula devoid of growth factor to induce glucose transport similar to EGF when compared to untreated controls, an effect which may be a response to stress-induced release of endogenous glucocorticoids.[194]

The effects of EGF on the activity of intestinal brushborder enzyme activities have been reported from several laboratories. Both systemic and enteral administration of EGF have been shown to enhance various enzyme activities in rabbits, rats, mice, and piglets.[172,177,195–198] Orogastric administration of EGF to suckling rabbits from 3 to 18 days of age induced sucrase activity and attenuated lactase activity of the proximal and middle small intestine.[195] In mice and rats, systemic administration of pharmacologic doses of EGF stimulated increased sucrase activities in most studies.[172,191,197,199] Subcutaneous injection of EGF enhanced sucrase activity and mRNA expression in suckling rats by a mechanism that did not require endogenous glucocorticoid expression.[197,200] Surprisingly the simultaneous administration of sucrose, the sucrase substrate, to suckling rats enhanced the EGF effect regardless of whether the animals had undergone adrenalectomy or not.[200] Of note, the investigators demonstrated that in nonadrenalectomized animals subcutaneous EGF rapidly increased serum corticosterone levels.

Enhanced disaccharidase activity has not generally been produced by enteral administration of EGF. Addition of EGF to formula at concentrations expected from normal suckling increased DNA content; however, there was no effect on lactase, sucrase, or maltase activities.[144] In organ cultures of fetal mouse intestinal mucosa, EGF failed to stimulate sucrase activity but did enhance alkaline phosphatase, maltase, and trehalase.[201] Culture of suckling mouse jejunum with EGF did not alter disaccharidase activity, and the authors proposed that EGF might induce systemic changes in vivo that influence neonatal intestinal development.[202] While EGF-specific binding was not altered during the study, no EGF receptor signal transduction events, such as tyrosine phosphorylation, were investigated at the time of these studies. Interestingly, organ cultures of human jejunum treated with EGF demonstrated increased lactase and decreased sucrase, trehalase, and glucoamylase activities correlating inversely with EGF concentration.[175]

Because of the functional overlap in ligand binding to the EGF receptor and potential overlap in signal transduction pathways between various ErbB family members, it is unlikely that a complete understanding of the role of EGF receptor ligands in intestinal development will be achieved with the currently available models.[123,133–135] However, the findings by Miettinen and colleagues demonstrating developmental immaturity of the intestinal epithelium in the EGF receptor knockout mice provide the strongest evidence of an important regulatory role for this receptor family in intestinal development.[178]

TRANSFORMING GROWTH FACTOR β

Overview

The TGFβ superfamily comprises a large number of related peptides, including the TGFβs, activins, bone morphogenetic proteins (BMPs), and müllerian inhibiting substance, among others. The number of structurally-related peptides in the TGFβ superfamily is now greater than 40.[203] Although a biologic or structural relatedness is suggested by the similarity in the nomenclature of TGFα and TGFβ, this is not the case and merely indicates that each of these peptides was originally named because of its transforming activity on cells in culture. Transforming growth factor β has been rather extensively investigated for its role in the regulation of diverse processes in the gastrointestinal tract, including regulation of epithelial cell growth, modulation of cellular differentiation, and regulation of the intestinal immune system.

Transforming Growth Factor β Genes and Proteins

The mammalian TGFβ growth factor family consists of three closely-related members with nearly identical biologic activity. These are designated TGFβ1, β2, and β3 and are often referred to as TGFβ isoforms.[204,205] The genes for these three proteins have been localized to human chromosomes 19, 1, and 14 respectively.[206,207] All three mammalian TGFβ molecules are first synthesized and secreted as biologically inactive (latent) precursor polypeptides incapable of binding to cell-surface TGFβ receptors. Nearly all cell types synthesize and secrete TGFβ.

The biologically active form of TGFβ is a 25-kDa homodimer. The carboxyterminal 112 amino acids that make up the three mammalian TGFβ isoforms exhibit 70 to 75% conservation of sequence and 100% conservation of the nine cysteine residues, while the aminoterminal precursor sequences are markedly dissimilar.[208] The sequence for TGFβ1 is highly conserved in mammals. Activation of latent TGFβ is believed to be a major step in the regulation of TGFβ activity. Latent TGFβ consists primarily of the N-terminal TGFβ precursor sequence, termed the latency associated peptide, noncovalently associated with the mature, C-terminal TGFβ sequence. The latent TGFβ complex also includes a second gene product, the latent TGFβ binding protein, which is structurally unrelated to TGFβ and associates with the latent molecule by disulfide bridging. Mature, biologically active TGFβ is released from the latent complex by certain nonphysiologic phenomena such as extremes of pH but the physiologic mechanism operative in vivo is not clearly understood. Proteolytic activation by proteases such as plasmin has been extensively characterized in vitro,[209] but recent experimental data indicate that thrombospondin may be the most attractive physiologic activator in vivo.[210] The basis for this conclusion is that plasminogen-null animals do not replicate the abnormalities observed in TGFβ1-deficient mice, while thrombospondin-null mice closely resemble the phenotype of TGFβ-deficient mice (see below). It is believed that thrombospondin confers a conformational change in the latency-associated peptide, releasing mature TGFβ for binding to its receptor. Other factors contributing to the stability of latent TGFβ include binding to the mannose-6-phosphate-IGF-II receptor and transglutaminase-dependent crosslinking of TGFβ to matrix proteins. A great deal remains to be learned about the complex regulation of TGFβ activation.

Transforming Growth Factor β Receptors

Transforming growth factor β receptors (TGFβR) were originally classified as types I (~53 kD), II (~70 kD), and III (~300 kD) on the basis of (^{125}I)-TGFβ crosslinking to cell-surface membranes. Each of these has been cloned in recent years.[204,205,211] All three isoforms of TGFβ bind to receptor types I, II, and III albeit with modest differences in affinity. Other members of the TGFβ superfamily bind to structurally-related cell surface receptors but these will not be further considered herein. Each of the three TGFβ receptors has an extracellular ligand-binding domain, a transmembrane sequence, and a cytoplasmic sequence. The TGFβRI and TGFβRII contain cytoplasmic serine-threonine kinase domains, indicating that these two receptors are responsible for signal transduction by TGFβ.[212,213] Multiple TGFβRI receptors have been cloned and characterized, including ALK-5,[213] Tsk7L,[214] and TSR-1[215] among others.[216,217] A single TGFβRII receptor has been identified.[212] Transforming growth factor β receptor III (betaglycan) is a heavily glycosylated, large molecular-weight proteoglycan without a recognizable intracellular signaling domain,[218] suggesting that this receptor may function as a ligand reservoir or to facilitate binding to TGFβRI and II.[219]

The TGFβRII exists as a constitutively autophosphorylated homodimer, independent of the presence of TGFβ. Transforming growth factor β receptor I also forms ligand-independent homodimers. Current understanding supports binding of TGFβ with the extracellular domain of homodimeric TGFβRII, which possesses the constitutively active, cytoplasmic serine-threonine kinase responsible for receptor autophosphorylation of TGFβRII and phosphorylation of TGFβRI.[220-222] Ligand binding recruits TGFβRI into a tetrameric receptor complex that results in transphosphorylation and activation of TGFβRI. Thus, the preponderance of evidence indicates TGFβ binds TGFβRI only in the presence of the TGFβRII. The TGFβRI serine-threonine kinase transiently phosphorylates and activates a family of unique intracellular signaling molecules, designated Smads, which then translocate to the nucleus and regulate the transcriptional machinery, as described below.[216] A differential contribution of type I and II receptors to the diverse biologic actions of TGFβ has been proposed.[223-225] Studies by Chen and co-workers suggest the type II receptor may mediate growth inhibition and the type I receptor extracellular matrix deposition.[223] In support of this, the Tsk7L type I receptor appears to mediate the epithelial-to-mesenchymal transition in mammary epithelial cells.[224] Precisely how these observations on differential receptor responses will ultimately be integrated with the model for heteromeric signaling is uncertain. Some have postulated that signaling may be regulated by a "critical ratio" of binding to the type I and II receptors.[226]

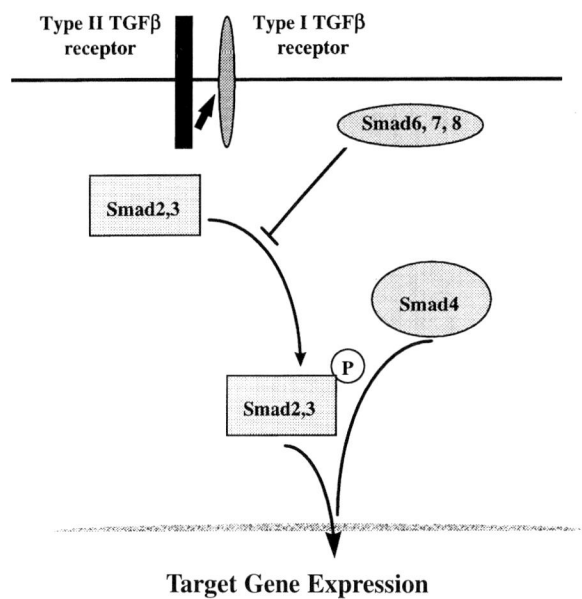

FIGURE 3-3. TGFβ-mediated signal transduction.

Transforming Growth Factor β–Mediated Intracellular Signaling

The intracellular signaling pathways used by proteins in the TGFβ superfamily and family of serine-threonine kinase receptors have been recently identified in mammalian systems.[216,227] These proteins were discovered on the basis of their homology with related peptides in *Drosophila* (MAD proteins) and *Caenorabditis elegans* (sma proteins). The nomenclature used in these invertebrate species was merged to provide the mammalian term: Smad. Eight Smad proteins, designated Smad1 to 8, have been isolated to date. These peptides are highly conserved across species but bear no known structural homology with more extensively characterized signaling proteins. There are no recognizable structural motifs to suggest function. In mammalian cells, activation of the TGFβRI by TGFβ results first in a physical association between Smad2 and Smad3, followed by receptor-dependent phosphorylation of both Smad2 and Smad3. Subsequently Smad4, which is not phosphorylated, associates with Smad2 and Smad3, and the heteromeric complex translocates to the nucleus (Figure 3-3). Transcriptional activation domains in each Smad protein have been identified. Smad6 and Smad7 antagonize TGFβ signaling. This is believed to occur by disruption of the association between Smad2, Smad3, and the type I receptor.[228] Smad8 has only recently been identified. Coincident with their discovery, Smad proteins were considered likely candidates for status as tumor suppressor genes by virtue of the fact they transduce growth inhibitory signals. This appears to be the case in a small percentage of colorectal tumors.[229,230] Very recently, germline mutations in Smad4 have been described in certain kindreds with juvenile polyposis coli, a preneoplastic condition.[231]

Biologic Actions of Transforming Growth Factor β Relevant to the Gastrointestinal Tract

Transforming growth factor β has been most extensively studied as an autocrine inhibitor of epithelial cell growth. Conversely, under certain conditions TGFβ is a growth stimulator for fibroblastic cells. This is believed to occur by induction of secondary mitogenic growth factors. Transforming growth factor β also induces extracellular matrix formation, and prominent effects on the immune system are observed. Selected observations relevant to the gastrointestinal tract are below.

Inhibition of Cell Growth

All the TGFβ isoforms are potent, reversible growth inhibitors in epithelial cells, including those of the gastrointestinal tract.[232] Under certain experimental conditions TGFβ may also stimulate a limited differentiation in intestinal epithelial cells.[93] Transforming growth factor β acts in the mid and late G1 phase of the cell cycle to inhibit critical cellular events required for G1 traverse and S-phase entry (DNA synthesis). Although there appears to be variability according to cell type under study, alterations in proto-oncogene expression (for example, c-myc, c-jun), inhibition of cyclin-dependent kinase activities (for example, cyclin D, cyclin E, cyclin A and their respective catalytic partners, the cyclin-dependent kinases, cdk2, cdk4, and cdk6) and induction of cyclin-dependent kinase inhibitors (for example, p21) have all been reported in a variety of cell types. In cultured intestinal epithelial cells, downregulation of cyclin D1 expression appears to be a key step in G1 arrest induced by TGFβ.[233]

The contribution of the TGFβ-related peptide family to regulation of intestinal growth in vivo is not well-understood despite finding mRNA and protein for all three

TGFβ isoforms in the intestinal mucosa. Studies have attempted to extrapolate function based on distribution of TGFβ mRNA or protein along the intestinal epithelial CV axis.[150,234,235] Conflicting conclusions and disparate hypotheses regarding possible roles for TGFβ in the regulation of intestinal epithelial proliferation and differentiation have been proposed. For example, a finding of TGFβ mRNA expression predominantly in the crypt[150] prompted a hypothesis that TGFβ modulates growth by acting as a brake on proliferation of crypt cells. Alternatively, it has been proposed, on the basis of localization of mRNA and protein predominantly at the villus tip,[234,235] that TGFβ may function by arresting growth and maintaining the terminally differentiated phenotype as enterocytes approach the villus tip. Another potential source of TGFβ during development is the large amount found in human milk and the occurrence of TGFβ in amniotic fluid.[236,237]

Recently, expression of TGFβRII in the murine small intestine and colonic epithelium was reported in a distribution nearly identical to ligand; that is, increased expression in the differentiated compartment and little or no expression in the proliferative compartment.[235] Collectively, these data support the view that the TGFβ pathway is a major autocrine and/or paracrine inhibitory axis in the intestinal epithelium. In support of this, loss of the TGFβRII appears to be a significant mechanism by which intestinal epithelial cells escape normal growth constraints leading to transformation.[238]

Induction of Extracellular Matrix Formation

One of the most striking effects of TGFβ is modulation of genes regulating extracellular matrix deposition. The end result is a prominent increase in matrix formation. This occurs by *increased* synthesis of extracellular matrix proteins and proteinase inhibitors, *decreased* synthesis of matrix degrading activities, and modulation of matrix receptors and binding proteins. Examples include stimulation of collagen, fibronectin, and plasminogen activator inhibitor and integrin synthesis and inhibition of plasminogen, collagenase, and elastase activities.[239] Interestingly, in many cell types the effects of TGFβ on cellular proliferation are dissociated from effects on induction of matrix, indicating the presence of diverse signaling pathways. The effect of TGFβ on extracellular matrix synthesis appears to have clinical significance, as a large number of fibrotic diseases are associated with increased TGFβ activity, and TGFβ increases wound healing in several models, including incisional wounds in the gastrointestinal tract.[240,241]

Effect on Immune Function

The effects of TGFβ on the immune system are complex but appear to be particularly important because of the prominent inflammation observed in the gastrointestinal mucosa of TGFβ deficient knockout mice (see below). Transforming growth factor β is produced by many immune system cells, including T cells, B cells, macrophages, NK cells, and others. Almost every aspect of immune function, including proinflammatory and immunosuppressive activities, is influenced by TGFβ action.[242] For example, antigen-presenting dendritic cells require TGFβ for differentiation from precursor cell types to the functional phenotype in vitro and in vivo.[243] The development of thymic precursors is also regulated by autocrine and paracrine TGFβ pathways.[242] One of the most prominent effects of TGFβ on immune cell function is its activity as an IgA switch-inducing factor in naive B cells. Transforming growth factor β induces IgA⁻ B cells to initiate IgA synthesis and secretion, an observation of particular importance in the gastrointestinal tract since IgA is the dominant isotype in the gastrointestinal tract.[244]

Transforming Growth Factor β Knockout and Transgenic Models

The prominent effects of TGFβ on cellular proliferation, migration, and matrix deposition have long stimulated interest in the effects of TGFβ on embryogenesis. Developmental patterns of TGFβ expression have been reported in nearly all organs, including the intestine. Early studies in mice showed the presence of immunoreactivity in the intestine for all three TGFβ isoforms. Expression was first detected in midgestation and occurred primarily in mature epithelial cells.[245] Targeted disruption of TGFβ1 was accomplished nearly simultaneously by several investigators.[246–248] Embryonic lethality was observed in approximately one-half of these animals, perhaps due to defective yolk sac vasculogenesis.[249] In the remaining TGFβ null mice, no development defect was observed at birth. It was hypothesized that redundancy in the TGFβ family "rescued" the normal phenotype and that the presence of placental or mammary gland-derived TGFβ compensated for loss of TGFβ1 expression. Two to 3 weeks after birth, homozygous TGFβ deficient animals developed a rapid-onset, fatal, wasting syndrome characterized by massive infiltration of multiple organs with mixed inflammatory cells. Inflammatory lesions were most prominent in the heart and lungs, but striking abnormalities were also observed in the gastric mucosa. The small bowel and colon were less involved. Peyer's patches were small. These studies suggested an important role for TGFβ1 in immune homeostasis, and subsequent work suggested that the inflammation is, at least in part, due to an autoimmune process. The degree of inflammation and wasting is ameliorated by modulating leukocyte adhesion with synthetic fibronectin peptides, emphasizing the aberrant nature of adhesive interactions in TGFβ1 deficiency.[250] No overt abnormalities in gastrointestinal development are observed in TGFβ2 and TGFβ3 knockout mice, although the latter have a defect in palate formation.

Overexpression of TGFβ in the liver of transgenic mice has been reported to cause hepatic fibrosis and atrophy of the pancreas.[251] Overexpression in the pancreas causes chronic pancreatitis and fibrosis.[252] An attractive alternate approach for determination of the roles for TGFβ in development has been the study of mice with a dominant-negative TGFβRII transgene. This approach circumvents the "problem" of ligand redundancy and also permits the use of tissue-specific promoters or inducible constructs. A dominant-negative TGFβRII under control of a MT promoter resulted in fibrosis of the pancreas along with macrophage inflammation, neoangiogenesis, and defective acinar cell differentiation.[253] There were no discernible effects on the liver. The effects on other gastrointestinal structures were not commented on.

FUTURE DIRECTIONS

In this chapter we have attempted to introduce the reader to selected recent developments in the understanding of growth factor regulation of the developing intestine. We have not reviewed the emerging evidence that cytokines such as tumor necrosis factor α, interferon γ, and interleukin-2 may directly regulate intestinal epithelial cell growth, development, and migration.[254–258]

While significant advances in molecular biology have been applied to the study of intestinal development, particularly through the use of transgenic mice, it is now clear there are limitations to the amount of information that can be gained from the intact animal. The genetic background of the animal studied may or may not permit a definitive understanding of the role of a receptor-ligand in this process, as evidenced by the EGF receptor knockout studies.[178–180] Investigators have unsuccessfully attempted to isolate multipotent intestinal stem cells for in vitro study. Such reagents would provide a complementary approach to the whole-animal studies of intestinal development and permit the development of a consensus regarding the hierarchy of growth factors and hormones during intestinal development.

REFERENCES

1. Walsh JW, Dockray GJ. Gut peptides. In: Martini L, editor. Comprehensive endocrinology. New York: Raven Press; 1994. p. 884.
2. Henning SJ, Rubin DC, Shulman RJ. Ontogeny of the intestinal mucosa. In: Johnson LR, editor. Physiology of the gastrointestinal tract. Vol. 1. New York: Raven Press; 1994. p. 571–610.
3. Henning SJ. Plasma concentrations of total and free corticosterone during development in the rat. Am J Physiol 1978;235:5.
4. McEwan IJ, Wright APH, Gustafsson J-A. Mechanism of gene expression by the glucocorticoid receptor: role of protein-protein interaction. Bioessays 1997;19:153–60.
5. Funder JW. Glucocorticoid receptors. J Steroid Biochem Mol Biol 1992;43:389–94.
6. Henning SJ, Ballard PL, Kretchmer N. A study of the cytoplasmic receptors for glucocorticoids in intestine of pre- and postweanling rats. J Biol Chem 1975;250:2073–9.
7. Lentze MJ, Colony PC, Trier JS. Glucocorticoid receptors in isolated intestinal epithelial cells in rats. Am J Physiol 1985;249:G58–65.
8. Costa A, Rocci MP, Arisio R, et al. Glucocorticoid receptors immunoreactivity in tissue of human embryos. J Endocrinol Invest 1996;19:92–8.
9. Cole TJ, Blendy JA, Monaghan P, et al. Targeted disruption of the glucocorticoid receptor gene blocks adrenergic chromaffin cell development and severely retards lung maturation. Genes Dev 1995;9:1608–21.
10. Doell RG, Kretchmer N. Intestinal invertase: precocious development of activity after injection of hydrocortisone. Science 1964;143:42–4.
11. Nanthakumar NN, Henning SJ. Ontogeny of sucrase-isomaltase gene expression in rat intestine: responsiveness to glucocorticoids. Am J Physiol 1993;264:G306–11.
12. Martin GR, Henning SJ. Enzymic development of the small intestine: are glucocorticoids necessary? Am J Physiol 1984;246:G695–9.
13. Henning SJ. Ontogeny of enzymes in the small intestine. Annu Rev Physiol 1985;47:231–45.
14. Yeh KY, Yeh M, Holt PR. Intestinal lactase expression and epithelial cell transit in hormone-treated suckling rats. Am J Physiol 1991;260:G379–84.
15. D'Agostino J, Henning SJ. Role of thyroxine in coordinate control of corticosterone and CBG in postnatal development. Am J Physiol 1982;242:E33–9.
16. D'Agostino J, Henning SJ. Postnatal development of corticosteroid-binding globulin: effect of thyroxine. Endocrinology 1982;111:1476–82.
17. McDonald MC, Henning SJ. Synergistic effects of thyroxine and dexamethasone on enzyme ontogeny in rat small intestine. Pediatr Res 1992;32:306–11.
18. Little JM, Lester R. Ontogenesis of intestinal bile salt absorption in the neonatal rat. Am J Physiol 1980;239:G319–23.
19. Barnard JA, Ghishan FK, Wilson FA. Ontogenesis of taurocholate transport by rat ileal brush border membrane vesicles. J Clin Invest 1985;75:869–73.
20. Barnard JA, Ghishan FK. Methylprednisolone accelerated the ontogeny of sodium-taurocholate cotransport in rat ileal brush border membranes. J Lab Clin Med 1986;108:549–55.
21. Heubi JE, Gunn TD. The role of glucocorticoids in postnatal development of ileal active bile salt transport. Pediatr Res 1985;19:1147–51.
22. Shneider BL, Dawson PA, Christie DM, et al. Cloning and molecular characterization of a rat ileal sodium-dependent bile acid transporter. J Clin Invest 1995;95:745–54.
23. Nowicki MJ, Shneider BL, Paul JM, Heubi JE. Glucocorticoids upregulated taurocholate transport by ileal brush border membrane. Am J Physiol 1997;36:G197–203.
24. Shneider BL, Setchell KDR, Crossman MW. Fetal and neonatal expression of the apical sodium-dependent bile acid transporter in the rat ileum and kidney. Pediatr Res 1997;42:189–94.
25. Christie DM, Dawson PA, Thevananther S, Shneider BL. Comparative analysis of the ontogeny of a sodium-dependent bile acid transporter in rat kidney and ileum. Am J Physiol 1996;271:G377–85.
26. deBelle RS, Vaupshas V, Vitullo BB, et al. Intestinal absorption of bile salts: immature development in the neonate. J Pediatr 1979;94:472–6.
27. Tutton PJM, Barkla DH. Steroid hormones as regulators of the proliferative activity of normal and neoplastic intestinal epithelial cells [review]. Anticancer Res 1988;8:451–6.
28. Sandle GI, Binder HJ. Corticosteroids and intestinal ion transport. Gastroenterology 1987;93:188–96.
29. Meneely R, Ghishan FK. Intestinal maturation in the rat: the effect of glucocorticoids on sodium, potassium, water and glucose absorption. Pediatr Res 1982;16:776–8.
30. Lee S, Szkachetka S, Christakos S. Effect of glucocorticoids and 1,25-dihydroxyvitamin D3 on the developmental expression of the rat intestinal vitamin D receptor gene. Endocrinology 1991;129:396–401.
31. Walsh MJ, LeLeiko NS, Sterling KM. Regulation of types I, III and IV procollagen mRNA synthesis in glucocorticoid-mediated intestinal development. J Biol Chem 1987;262:10814–18.
32. Shi YB. Cell-cell and cell-ECM interactions in epithelial apoptosis and cell renewal during frog intestinal development. Cell Biochem Biophys 1995;27:179–202.
33. LoPresti JS, Singer PA. Physiology of thyroid hormone synthesis, secretion and transport. In: Falk SA, editor. Thyroid disease: endocrinology, surgery, nuclear medicine, and radiotherapy. Philadelphia: Lippincott-Raven Publishers; 1997. p. 29.
34. Becker KB, Stephens KC, Davey JC, et al. The type 2 and type 3 iodothyronine deiodinases play important roles in coordinating development in *Rana catesbeiana* tadpoles. Endocrinology 1997;138:2989–97.

35. Shi YB, Liang VC, Parkison C, Cheng SY. Tissue-dependent developmental expression of a cytosolic thyroid hormone protein gene in *Xenopus*: its role in the regulation of amphibian metamorphosis. FEBS Letters 1994;355:61–4.
36. Nguyen TT, DiStefano JJ III, Yamada H, Yeh YM. Steady state organ distribution and metabolism of thyroxine and 3,5,3′-triiodothyronine in intestines, liver, kidneys, blood and residual carcass of the rat in vivo. Endocrinology 1993;133:2973–83.
37. Apriletti JW, Ribeiro RCJ, Wagner RL, et al. Molecular and structural biology of thyroid hormone receptors. Clin Exp Pharmacol Physiol 1998;25:S2–11.
38. Wong R, Zhu XG, Pineda MA, et al. Cell type-dependent modulation of the dominant negative action of human mutant thyroid hormone beta 1 receptors. Mol Med 1995;1:306–19.
39. Hodin RA, Meng S, Chamberlain SM. Thyroid hormone responsiveness is developmentally regulated in the rat small intestine: a possible role for the alpha-2 receptor variant. Endocrinology 1994;135:564–8.
40. Ishizuya-Oka A, Shimozawa A. Induction of metamorphosis by thyroid hormone in anuran small intestine cultured organotypically in vitro. In Vitro Cell Dev Biol Anim 1991;27A: 853–7.
41. Su Y, Shi Y, Stolow MA, Shi YB. Thyroid hormone induces apoptosis in primary cell cultures of tadpole intestine: cell type specificity and effects of extracellular matrix. J Cell Biol 1997;15:1533–43.
42. Su Y, Shi YB. Cyclosporin A but not FK506 inhibits hormone-induced apoptosis in tadpole intestinal epithelium. FASEB J 1997;11:559–65.
43. Cohn SM, Simon TC, Roth KA, et al. Use of transgenic mice to map cis-acting elements in the intestinal fatty acid binding protein gene (Fabpi) that controls its cell lineage-specific and regional patterns of expression along the duodenal-colonic and crypt-villus axes of the gut epithelium. J Cell Biol 1992;119:27–44.
44. Shi YB, Hayes WP. Thyroid hormone-dependent regulation of the intestinal fatty acid-binding protein gene during amphibian metamorphosis. Dev Biol 1994;161:48–58.
45. Ishizuya-Oka A, Ueda S, Damjanovski S, et al. Anteroposterior gradient of epithelial transformation during amphibian intestinal remodeling: immunohistochemical detection of intestinal fatty acid-binding protein. Dev Biol 1997;192:149–61.
46. Ishizuya-Oka A, Shimozawa A. Inductive action of epithelium on differentiation of intestinal connective tissue of *Xenopus laevis* tadpoles during metamorphosis in vitro. Cell Tissue Res 1994;277:427–36.
47. Wang J, Whetsell M, Klein JR. Local hormone networks and intestinal T cell homeostasis. Science 1997;275:1937–9.
48. Patterton D, Hayes WP, Shi YB. Transcriptional activation of the matrix metalloproteinase gene stromelysin-3 coincides with thyroid hormone-induced cell death during frog metamorphosis. Dev Biol 1995;167:252–62.
49. Stolow MA, Shi YB. *Xenopus* sonic Hedgehog as a potential morphogen during embryogenesis and thyroid hormone-dependent metamorphosis. Nucleic Acids Res 1995;23:2555–62.
50. Stolow MA, Bauzon DD, Li J, et al. Identification and characterization of a novel collagenase in *Xenopus laevis*: possible roles during frog development. Mol Biol Cell 1996;7:1471–83.
51. Ishizuya-Oka A, Ueda S, Shi YB. Temporal and spatial regulation of a putative transcriptional repressor implicates it as playing a role in thyroid hormone-dependent organ transformation. Dev Genet 1997;20:329–37.
52. Liang VC, Sedgwick T, Shi YB. Characterization of the *Xenopus* homolog of an immediate early gene associated with cell activation: sequence analysis and regulation of its expression by thyroid hormone during amphibian metamorphosis. Cell Res 1997;7:179–93.
53. Zucker SN, Castillo G, Band Horowitz S. Down-regulation of the mdr gene by thyroid hormone during *Xenopus laevis* development. Mol Cell Endocrinol 1997;129:73–81.
54. Ingham PW. Transducing Hedgehog: the story so far. EMBO J 1998;17:3505–11.
55. Ishizuya-Oka A, Stolow MA, Ueda S, Shi YB. Temporal and spatial expression of an intestinal Na^+/PO_4 3-cotransporter correlates with epithelial transformation during thyroid hormone-dependent frog metamorphosis. Dev Genet 1997;20:53–66.
56. Tenore A, Fasano A, Gasparini N, et al. Thyroxine effect on intestinal Cl^-/HCO_3-exchange in hypo- and hyperthyroid rats. J Endocrinol 1996;151:431–7.
57. Kandasamy RA, Orlowski J. Genomic organization and glucocorticoid transcriptional activation of the rat Na^+/H^+ exchanger Nhe3 gene. J Biol Chem 1996;271:10551–9.
58. Pacha J. Ontogeny of Na^+ transport in rat colon. Comp Biochem Physiol A Physiol 1997;118:209–10.
59. Giannella RA, Orlowski J, Jump ML, Lingrel JB. $Na^{(+)}$-$K^{(+)}$-ATPase gene expression in rat intestine and Caco-2 cells: response to thyroid hormone. Am J Physiol 1993;265: G775–82.
60. Henning SJ. Functional development of the gastrointestinal tract. In: Johnson L, editor. Physiology of the gastrointestinal tract. Vol. 1. New York: Raven; 1987. p. 285.
61. Hodin RA, Chamberlain SM, Upton MP. Thyroid hormone differentially regulates rat intestinal brush border enzyme gene expression. Gastroenterology 1992;103:1529–36.
62. Hodin RA, Shei A, Morin M, Meng S. Thyroid hormone and the gut: selective transcriptional activation of a villus-enterocyte marker. Surgery 1996;120:138–43.
63. Fraichard A, Chassande O, Plateroti M, et al. The T3Rα gene encoding a thyroid hormone receptor is essential for postnatal development and thyroid hormone production. EMBO J 1997;16:4412–20.
64. LeRoith D. Insulin-like growth factor receptors and binding proteins. Baillieres Clin Endocrinol Metab 1996;10:49–73.
65. LeRoith D. Insulin-like growth factors. N Engl J Med 1997; 336:633–40.
66. Rubin R, Baserga R. Biology of disease: insulin-like growth factor-I receptor. Lab Invest 1995;73:311–31.
67. Jones JI, Clemmons DR. Insulin-like growth factors and their binding proteins: biological actions. Endocr Rev 1995; 16:3–34.
68. Nielsen FC. The molecular and cellular biology of insulin-like growth factor II. Prog Growth Factor Res 1992;4:257–90.
69. Sussenbach JS. The gene structure of the insulin-like growth factor family. Prog Growth Factor Res 1989;1:33–40.
70. Rotwein P, Pollock KM, Didier DK, Krivi GG. Organization and sequence of the human insulin-like growth factor I gene. J Biol Chem 1986;261:4828–32.
71. Lund PK. Insulin-like growth factors. In: Walsh JH, Dockray GJ, editors. Gut peptides: biochemistry and physiology. New York: Raven Press; 1994. p. 587.
72. Hoyt EC, Van Wyk JJ, Lund PK. Tissue and development specific regulation of a complex family of rat insulin-like growth factor I messenger ribonucleic acids. Mol Endocrinol 1988;2: 1077–86.
73. Han VKM, Lund PK, Lee DC, D'Ercole AJ. Expression of somatomedin/insulin-like growth factor messenger RNAs in the human fetus: identification, characterization and tissue distribution. J Clin Endocrinol Metab 1988;66:422–9.
74. Abbott AM, Bueno R, Pedrini MT, et al. Insulin-like growth factor I receptor gene structure. J Biol Chem 1992;267: 10759–63.
75. Siddle K, Soos MA, Field CE, Nave BT. Hybrid and atypical insulin/insulin-like growth factor I receptors. Horm Res 1994;41:56–65.

76. Izumi T, White MF, Takashi K, et al. Insulin like growth factor I rapidly stimulates tyrosine phosphorylation of a Mr 185000 protein in intact cells. J Biol Chem 1987;262:1282–7.
77. Stewart CEH, Rotwein P. Growth, differentiation and survival: multiple physiological functions for insulin-like growth factors. Physiol Rev 1996;76:1005–26.
78. Heinz-Erian P, Kessler U, Funk B, et al. Identification and in situ localization of the insulin-like growth factor-II/mannose-6-phosphate (IGF-II/M6P) receptor in the rat gastrointestinal tract: comparison with the IGF-I receptor. Endocrinology 1991;129:1769–78.
79. Adamo M, Lowe WL Jr, LeRoith D, Roberts CT Jr. Insulin-like growth factor I messenger ribonucleic acids with alternative 5′-untranslated regions are differentially expressed during development of the rat. Endocrinology 1989;124:2737–44.
80. Laburthe M, Rouyer-Fessard C, Gammeltoft S. Receptors for insulin-like growth factors I and II in rat gastrointestinal epithelium. Am J Physiol 1988;254:G457–62.
81. Ryan J, Costigan DC. Determination of the histological distribution of insulin like growth factor 1 receptors in the rat gut. Gut 1993;34:1693–7.
82. Brown AL, Graham DE, Nissley SP, et al. Developmental regulation of insulin-like growth factor II mRNA in different rat tissues. J Biol Chem 1986;261:13144–50.
83. Lund PK, Moats-Staats BM, Hynes MA, et al. Somatomedin-C/insulin-like growth factor-I and insulin-like growth factor-II mRNAs in rat fetal and adult tissues. J Biol Chem 1986;261:14539–44.
84. Termanini B, Nardi RV, Finan TM, et al. Insulin like growth factor I receptors in rabbit gastrointestinal tract. Characterization and autoradiographic localization. Gastroenterology 1990;99:51–60.
85. Schober DA, Simmen FA, Hadsell DL, Baumrucker CR. Perinatal expression of type I IGF receptors in porcine small intestine. Endocrinology 1990;126:1125–32.
86. Pillion DJ, Haskell JF, Atchison JA, et al. Receptors for IGF-I, but not for IGF-II, on proximal colon epithelial cell apical membranes. Am J Physiol 1989;257:E27–34.
87. Pillion DJ, Grizzle WE, Yang M, et al. Expression of IGFII/Man-6-P receptors on rat, rabbit and human colon epithelial cells. Am J Physiol 1993;264:R1101–10.
88. Rouyer-Fessard C, Gammeltoft S, Laburthe M. Expression of two types of receptor for insulin like growth factors in human colonic epithelium. Gastroenterology 1990;98:703–8.
89. Park JH, Vanderhoof JA, Blackwood D, Macdonald RG. Characterization of type I and type II insulin-like growth factor receptors in an intestinal epithelial cell line. Endocrinology 1990;126:2998–3005.
90. Sklar MM, Kiess W, Thomas CL, Nissley SP. Developmental expression of the tissue insulin-like growth factor II/mannose 6 phosphate receptor in the rat. J Biol Chem 1989;264:16733–8.
91. Young GP, Taranto TM, Jonas HA, et al. Insulin-like growth factors and the developing and mature rat small intestine: receptors and biological actions. Digestion 1990;46:240–52.
92. Conteas CN, McMorrow B, Luk GD. Modulation of epidermal growth factor-induced cell proliferation and receptor binding by insulin in cultured intestinal epithelial cells. Biochem Biophys Res Commun 1989;161:414–19.
93. Kurokowa M, Lynch K, Podolsky DK. Effects of growth factors on an intestinal epithelial cell line: transforming growth factor β inhibits proliferation and stimulates differentiation. Biochem Biophys Res Comm 1987;142:775–82.
94. Duncan MD, Koramn LY, Bass B. Epidermal growth factor primes intestinal epithelial cells for proliferative effect of insulin-like growth factor I. Dig Dis Sci 1994;39:2197–201.
95. Donovan SM, Hintz RL, Rosenfeld RG. Insulin-like growth factors I and II and their binding proteins in human milk: effect of heat treatment on IGF and IGF-binding protein stability. J Pediatr Gastroenterol Nutr 1991;13:242–53.
96. Chaurasia OP, Marcuard SP, Seidel ER. Insulin-like growth factor I in human gastrointestinal exocrine secretions. Regul Pept 1994;50:113–19.
97. Phillips AF, Rao R, Anderson GG, et al. Fate of insulin-like growth factors I and II administered orogastrically to suckling rats. Pediatr Res 1995;37:586–92.
98. Burrin DG, Wester TJ, Davis TA, et al. Orally administered IGF-I increases intestinal mucosal growth in formula-fed neonatal pigs. Am J Physiol 1996;270:R1085–91.
99. Trahair JF, Wing SJ, Owens PC. Regulation of gastrointestinal growth in fetal sheep by luminally administered insulin-like growth factor I. J Endocrinol 1997;152:29–38.
100. Potten CS, Owen G, Hewitt D, et al. Stimulation and inhibition of proliferation in the small intestinal crypts of the mouse after in vivo administration of growth factors. Gut 1995;36:864–73.
101. Steeb C-B, Trahair JF, Tomas FM, Read LC. Prolonged administration of IGF peptides enhances growth of gastrointestinal tissues in normal rats. Am J Physiol 1994;266:G1090–8.
102. Steeb C-B, Trahair JF, Read LC. Administration of insulin-like growth factor-I (IGF-I) peptides for three days stimulates proliferation of the small intestinal epithelium in rats. Gut 1995;37:630–8.
103. Steeb C-B, Shoubridge CA, Tivey DR, Read LC. Systemic infusion of IGF-I or LR^{3}IGF-I stimulates organ growth and proliferation of gut tissues in suckling rats. Am J Physiol 1997;272:G522–33.
104. Mantell MP, Ziegler TR, Adamson WT, et al. Resection-induced colonic adaptation is augmented by IGF-I and associated with upregulation of colonic IGF-I mRNA. Am J Physiol 1995;269:G974–80.
105. Vanderhoof JA, McCusker RH, Clark R, et al. Truncated and native insulin-like growth factor I enhance mucosal adaptation after jejunoileal resection. Gastroenterology 1992;102:1949–56.
106. Peterson CA, Ney DM, Hinton PS, Carey HV. Beneficial effects of insulin-like growth factor I on epithelial structure and function in parenterally fed rat jejunum. Gastroenterology 1996;111:1501–8.
107. Chen K, Okuma T, Okamuar K, et al. Insulin-like growth factor I prevents gut atrophy and maintains intestinal integrity in septic rats. JPEN J Parenter Enteral Nutr 1997;19:119–24.
108. Inaba T, Saito H, Fukushima R, et al. Insulin-like growth factor I has beneficial effects, whereas growth hormone has limited effects on postoperative protein metabolism, gut integrity, and splenic weight in rats with chronic mild liver injury. JPEN J Parenter Enteral Nutr 1997;21:55–62.
109. Ulshen MH, Dowling RH, Fuller CR, et al. Enhanced growth of small bowel in transgenic mice overexpressing bovine growth hormone. Gastroenterology 1993;104:973–80.
110. Parrizas M, Saltiel AR, LeRoith D. Insulin-like growth factor inhibits apoptosis using the phosphatidylinositol 3-kinase and mitogen-activated protein kinase pathways. J Biol Chem 1997;272:154–61.
111. Matthews RJ, Bowne DB, Flores E, Thomas ML. Characterization of hematopoietic intracellular protein tyrosine phosphatases: description of a phosphatase containing an SH2 domain and another enriched in proline-, glutamic acid-, serine-, and threonine-rich sequences. Mol Cell Biol 1992;12:2396–405.
112. Ohneda K, Ulshen MH, Fuller CR, et al. Enhanced growth of small bowel in transgenic mice expressing human insulin-like growth factor. Gastroenterology 1997;112:444–54.

113. Ward A, Bates P, Fisher R, et al. Disproportionate growth in mice with *Igf*-2 transgenes. Proc Natl Acad Sci U S A 1994; 91:10365–9.
114. Wolf E, Kramer R, Blum WF, et al. Consequences of postnatally elevated insulin-like growth factor-II in transgenic mice: endocrine changes and effects on body and organ growth. Endocrinology 1994;135:1877–86.
115. Underwood LE, Clemmons DR, Maes M, et al. Regulation of somatomedin C/insulin-like growth factor I by nutrients. Horm Res 1986;24:166–76.
116. Winesett DE, Ulshen MH, Hoyt EC, et al. Regulation and localization of the insulin-like growth factor system in small bowel during altered nutrient status. Am J Physiol 1995; 268:G631–40.
117. Ziegler TR, Almahfouz A, Pedrini MT, Smith RJ. A comparison of rat small intestinal insulin and insulin-like growth factor I receptors during fasting and refeeding. Endocrinology 1995;136:5148–54.
118. Guo Y-S, Townsend CM Jr, Jin G-F, et al. Differential regulation of TGF-β1 and insulin of insulin-like growth factor binding protein-2 in IEC-6 cells. Am J Physiol 1995;268: E1199–204.
119. Oguchi S, Walker WA, Sanderson IR. Profile of IGF-binding proteins secreted by intestinal epithelial cells changes with differentiation. Am J Physiol 1994;267:G843–50.
120. Wood TL. Gene-targeting and transgenic approaches to IGF and IGF binding protein function. Am J Physiol 1995;269: E613–22.
121. Liu J-P, Baker J, Perkins AS, et al. Mice carrying null mutations of the genes encoding insulin-like growth factor (Igf-1) and type 1 IGF receptor (Igfr). Cell 1993;75:59–72.
122. Baker J, Liu J-P, Robertson EJ, Efstratiadis A. Role of insulin-like growth factors in embryonic and postnatal growth. Cell 1993;75:73–82.
123. Ullrich A, Schlessinger J. Signal transduction by receptors with tyrosine kinase activity. Cell 1990;61:203–12.
124. Cohen S. Isolation of a mouse submaxillary gland protein accelerating incisor eruption and eyelid opening in the newborn animal. J Biol Chem 1962;237:1555–62.
125. Carpenter G, Wahl MI. The epidermal growth factor family. In: Sporn M, Roberts A, editors. Handbook of experimental pharmacology. Vol. 95/I. Peptide growth factors and their receptors I. Vol. I. Heidelberg: Springer-Verlag; 1990. p. 69.
126. Carpenter G, Cohen S. Epidermal growth factor. J Biol Chem 1990;265:7709–12.
127. Brissenden JE, Derynck R, Francke U. Mapping of transforming growth factor α gene on human chromosome 2 close to the breakpoint of the Burkitt's lymphoma t(2:8) variant. Cancer Res 1985;45:5593–7.
128. Brissenden JE, Ullrich A, Francke U. Human chromosomal mapping of genes for insulin-like growth factors I and II and epidermal growth factor. Nature 1984;310:781–4.
129. Bell GI, Fong NM, Stempie NM, et al. Human epidermal growth factor precursor: cDNA sequence, expression in vitro and gene organization. Nucleic Acids Res 1986;14:8427–46.
130. Derynck R, Roberts AB, Winkler ME, et al. Human transforming growth factor-α: precursor sequence, gene structure, and heterologous expression. Cancer Cells 1985;3:79–86.
131. Haley J, Whittle N, Bennett P, et al. The human EGF receptor gene: structure of the 110kb locus and identification of sequences regulating its transcription. Oncogene Res 1987;1:375–96.
132. Carpenter G. Receptor tyrosine kinase substrates: *src* homology domains and signal transduction. FASEB J 1992;6:3283–9.
133. Alimandi M, Wang L, Bottaro D, et al. Epidermal growth factor and betacellulin mediate signal transduction through co-expressed ErbB2 and ErbB3 receptors. EMBO J 1997;16: 5608–17.
134. Tzahar E, Pinkas-Kramarski R, Moyer JD, et al. Bivalence of EGF-like ligands drives the ErbB signaling network. EMBO J 1997;16:4938–50.
135. Heldin CH. Dimerization of cell surface receptors in signal transduction. Cell 1995;80:213–23.
136. Konturek JW, Bielanski W, Konturek SJ, et al. Distribution and release of epidermal growth factor in man. Gut 1989;30:1194–200.
137. Wright NA, Pike C, Elia G. Induction of a novel epidermal growth factor-secreting cell lineage by mucosal ulceration in human gastrointestinal stem cells. Nature 1990;343:82–5.
138. Hermiston ML, Gordon JI. Inflammatory bowel disease and adenomas in mice expressing a dominant negative N-cadherin. Science 1995;270:1203–7.
139. Miettinen PJ, Perheentupa J, Otonkoski T, et al. EGF- and TGF-α-like peptides in human fetal gut. Pediatr Res 1989;26:25–30.
140. Playford RJ, Woodman AC, Clark P, et al. Effect of luminal growth factor preservation on intestinal growth. Lancet 1993;341:843–8.
141. Playford RJ, Marchbank T, Calnan DP, et al. Epidermal growth factor is digested to smaller, less active forms in acidic gastric juice. Gastroenterology 1995;108:92–101.
142. Thornburg W, Rao RK, Matrisian LM, et al. Effect of maturation on gastrointestinal absorption of epidermal growth factor in rats. Am J Physiol 1987;253:G68–71.
143. Schaudies RP, Grimes J, Davis D, et al. EGF content in the gastrointestinal tract of rats: effect of age and fasting/feeding. Am J Physiol 1989;256:G856–61.
144. Pollack PF, Goda T, Colony PC, et al. Effects of enterally fed epidermal growth factor on the small and large intestine of the suckling rat. Regul Peptides 1987;17:121–32.
145. Carpenter G. Epidermal growth factor is a major growth-promoting agent in human milk. Science 1980;210:198–9.
146. Beardmore JM, Richards RC. Concentrations of epidermal growth factor in mouse milk throughout lactation. J Endocrinol 1983;96:287–92.
147. Moran JR, Courtney ME, Orth DN, et al. Epidermal growth factor in human milk: daily production and diurnal variation during early lactation in mothers delivering at term and at premature gestation. J Pediatr 1983;103:402–4.
148. Okada M, Ohmura E, Kamiya Y, et al. Transforming growth factor (TGF)-α in human milk. Life Sci 1991;48:1151–6.
149. Dvorak B, Koldovsky O. The presence of transforming growth factor-α in the suckling rat small intestine and pancreas and the absence in rat milk. Pediatr Res 1994;35: 348–53.
150. Koyama S, Podolsky DK. Differential expression of transforming growth factors α and β in rat intestinal epithelial cells. J Clin Invest 1989;83:1768–73.
151. Thomas DM, Nasim MM, Gullick WJ, Alison MR. Immunoreactivity of transforming growth factor alpha in the normal adult gastrointestinal tract. Gut 1992;33:628–31.
152. Hormi K, Lehy T. Developmental expression of transforming growth factor-α and epidermal growth factor receptor proteins in the human pancreas and digestive tracts. Cell Tissue Res 1994;278:439–50.
153. Miettinen PJ. Transforming growth factor-α and epidermal growth factor expression in human fetal gastrointestinal tract. Pediatr Res 1993;33:481–6.
154. Dvorak B, Holubec H, LeBouton AV, et al. Epidermal growth factor and transforming growth factor-α mRNA in rat small intestine: in situ hybridization study. FEBS Lett 1994;352:291–5.
155. Podolskly DK. Regulation of intestinal epithelial proliferation: a few answers, many questions. Am J Physiol 1993;27: G179–86.

156. Barnard JA, Beauchamp RD, Russell WE, et al. Epidermal growth factor-related peptides and their relevance to gastrointestinal pathophysiology. Gastroenterology 1995;108:564–80.
157. Toyoda S, Lee P-C, Lebenthal E. Interaction of epidermal growth factor with specific binding sites of enterocytes isolated from rat small intestine during development. Biochim Biophys Acta 1986;886:295–301.
158. Scheving LA, Shiurba RA, Nguyen TD, Gray GM. Epidermal growth factor receptor of the intestinal enterocyte—localization to laterobasal but not brush border membrane. J Biol Chem 1989;264:1735–41.
159. Thompson JF. Specific receptors for epidermal growth factor in rat intestinal microvillus membranes. Am J Physiol 1988;254:G429–35.
160. Beauchamp RD, Barnard JA, McCutchen CM, et al. Localization of transforming growth factor α and its receptor in gastric mucosal cells. J Clin Invest 1989;84:1017–23.
161. Borlinghaus P, Wieser S, Lamerz R. Epidermal growth factor, transforming growth factor-α, and epidermal growth factor receptor content in normal and carcinomatous gastric and colonic tissue. Clin Invest 1993;71:903–7.
162. Menard D, Pothier P. Radioautographic localization of epidermal growth factor receptors in human fetal gut. Gastroenterology 1991;101:640–9.
163. Playford RJ, Hanby AM, Gschmeissner S, et al. The epidermal growth factor receptor (ERF-R) is present on the basolateral, but not the apical, surface of the enterocytes in the human gastrointestinal tract. Gut 1996;39:262–6.
164. Thompson JF, Van Den Berg M, Stokkers CF. Developmental regulation of epidermal growth factor receptor kinase in rat intestine. Gastroenterology 1994;107:1278–87.
165. Gallo-Payet N, Hugon JS. Epidermal growth factor receptors in isolated adult mouse intestinal cells: studies *in vivo* and in organ culture. Endocrinology 1985;116:194–201.
166. Barnard JA, Polk WH, Moses HL, Coffey RJ. Production of transforming growth factor-α by normal rat small intestine. Am J Physiol 1991;261:C994–1000.
167. Polk DB. Ontogenic regulation of PLCγ1 activity and expression in the rat small intestine. Gastroenterology 1994;107:109–16.
168. Gallo-Payet N, Pothier P, Hugon JS. Ontogeny of EGF receptors during postnatal development of mouse small intestine. J Pediatr Gastroenterol Nutr 1987;6:114–20.
169. Scheving LA, Yeh YC, Tsai TH, Scheving LE. Circadian phase-dependent stimulatory effects of epidermal growth factor on deoxyribonucleic acid synthesis in the duodenum, jejunum, ileum, caecum, colon, and rectum of the adult male mouse. Endocrinology 1980;106:1498–503.
170. Berseth CL. Enhancement of intestinal growth in neonatal rats by epidermal growth factor in milk. Am J Physiol 1987;253:G662–5.
171. Berseth CL, Go VLW. Enhancement of neonatal somatic and hepatic growth by orally administered epidermal growth factor in rats. J Pediatr Gastroenterol Nutr 1988;7:889–93.
172. Malo C, Menard D. Influence of epidermal growth factor on the development of suckling mouse intestinal mucosa. Gastroenterology 1982;83:28–35.
173. Arsenault P, Menard D. Stimulatory effects of epidermal growth factor on deoxyribonucleic acid synthesis in the gastrointestinal tract of the suckling mouse. Comp Biochem Physiol 1987;86B:123–7.
174. Walker-Smith JA, Phillips AD, Walford N, et al. Intravenous epidermal growth factor/urogastrone increases small-intestinal cell proliferation in congenital microvillous atrophy. Lancet 1985;8466:1239–40.
175. Menard D, Arsenault P, Pothier P. Biologic effects of epidermal growth factor in human fetal jejunum. Gastroenterology 1988;94:656–63.
176. Challacombe DN, Wheeler EE. Trophic action of epidermal growth factor on human duodenal mucosa cultured in vitro. Gut 1991;32:991–3.
177. Goodlad RA, Raja KB, Peters TJ, Wright NA. Effects of urogastrone-epidermal growth factor on intestinal brush border enzymes and mitotic activity. Gut 1991;32:994–8.
178. Miettinen PJ, Berger JE, Meneses J, et al. Epithelial immaturity and multiorgan failure in mice lacking epidermal growth factor receptor. Nature 1995;376:337–41.
179. Sibilla M, Wagner EF. Strain-dependent epithelial defects in mice lacking the EGF receptor. Science 1995;269:234–8.
180. Threadgill DW, Dlugosz AA, Hansen LA, et al. Targeted disruption of mouse EGF receptor: effect of genetic background on mutant phenotype. Science 1995;269:230–4.
181. Honegger AM, Schmidt A, Ullrich A, Schlessinger J. Evidence for epidermal growth factor (EGF)-induced intermolecular autophosphorylation of the EGF receptors in living cells. Mol Cell Biol 1990;10:4035–44.
182. Moroni MC, Willingham MC, Beguinot L. EGF-R antisense RNA blocks expression of the epidermal growth factor receptor and supresses the transforming phenotype of a human carcinoma cell line. J Biol Chem 1992;267:2714–22.
183. Goodlad RA, Savage AP, Lenton W, et al. Does resection enhance the response of the intesine to urogastrone-epidermal growth factor in the rat? Clin Sci 1988;75:121–6.
184. Read LC, Ford WDA, Filsell OH, et al. Is orally-derived epidermal growth factor beneficial following premature birth or intestinal resection? Endocrinol Exp 1986;20:199–207.
185. Chaet MS, Arya G, Ziegler MM, Warner BW. Epidermal growth factor enhances intestinal adaptation after massive small bowel resection. J Pediatr Surg 1994;29:1035–9.
186. O'Loughlin E, Winter M, Shun A, et al. Structural and functional adaptation following jejunal resection in rabbits: effect of epidermal growth factor. Gastroenterology 1994;107:87–93.
187. Helmrath MA, Shin CE, Erwin CR, Warner BW. Epidermal growth factor upregulates the expression of its own intestinal receptor after small bowel resection. J Pediatr Surg 1998;33:229–34.
188. Helmrath MA, Erwin CR, Warner BW. A defective EGF-receptor in waved-2 mice attenuates intestinal adaptation. J Surg Res 1997;69:76–80.
189. Opleta-Madsen K, Hardin J, Gall DG. Epidermal growth factor upregulates intestinal electrolyte and nutrient transport. Am J Physiol 1991;260:G807–14.
190. Hardin JA, Buret A, Meddings JB, Gall DG. Effect of epidermal growth factor on enterocyte brush-border surface area. Am J Physiol 1993;264:G312–8.
191. Oka Y, Ghishan FK, Greene HL, Orth DN. Effect of mouse epidermal growth factor/urogastrone on the functional maturation of rat intestine. Endocrinology 1983;112:940–4.
192. Bruns DE, Krishnan AV, Feldman D, et al. Epidermal growth factor increases intestinal calbindin-D_{9k} and 1,25-dihydroxyvitamin D receptors in neonatal rats. Endocrinology 1989;125:478–85.
193. Schwartz MZ, Storozuk RB. Influence of epidermal growth factor on intestinal function in the rat: comparison of systemic infusion versus luminal perfusion. Am J Surg 1988;155:18–22.
194. Green HL, Moore MC, Said HM, et al. Intestinal glucose transport in suckling rats fed artifical milk with and without added epidermal growth factor. Pediatr Res 1987;21:404–8.
195. O'Loughlin EV, Chung M, Hollenberg M, et al. Effect of epidermal growth factor on ontogeny of the gastrointestinal tract. Am J Physiol 1985;249:G674–8.
196. Calvert R, Beaulieu J-F, Menard D. Epidermal growth factor accelerates the maturation of fetal mouse intestinal mucosa in utero. Experientia 1982;38:1096–7.

197. Foltzer-Jourdainne C, Garaud J-C, Nsi-Emvo E, Raul F. Epidermal growth factor and the maturation of intestinal sucrase in suckling rats. Am J Physiol 1993;265:G459–66.
198. James PS, Smith MW, Tivey DR, Wilson TJG. Epidermal growth factor selectively increases maltase and sucrase activities in neonatal piglet intestine. J Physiol 1987;393:583–94.
199. Harada E, Hashimoto Y, Syuto B. Epidermal growth factor accelerates the intestinal cessation of macromolecular transmission in the suckling rat. Comp Biochem Physiol A 1990;97:201–4.
200. Emvo EN, Raul F, Koch B, et al. Sucrase-isomaltase gene expression in suckling rat intestine: hormonal, dietary, and growth factor control. J Pediatr Gastroenterol Nutr 1996;23:262–9.
201. Beaulieu JF, Menard D, Calvert R. Influence of epidermal growth factor on the maturation of the fetal mouse duodenum in organ culture. J Pediatr Gastroenterol Nutr 1985;4:476–81.
202. Menard D, Arsenault P, Gallo-Payet N. Epidermal growth factor does not act as a primary cue for inducing developmental changes in suckling mouse jejunum. J Pediatr Gastroenterol Nutr 1986;5:949–55.
203. Derynck R, Feng X-H. TGF signaling. Biochim Biophys Acta 1997;1333:F105–50.
204. Massague J, Attisano A, Wrana JL. The TGF family and its composite receptors. Trends Cell Biol 1994;4:172–8.
205. Kingsley DM. The TGF-β superfamily: new members, new receptors, and new genetic tests of function in different organisms. Genes Dev 1994;8:133–46.
206. Barton DE, Foellmer BE, Du J, et al. Chromosomal locations of TGF-βs2 and 3 in the mouse and human. Oncogene Res 1988;3:323–31.
207. Fujii D, Brissenden JE, Derynck R, Francke U. Transforming growth factor-β gene maps to human chromosome 19 long arm and to mouse chromosome 7. Somat Cell Mol Genet 1986;12:281–8.
208. Derynck R, Lindquist PB, Lee A, et al. A new type of transforming growth factor-β, TGF-β3. EMBO J 1988;7:3737–43.
209. Lyons RM, Gentry LE, Purchio AF, Moses HL. Mechanism of activation of latent recombinant transforming growth factor-β1 by plasmin. J Cell Biol 1990;110:1361–7.
210. Crawford SE, Stellmach V, Murphy-Ullrich JE, et al. Thrombospondin-1 is a major activator of TGFβ1 in vivo. Cell 1998;93:1159–70.
211. Lin HY, Lodish HF. Receptors for the TGF-β superfamily: multiple polypeptides and serine/threonine kinases. Trends Cell Biol 1993;3:14–9.
212. Lin HY, Wang X-F, Ng-Eaton E, et al. Expression of cloning of the TGF type II receptor, a functional transmembrane serine/threonine kinase. Cell 1992;68:775–85.
213. Franzen P, ten Dijke P, Ichijo H, et al. Cloning of a TGF type I receptor that forms a heteromeric complex with the TGF type II receptor. Cell 1993;75:1–20.
214. Ebner R, Chen R-H, Shum L, et al. Cloning of a type I TGF-β receptor and its effect on TGF-β binding to the type II receptor. Science 1993;260:1344–8.
215. Attisano L, Carcamo J, Ventura F, et al. Identification of human activin and TGF type I receptors that form heteromeric kinase complexes with type II receptors. Cell 1993;75:671–80.
216. Attisano L, Wrana JL. Signal transduction by members of the transforming growth factor β-superfamily. Cytokine Growth Factor Rev 1996;7:327–39.
217. Lin HY, Moustakas A. TGF receptors. Structure and function. Cell Mol Biol 1994;40:337–49.
218. Lopez-Casillas F, Cheifez S, Doody J, et al. Structure and expression of the membrane proteoglycan betaglycan, a component of the TGF receptor system. Cell 1991;64:785–95.
219. Lopez-Casillas F, Wrana JL, Massague J. Betaglycan presents ligand to the TGFβ signaling receptor. Cell 1993;73:1435–44.
220. Laiho M, Weiss FMB, Boyd FT, et al. Responsiveness to transforming growth factor ß restored by genetic complementation between cells defective in TGF receptors I and II. J Biol Chem 1991;266:9108–12.
221. Geiser AG, Burmester JK, Webbink R, et al. Inhibition of growth by transforming growth factor β following fusion of two nonresponsive human carcinoma cell lines: implication of the type II receptor in growth inhibitory responses. J Biol Chem 1992;267:2588–93.
222. Okadome T, Yamashita H, Franzen P, et al. Distinct roles of the intracellular domains of transforming growth factor β and type I and type II receptors in signal transduction. J Biol Chem 1994;269:30753–6.
223. Chen R-H, Ebner R, Derynck R. Inactivation of the type II receptor reveals two receptor pathways for the diverse TGF-β activities. Science 1993;260:1335–8.
224. Miettinen PJ, Ebner R, Lopez AR, Derynck R. TGFβ induced transdifferentiation of mammary epithelial cells to mesenchymal cells: involvement of type I receptors. J Cell Biol 1994;127:2021–36.
225. Zhao J, Buick RN. Regulation of transforming growth factor β receptors in H-ras oncogene-transformed rat intestinal epithelial cells. Cancer Res 1995;55:6181–8.
226. Mulder KM, Segarini PR, Morris SL, et al. Role of receptor complexes in resistance or sensitivity to growth inhibition by TGFβ in intestinal epithelial cell clones. J Cell Physiol 1993;154:162–74.
227. Heldin C-H, Miyazono K, ten Dijke P. TGF signalling from cell membrane to nucleus through SMAD proteins. Nature 1997;390:465–71.
228. Hayashi H, Abdollah S, Qiu Y, et al. The MAD-related protein Smad7 associates with the TGFβ receptor and functions as an antagonist of TGFβ signaling. Cell 1997;89:1165–73.
229. Eppert K, Scherer SW, Ozcelik H, et al. MADR2 maps to 18q21 and encodes a TGFβ-related MAD-related protein that is functionally mutated in colorectal carcinoma. Cell 1996;86:543–52.
230. Takagi Y, Kohmura H, Futamura M, et al. Somatic alterations of the DPC4 gene in human colorectal cancers in vivo. Gastroenterology 1996;111:1369–72.
231. Howe JR, Roth S, Ringold JC, et al. Mutations in the SMAD4/DPC4 gene in juvenile polyposis. Science 1998;280:1086–8.
232. Barnard JA, Lyons RM, Moses HL. The cell biology of transforming growth factor β. Biochim Biophys Acta 1990;1032:79–87.
233. Ko TC, Sheng HM, Reisman D, et al. Transforming growth factor beta inhibits cyclin D1 expression in intestinal epithelial cells. Oncogene 1995;10:177–84.
234. Barnard JA, Beauchamp RD, Coffey RJ, Moses HL. Regulation of intestinal epithelial cell growth by transforming growth factor typeβ. Proc Natl Acad Sci U S A 1989;86:1578–82.
235. Barnard JA, Warwick GJ, Gold LI. Localization of transforming growth factor β isoforms in the normal murine small intestine and colon. Gastroenterology 1993;105:67–73.
236. Saito S, Yoshida M, Ichijo M, et al. Transforming growth factor-beta (TGFβ) in human milk. Clin Exp Immunol 1993;94:220–4.
237. Lang AK, Searle RK. The immunomodulatory activity of human amniotic fluid can be correlated with TGFβ1 and TGFβ2 activity. Clin Exp Immunol 1994;97:158–63.
238. Markowitz SD, Roberts AB. Tumor suppressor activity of the TGF-β pathway in human cancers. Cytokine Growth Factor Rev 1996;7:93–102.

239. Grande JP. Role of transforming growth factor-β in tissue injury and repair. Proc Soc Exp Biol Med 1997;214:27–40.
240. Mustoe TA, Landes A, Cromack DT. Differential acceleration of healing of surgical incisions in the rabbit gastrointestinal tract by platelet-derived growth factor and transforming growth factor, type β. Surgery 1990;108:324–30.
241. Border WA, Nobel NA. Transforming growth factor beta in tissue fibrosis. N Engl J Med 1994;331:1286–92.
242. Litterio JJ, Roberts AB. TGF β: a critical modulator of immune cell function. Clin Immunol Immunopathol 1997;84:244–50.
243. Strobl H, Riedel E, Scheinecker C, et al. TGFβ1 promotes *in vitro* development of dendritic cells from CD34+ hemopoietic progenitors. J Immunol 1996;157:1499–507.
244. van Vlasselaer P, Punnonen J, de Vries JE. Transforming growth factor β directs IgA switching in human B cells. J Immunol 1992;148:2062–7.
245. Pelton RW, Saxena B, Jones M, et al. Immunohistochemical localization of TGFβ1, TGFβ2, and TGFβ3 in the mouse embryo: expression pattern suggests multiple roles in embryonic development. J Cell Biol 1991;115:1091–105.
246. Shull MM, Ormsby I, Kier AB, et al. Targeted disruption of the mouse transforming growth factor-β1 gene results in multifocal inflammatory disease. Nature 1992;359:693–9.
247. Kulkarni AB, Huh C-G, Becker D, et al. Transforming growth factor β1 null mutation in mice causes excessive inflammatory response and early death. Proc Natl Acad Sci U S A 1993;90:770–4.
248. Kulkarni AB, Ward JM, Yaswen L, et al. Transforming growth factor-β1 null mice: an animal model for inflammatory disorders. Am J Pathol 1995;146:264–75.
249. Dickson MC. Transforming growth factor β1 is essential for hematopoiesis and endothelial differentiation *in vivo*. Development 1995;121:1845–54.
250. Hines KL, Kulkarni AB, McCarthy JB, et al. Synthetic fibronectin peptides interrupt inflammatory cell infiltration in transforming growth factor β1 knockout mice. Proc Natl Acad Sci U S A 1994;91:5187–91.
251. Sanderson N, Factor V, Nagy P, et al. Hepatic expression of mature transforming growth factor beta 1 in transgenic mice results in multiple tissue lesions. Proc Natl Acad Sci U S A 1995;92:2572–6.
252. Lee M-S, Gu D, Feng L, et al. Accumulation of extracellular matrix and developmental dysregulation in the pancreas by transgenic production of transforming growth factor beta 1. Am J Pathol 1995;147:53–67.
253. Bottinger EP, Jakubczak JL, Roberts ISD, et al. Expression of a dominant-negative mutant TGF-β type II receptor in transgenic mice reveals essential roles for TGF-β in regulation of growth and differentiation in the exocrine pancreas. EMBO J 1997;16:2621–33.
254. Ziambaras T, Rubin DC, Perlmutter DH. Regulation of sucrase-isomaltase gene expression in human intestinal epithelial cells by inflammatory cytokines. J Biol Chem 1996;271:1237–42.
255. Kaiser GC, Polk DB. Tumor necrosis factor alpha regulates proliferation in a mouse intestinal cell line. Gastroenterology 1997;112:1231–40.
256. Thompson FM, Mayrhofer G, Cummins AG. Dependence of epithelial growth of the small intestine on T-cell activation during weaning in the rat. Gastroenterology 1996;111:37–44.
257. Lollini P, D'Errico A, DeGiovanni C, et al. Systemic effects of cytokines released by gene-transduced tumor cells: marked hyperplasia induced in small bowel by interferon transfectants through host lymphocytes. Int J Cancer 1995;61:425–30.
258. Dignass AU, Podolsky DK. Interleukin 2 modulates intestinal epithelial cell function *in vitro*. Exp Cell Res 1996;225:422–9

CHAPTER 4

Role of Cytokeratins in Epithelial Cell Development

Andrea Quaroni, PhD

David Calnek, PhD

The absorptive epithelium of the small intestine undergoes a process of cellular renewal in which the functional enterocytes are constantly replenished by proliferative precursor cells in the crypts of Lieberkühn, differentiate in the upper region of the crypts, migrate toward the villus tips, and are finally shed into the lumen.[1] Accompanying differentiation are significant changes in cellular morphology and ultrastructure, as well as in expression of enzymes and transport mechanisms required for nutrient absorption. Classic structural features of the polarized absorptive villus cells include distinct apical and basolateral membrane domains separated by tight junctional complexes, an extensive and highly ordered brushborder region at their apical or luminal aspect, and an extensive cytoplasmic network of intermediate-sized filaments (also called tonofilaments) that are particularly abundant at the subapical and basal aspects of the cells. The brushborder region exhibits two distinct zones: the microvillar digitations containing bundled actin filaments, and the underlying terminal web containing several distinct types of filaments.[2] The subapical intermediate filaments (IF) are composed of specific cytokeratins associated with the desmosomes and the terminal web.[3] Collectively these structures contribute to the cytoplasmic organization and cytoskeletal architecture of the intestinal epithelial cell.

Marked ultrastructural differences exist between proliferative crypt cells and absorptive villus cells. While the luminal aspect of the crypt cells is covered by numerous microvilli, these are shorter, wider, and more irregular in shape and distribution than those of the villus cells.[4] In addition, no well-developed terminal web is present in the undifferentiated crypt cells: instead, the bundles of actin microfilaments comprising the core of the microvilli penetrate into the cell cytoplasm to a depth of 3 to 5 μm, and cellular organelles are present in the upper portion of the apical cytoplasm.[4,5] Detailed studies[5] have demonstrated that actin, villin, myosin, tropomyosin, and spectrin are already concentrated in the luminal cytoplasm of the stem cells, present at the bottom of the crypts and displaying relatively few and short microvilli. Thus, brushborder formation may involve reorganization of existing cytoskeletal proteins induced by an as-yet-unidentified cellular component. The terminal web becomes organized as a structure detectable at the ultrastructural level somewhat later, as the newly differentiated cells reach the top of the crypts.

The IF composition of the intestinal epithelium was initially studied by Franke's group: three keratins were identified that are characteristic of simple epithelia in general, including a single type II component (CK8) and two type I proteins (CK18 and CK19).[3,6] Subsequent studies[7,8] have revealed the presence of a new type I cytokeratin (K20-21) that exhibits a remarkable cell and tissue-specific distribution and is primarily expressed by differentiated intestinal epithelial cells in both small and large intestines. This suggests that keratin tonofilaments may have important functional role(s) in the intestinal epithelium, and this novel cytokeratin may be necessary for the structural organization of the small-intestinal absorptive cells and surface colonic epithelial cells.

The developmentally regulated assembly of the brushborder and terminal web in fetal intestinal cells bears many similarities to the analogous processes taking place during crypt cell differentiation in adult animals.[5,9] In fetal rats, the first stage of maturation is characterized by the formation of a stratified epithelium, up to 10 cells thick, around 15 days of gestation (dg),[10,11] that persists until 18 dg. During this period, the cells facing the lumen are covered with a few microvilli of variable length, and junctional complexes are rare. The transition from stratified to single epithelium occurring at 18 to 19 dg is accompanied by formation of the villi, and represents a major step in the maturation of the intestinal mucosa. Assembly of the brushborder cytoskeleton and of the apical terminal web are, therefore, relatively late events in fetal intestinal maturation, and have been studied in detail in chicks[12] and mice.[13,14] They have been described as gradual and complex processes, characterized in the chick by the apical redistribution of actin-binding proteins occurring a few days before the appearance of adult-type microvilli[12] on the luminal surface of the enterocytes. In both chick and mouse embryos, villin and fimbrin become concentrated in the apical cytoplasm asynchronously,[12,13] but in all cases the terminal web cytoskeleton is assembled later in development,[13,15] when the differentiation-related cytokeratin K20-21 also starts to be expressed. Thus, this process represents a complementary in vivo model system to investigate the possible roles of different cytoskeletal proteins in assembly and function of the cytoskeletal network.

CYTOSKELETON IN INTESTINAL CELLS

Enterocytes are highly polarized, tall columnar cells that can be easily recognized by their luminal surface specializations, collectively known as the brushborder. Chicken enterocytes located on the upper third of villi have been estimated to contain approximately 1200 microvilli per cell.[16] Among different species, the brushborder microvilli range between 0.5 and 1.5 μm in length, and 0.1 μm in width.[17] It is believed that the brushborder increases the apical surface area by as much as 14- to 40-fold.[18] Electron microscopic analysis also has revealed that a complex filamentous surface coat, or glycocalyx, covers and attaches directly to the microvillus membrane.[17,19] The glycocalyx has been proposed to help protect the luminal cell surface.[17]

All intestinal epithelial cells have very extensive junctional complexes located at the apical margin of the lateral membrane.[20] Three types of cellular junctions, oriented in an apical-to-basal arrangement, comprise the complex: zonula occludens (tight junction), zonula adherens (belt desmosome), and macula adherens (spot desmosome). The lateral membranes between two adjacent epithelial cells become closely associated along the junctional complex, especially at the level of the tight junction. This suggests that the junctional complex is important, at least in part, in cell-cell attachment or adhesion.

The brushborder cytoskeleton has been divided into two structurally and functionally distinct domains: the microvillus core, and the terminal web. The brushborders of the chicken and some mammals (mouse, rat, and human) are quite similar in terms of composition, organization, and assembly.[21] These observations suggest a conserved brushborder function between the avian and mammalian intestine. The estimated number of core filaments appears to vary between species, but remains constant within the same species, ranging between 10 and 50 per cell.[22] Rat intestinal microvilli were estimated to consist of about 50 core filaments,[23] compared with 15 to 20 in adult chickens,[22] and approximately 15 in 10-day-old chicks.[16] The microvillus core filaments are organized into loose, hexagonally packed arrangements that appear to terminate at electron-dense material at each microvillus tip and run down to the base of the terminal web.[23,24]

The ultrastructure of the terminal web of absorptive cells in the small intestine of the chicken, mouse, and rat and in the colon of the mouse has been examined by several groups.[23,25–29] At the level of the electron microscope, the terminal web was described as appearing to extend out to the zonula adherens or belt desmosome as a dense layer of material subjacent to, and in a plane parallel with, the luminal cell surface.[23] The rootlets of the microvillus cores, the most obvious feature of the terminal web, were demonstrated to embed between interconnecting filaments of the terminal web, and terminate at the level of the zonula adherens junction. Further ultrastructural examination of the terminal web demonstrated that it could be divided into three distinct zones defined on the basis of the kinds and densities of filaments.[26] The apical, intermediate, and basal zones of the terminal web reside in the plane of the zonula occludens (tight), zonula adherens (belt desmosome), and macula adherens (spot desmosome) junctions, respectively. Impressive quick-freeze, deep-etch rotary shadow replicas of mouse brushborders clearly demonstrated, in three dimensions, that the actin core rootlets penetrating the terminal web remain tightly bundled without any evidence of splaying at their ends.[27–30]

Electron microscopic analysis had revealed that populations of intermediate filaments were found to concentrate in the basal zone of the terminal web,[26] as well as in interconnecting spot desmosomal plaques along the lateral membrane of villus cells.[4] Several years later, isolated brushborder preparations of rat intestinal absorptive cells were found to contain desmosome-associated tonofilaments.[31] Fodrin, a spectrin-related protein, was shown to interconnect core rootlets at all levels of the terminal web, and among other things connect the rootlets with a concentrated population of intermediate filaments in the basal zone of the terminal web.[28] This result acknowledged the presence of cytokeratins directly associating with a specific terminal web protein, and provided the first indication that they may be important in facilitating vertical stability to the core rootlets and possibly the entire brushborder cytoskeleton.

Electron microscopic examinations have afforded a wealth of information regarding ultrastructural differences between undifferentiated crypt cells and differentiated villus cells. The major changes accompanying fine structural development of maturing enteroctyes have been extensively studied, and include a gradual increase in the total cell size, appearance of several highly ordered and well-developed microvilli[32] and terminal web,[23,25,33,34] exclusion of cell organelles within the brushborders, elaboration of lateral membrane interdigitations, appearance of smooth endoplasmic reticulum, an increase in rough endoplasmic reticulum, better-developed Golgi system, an increase in the number of mitochondria, and a shifting of the nucleus to a more central location.[35]

Biochemic Composition of the Brushborder Cytoskeleton

Significant progress in cellular and subcellular fractionation techniques has allowed excellent separation and isolation of relatively uncontaminated populations of crypt and villus cells,[36] as well as of luminal membranes.[37,38] Isolated brushborders have been extensively used as a model system from which to investigate the physiologic and biochemic nature of the brushborder membrane and actin-based cytoskeleton of mature enterocytes.[39,40]

The core filaments supporting the microvilli were found to consist of filamentous actin,[41] composed of both β and γ isoforms,[40] and uniformly polarized with their "barbed" or fast-growing ends facing the tips of the microvilli.[42] The actin core filaments and microvillus membrane are laterally crossbridged by protein complexes, composed of 110- and 17-kDa proteins.[43] Immunologic means were employed to identify the 17-kDa protein as calmodulin (CM).[44] The 110-kDa protein was shown to be a member of the myosin I family,[45] a group of small myosins lacking a tail but possessing a lipid binding domain.[46] In addition to helping provide structural support between the brushborder membrane and microvillus actin core, and possibly acting to buffer free calcium ions, other functions of the complex remain elusive.

Two major cytoskeletal proteins that act to bundle F-actin in a Ca^{2+}-dependent and -independent manner are the 95-kDa villin[47–49] and the 68-kDa fimbrin,[50,51] respectively. A minor protein found within the microvillus core is the 80-kDa protein ezrin.[52]

In addition to actin, immunolocalization studies indicate the presence of villin, fimbrin, and BB myosin I within the terminal web core rootlets.[53,54] Other major rootlet proteins such as fodrin,[28] α-actinin,[53,55] myosin,[53] tropomyosin,[55] and caldesmon[55] appear to associate only with the surface of the rootlets. Immunolocalization of cytokeratins in frozen sections of the adult rat intestinal epithelium revealed complex filamentous arrays that were not observed in the microvilli but were concentrated in the terminal web and basal regions.[6] Cytokeratin filaments appeared to anchor themselves to spot desmosomes along the apical skeletal disc. The great intensity in, and the complexity of, immunofluorescence staining patterns of cytokeratin filaments in the intestinal epithelium demonstrated that they are major elements within these cells. Two-dimensional Western blots resolving desmosome-associated tonofilaments, derived from adult rat intestinal brushborders, showed the presence of keratins 8 and 19, together with a small abundance of keratin 18.[3] These results suggest that these keratins might be important in helping to reinforce and stabilize the cell shape and adhesion mediated by spot desmosomes. They also suggest that keratins 8, 18, and 19 might be involved in the vertical stabilization of the overall brushborder architecture, where they make close associations with the basal zone of the terminal web.

Although microvilli are present on the surface of both undifferentiated crypt cells and villus cells, there are significant differences in their structure and organization. The total length of the microvillus core filaments for both cells is the same, and it has been suggested that elongation of the microvilli occurs by addition of membrane at their base.[5] Straightening of the microvilli as crypt cells migrate toward the base of the villi could be accomplished through the expression and localization of myosin in the terminal web, since a high level of inter-rootlet crosslinking occurs as these cells mature. In crypt cells the terminal web is essentially rudimentary while the adherens junction is well formed, but by the time these cells have migrated to the base of the villus they have nearly completed assembling functionally mature brushborders. It was shown that most microvillus core proteins are synthesized well before the appearance of microvilli, unlike terminal web components.[21] Elements of the terminal web are typically expressed concomitantly with terminal web formation. The reason for this is unclear, but it may be vitally important for the cell to temporally separate the expression of these two sets of cytoskeletal proteins in order to prevent the assembly of anomalous and disruptive structures. In vivo pulse labeling of intestinal epithelial cells with radioactive amino acids has demonstrated that the brushborder cytoskeleton undergoes steady-state turnover of its constituent proteins.[56] Turnover of brushborder cytoskeletal proteins could function to maintain normal length and stability of microvilli.[56] Several potential physiologic functions can be attributed to such processes. A primary role of the brushborder cytoskeleton is to help establish and maintain the enlarged apical surface area. The brushborder cytoskeleton, in conjunction with the junctional complex, is known also to influence paracellular permeability[57,58] in a manner that might facilitate nutrient transport across the epithelium. The brushborder is also the site of Ca^{2+} absorption. Brushborder calmodulin, as well as calbindin, might help protect the integrity of the brushborder cytoskeleton by buffering high levels of free Ca^{2+} that cause villin-activated actin core solation. The expression patterns of mRNAs (messenger RNAs) encoding brushborder cytoskeletal proteins are varied. The mRNA species encoding actin, myosin II, and nonerythroid spectrin (fodrin and TW260-240) appear to remain constant with respect to the crypt-villus (CV) axis. On the other hand, mRNA species encoding tropomyosin, villin, and calmodulin tend to increase in concentration as intestinal epithelial cells mature.[5,13] Apparently, during enterocyte maturation it is the reorganization of these brushborder cytoskeletal proteins, and not their initial gene expression, that is predominantly regulated.[5]

CYTOKERATINS: STRUCTURE, COMPOSITION, AND TISSUE-SPECIFIC KERATIN GENE EXPRESSION

Intermediate filaments are a major constituent of the cytoskeleton of most vertebrate cells. Presently, there are five classes of intermediate filaments that are known to exist: type I keratins; type II keratins; type III (vimentin, desmin, glial filaments); type IV (neural filaments); and type V (lamins). All intermediate filaments share a common overall secondary structural design. They all possess a highly conserved α-helical central rod domain that is almost invariably 310 amino acids in length, and is flanked by nonhelical amino- and carboxy-terminal extensions that show great divergence in size and sequence. Research in the last 15 years has shown that keratins, also termed cytokeratins, prekeratins, or tonofilaments, are expressed in virtually all epithelia, with few exceptions.[59] Of all epithelia studied, only those found in the lens and retina lack keratin synthesis. To date, as many as 20 different human cytokeratins have been cataloged as distinct gene products.[60] Presently, the nomenclature adopted for homologous keratins derived from different animals is based on the indexing of human keratins, but earlier nomenclature varied making it more difficult to compare keratin homologs in different species. Not only do cytokeratins display epithelial-type specific expression (stratified versus simple), but they also appear to exhibit changes in their expression patterns among cells of the same epithelium during different periods of development and differentiation.[59] Hence, by studying keratin expression patterns during differentiation and development, an understanding of the potential function(s) of keratins could be advanced. Additionally, some of the basic regulatory mechanisms underlying differentiation could be further elucidated by examining all levels of keratin gene expression.

Classification of Keratins

Converging evidence from several laboratories using different approaches has resulted in classification of keratins into two separate subfamilies. Initially, this was based on both molecular and immunologic approaches. Southern blot analysis of restriction-enzyme digested human genomic DNA using two distinct epidermal keratin cDNA (complementary or copy DNA) probes demonstrated two different hybridization patterns that comprised about 10 fragments each.[61] Keratin mRNAs also showed the ability to hybridize to one, but not both, of two cloned epidermal keratin cDNAs encoding 50- and 56-kDa keratins.[62] The predicted amino acid sequences of the 50- and the 56-kDa keratins were compared to the amino acid sequences of the two distinct types of wool keratins and were shown to be highly homologous, with only one of the two types.[63,64] Working solely at the level of the keratin proteins, a keratin subfamily was defined on the basis of tryptic peptide maps of closely related members of the relatively large and basic keratins.[65] Monoclonal antibody studies also delineated two keratin subfamilies according to their immunoreactivity characteristics on one-dimensional Western blots.[66] A more thorough classification of epidermal keratins defined keratin subfamilies A and B in terms of their AE1-AE3 monoclonal antibody cross-reactivities, isoelectric points, and cellular differentiation pathways.[67] Subfamily A keratins, which demonstrated immunoreactivity with the AE1 monoclonal antibody on two-dimensional Western blots, were relatively acidic and smaller in size than subfamily B keratins. Subfamily B keratins were recognized by AE3 monoclonal antibodies and displayed relatively neutral-basic charges. The present keratin nomenclature is based on significant differences between the amino acid sequences of the α-helical domains of type I and type II wool keratins. Consequently, subfamily A keratins are now referred to as type I keratins, and subfamily B keratins are referred to as type II keratins.

Rules for Keratin Expression

Careful examination of keratin expression patterns of most epithelia has revealed consistent trends or "rules" that appear to dictate keratin synthesis. These rules were used to develop a unifying model for most, if not all, mammalian keratins.[68] At least one member of each keratin subfamily is expressed in all epithelial tissues.[59,60,66,69] Terminally differentiating epithelial cells appear to express type I and type II keratin partners in balanced ratios so as not to disrupt intermediate filament formation.[70] Part of the unifying model of keratin expression proposed by Sun et al.[68] illustrated the close resemblance of the two keratin subfamilies in terms of their relative size distributions. The size differential between the smallest and largest members within each subfamily in humans is approximately 15 to 16 kDa. Keratins having identical size rankings between subfamilies were coexpressed as preferred keratin pairs. It had also been noticed by Sun et al.[68] that the type II partner in a coordinately expressed keratin pair was always larger than its type I counterpart, most often by an allowance of 7 to 11 kDa. The functional significance of these results is unclear at the present, but they may possibly explain the evolution of complex epithelia derived from primitive simple epithelia, as recapitulated during embryonic development of the epidermis.[68] Direct relationships between epithelial cell types (stratified versus simple), and their specific programs of differentiation (keratinization versus nonkeratinization), and the coexpression of preferred keratin pairs was realized.[68] All stratified epithelia, and cell cultures derived therefrom, express in varying degrees the keratin "pair" K5 and K14 (K5-K14), which are known to be keratinocyte-specific markers.[66] Highly proliferative stratified epithelia, found in sites of epidermal diseases, keratinocyte cultures, or regenerating corneal epithelium, express K6-K16, and K17 as markers for hyperproliferation.[71] However, others have suggested that the expression of the keratin K6-K16 pair during rapid cell growth is not directly linked with DNA synthesis.[71] Corneal-, esophageal-, skin-, and palm-and-sole-type programs of differentiation all have their own characteristic sets of coordinately expressed keratin pairs.[31,60,68]

While a single cell-layered epithelium is considered simple in terms of tissue design, it also reflects simple patterns of keratin expression.[60,66,72] Characteristically, simple epithelia, like those found in the small intestine and colon, synthesize the smallest existing keratins known from each subfamily, the 52-kDa keratin 8 (K8) (type II) and its type I partners, the 40-kDa keratin 19 (K19) and the 45-kDa keratin 18 (K18).[68] According to immunoblot studies, K7, a 54-kDa type II cytokeratin, displayed a restricted distribution among simple epithelial cells such as glandular and mesothelial epithelial cells.[60] Carcinomas derived from simple epithelia most often reflect keratin expression profiles very similar to their normal tissue counterparts.[69] Only the K8-K18 pair, however, has been considered the simple epithelial-specific marker.[68]

Assembly of Keratin Intermediate Filaments

By defining the requirements necessary for 10-nm keratin filament formation, we may arrive at a fuller understanding of their structure and function. However, the mechanisms contributing to filament assembly are complex and not yet completely understood. The sequence of events leading to higher-order structures, such as protofilaments (2- to 3-nm diameter) and protofibrils (4.5-nm diameter) and 10-nm intermediate filaments, is essentially unknown.

While other classes of intermediate filaments (vimentin, desmin, etc.) are formed from homopolymers, cytokeratin filaments require the presence of equimolar amounts of type I and type II keratins in vitro.[73,74] The basic subunit of these obligatory heteropolymers is a coiled-coil heterodimer aligned parallel and in register.[74–77] Heterodimers, composed of keratins K5 and K14, appeared to be arranged in an anti-parallel and unstaggered manner in tetramers.[76] However, there remains some controversy as to the actual keratin orientation in tetramers.

The early steps in filament formation appear to first quickly form heterodimers and then heterotetramers as the most stable building block of intermediate filaments. The coexistence of a number of distinct higher-ordered structures, under very strong denaturing conditions, indicates that several associations take place at the same time.[76] Proteolytic fragments of keratins that retain their central rod domain can still assemble into heterotypic oligomers, but not normal 10-nm filaments.[78] This suggests that the rod domain is capable of lower-ordered structure assembly but not regular filament formation. Carboxy-tailless mutants of keratins have been shown to assemble into regular intermediate filaments in vitro, and in transfected mouse 3T3-L1 cells.[75,79] Interestingly, tailless mutants of type I and type II keratins were found to accumulate as intermediate filament bundles, not only in the cytoplasm, but also in the nucleus.[79] This report also demonstrated that the amino-headless keratin mutants transfected into 3T3-L1 cells were expressed and localized in the cytoplasm, but did not form intermediate filaments. The data collected from these studies indicate that the amino-terminal extensions of keratins are necessary for proper filament formation. Additionally, the carboxy-tail extension appears required for correct cytoplasmic localization. Site-directed mutagenesis of the consensus motif found at the end of coil 2b domain in all intermediate filaments demonstrated that tetramer formation was unaffected.[80] However, these mutant keratins assembled into large, dense aggregates instead of regular intermediate filaments. These results suggest that this particular consensus sequence is necessary for proper filament formation. A 20-residue peptide, whose sequence represents the consensus sequence of the carboxy-terminal end of coil 2b of the rod domain, when added in a large molar excess, was shown to inhibit keratin filament formation, and disassemble pre-existing filaments.[81] It was suggested also that this consensus sequence is essential for instructing proper filament alignment and stabilization of adjacent tetramers and/or protofilaments.

A number of skin-blistering diseases have been shown to express keratin polypeptide mutants. Two distinct mutations were observed in the carboxy-terminal consensus motif at the end of the coil 2b segment of the rod domain in keratins K1 and K5.[82,83] A mutation found at the junction of the amino-head extension region and the coil 1a segment of the rod domain of keratin K10 was observed in another patient afflicted by a skin-blistering disease.[83] The results from these studies demonstrate that these keratin mutations cause severe perturbations in keratin filament assembly that lead to cytolysis, and release of the epidermis from its substratum. These studies were the first to provide strong evidence that the primary function of intact keratin intermediate filament networks is to provide mechanical stability to epidermal cells.

Post-translational Modifications of Cytokeratins

Cytokeratins undergoing postsynthetic modifications have been recognized since the early 1980s. At this time the best-characterized post-translational modification of keratins appears to be their phosphorylation.[84-88] The functional role(s) of cytokeratin phosphorylation is not well understood, but the phosphorylation of cytokeratins,[85] in addition to vimentin,[89] desmin,[90] neurofilaments,[91] and nuclear lamins,[92] appears to be important in controlling their organization in cells, especially during mitosis.

There is evidence that cytokeratins, unlike other intermediate filaments, may not be as stable as originally envisioned, as suggested by the acrylamide-regulated aggregation of keratin filaments in cultured PtK1 cells, possibly due to their dephosphorylation.[93] Normal keratin filament organization is restored upon removal of acrylamide, concomitant with rephosphorylation of keratins. These results indicate that the phosphorylation status of keratins can drastically modulate their cellular organization. Another study provided evidence that phorbol acetate stimulation of protein kinase C (PKC) may enhance the phosphorylation of keratins K8 and K18 in HT-29 cells.[94] Biochemic and immunologic data demonstrated that keratins K8 and K18 in these cells are physically associated with, and phosphorylated (in a calcium-independent manner) by, a 40-kDa catalytic subunit of PKC ε-related kinase.[88] The functional significance of this process is, however, still unclear.

Metabolic labeling studies in which the human colonic tumor cell line HT-29 was treated with [^{3}H]glucosamine demonstrated that cytokeratins K8 and K18 are glycosylated at several sites with single O-linked N-acetylglucosamine molecules.[95] A relatively greater turnover rate of the O-linked N-acetylglucosamine moieties associated with keratins K8 and K18 suggests a possible active functional role(s).[95] It was speculated that glycosylation may block serine/threonine phosphorylation on these keratins. Limited proteolysis has been recognized as another form of post-translational modification typical of cytokeratins.[96-98] Rat intestinal brushborder cytokeratins separated by two-dimensional gel electrophoresis demonstrated limited proteolysis of keratin K8 (component A), whose derived subfragments were identified by immunoblotting.[96] The functional significance of cytokeratin proteolysis is currently unknown. It might function as a basic mechanism for turning over the steady state level of keratins.

Regulation of Cytokeratin Gene Expression

In order to guarantee tissue- and cell type–specific expression, there must be highly coordinated and tightly regulated mechanisms controlling the precise expression patterns of keratin genes. Differentially regulated keratin mRNAs of different epithelia are derived from distinct genes.[61,62] The regulatory elements that help control keratin gene expression are gradually being elucidated. Therefore, it is essential to determine the molecular mechanisms that regulate the expression of these genes if we are to understand how committed programs of differentiation arise, particularly in the intestine. Two recent reports revealed a number of possible regulatory elements in the mouse gene that encodes the equivalent of human keratin K8.[99,100] A CpG dinucleotide cluster region located around the first exon of the mouse keratin K8 gene appears to be hypomethylated in PYS-2 endodermal cells. Retinoic acid-treated F9 embryonic carcinoma cells express this gene while BALB-C 3T3 cells, which are devoid of keratin K8 gene expression, exhibit a hypermethylation state in these CpG clusters. The correlation between the state of methylation and keratin K8 expression strongly suggests that a general gene regulatory mechanism is operative. Whether this type of gene regulation is widespread among all keratin genes is not known. Other potential cis-regulatory sequences associated with the keratin K8 gene, including polyoma enhancer motifs (PEA1 and PEA3) and AP-1 elements have been shown to exist.[100] A 31 downstream enhancer element, homologous to the PEA3 motif of the polyoma virus alpha enhancer core, was found to activate the mouse keratin K8 gene promoter.[101] These findings indicate that one of the possible regulatory mechanisms controlling mouse keratin K8 gene expression is a 31bp downstream enhancer.

Several studies have shown that molecular mechanisms involved in simple epithelial keratin gene regulation can be influenced by exogenous factors in vitro. Retinoic acid promotes differentiation and enhances the expression of simple epithelial keratins K8 and K18 in F9 cells.[99,102,103] Retinoid-mediated transcriptional activity of keratin K7, K8, K18, and K19 was enhanced in cultured simple epithelial cells of embryonic mesodermal origin, such as human mesothelial LP9 cells[104] and potoroo kidney PtK2 cells.[105] Retinoids in the presence of intercellular interactions were shown to be essential in enhancing keratin transcription as well as an epithelioid morphology in LP-9 cells.[104]

Previous work has shown that dexamethasone in the presence of insulin selectively stimulates keratin K8 and K18 synthesis in cultured rat hepatocytes. After a 48-hour exposure to insulin and dexamethasone, EGF administration first caused rapid and selective phosphorylation of keratin K8, then a rearrangement of K8-K18 filaments, followed by synthesis of DNA several hours later in cultured rat hepatocytes.[106] EGF appears to have a direct affect on cytokeratin post-translational modification and organization in cultured rat hepatocytes. From these results it was proposed that phosphorylation of K8 and subsequent rearrangement of K8-containing filaments are part of the cascade of events prior to DNA synthesis in EGF-stimulated rat hepatocytes. Thyroid hormone, triiodothyronine (T3), has been demonstrated to induce the expression of the 63-kDa keratin gene during Xenopus laevis development in vitro and in vivo in a two-step process.[107,108] Initial activation of the 63-kDa keratin genes does not appear to depend on T3, but high-level expression following activation does. Larval epidermal cells of Xenopus laevis treated for 4 days with T3 produced a nine-fold increase in the abundance of the 63-kDa keratin mRNA, while T3 plus hydrocortisone (HC) stimulated it 18-fold.[109] These results suggest a synergistic effect of T3 and HC on keratin expression at the level of the mRNA. Only sparse evidence is available to demonstrate that extracellular matrix components can direct specific changes in keratin expression in cultured mesothelial[110] and conjunctival[111] cells. For example, K12, the corneal-specific type I keratin, is expressed in conjunctival cells that are maintained on a corneal substrate in the presence of a basement membrane.

INTESTINAL CYTOKERATINS: COMPOSITION AND DISTRIBUTION

The cellular organization of intestinal IFs and their keratin composition were first analyzed biochemically by Franke's group, which identified K8, K18, and K19 as their main components.[3,6] This seminal study stressed the importance of IFs in the structural organization of absorptive villus cells and in providing a link with desmosomal junctions, similar to what had been observed in most other "simple" epithelia. Evidence for significant differences in keratin composition among intestinal cell types, and their potential association with cell differentiation, was first obtained by immunofluorescence staining with a panel of monoclonal antikeratin antibodies, four of which (RK4, CaCo3-28, RK7, RK5) were found to be specific, respectively, for K8, K18, K19, and a newly identified member of the type I keratin subfamily.[7] Screening of an intestinal cDNA library with these monoclonal antibodies (mAbs) provided conclusive evidence for the identity of the cytokeratins recognized, and led to the molecular characterization of K21, a keratin primarily expressed in the GI epithelium.[8] This new keratin was later found to be the rat homolog of human K20, for which only very limited sequence information had been previously provided.[112] Thus, K20 and K21 are now recognized as products of the same gene, leading to their designation as K20-21.

Indirect immunofluorescence staining of intestinal frozen sections has demonstrated interesting compositional differences in keratin IFs along the CV axis in small intestine, and between crypt and surface epithelium in the large intestine, that are illustrated in Figures 4-1 and 4-2. In both segments of intestine all epithelial cells were stained with mAbs specific for K8 and K19. Surprisingly, K18 (the most common K8

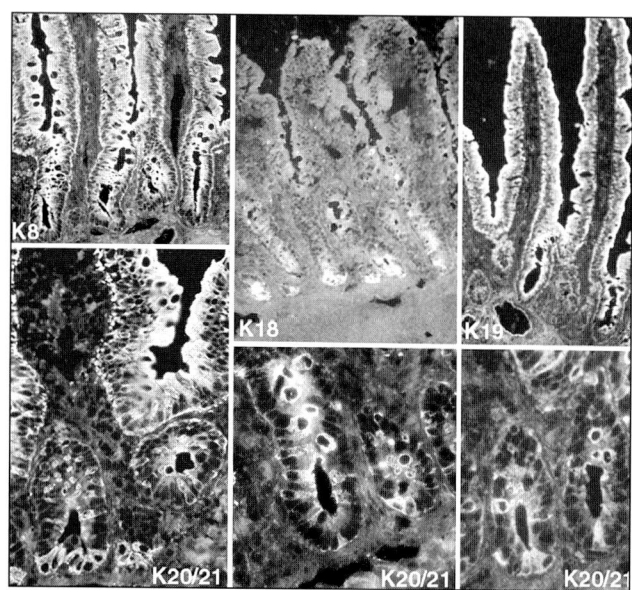

FIGURE 4-1. Distribution of cytokeratins in adult rat small intestine. Frozen sections were fixed with 2% formaldehyde and stained by the double-label immunofluorescence technique with monoclonal antibodies RK4 (specific for cytokeratin K8), RK5 (specific for cytokeratin K20-21), CaCo3-28 (specific for cytokeratin K18), and RK7 (specific for cytokeratin K19).

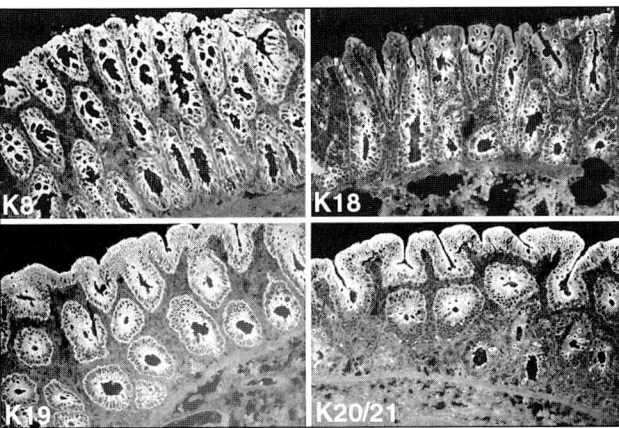 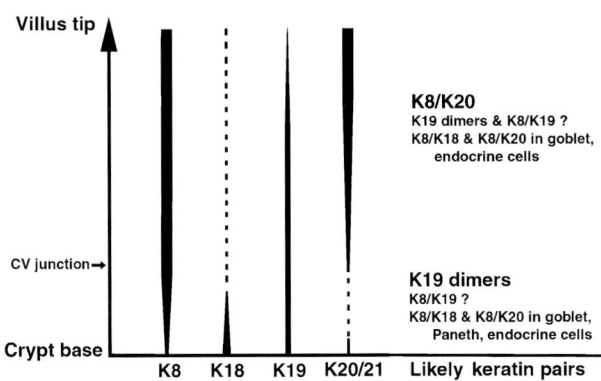

FIGURE 4–2. Cytokeratin expression in adult rat colon. Frozen sections were fixed with 2% formaldehyde and stained by the double-label immunofluorescence technique with monoclonal antibodies RK4 (specific for cytokeratin K8), RK5 (specific for cytokeratin K20-21), CaCo3-28 (specific for cytokeratin K18), and RK7 (specific for cytokeratin K19).

FIGURE 4–3. Changes in cytokeratin expression along the CV axis in adult rat small intestine. Thickness of the bands is meant to convey a relative semiquantitative evaluation of the cellular concentration of each keratin subunit. Dotted lines represent expression only in selected cell types (K18 in Paneth's, enteroendocrine, goblet cells, but not proliferative crypt cells and absorptive villus cells; K20-21 only in differentiated cell types in the crypts). Likely keratin pairs present in crypt or villus cells are listed to the right.

partner in most "simple" epithelia) was found not to be present in absorptive villus cells (see Figure 4–1) or in surface colonic epithelial cells (see Figure 4–2), its distribution being restricted to Paneth's and enteroendocrine cells in the small intestine, and to most crypt cells in the colon. In contrast, K20-21 was localized exclusively in the differentiated intestinal cells, including the absorptive and goblet cells present on the villi, and Paneth's, goblet, and endocrine cells in the crypts (see Figure 4–1). Interestingly, while staining for K8 and K20-21 in absorptive villus cells was localized primarily at the periphery of the cells (luminal, lateral, and basal aspects), the same cells stained for K19 showed in addition a fibrillar pattern in the central regions of the cells' cytoplasm. This indicates that cytokeratin filaments of different composition may coexist in such cells, including filaments composed of K19 alone, or with a different partner from K8.[7] Biochemical analysis performed by two-dimensional slab gel electrophoresis and Western blot[7] confirmed the existence of important compositional differences between keratin IFs present in crypt and villus cells. In villus fractions, K8 (present as two major isoelectric variants) was the most abundant, and K20-21 was identified as two spots differing both in Mr and pI, indicative of extensive post-translational processing. In crypt cell fractions, K19 far surpassed K8 in abundance, and K20-21 was either absent or produced a very faint spot, consistent with its expression only in goblet, Paneth's, and enteroendocrine cells. (Cells analyzed were from the rat proximal jejunum, where Paneth's cells are least abundant.) These results are summarized in a diagram in Figure 4–3, where the likely subunit composition of keratin heterodimers in CV cells is indicated. Taken together, these findings imply that keratin gene expression is surprisingly well-regulated during differentiation of the adult intestinal epithelium, and the presence of keratin tonofilaments of distinct composition may be crucial for the proper function of different cell types.

Examination of the distribution of intestinal keratin mRNAs by in situ hybridization provided evidence for a primary regulation of keratin gene expression at the transcriptional level, with the important exception of K19.[113] The radioactive K8 riboprobe led to deposition of silver grains in epithelial cells along the entire CV axis, but the intensity of the stain was much greater in the crypts and in the lower villus regions, declining markedly toward the tips of the villi. This is in accordance with the marked decline in mRNA synthesis and overall mRNA levels in differentiated intestinal cells after leaving the lower regions of the villi.[114] Some cells in the lamina propria, most likely smooth muscle cells, also appeared to transcribe some K8 mRNA. This finding appears to confirm reports demonstrating low-level expression of simple epithelial keratins in smooth muscle cells from various tissues.[115,116] With the K21 riboprobe a strong signal was only observed starting at the top of the crypts, where differentiated cells are known to be first produced. Although the intensity of the reaction decreased slightly toward the tips of the villi, this gradient of mRNA abundance was not as pronounced as that observed with the K8 riboprobe. The K18 riboprobe localized its corresponding mRNA exclusively in the region of the crypts, and the intensity of the deposition of silver grains was strongest at the bottom of the crypts, in accordance with the immunofluorescence staining pattern for K18 (see Figure 4–1). Surprisingly, in situ hybridization using the K19 riboprobe led to staining only in the region of the crypts, in clear contrast with the corresponding K19 protein distribution over the entire intestinal epithelium (see Figures 4–1 and 4–2). This indicates that differentiated villus cells do not transcribe K19 mRNA, or rapidly degrade it, and likely are not synthesizing significant amounts of K19 protein. These findings provide strong evidence for a negative transcriptional control mechanism repressing K19 gene expression in villus cells, and suggest that the K19-containing IFs detected in these cells are primarily inherited from the proliferative crypt cells from which they originated.

EARLY INTESTINAL DEVELOPMENT AND CHANGES IN CYTOKERATIN EXPRESSION

Villus Formation during Fetal Development

The last 7 days of a 21- to 22-day gestational period of the fetal rat are marked by rapid and complex intestinal tissue remodeling and processes leading to the formation of true villi. The sequence of structural changes during fetal rat growth has been reported in detail.[10,11,117,118] At day 13, the epithelium consists of a highly undifferentiated single cell layer. This subsequently undergoes stratification into six to eight cell layers during the next 4 days. By day 17, the initial sign of villus formation appears: the presence of secondary lumina. These are small gaps formed between adjacent stratified epithelial cells that exhibit numerous microvilli at their surface. Villus formation is even more evident on day 18, and is characterized by an increase in the number and size of secondary lumina, their fusion with the main lumen to properly orient the villus axis,[118] elaborate rearrangement of junctional complexes,[119] upward growth of the surrounding mesenchyme toward the lumen to become the presumptive lamina propria,[118] the formation of the brushborder on the apical aspect of luminal cells,[11] and the expression of new brushborder enzymes.[120,121]

Cytodifferentiation becomes apparent on day 19 when absorptive cells, characterized by numerous and well-organized microvilli, are interspersed by highly developed enteroendocrine cells.[118] Only partially differentiated goblet cells are present at this time. By day 20, a well-developed terminal web underlies a functional microvillus membrane and cytoskeletal core in the absorptive villus cells. At approximately days 21 to 22, despite the lack of crypts of Lieberkühn, the epithelium establishes a restricted region of proliferation which is now found predominantly among those epithelial cells lining the bottom third of each villus.[122] Early reports first recognized that morphogenic processes of the intestinal epithelium generally follow a temporal-spatial gradient created along the anteroposterior axis of the intestine.[10,117,123] For example, the initial appearance of forming villi in the duodenum (day 18) precedes that found in the ileum (days 19 to 20). Later reports further defined regional biochemic differences in brushborder enzymatic activities of the fetal mouse[124] and guinea pig.[125] These data strongly suggest that biochemic differences occurring during fetal intestinal development are highly coordinated with morphogenesis of this tissue. Regional differences established in the fetus have been shown to persist along the proximal-to-distal axis of the adult intestine.[126] It seems likely that development of the intestine depends on a gradient of morphogenic signals, not yet identified, that are generated, at least in part, by surrounding cells that probably bring about changes in epithelial cell gene expression.

Crypt Formation

The timing of crypt formation during development differs among various species. In humans, primordial crypts are first observed between weeks 11 and 12 of gestation. They become well-developed by the end of the twelfth week of gestation.[127] In rats and mice the crypts form from cells lining the intervillous region within the first week after birth.[118] There appear to be regional differences with regard to the initial appearance of crypts along the proximal-distal axis. Crypt formation first appears in the duodenum, then about 1 week later in the ileum of human fetuses.[127]

Keratin Expression

Expression and distribution of intermediate filaments composed of cytokeratins K8, K19, and K20-21 during pre- and postnatal development of rat intestine were studied by immunofluorescence staining with the keratin-type specific mAbs RK4, RK7, and RK5, respectively,[128] and the key results obtained are illustrated in Figures 4–4 and 4–5. Around 15 dg, when a stratified undifferentiated epithelium is present, the most intense staining of the epithelium was observed with RK7, specific for K19 (see Figure 4–4); staining for K8 was also observed, but it was considerably weaker. Biochemical analysis, performed by two-dimensional slab gel electrophoresis and immunoblotting[128] confirmed and extended these results: in samples of water-insoluble filaments obtained from total fetal intestines at days 16 to 18, K19 (present as two to three isoelectric variants) was by far the most abundant cytokeratin. Expression of K20-21 was first observed by immunofluorescence staining at days 17 to 18 (see Figure 4–4), depending on the location of the segment of intestine along the proximal-distal axis; biochemically, two to three K20-21 isoelectric variants were first detected at day 18, reaching maximal expression by days 20 to 21.[128] At the same time, the relative abundance of K8 increased markedly, becoming the most abundant keratin species. Immediately after birth the total cytokeratin pattern on two-dimensional blots increased dramatically in complexity, a clear sign of extensive post-translational modifications, likely including phosphorylation, glycosylation, and proteolytic processing-degradation, most evident in K8- and K19-related polypeptides.[128]

Northern blot analysis of the corresponding cytokeratin mRNAs, including K18, and in situ hybridization with riboprobes, extended the immunofluorescence and blotting data. Low but comparable levels of K8 and K19 mRNAs were

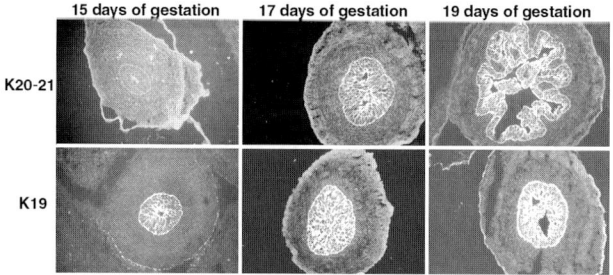

FIGURE 4–4. Expression and cellular distribution of keratins K19 and K20-21 in rat small intestine during fetal development. Frozen sections were fixed with 2% formaldehyde and stained by the double-label immunofluorescence technique with monoclonal antibodies RK5 (specific for cytokeratin K20-21) and RK7 (specific for cytokeratin K19).

detected at day 16,[128] and were localized over the entire epithelium.[113] This was in partial contrast with the results obtained by two-dimensional gel analysis of cytoskeletal proteins obtained from the same tissue, in which K19 was present in much larger amounts than K8. This finding is evidence for regulation of keratin polypeptides expression, already at this stage of intestinal development, at the post-transcriptional level or by differential degradation. The K18 mRNA was detected in significant amounts at day 16 (the earliest group of specimens obtained in sufficient amounts for Northern blot), and increased markedly in abundance toward the end of the gestational period. Soon after birth, K18 mRNA started to decline rapidly in abundance, to become barely detectable in adult intestinal specimens.[128] The K20-21 mRNA was first detected by Northern blot at day 18. Underscoring the initial cytodifferentiation of the intestinal epithelium toward the end of gestation, after formation of the villi (at day 20) K8 and K20-21 mRNAs were expressed by the entire epithelium, whereas K18 and K19 mRNAs were localized to the cells present at the base of the villi.[113] Such a differential expression of keratin genes, essentially identical to that observed along the CV axis in adult intestine[113] is remarkable, considering that discernible crypts are not present until after birth. It represents the clearest evidence for the importance of proper intermediate filaments formation to the function of proliferative and differentiated intestinal epithelial cells. It should be noted that the localization of K19 mRNA specifically at the base of the forming fetal villi represents the earliest reported sign of spatial cellular specialization in the development of the intestinal epithelium: markers of differentiation such as lactase, maltase, or aminopeptidase N were detected over the entire epithelium until day 20.[128] This finding also indicates that synthesis of new K19 is incompatible with the organization or function of differentiated intestinal cells, to the point that K19 gene transcription is inhibited and previously transcribed mRNA is rapidly degraded as soon as the cells start to differentiate.

Summarizing these data (see Figure 4–5), the cytokeratin expression patterns observed during fetal development of the rat small intestine parallel closely the process of differentiation in adult tissue. The K19, being by far the major component detected at the biochemical level during the earliest stages of development (and in the adult crypt cells), must have been able to form homodimers, since it was found in water-insoluble cytoskeletal filaments extensively extracted with detergents and low-high salt solutions. The K19 expression has been observed in several other simple and stratified epithelia, but never as the major type I keratin present.[60] Normally, unpaired type I or type II keratins are not synthesized in considerable quantities,[70] do not incorporate appreciably into pre-existing keratin filaments, and are rapidly degraded by proteolytic enzymes.[98,129–132] In contrast, the unbalanced expression of K19 in the undifferentiated intestinal epithelium appeared to be stable, without signs of extensive degradation. It should be noted, however, that K19 differs from all other IF proteins because of the absence of a globular tail domain, replaced by a continuation of the α-helical character through a short stretch of 13 amino acids.[133] It has been suggested that its primary role may be to correct type I-type II imbalances,[134] potentially

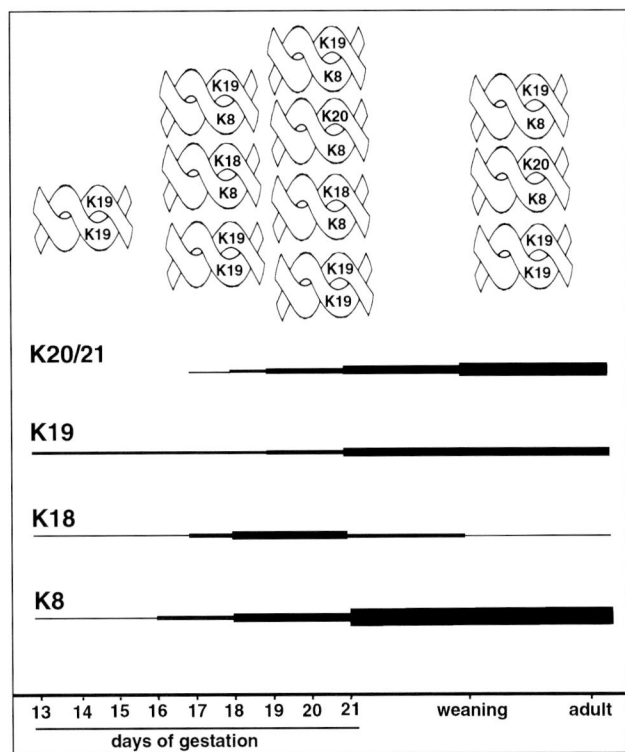

FIGURE 4–5. Changes in cytokeratin expression during fetal and postnatal development of rat small intestine. Thickness of the bands is meant to convey a relative semiquantitative evaluation of the cellular concentration of each keratin subunit. Major keratin pairs expressed at key developmental stages are indicated at the top of the figure.

resulting in the formation of short polymers. While in vitro studies have been unable to demonstrate qualitative differences between filaments formed with keratin pairs K8-K18 and K8-K19, in living cells the network formed by K8-K18 was morphologically superior to the irregular and discontinuous one formed by K8 and K19.[135] Such differences may be vitally important in cells characterized by continuous and rapid growth, such as early fetal intestinal cells and adult crypt cells. It can be concluded that, within such rapidly dividing cells, the form in which keratin IFs are organized may be under special constraints, and require the presence of relatively short or incomplete filaments that can be, at least partially, disassembled when the cells divide.

Even though the fetal intestinal epithelium undergoes a short period of stratification, it does not express cytokeratin patterns typical of other stratified epithelia. By ensuring a continuation of simple epithelial cytokeratin patterns expressed in the stratified epithelium of the fetal rat intestine, this tissue might secure a committed pathway leading to a simple differentiated epithelial phenotype. Alternatively, stabilization of the stratified epithelial phenotype might require, at least in part, those patterns of keratins characteristic of other stratified epithelia, such as the epidermis, and thus be incompatible with the subsequent maturation of the intestine.

Regulation of K20-21 expression appears to be primarily at the level of gene transcription, since its protein and mRNA patterns were similar in adult[113] and in fetal[128] rat intestine. In the absorptive villus cells of the adult rat, and in the upper villus cells of the developing fetal intestine around day 20, expression of K20-21 and of K18 appeared to be inversely related, so that in the adult, K18 mRNA was exclusively detected in the region of the crypts and the protein was specifically localized in the Paneth's, enteroendocrine, and goblet cells.[113] Since all differentiated intestinal cells originate from the same immortal stem cell, this finding suggests that K18 gene transcription is specifically suppressed in cells that become committed to the absorptive cell lineage in adult intestine, but not in the differentiated cells present during late gestation and the first 1 to 2 weeks after birth (see Figure 4–5). It should be noted that the absorptive villus cells are the only ones to display a well-organized brush-border and terminal web, and that the other differentiated intestinal cell types coexpress K18 and K20-21. It appears likely, therefore, that for the function and/or structural organization of the absorptive cells, the presence of K20-21 and the absence of K18 are equally important, possibly because as these cells differentiate they require the assembly of new keratin filaments exclusively formed by the K8-K20 heterodimer. The timely activation of the K20-21 gene during fetal development when the brushborder cytoskeleton, and in particular the terminal web, are first assembled is strong indication for a potential specific function of this keratin subunit in the organization of the apical cytoplasmic network. At the same time in the rat, and at comparable stages of development in chicks and mice, other important cytoskeletal proteins (such as villin, BB myosin I, spectrin, caldesmon, and TW 260-240) have been found to appear, or to undergo significant changes in cellular distribution.[12–14,21] Keratin filaments composed of K8 and K20-21 may provide a crucial link between actin-based microvillar cores, the terminal web filaments, and intermediate filaments that are interwoven with them.

CONCLUSION AND ISSUES FOR FUTURE INVESTIGATION

Intestinal epithelial cells undergo elaborate structural and functional changes while they mature so that they can optimize nutrient digestion and absorption. Paramount in helping establish and maintain these changes is the presence of complex systems of cytoskeletal proteins, especially those found associated with the actin-based cytoskeleton that facilitates luminal brushborder formation. Many of the major brushborder cytoskeletal proteins have been identified, and are well-characterized in terms of their biochemical function. Cytokeratin intermediate filaments are produced in relatively large amounts by intestinal epithelial cells. In these cells, cytokeratin-containing filaments organize as a complex, dense meshwork at the base of the brushborder, along the cortical cytoplasm of the lateral membrane, interconnecting spot desmosomes, and as a concentrated population in the basal cytoplasm, presumably associated with adhesive proteins.

The primary function of cytokeratins was clearly illustrated in the epidermis, based on mutational studies and investigation of naturally-occurring diseases caused by keratin gene alterations. Properly assembled cytokeratin networks are required to protect the integrity of the tissue and provide mechanical stability of its constituent cells by preventing tissue detachment from the extracellular matrix. Cytokeratin filaments are believed to perform similar functions in differentiated intestinal epithelial cells, but direct evidence is still lacking, and this represents a major area of future investigation.

The work done to date has identified and characterized the major keratin gene products expressed in the intestine, their differentiation, and developmentally regulated changes in their expression and organization. There is also limited evidence that turnover of cytokeratin mRNAs and polypeptides may be important in their proper function in intestinal cells. The complexity of keratin-related polypeptides detected on two-dimensional gels, particularly in samples from adult CV cells, has been interpreted as evidence for extensive post-translational modification involving phosphorylation and partial proteolysis; but their physiologic role (if any) in the intestine has yet to be addressed.

Because expression of specific cytokeratin genes has been found to be highly regulated during maturation and differentiation of intestinal epithelial cells, it is likely that each cytokeratin has a distinctive function(s). Only one type II cytokeratin, K8, has been detected in the intestinal epithelium, and its marked increase in abundance between day 15 and birth (and with differentiation at the CV junction in adult intestine) is likely to accommodate corresponding increases in the amounts of type I keratin subunits, so that proper heteropolymer filament assembly can rapidly take place as the epithelium grows in overall size. Its primary type I partners, K18 or K19 in fetal and crypt cells, and K20-21 in adult villus cells, should contribute subtle but potentially important differences in filament length, stability, and function. A key unresolved issue is the nature of the link between keratin tonofilaments and actin-based microvillar rootlets described by SEM in the terminal web of the villus cells. It is generally assumed that specificity and function of different keratin gene products is largely dictated by their amino- and carboxyterminal globular extensions; and here is where the importance of the intestine-specific K20-21 may reside. The timing of its expression during fetal maturation, and with differentiation of absorptive villus cells, indicates that this type I cytokeratin may play a crucial role in organization and assembly of the terminal web; but no direct evidence for such a function has been obtained to date.

K19, the most abundant cytokeratin subunit in early fetal cells and in proliferative crypt cells, appears to play a special role in the intestine. Its very tight regulation, and its unique nature (absence of a true carboxyterminal globular extension), with the potential to form short homopolymeric filaments, may be crucial to the rapid renewal rate of such cells.

A surprising feature of the intestinal epithelium is the apparently minor role played by K18-containing keratin filaments. The K8-K18 heterodimers represent by far the most common intermediate filament component in most other "simple" epithelia and in cultured epithelial cells. Instead, in the intestine they are expressed in significant amounts only during a short period of development: in the rat, from 17 to 18 days of gestation to weaning. Thereafter, K8-K18 dimers are rigorously excluded from absorptive villus cells, while present in Paneth's, enteroendocrine, and at least some goblet cells. In the large intestine, K18 is distributed over the entire crypts, but absent in the surface epithelium. Such a tightly regulated expression, that must include selective degradation of K18 filaments as colonic crypt cells reach the surface, is likely to have an important physiologic function.

Future studies will be essential to fully characterize the nature of the molecular mechanisms controlling intestinal keratin gene expression if we are to understand how committed programs of cellular differentiation arise in intestinal epithelial cells. Identification and characterization of the cis- and trans-acting factors that govern developmental-, regional-, and cell type–specific expression of intestinal cytokeratins will be important not only to reveal regulatory mechanisms that specifically affect the intestine, but also those that might affect a wide range of tissues.

REFERENCES

1. Cheng H, Leblond CP. Origin, differentiation and renewal of the four main epithelial cell types in the mouse small intestine. I. Columnar cell. Am J Anat 1974;141:461–80.
2. Mooseker MS. Organization, chemistry, and assembly of the cytoskeletal apparatus of the intestinal brush border. Annu Rev Cell Dev Biol 1985;1:209–41.
3. Franke WW, Winter S, Grund C, et al. Isolation and characterization of desmosome-associated tonofilaments from rat intestinal brush border. J Cell Biol 1981;90:116–27.
4. Trier JS. Studies on small intestinal crypt epithelium. I. The fine structure of the crypt epithelium of the proximal small intestine of fasting humans. J Cell Biol 1963;18:599–620.
5. Fath KR, Obenauf SD, Burgess DR. Cytoskeletal protein and mRNA accumulation during brush border formation in adult chicken enterocytes. Development 1990;109:449–59.
6. Franke WW, Appelhans B, Schmid C, et al. The organization of cytokeratin filaments in the intestinal epithelium. Eur J Cell Biol 1979;19:255–68.
7. Quaroni A, Calnek D, Quaroni E, et al. Keratin expression in rat intestinal crypt and villus cells. Analysis with a panel of monoclonal antibodies. J Biol Chem 1991;266:11923–31.
8. Chandler JS, Calnek D, Quaroni A. Identification and characterization of rat intestinal keratins. J Biol Chem 1991;266: 11932–8.
9. Heintzelman MB, Mooseker MS. Assembly of the brush border cytoskeleton: changes in the distribution of microvillar core proteins during enterocyte differentiation in adult chicken intestine. Cell Motil Cytoskeleton 1990;15:12–22.
10. Kammeraad A. The development of the gastrointestinal tract of the rat. I. Histogenesis of the epithelium of the stomach, small intestine and pancreas. J Morphol 1942;70:323–51.
11. Dunn S. The fine structure of the absorptive epithelial cells of the developing small intestine of the rat. J Anat 1967;101:57–67.
12. Shibayama T, Carboni JM, Mooseker MS. Assembly of the intestinal brush border: appearance and redistribution of microvillar core proteins in developing chick enterocytes. J Cell Biol 1987;105:355–44.
13. Ezzell RM, Chafel MM, Matsudaira PT. Differential localization of villin and fimbrin during development of the mouse visceral endoderm and intestinal epithelium. Development 1989;106:407–19.
14. Maunoury R, Robine S, Prignault E, et al. Villin expression in the visceral endoderm and in the gut anlage during early mouse embryogenesis. EMBO J 1988;7:3321–9.
15. Chambers C, Grey RD. Development of the structural components of the brush border in absorptive cells of the chick intestine. Cell Tissue Res 1979;204:387–405.
16. Stidwell RP, Burgess DR. Regulation of intestinal brush border microvillus length during development by the G- to F-actin ratio. Dev Biol 1986;114:381–8.
17. Madara JL, Trier JS. Functional morphology of the mucosa of the small intestine. In: Johnson LR, editor. Physiology of the gastrointestinal tract. 2nd ed. New York: Raven Press; 1987. p. 1209–51.
18. Trier JS, Rubin CE. Electron microscopy of the small intestine: a review. Gastroenterology 1965;49:574–603.
19. Ito S. The enteric surface coat on cat intestinal microvilli. J Cell Biol 1965;27:475–91.
20. Farquhar MG, Palade GE. Junctional complexes in various epithelia. J Cell Biol 1963;17:375–412.
21. Heintzelman MB, Mooseker MS. Assembly of the intestinal brush border cytoskeleton. Curr Top Dev Biol 1992;26:93–122.
22. Burgess DR. The brush border: a model for structure, biochemistry, motility, and assembly of the cytoskeleton. Adv Cell Biol 1987;1:31–58.
23. Brunser O, Luft JH. Fine structure of the apex of absorptive cells from rat small intestine. J Ultrastr Res 1970;31:291–311.
24. Mukerjee TM, Staehelin LA. The fine structural organization of the brush border of intestinal epithelial cells. J Cell Sci 1971;8:573–99.
25. Paylay SL, Karlin LJ. An electron microscopic study of the intestinal villus. II. The pathway of fat absorption. J Biophys Biochem Cytol 1959;5:373–84.
26. Hull BE, Staehelin LA. The terminal web. A reevaluation of its structure and function. J Cell Biol 1979;81:67–82.
27. Hirokawa N, Tilney LG, Fujiwara K, Heuser JE. Organization of actin, myosin, and intermediate filaments in the brush border of intestinal epithelial cells. J Cell Biol 1982;94:425–43.
28. Hirokawa N, Cheney RE, Willard M. Location of a protein of the fodrin-spectrin-TW260/240 family in the mouse intestinal brush border. Cell 1983;32:953–65.
29. Hirokawa N, Keller III TCS, Chasan R, Mooseker MS. Mechanism of brush border contractility studied by the quick-freeze, deep-etch method. J Cell Biol 1983;96:1325–36.
30. Hirokawa N, Heuser JE. Quick-freeze, deep-etch visualization of the cytoskeleton beneath surface differentiations of intestinal epithelial cells. J Cell Biol 1981;91:399–409.
31. Franke WW, Schiller DL, Moll R, et al. Diversity of cytokeratins: differentiation-specific expression of cytokeratin polypeptides in epithelial cells and tissues. J Mol Biol 1981;153:933–59.
32. Granger B, Baker RF. Electron microscope investigation of the striated border of intestinal epithelium. Anat Rec 1950;107:423–41.
33. Puchtler H, Leblond CP. Histochemical analysis of cell membranes and associated structures as seen in the intestinal epithelium. Am J Anat 1958;102:1–31.
34. McNabb JD, Sandborn E. Filaments in the microvillus border of intestinal cells. J Cell Biol 1964;22:701–4.
35. van Dongen JM, Visser WJ, Daems WT, Galjaard H. The relation between cell proliferation, differentiation and ultrastructural development in rat intestinal epithelium. Cell Tissue Res 1976;174:183–99.
36. Weiser MM. Intestinal epithelial cell surface membrane glycoprotein synthesis. I. An indicator of cellular differentiation. J Biol Chem 1973;248:2536–41.
37. Hopfer U, Nelson K, Perrotto J, Isselbacher KJ. Glucose transport in isolated brush border membranes from rat small intestine. J Biol Chem 1973;248:25–32.
38. Kessler M, Acuto O, Storelli C, et al. A modified procedure for the rapid preparation of efficiently transporting vesicles from small intestinal brush border membranes. Biochim Biophys Acta 1978;506:136–54.

39. Miller D, Crane RK. A procedure for the isolation of the epithelial brush border membrane of hamster small intestine. Anal Biochem 1961;2:284–6.
40. Bretscher A, Weber K. Purification of microvilli and an analysis of the protein components of the microfilament core bundle. Exp Cell Res 1978;116:397–407.
41. Tilney LG, Mooseker MS. Actin in the brush border of epithelial cells of the chicken intestine. Proc Natl Acad Sci U S A 1971;68:2611–5.
42. Mooseker MS, Tilney LG. The organization of an actin filament-membrane complex: filament polarity and membrane attachment in the microvilli of intestinal epithelial cells. J Cell Biol 1975;67:725–43.
43. Matsudaira PT, Burgess DR. Identification and organization of the components in the isolated microvillus cytoskeleton. J Cell Biol 1979;83:667–73.
44. Howe CL, Mooseker MS, Graves TA. Brush-border calmodulin. J Cell Biol 1980;85:916–23.
45. Mooseker MS, Coleman TR. The 110-kD protein-calmodulin complex of the intestinal microvillus (brush border myosin I) is a mechanoenzyme. J Cell Biol 1989;108:2395–400.
46. Hayden SM, Wolenski JS, Mooseker MS. Binding the brush border myosin I to phospholipid vesicles. J Cell Biol 1990;111:443–51.
47. Bretscher A, Weber K. Villin is a major protein of the microvillus cytoskeleton which binds both G- and F-actin in a calcium-dependent manner. Cell 1980;20:839–47.
48. Mooseker MS, Graves TA, Wharton KA, et al. Regulation of microvillus structure: calcium-dependent solation and crosslinking of actin filaments in the microvilli of intestinal epithelial cells. J Cell Biol 1980;87:809–22.
49. Matsudaira PT, Burgess RD. Organization of the cross-filaments in intestinal microvilli. J Cell Biol 1982;92:657–64.
50. Bretscher A. Fimbrin is a cytoskeletal protein that cross-links F-actin in vitro. Proc Natl Acad Sci U S A 1981;78:6849–53.
51. Glenney JR, Kaulfus P, Matsudaira P, Weber K. F-actin binding and bundling properties of fimbrin, a major cytoskeletal protein of the microvillus core filaments. J Biol Chem 1981;256:9283–8.
52. Bretscher A. Purification of an 80K protein that is a component of the isolated microvillus cytoskeleton, and its localization in nonmuscle cells. J Cell Biol 1983;97:425–32.
53. Drenckhahn D, Dermietzel R. Organization of the actin filament cytoskeleton in the intestinal brush border: a quantitative and qualitative immunoelectron microscope study. J Cell Biol 1988;107:1037–48.
54. Coudrier E, Reggio H, Louvard D. Immunolocalization of the 110,000-dalton molecular weight cytoskeletal protein of intestinal microvilli. J Mol Biol 1981;152:49–64.
55. Bretscher A, Lynch W. Identification and localization of immunoreactive forms of caldesmon in smooth and nonmuscle cells: a comparison with the distribution of tropomyosin and alpha-actinin. J Cell Biol 1985;100:1656–63.
56. Stidwell RP, Wysolmerski T, Burgess DR. The brush border cytoskeleton is not static: in vivo turnover of proteins. J Cell Biol 1984;98:641–5.
57. Madara JL, Barenberg D, Carlson S. Effects of cytochalasin D on occluding junctions of intestinal absorptive cells: further evidence that the cytoskeleton may influence paracellular permeability and junctional charge selectivity. J Cell Biol 1986;102:2125–36.
58. Madara JL. Intestinal absorptive cell tight junctions are linked to cytoskeleton. Am J Physiol 1987;253:C171–5.
59. O'Guin WM, Schermer A, Lynch M, Sun TT. Differentiation-specific expression of keratin pairs. In: Goldman RD, Steinert PM, editors. Cellular and molecular biology of intermediate filaments. New York: Plenum Publishing; 1990. p. 301–34.
60. Moll R, Franke WW, Schiller DL, et al. The catalog of human cytokeratins: patterns of expression in normal epithelia, tumors and cultured cells. Cell 1982;31:11–24.
61. Fuchs E, Coppock H, Green H, Cleveland DW. Two distinct classes of keratin genes and their evolutionary significance. Cell 1981;17:75–84.
62. Kim KH, Rheinwald JG, Fuchs E. Tissue specificity of epithelial keratins: differential expression of mRNAs from two multigene families. Mol Cell Biol 1983;3:495–502.
63. Hanokoglu I, Fuchs E. The cDNA sequence of a human epidermal keratin: divergence of sequence but conservation of structure among intermediate filament proteins. Cell 1982;31:243–52.
64. Hanokoglu I, Fuchs E. The cDNA sequence of a type II cytoskeletal keratin reveals constant and variable domains among keratins. Cell 1983;33:915–24.
65. Schiller DL, Franke WW, Geiger B. A subfamily of relatively large and basic cytokeratin polypeptides as defined by peptide mapping is represented by one of several polypeptides in epithelial cells. EMBO J 1982;6:761–9.
66. Tseng SCG, Jarvinen MJ, Nelson WG, et al. Correlation of specific keratins with different types of epithelial differentiation: monoclonal antibody studies. Cell 1982;30:361–72.
67. Eichner R, Bonitz P, Sun TT. Classification of epidermal keratins according to their immunoreactivity, isoelectric point, and mode of expression. J Cell Biol 1984;98:1388–96.
68. Sun TT, Eichner R, Schermer A, et al. Classification, expression, and possible mechanisms of evolution of mammalian epithelial keratins: a unifying model. In: Levine A, Topp W, Vande Woude G, Watson JD, editors. The cancer cell. Vol 1. The transformed phenotype. Cold Spring Harbor (NY): Cold Spring Harbor Symposia; 1984. p. 169–76.
69. Cooper D, Schermer A, Sun TT. Classification of human epithelia and their neoplasms using monoclonal antibodies to keratins: Strategies, applications, and limitations. Lab Invest 1985;52:243–56.
70. Kim KH, Marchuk D, Fuchs E. Expression of unusually large keratin during terminal differentiation: balance of type I and type II is not disrupted. J Cell Biol 1984;99:1872–7.
71. Schermer AJ, Jester V, Hardy C, et al. Transient synthesis of K6 and K16 keratins in regenerating rabbit corneal epithelium: keratin markers for an alternative pathway of keratinocyte differentiation. Differentiation 1989;42:103–10.
72. Leube RE, Bosch FX, Romano V, et al. Cytokeratin expression in simple epithelia. III. Detection of mRNAs encoding human cytokeratins nos. 8 and 18 in normal and tumor cells by hybridization with DNA sequences in vitro and in situ. Differentiation 1986;33:69–85.
73. Franke WW, Schiller DL, Hatzfeld M, Winter S. Protein complexes of intermediate-sized filaments: melting of cytokeratin complexes in urea reveals different polypeptide separation characteristics. Proc Natl Acad Sci U S A 1983;80:7113–7.
74. Hatzfeld M, Franke WW. Pair formation and promiscuity of cytokeratins: formation in vitro of heterotypic complexes and intermediate-sized filaments by homologous and heterologous recombinations of purified polypeptides. J Cell Biol 1985;101:1826–41.
75. Hatzfeld M, Weber K. Tailless keratins assemble into regular intermediate filaments in vitro. J Cell Sci 1990;97:317–24.
76. Coulombe PA, Fuchs E. Elucidating the early stages of keratin filament assembly. J Cell Biol 1990;111:153–69.
77. Steinert PM. The two-chain coiled-coil molecule of native epidermal keratin intermediate filaments is a type I-type II heterodimer. J Biol Chem 1990;265:8766–74.
78. Hatzfeld M, Maier G, Franke WW. Cytokeratin domains involved in heterotypic complex formation determined by in-vitro binding assays. J Mol Biol 1987;197:237–55.

79. Bader BL, Magin TM, Freudenmann M, et al. Intermediate filaments formed de novo from tail-less cytokeratins in the cytoplasm and in the nucleus. J Cell Biol 1991;115:1293–307.
80. Hatzfeld M, Weber K. Modulation of keratin intermediate filament assembly by single amino acid exchanges in the consensus sequence at the C-terminal end of the rod domain. J Cell Sci 1991;99:351–62.
81. Hatzfeld M, Weber K. A synthetic peptide representing the consensus sequence motif at the carboxy-terminal end of the rod domain inhibits intermediate filament assembly and disassembles preformed filaments. J Cell Biol 1992;116:157–66.
82. Lane EB, Rugg EL, Navsaria H, et al. A mutation in the conserved termination peptide of keratin 5 in hereditary skin blistering. Nature 1992;356:244–46.
83. Rothnagel JA, Dominey AM, Dempsey LD, et al. Mutations in the rod domain of keratins I and 10 in epidermolytic hyperkeratosis. Science 1992;257:1128–30.
84. Steinert PM, Wantz ML, Idler WW. 0-Phosphoserine content of intermediate filament subunits. Biochemistry 1982;21:177–83.
85. Celis JE, Larson PM, Fey SJ, Celis A. Phosphorylation of keratin and vimentin polypeptides in normal and transformed mitotic human epithelial amnion cells: behavior of keratin and vimentin filaments during mitosis. J Cell Biol 1983;97:1429–34.
86. Gilmartin ME, Mitchell J, Vidrich A, Freedberg IM. Dual regulation of intermediate phosphorylation. J Cell Biol 1984;98:1144–9.
87. Eckert BS, Yeagle PL. Modulation of keratin intermediate filament distribution in vivo by induced changes in cyclic AMP-dependent phosphorylation. Cell Motil Cytoskeleton 1990;17:291–300.
88. Omary MB, Baxter GT, Chou CF, et al. PKC epsilon-related kinase associates with phosphorylates cytokeratin 8 and 18. J Cell Biol 1992;117:583–93.
89. Inakagi M, Nishi Y, Nishizawa K, et al. Site-specific phosphorylation induces disassembly of vimentin filaments in vitro. Nature 1987;328:649–52.
90. Inakagi M, Gonda Y, Matsuyama M, et al. Intermediate filamentary constitution in vitro. The role of phosphorylation on the assembly-disassembly of desmin. J Biol Chem 1988;263:5970–8.
91. Gonda Y, Nishizawa K, Ando S, et al. Involvement of protein kinase C in the regulation of assembly-disassembly of neurofilaments in vitro. Biochem Biophys Res Commun 1990;167:1316–25.
92. Ottaviano Y, Gerace L. Phosphorylation of the nuclear lamins during interphase and mitosis. J Biol Chem 1985;260:624–32.
93. Eckert BS, Yeagle PL. Acrylamide treatment of PtK1 cells causes dephosphorylation of keratin polypeptides. Cell Motil Cytoskeleton 1988;6:15–24.
94. Chou CF, Omary MB. Phorbol acetate enhances the phosphorylation of cytokeratins 8 and 18 in human colonic epithelial cells. FEBS Lett 1991;282:200–4.
95. Chou CF, Smith AJ, Omary MB. Characterization and dynamics of O-linked glycosylation of human cytokeratin 8 and 18. J Biol Chem 1992;267:3901–6.
96. Schiller DL, Franke WW. Limited proteolysis of cytokeratin A by an endogenous protease: removal of positively charged terminal sequences. Cell Biol Int Rep 1983;7:3.
97. Bowdin PE, Quinlan RA, Breitkreutz D, Fusenig NE. Proteolytic modification of acidic and basic keratins during terminal differentiation of mouse and human epidermis. Eur J Biochem 1984;142:29–36.
98. Katagata Y, Aso K. The presumption of proteolytic enzymes related to the formation of intermediates during the terminal differentiation. FEBS Lett 1988;230:151–4.
99. Oshima RG, Trevor K, Shevinsky LH, et al. Identification of the gene coding for the Endo B murine cytokeratin and its methylated, stable inactive state in mouse nonepithelial cells. Genes Dev 1988;2:505–16.
100. Tamai Y, Takemoto Y, Matsumoto M, et al. Sequence of the Endo A gene encoding mouse cytokeratin and its methylated state in the CpG-rich region. Gene 1991;104:169–76.
101. Takemoto Y, Fujimura Y, Matsumoto M, et al. The promoter of the endo A cytokeratin gene is activated by a 31 downstream enhancer. Nucleic Acids Res 1991;19:2761–5.
102. Oshima RG. Identification and immunoprecipitation of cytoskeletal proteins from murine extra-embryonic endodermal cells. J Biol Chem 1981;256:8124–33.
103. Trabor JM, Oshima RG. Identification of mRNA species that code for extra-embryonic endodermal cytoskeletal proteins in differentiated derivatives of murine embryonal carcinoma cells. J Biol Chem 1982;257:8771–4.
104. Kim KH, Stellmach V, Javors J, Fuchs E. Regulation of human mesothelial cell differentiation: opposing roles of retinoids and epidermal growth factor in the expression of intermediated filament proteins. J Cell Biol 1987;105:3039–51.
105. Glass C, Fuchs E. Isolation, sequence, and differential expression of a human K7 gene in simple epithelial cells. J Cell Biol 1988;107:1337–50.
106. Baribault H, Blouin R, Bourgon L, Marceau N. Epidermal growth factor-induced selective phosphorylation of cultured rat hepatocyte 55-kD cytokeratin before filament reorganization and DNA synthesis. J Cell Biol 1989;109:1665–76.
107. Mathisen PM, Miller L. Thyroid hormone induction of keratin genes: a two-step activation of gene expression during development. Genes Dev 1987;1:1107–17.
108. Mathisen PM, Miller L. Thyroid hormone induces constitutive keratin gene expression during Xenopus laevis development. Mol Cell Biol 1989;9:1823–31.
109. Shimizu-Nishikawa K, Miller L. Hormonal regulation of adult type keratin gene expression in larval epidermal cell of the frog Xenopus laevis. Differentiation 1992;49:77–83.
110. Mackay AM, Tracy RP, Craighead JE. Cytokeratin expression in rat mesothelial cells in vitro is controlled by the extracellular matrix. J Cell Sci 1990;95:97–107.
111. Kurpakus MA, Stock EL, Jones JCR. The role of the basement membrane in differential expression of keratin proteins in epithelial cells. Dev Biol 1992;150:243–55.
112. Moll R, Schiller DL, Franke WW. Identification of protein IT of the intestinal cytoskeleton as a novel type I cytokeratin with unusual properties and expression patterns. J Cell Biol 1990;111:567–80.
113. Calnek D, Quaroni A. Differential localization by in situ hybridization of distinct keratin mRNA species during intestinal epithelial cell development and differentiation. Differentiation 1993;53:95–104.
114. Uddin M, Altmann GG, Leblond CP. Radioautographic visualization of differences in the pattern of [3H]uridine and [3H]orotic acid incorporation into the RNA of migrating columnar cells in the rat small intestine. J Cell Biol 1984;98:1619–29.
115. Bader BL, Jahn L, Franke WW. Low level expression of cytokeratins 8, 18, and 19 in vascular smooth muscle cells of human umbilical cord and in cultured cells derived therefrom, with an analysis of the chromosomal locus containing cytokeratin 19. Eur J Cell Biol 1988;47:300–19.
116. Gown AM, Boyd HC, Chang Y, et al. Smooth muscle cells can express cytokeratins of simple epithelium. Am J Pathol 1988;132:223–32.
117. Hilton WA. The morphology and development of intestinal fold and villi in vertebrates. Am J Anat 1902;1:459–505.
118. Mathan M, Moxey PC, Trier JS. Morphogenesis of fetal rat duodenal villi. Am J Anat 1976;146:73–92.

119. Madara JL, Neutra M, Trier JS. Junctional complexes in fetal rat small intestine during morphogenesis. Dev Biol 1981;86:170–8.
120. Quaroni A. Development of fetal rat intestine in organ and monolayer culture. J Cell Biol 1985;100:1611–22.
121. Quaroni A. Pre- and postnatal development of differentiated functions in rat intestinal epithelial cells. Dev Biol 1985;111:280–92.
122. Hermos JA, Mathan M, Trier JS. DNA synthesis and proliferation by villous epithelial cells in fetal rats. J Cell Biol 1971;50:255–8.
123. Helander HF. Morphological studies on the development of the rat colonic mucosa. Acta Anat (Basel) 1973;85:153–76.
124. Calvert R, Malka D, Menard D. Establishment of regional differences in brush border enzymatic activities during the development of the fetal mouse small intestine. Cell Tissue Res 1981;214:97–106.
125. Bailey DS, Cook A, McAllister G, et al. Structural and biochemical differentiation of the mammalian small intestine during foetal development. J Cell Sci 1984;72:195–212.
126. Gordon JI. Intestinal epithelial cell differentiation: new insights from chimeric and transgenic mice. J Cell Biol 1989;108:1187–94.
127. Moxey PC, Trier JS. Specialized cell types in the human fetal small intestine. Anat Rec 1978;191:269–86.
128. Calnek D, Quaroni A. Changes in keratin expression during fetal and postnatal development of intestinal epithelial cells. Biochem J 1992;285:939–46.
129. Domenjoud L, Jorcano JL, Breuer B, Alonso A. Synthesis and fate of keratins 8 and 18 in nonepithelial cells transfected with cDNA. Exp Cell Res 1988;179:352–61.
130. Kulesh DA, Oshima RG. Cloning the human keratin 18 and its expression in nonepithelial mouse cells. Mol Cell Biol 1988;8:1540–50.
131. Knapp AC, Franke WW. Spontaneous losses of control of cytokeratin gene expression in transformed non-epithelial human cells occurring at different levels of regulation. Cell 1989;59:67–79.
132. Kulesh DA, Cecena G, Darmon YM, et al. Posttranslational regulation of keratins: degradation of mouse and human keratins 18 and 8. Mol Cell Biol 1989;9:1553–65.
133. Bader BL, Magin TM, Hatzfeld M, Franke WW. Amino acid sequence and gene organization of cytokeratin no. 19, an exceptional tail-less intermediate filament protein. EMBO J 1986;5:1865–75.
134. Eckert RL. Sequence of the human 40-kDa keratin reveals an unusual structure with very high sequence identity to the corresponding bovine keratin. Proc Natl Acad Sci U S A 1988;85:1114–18.
135. Lu X, Lane EB. Retrovirus-mediated transgenic keratin expression in cultured fibroblasts. Cell 1990;62:681–96.

CHAPTER 5

Development of Endocytosis in the Intestinal Epithelium

Jean M. Wilson, PhD

James E. Casanova, PhD

The intestinal epithelium forms a barrier that provides for the selective passage of macromolecules between the lumen and the serosal surface; paracellular transport of macromolecules and pathogens is limited by the presence of tight junctions between the cells of the epithelium. Therefore, macromolecules that cross this barrier often do so via membrane-bound vesicles. The ability of the epithelial barrier to allow some macromolecules to cross while selectively excluding antigens or pathogens is critical to normal function.[1,2] Also, during development, the immature intestine goes through a phase in which the enterocytes are highly endocytic, and the increased susceptibility of preterm as well as term neonates to enteric infection and allergies[2] may reflect increased endocytic activity of these cells. Understanding the mechanisms of endocytosis and selective transepithelial transport will enhance our understanding of the intestinal barrier and provide strategies for the prevention of opportunistic infection and inappropriate antigen transport, as well as for efficient vaccine and drug delivery. In addition, it will provide insight into the development of immunity at the mucosal surface.

In this chapter, we will describe the current knowledge of endocytic pathways in epithelial cells of the intestine as well as other organs, since endocytosis in the gastrointestinal tract shares many features with endocytosis in other cell types of the body. We will then describe the developmental changes in endocytosis that occur during maturation of enterocytes.

ENDOCYTOSIS

Endocytosis is the process by which surface-bound ligands and fluid-phase macromolecules are internalized by eukaryotic cells.[3] These internalized macromolecules may be required for cellular metabolism or, in the case of hormones, may themselves alter cellular metabolic processes. The endocytic process is mediated by specialized invaginations of the plasma membrane that pinch off to form vesicles. One of the best-characterized mechanisms for uptake at the plasma membrane is via clathrin-coated pits and vesicles.[4] Clathrin-coated pits are sites where receptors and ligands are concentrated prior to internalization. The clathrin coat assembles on the cytoplasmic side of the membrane and is composed of heavy and light chains of the protein clathrin. These clathrin coats also contain a set of proteins called adaptors or, collectively, the AP-2 complex; the adaptor proteins are thought to provide the link between proteins of the plasma membrane and the clathrin coat.[5] Using affinity chromatography and the yeast two-hybrid system,[6-8] a subset of adaptor proteins has been found to directly interact with the cytoplasmic domains of receptors and thus may provide the mechanism for the concentration of receptors in the clathrin-coated pit.

Caveolae are another type of vesicle involved in uptake at the plasma membrane.[9] Initially identified as flask-shaped membrane invaginations in endothelial cells and adipocytes,[10] their importance in endocytosis in other cell types remains controversial. Caveolae are characterized by the presence of the coat protein caveolin, and are enriched in cholesterol.[11,12] In nonintestinal cells, caveolae have been implicated in the uptake of folate[13] and have been shown to concentrate the GM_1 ganglioside, which is the binding site for cholera toxin and the *Escherichia coli* heat-labile toxin.[14] In intestinal epithelial cells, cholera toxin binds to the GM_1 ganglioside at the apical plasma membrane and is internalized, and the A_1- subunit is transported to the basolateral membrane, where adenylate cyclase is stimulated.[15-18] Although a role for vesicular transport of cholera toxin in intestinal cells has been suggested,[19] the role of caveolae in this process remains to be determined. In fact, although caveolin has been found in the renal cell line Madin-Darby Canine Kidney (MDCK),[20] the role of caveolae in endocytosis and trafficking in enterocytes is completely uncharacterized and is an area that requires further research.

Although there is a lot of information in many cell types about uptake by clathrin- or caveolin-coated vesicles, another pathway exists for the uptake of molecules in the fluid phase that occurs by an as-yet-uncharacterized mechanism.[21] The importance of this pathway in mammalian cells is demonstrated by the use of temperature-sensitive mutants that are defective in clathrin-mediated endocytosis.[22] In these mutants, shifting cells to the nonpermissive temperature inhibits receptor-mediated endocytosis; however, endocytosis of fluid-phase materials returns to normal levels within 30 minutes of the shift to nonpermissive temperature. Experiments with yeast[23] and, more recently, mammalian cells[24] suggest that this pathway is regulated by the actin cytoskeleton. The importance of this pathway in the normal development and function of the intestine remains to be elucidated.

ENDOCYTOSIS IN POLARIZED CELLS

In epithelia, endocytosis occurs from both the apical and basolateral membranes, and the routes of membrane trafficking are illustrated in Figure 5–1. Uptake from the basolateral domain allows the cells to internalize an array of substances from the blood, including transferrin, low-density lipoprotein (LDL), and, in some cells, IgA. Substances that can be taken up from the apical domain include vitamins and growth factors.[25–30] Interestingly, there are differences in both the rates of endocytosis from apical and basolateral membranes as well as their sensitivities to a variety of pharmacologic agents. First, the fungal metabolite cytochalasin D, which acts by inducing the disassembly of actin filaments, preferentially inhibits endocytosis from the apical membrane but not the basolateral membrane in MDCK cells[31] and in the human intestinal cell line CaCo-2.[32] This selective effect occurs despite the fact that the actin cytoskeleton is disrupted at both poles of the cell. Furthermore, cytochalasin D inhibits both clathrin-mediated and clathrin-independent endocytic routes at the apical pole.[31] Second, it has been observed that clathrin-coated pits mature into vesicles more slowly at the apical surface (~6 to 8 minutes) than at the basolateral surface (1.1 to 1.5 minutes) of MDCK cells.[33] Third, it has been shown that mastoparan, a component of wasp venom that activates members of the G_i class of heterotrimeric G proteins, specifically stimulates apical endocytosis in a clathrin-independent fashion.[34]

Despite these mechanistic differences, the fundamental machinery of clathrin and adaptors is thought to be the same at both poles of the cell. The observed differences may, therefore, be due to as-yet-uncharacterized regulatory factors, or to biophysical differences related to the actin cytoskeleton or membrane phospholipid composition. Nonetheless, once internalization is complete, the endocytic pathways originating from either pole of the cell can converge, resulting in mixing of internalized macromolecules.[35–39]

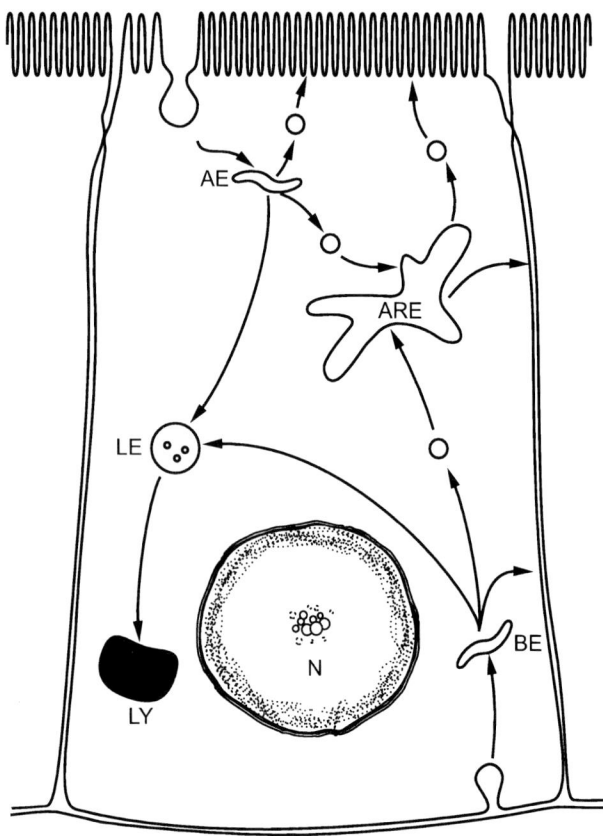

FIGURE 5–1. Endocytic pathways in polarized epithelial cells. Endocytosis occurs at the apical (luminal) and basolateral (serosal) surfaces. After endocytosis, vesicles fuse with apical endosomes (AE) or basolateral endosomes (BE). Macromolecules can be recycled back to their respective plasma membrane domains or be targeted to the apical recycling endosome (ARE) or the late endosomes (LE). Macromolecules that are to be transcytosed (such as IgA or growth factors) are targeted from the apical recycling endosome to the opposite plasma membrane domain. Macromolecules that are destined to be degraded are targeted from the late endosomes to the lysosomes (LY).

ENDOCYTIC PATHWAYS

Sorting, recycling, and targeting of endocytosed materials are mediated by a series of morphologically and functionally heterogeneous membrane-bound compartments known collectively as endosomes.[40–43] Although some components of endosomes have been shown to be derived from the plasma membrane, endosomes contain proteins that are unique to this organelle, including endotubin, an apical endosomal protein found in developing intestine.[44–47]

Sorting endosomes are located in the periphery of the cell, and are the first endosomal compartment entered by internalized ligands and receptors.[48,49] These endosomes have a mildly acidic pH which promotes the dissociation of a variety of receptor-ligand complexes.[50] In most cases, free ligands (or other fluid-phase contents) and membrane proteins targeted for degradation (e.g., epidermal growth factor receptors) are segregated from recycling membrane constituents for transport to the lysosomes; hence, the designation "sorting endosomes." Ultrastructural studies indicate that sorting endosomes are often tubulovesicular in nature, with a cisternal element containing fluid-phase markers and tubular extensions containing recycling proteins. The sorting endosomes have also been referred to as CURL (Compartment for Uncoupling of Receptor and Ligand),[40] and it has been hypothesized that the observed tubulovesicular morphology provides an optimal geometric configuration for sorting of soluble and membrane-bound cargo.[48,51]

After sorting has occurred, the cisternal elements of sorting endosomes are thought to separate from the tubular elements and undergo a process of maturation into late endosomes, which involves the selective removal of some proteins and the import of others.[43,52] Late endosomes have a pH of 5 to 6 and are the site at which newly synthesized lysosomal enzymes are targeted from the Golgi apparatus to the endocytic pathway. These endosomes are characterized by the presence of mannose-6-phosphate receptor (the carrier protein for soluble lysosomal hydrolases), lysosomal hydrolases themselves (e.g., cathepsins), and lysosomal membrane proteins.[53–57]

Finally, lysosomes are the terminal destination in the endocytic pathway. Late endosomes can fuse with pre-existing lysosomes that have an acidic pH of 5.0 to 5.5 and contain active lysosomal enzymes.[54] The membranes of lysosomes contain specialized membrane proteins that are highly glycosylated, with carbohydrate residues comprising up to 75 percent of their molecular weight.[55–58] The function of these membrane proteins is not known, but it has been suggested that they may protect the lysosomal membrane from proteases and lipases present within the lumen of the lysosome.[58]

In contrast to the degradative pathway, recycling receptors and membrane lipids that have been concentrated in the tubular extensions of the sorting endosomes are routed to a second endosomal compartment (referred to as the recycling endosome) and subsequently returned to the cell surface.[48,59,60] The recycling compartment is located in close proximity to the centrioles in most cells and requires an intact microtubule network to retain this localization.[61] The recycling endosomes are primarily tubular in structure, although cisternae have been observed.

In epithelial cells the recycling endosomes are also concentrated in the region of the centrioles, which are located in the cytoplasm at the extreme apical pole of the cell.[62,63] Unlike their counterpart in nonpolarized cells, which appears to simply package recycling proteins for transport back to the cell surface, epithelial recycling endosomes seem to serve as a major intersection for endocytic and transcytotic trafficking in these cells and, thus, also perform a sorting function. It has been shown that membrane proteins internalized from both apical and basolateral poles of the cell can be colocalized in this region within 10 minutes of internalization.[62,63] Even endocytosed transferrin receptors, which are recycled to the basolateral pole with very high efficiency, can pass through the apical recycling endosomes before returning to the basolateral surface.[63] In contrast, transcytosing polymeric immunoglobulin receptor (pIgR)/IgA complexes, which are also internalized from the basolateral membrane, are sorted from transferrin receptors in this compartment and then transported to the apical surface, where ligand is released.

REGULATION OF ENDOCYTIC PATHWAYS

The processes of internalizing, sorting, and packaging of proteins and targeting them to their appropriate subcellular destinations require a complex cellular machinery that is tightly regulated. A common feature of these processes appears to be the participation of GTPases that, by acting as molecular switches, control the assembly and disassembly of coat protein complexes responsible for carrier vesicle formation, targeting, and fusion.[64] At least five families of GTPases have been shown to function in some aspect of vesicular transport, including the dynamins, ADP-ribosylation factors (ARFs), Sar1, rab-ypt, and certain members of the rho-rac-cdc42 family. Although each of these families serves a different function in membrane trafficking, they share at least one mechanistic feature: they exist in two interconvertible conformational states, one inactive (GDP-bound) and one active (GTP-bound). Typically, generation of the active form requires the displacement of bound GDP by GTP, a reaction stimulated by specific guanine nucleotide exchange factors (GEFs). Similarly, hydrolysis of bound GTP requires the activity of isoform-specific GTPase-activating proteins (GAPs).

DYNAMINS

Dynamins constitute a family of at least three closely related proteins of approximately 100 kD that appear to function in the formation of clathrin-coated vesicles. These proteins are characterized by the presence of an NH2-terminal GTP-binding domain, a pleckstrin homology (PH) domain, a coiled-coil domain, and a C-terminal proline-arginine-rich domain (PRD).[65,66] GTPase activity of dynamins is stimulated by interaction with microtubules,[67,68] acidic phospholipids,[69,70] or SH3-domain-containing proteins such as Grb-2[71,72] with the proline-arginine-rich domain, or by the binding of inositol phospholipids to the pleckstrin homology domain.[73] Enhanced GTPase activity appears to correlate with self-assembly of the protein into polymers.[69,74]

The role of dynamins in endocytosis was first discovered by analysis of the *Drosophila* mutant shibire. Flies with temperature-sensitive shibire alleles become paralyzed at the restrictive temperature due to a failure to internalize synaptic vesicle components following neurotransmitter release. Electron micrographs of nerve terminals revealed the presence of elongated, clathrin-coated tubules emanating from the synaptic membrane, suggesting that the formation of endocytic vesicles from clathrin-coated invaginations was impaired. Subsequent cloning of the shibire gene revealed that it was highly homologous to Dynamin I, which had originally been isolated as a microtubule-associated protein from rat brain.[75] Using permeabilized mammalian synaptosomes, it was subsequently shown that the GTPase activity of dynamin was required for the pinching off of coated buds to form vesicles; in the presence of nonhydrolyzable GTP analogs, clathrin-coated tubules were observed that were remarkably similar in structure to those observed in the *Drosophila* shibire mutants.[76] Similarly, expression of mutant dynamins deficient in GTP binding in cultured cells has been shown to completely inhibit clathrin-mediated endocytosis.[22]

As described above, there are at least three mammalian isoforms of dynamin, which are differentially expressed. Dynamin I is expressed exclusively in the brain. Dynamin II is ubiquitously expressed, suggesting that it mediates clathrin-dependent endocytosis in most cells. Dynamin III is predominantly expressed in testis; its function there is unknown.

As Dynamin II is the only known isoform in epithelial tissues, it is presumed to function at both poles of the cell in the formation of clathrin-coated vesicles. However, since the GTPase activity of the protein is subject to regulation by both phospholipids and interacting proteins, it is possible that dynamin activity is differentially regulated depending on its microenvironment. Interestingly, localization of dynamin in the intestine of the nematode *C. elegans* indicates that it is concentrated at the apical pole of the cell.[77] Therefore, there may be as-yet-uncharacterized isoforms of dynamin that regulate endocytosis from the different plasma membrane domains.

RABS

Unlike dynamins, which participate in vesicle formation, rabs appear to function in vesicle docking and/or fusion with target membranes.[64,78] Each step in vesicular transport requires the function of one or more specific rabs, which are thought to provide target specificity to the docking reaction. Mammalian rabs comprise a family of more than 30 members, many of which have counterparts in yeast, where they are called ypt1, -2, -3, etc. All rab-ypt proteins are small (25 to 30 kD), similar in structure to the small GTP-binding protein ras, and are covalently modified at their C-termini by the addition of two isoprenyl groups. This modification is essential to rab function, presumably facilitating the interaction of these proteins with membranes.

In the endocytic pathway, rab4 and rab5 have been localized to early (sorting) endosomes, although they have distinct functions. Rab5 regulates the fusion of endocytic vesicles with endosomal membranes[44] as well as homotypic endosome-endosome fusion[79,80] whereas rab4 regulates the recycling of membrane components from the endosome back to the plasma membrane.[46] Rab7, rab9, and rab24 have been identified on the membranes of late endosomes, and rab7 has been shown to be necessary for the transport of cargo, from the early endosomal compartment to late endosomes.[81] Recently, rab11 has been localized to pericentriolar recycling endosomes in BHK-21 cells and is thought to function in the transport of membrane constituents from sorting endosomes to the recycling compartment.[82] In epithelial tissues, rab11 has been localized to vesicular structures in the apical cytoplasm that, by analogy with non-polarized cells, may represent the recycling endosomal compartment. Immunofluorescent staining with anti-rab11 antibodies has resulted in prominent staining in parietal cells and surface mucous cells of the stomach, ileal and colonic enterocytes, hepatocytes, renal tubule epithelia, glandular cells of the prostate, pancreatic acinar cells, and the squamous epithelia of the skin and esophagus.[83]

The majority of mammalian rabs are ubiquitously expressed among cell types, presumably because they regulate transport pathways that are common to all cells. However, some rabs exhibit a more restricted tissue distribution. Rab3A is located on the small synaptic vesicles of neuronal cells, while rab3D is enriched in adipose tissue and the secretory granules of endocrine and exocrine cells.[84] In addition, several rabs have been identified that are expressed exclusively in epithelia, suggesting that they regulate vesicular transport pathways unique to epithelial cells. For example, rab17 is expressed in the epithelial cells of the kidney and intestine and is localized to the basolateral plasma membrane as well as to apical tubules.[85] Its function in these cells has yet to be determined. Recently a second epithelial-specific rab, rab25, was cloned from a gastric parietal cell library and has been found to be highly expressed in gastrointestinal mucosa, kidney, and lung.[86] In parietal cells, rab25 has been localized to a complex network of tubulovesicles underlying the apical membrane. These tubulovesicles are storage sites for H^+,K^+ ATPase which are inserted into the apical membrane in response to hormonal cues. This compartment is, therefore, likely to represent a modified recycling endosome that is responsive to second messengers.

ACUTE REGULATION OF ENDOCYTOSIS

The GTPases described above, along with other components of the endocytic machinery, regulate the formation and fusion of carrier vesicles in a constitutive manner; that is, they function continuously at a basal rate, regardless of extracellular influences. Superimposed on this constitutive activity is an additional level of regulation that is controlled by second messengers. Although there is considerable evidence in the literature of endocytic modulation by second messengers, the data are somewhat confusing and, in some cases, contradictory. Moreover, some aspects of regulation appear to be cell type specific. For example, cAMP agonists have been shown to stimulate apical endocytosis in the renal cell line MDCK[34] but to inhibit apical endocytosis in a different renal tubule line, OK.[87] Also, inhibition of endocytosis by cAMP agonists was observed in the crypt-like human cell line T84,[88] as well as in Ussing chamber experiments with segments of rat ileum.[89] Similarly, protein kinase C agonists have been shown to inhibit endocytosis in OK cells[87] but to stimulate endocytosis in ileum enterocytes.[89] In this regard, both mastoparan and aluminum fluoride, thought to be activators of heterotrimeric G proteins, have been shown to stimulate apical endocytosis in MDCK cells.[34] It is important to note that the specificity of both these reagents for heterotrimeric G proteins has been questioned, and more detailed experiments will be required to resolve this issue.

The underlying mechanisms of endocytic regulation by second messengers and/or kinases are poorly understood. In some cases, endocytosis of specific proteins may be regulated by direct phosphorylation of the protein itself. For example, the endocytic rate of the cystic fibrosis transmembrane conductance regulator (CFTR) appears to be negatively regulated by phosphorylation by both protein kinase A and protein kinase C.[90] In other cases, regulation may derive from effects on the endocytic machinery rather than phosphorylation of endocytosed proteins. Such results highlight the complexity of the regulation of endocytosis in epithelial cells, which will require further investigation to resolve its intricacies.

INTESTINAL BARRIER

Epithelial cells of the gastrointestinal tract serve as a selective barrier to the diffusion of macromolecules between the intestinal lumen and the serum. Still, endocytosis of luminal macromolecules occurs (Figure 5–2), and the transepithelial transport of a subset of macromolecules is required for some intestinal functions, particularly those related to development and mucosal immunity.

The developing intestine possesses a great capacity for the endocytosis of macromolecules present in swallowed fluids, and the absorptive enterocytes are highly specialized for the uptake and processing of these materials.[91,92] In fact, the sorting capabilities of endosomes were first demonstrated in the enterocytes of the neonatal rat jejunum.[93] Passive immunity is conferred upon the neonate by the selective binding of maternal IgG, present in milk, to F_c receptors associated with B_2-microglobulin on the enterocyte apical plasma membrane.[94,95] The receptor-ligand complex is subsequently internalized and delivered to the apical endosomal compartment along with other nonspecifically absorbed macromolecules.[93] In the apical endosomes, the IgG is sorted to coated vesicles, which are then targeted to the basolateral membrane. The acidic pH of endosomes is thought to be important in the stability of the F_c receptor-ligand complex, enabling the selective transfer of IgG to transepithelial transport vesicles while promoting the dissociation of other, lysosome-directed ligands.[96]

In addition to the specific transport of IgG or growth factors across the epithelium, antigens from pathogens and dietary sources can cross the epithelium in significant amounts; this transport is critical for the development of both mucosal immunity and tolerance. As mentioned previously, the developing intestine is more permeable to macromolecules and pathogens present in the lumen; however, the mechanism of transport of these agents remains unresolved. Although the enterocytes can transport molecules across the epithelial barrier,[97] another important route of antigen uptake is via the microfold or M-cells that overlay collections of lymphocytes called Peyer's patches.[98,99] Microfold cells have been shown to internalize and transport both fluid-phase and membrane-bound materials, as well as bacteria and viruses. Although M-cells are present in the human intestine as early as 16 weeks of gestation,[100] their role in immunity during fetal development has not been determined. Nonetheless, endocytosis of macromolecules by M-cells is thought to use the same molecular machinery as other cell types of the intestine, although specific cell-surface receptors or regulatory factors that affect antigen sampling from the lumen remain undefined.

Transepithelial transport occurs in two directions. Transport of IgG occurs from the apical plasma membrane to the basolateral membrane and provides the basis for passive immunity in many animals.[94] In contrast, the polymeric immunoglobulins IgA and IgM, which are the primary antibodies in mucosal secretions, must be transported from their site of synthesis in the lamina propria into mucosal secretions, where they have their effect. Thus, the transepithelial transport of IgA from the lamina propria to the intestinal lumen (basolateral to apical) is critical for the maintenance of mucosal immunity in all mammals. Upon

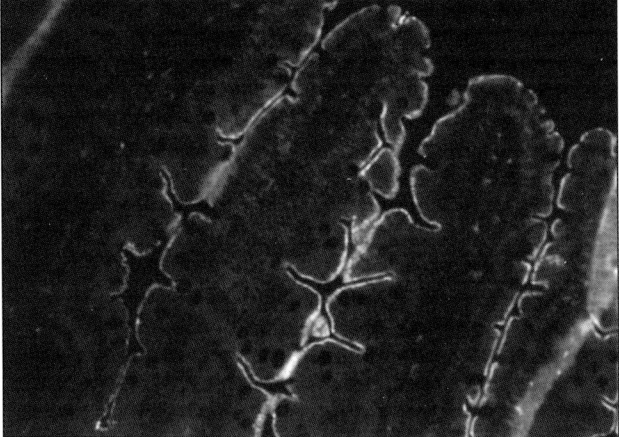

FIGURE 5–2. Apical endocytosis of a fluid-phase marker in rat jejunum. A ligated loop of adult rat small intestine was lumenally perfused with fluorescein-conjugated dextran for 30 minutes at 37°C. The loop was then opened, washed with saline solution, and fixed with paraformaldehyde-lysine-periodate fixative. Four-micron frozen sections were counterstained with Evans Blue (staining) to reveal tissue architecture. The granular staining in the apical margins of the cells is likely to represent early (sorting) and late endosomes. Because of the relatively short incubation with marker, lysosomes are not labeled. (Photo courtesy of Dr. Ivan Sabolic, Institute for Medical Research and Occupational Health, Zagreb, Croatia.)

binding to the pIgR at the basolateral membrane, receptor-ligand complexes are internalized in clathrin-coated vesicles and, along with other receptors and their respective ligands, enter a population of sorting endosomes.[101] Unlike many pH-sensitive ligands (e.g., low-density lipoprotein), IgA and IgM remain bound to the pIgR at endosomal pH. The receptor-ligand complexes are then packaged into transcytotic carrier vesicles and transported to the apical pole of the cell. It had previously been thought that these carrier vesicles fused directly with the apical plasma membrane; however, recent evidence indicates that IgA enters the apical recycling endosomes en route to the apical surface.[62,63] In this compartment, pIgR-ligand complexes are sorted from other, recycling receptors (e.g., transferrin receptor) and subsequently transported to the apical plasma membrane. Upon reaching the apical surface, the receptor is proteolytically cleaved, releasing the ligand as a complex with an extracellular receptor fragment, termed secretory component. Although this pathway has been described in detail and molecular signals that route the polymeric IgA receptor through the cell are identified,[102–105] the mechanism of sorting of this receptor is still unclear.

The transcytotic pathway appears to be subject to acute regulation by protein and lipid kinases. In a model epithelial cell system, transepithelial transport of IgA has been found to be stimulated by activation of both protein kinase C[106] and protein kinase A.[107] In both cases, kinase activation was observed to selectively affect a late stage in transport, presumably involving either exit from the apical recycling compartment, transport from the recycling compartment to the apical membrane, or fusion of carrier vesicles with the apical membrane. Further experiments will be required to distinguish between these possibilities. The stimulation of transcytosis by either PKC or PKA was not limited to IgA, in that enhanced transcytosis of transferrin[106] or of the galactose-binding lectin ricin[107] could also be demonstrated. These findings suggest that both kinases regulate the flow of membrane through the transcytotic pathway but do not affect the sorting of proteins into the transcytotic pathway. It should also be pointed out that these kinases act only to regulate the rate of transport; their activity is not required for constitutive transcytosis to occur. However, since some intestinal pathogens such as Vibrio cholerae secrete toxins that result in increased cellular levels of cAMP,[18] it will be important to determine the role of these changes in membrane trafficking during the disease process.

In contrast to the acute regulation of membrane trafficking by PKA and PKC, phosphorylation of certain inositol phospholipids has been shown to play an important role in postendocytic transport events and may regulate membrane-trafficking events in a constitutive fashion. Although the mechanism of action of these enzymes remains unclear, they have been shown to be important in a range of membrane-trafficking events. Phosphatidylinositol-3-kinases (PI 3Ks) constitute a family of phospholipid kinases which phosphorylate the inositol ring of the phospholipid at the D3 position but vary in their substrate specificity, mechanism of activation, and sensitivity to pharmacologic inhibitors.[108] Specifically, the activity of PI 3Ks appears to be required for transport of endocytosed cargo from sorting endosomes to either the lysosomal,[109,110] recycling,[110,111] or transcytotic pathways.[112] Importantly, in the latter study, transcytosis of IgA was inhibited 50% by the PI 3K inhibitor, wortmannin. While many isoforms of PI 3K are activated by signaling cascades originating at the cell surface, at least one isoform, vps34, which has been identified in both yeast and human cells, appears to be constitutively active. Since a variety of constitutive postendocytic transport processes are inhibited by PI 3K inhibitory drugs such as wortmannin, it is possible that vps34p is the dominant isoform in vesicular transport.

ENDOCYTIC COMPARTMENTS IN THE DEVELOPING INTESTINE

The roles of endocytosis of nutrients, growth factors, hormones, and gamma globulins in the growth and development of the fetus and neonate are subjects of intense interest. During development of the intestinal epithelium, a conversion occurs from a stratified to a simple columnar epithelium.[113,114] Introduction of tracers into the lumen of fetal gut prior to the conversion from a stratified to a simple epithelium shows that the surface cells of the stratified epithelium are capable of endocytosis of lumenal contents.[115] However, the majority of endocytic activity is seen after conversion to a simple columnar epithelium, when the enterocytes assemble an extensive endocytic complex in the apical cytoplasm. This apical endocytic complex is located just beneath the microvillus membrane and is composed of an extensive array of membrane tubules and vesicles (Figure 5–3). It is found in the enterocytes of a large number of species during

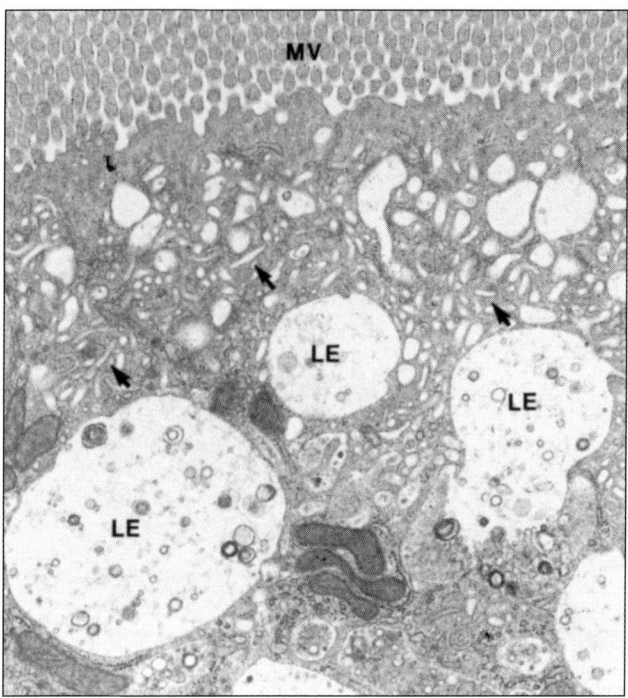

FIGURE 5–3. Apical endosomal complex of the developing ileum: electron microscopy of the apical region of the developing rat ileum. The extensive tubular early endosomes (arrows) are present just beneath the microvilli (MV). Late endosomes (LE) have typical vesicular inclusions.

development; in the pig, calf, and sheep it is present for a significant time in utero and persists for a short time after birth.[116,117] In the fetal human, this complex is present at 10 weeks of gestation and persists until at least 22 weeks gestational age.[118] In the rat, it assembles shortly before birth and persists until weaning at 17 to 20 days after birth. Endocytosis of lumenal contents into these endosomes has been shown to occur in the fetal intestine of the rat, monkey, and human.[115,118–120] In the human, rapid clearance of proteins from the amniotic fluid of the near-term fetus has been demonstrated,[121] and amniotic fluid contains significant amounts of a host of growth factors.[122–125] In the duodenum and jejunum of the rat, the apical endosomes have been shown to be important in the sorting and transepithelial transport of IgG present in milk.[93,96] In the ileum, these tubular endosomes are characterized by the presence of membrane arrays on their ectoplasmic surface and by the expression of a membrane glycoprotein called endotubin.[47,126–128] The membrane arrays are known to be composed of B-N-acetylglucosaminidase;[129] the reason for the dense and orderly arrangement of this normally lysosomal enzyme is unclear. Endotubin shares sequence similarity with the LDL-receptor-related family of proteins;[130,131] however, its function in the endosomes of developing intestine remains unknown. Since the ileum does not participate in IgG transport, the apical endosomes were originally suggested to comprise an elaboration of the apical plasma membrane invaginations and to serve only as a conduit to the lysosomes for the degradation of endocytosed milk components.[126,127,132] However,

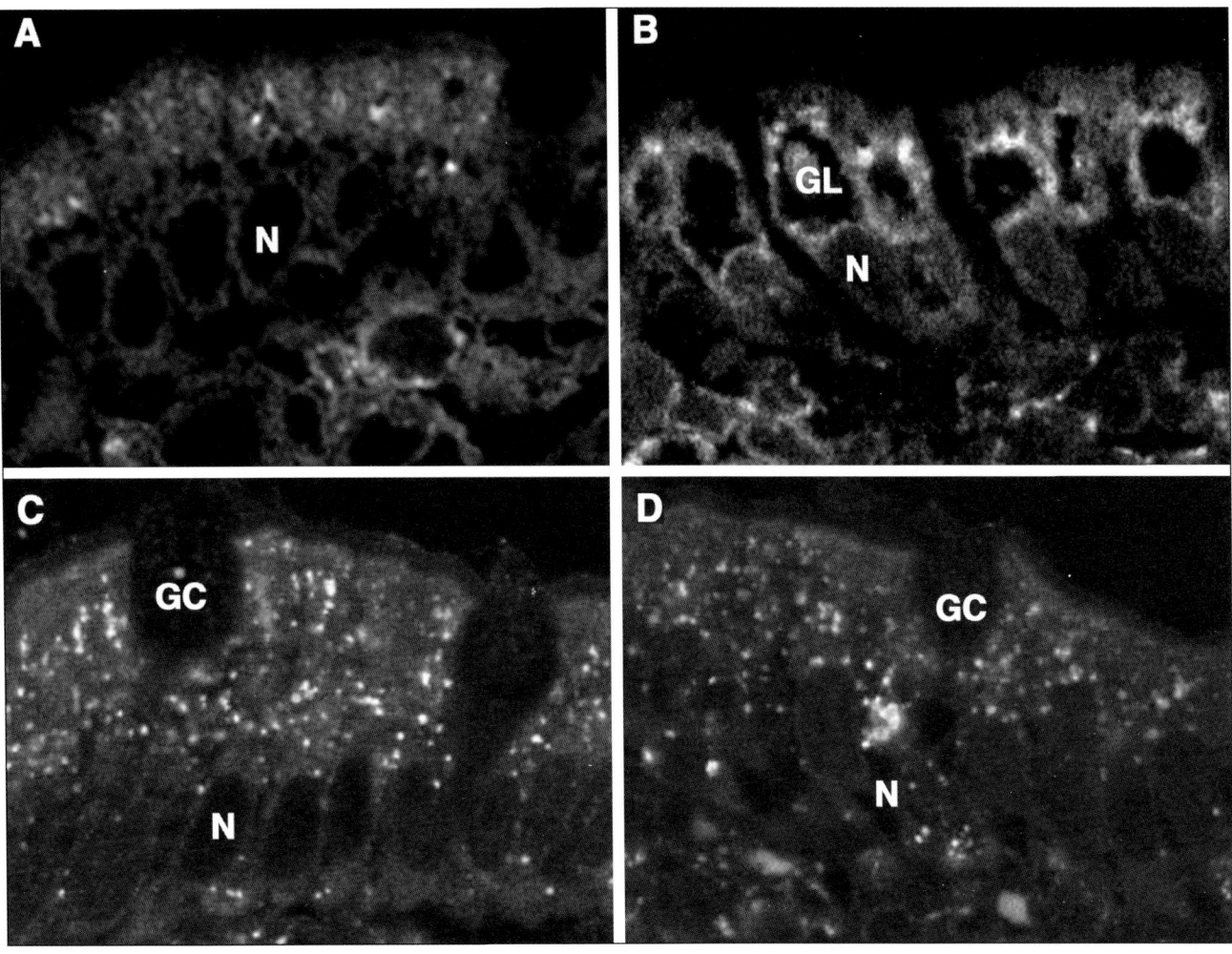

FIGURE 5–4. Lysosomal compartments in the developing and adult intestine. Sections of neonatal and adult intestine stained with an antibody against a lysosomal membrane protein (lgp120). In the neonatal jejunum (A), lysosomes are sparse and scattered through the apical cytoplasm. In the neonatal ileum (B), the giant lysosome (GL) fills the supranuclear cytoplasm. Smaller lysosomes are also present apical to the giant lysosome. In the adult jejunum (C) and ileum (D), lysosomes are numerous and are predominantly located in the apical cytoplasm. N = nucleus; GC = goblet cell.

the demonstration of two distinct endosomal compartments involved in the transfer of membrane-bound or fluid-phase macromolecules to the giant lysosome (see below) indicated that these membranes are capable of sorting internalized macromolecules.[133] Subsequently, it has been shown that growth factors such as NGF and EGF, which are present in salivary secretions, milk, and amniotic fluid,[134–136] can be selectively internalized by jejunal and ileal cells, transported across the epithelium, and released intact into the circulation.[28–30,137] As macromolecules that are taken up by fluid-phase endocytosis are directed primarily to lysosomes, it is clear that the cells of the developing intestine are actively sorting and targeting these macromolecules. This ability to effectively sort molecules such as growth factors may be critical for the development of the intestine as well as other organ systems.

In concert with the apical endosomal complex, the lysosomal compartment of the enterocytes also goes through extensive modifications during development (Figure 5–4). For example, there are many more lysosomes present in the adult jejunal enterocytes than in the enterocytes of the developing jejunum, perhaps reflecting the greater role of transepithelial transport in these immature enterocytes. The lysosomal compartment of the ileum undergoes a dramatic reorganization during development. A hallmark of the enterocytes of the developing ileum is a large supranuclear lysosomal vacuole that is called the giant lysosome. Because luminal proteases are relatively inactive in the rodent developing intestine, the giant lysosome is thought to carry out the bulk of the digestive processing of proteins and lipids present in milk. In the rat, the giant lysosome assembles rapidly on day 1 after birth and is present throughout the suckling period.[138] In the human, the presence of the giant lysosome is more variable but has been observed at 17 weeks gestational age.[118] Since most nutrition in the fetal human is derived from passage of materials across the placenta, the role of this lysosomal system in human intestinal development remains unknown.

However, as in the jejunum, the giant lysosome is replaced by many small lysosomes in the mature enterocyte. The factors that regulate these changes in the lysosomal compartments are unknown.

The importance of endocytosis and transport of macromolecules in the development of the intestine in the human fetus and neonate have become increasingly apparent. Although the majority of passive immunity is conferred transplacentally, receptors for gamma globulins have been detected in fetal intestinal epithelial cells,[139] and uptake of immunoglobulins has been detected in neonates.[140] In addition, human milk contains a number of hormones, including EGF, NGF, prolactin, and insulin,[134] and these substances may cross the intestine in biologically significant amounts. Growth of the human fetal intestine is stimulated by EGF,[141] and the selective transfer of biologically active molecules may play an important role in the pre- and postnatal development of the intestine. Therefore, endocytosis in the developing intestine may play a critical role in the growth and differentiation of the intestine, as well as other organ systems. However, the immature intestine may not discriminate well between substances necessary for growth and development and those that are pathogenic. Premature infants are more susceptible to intestinal infection by a variety of agents, and this may be due to the greater endocytic capacity and/or increased transepithelial transport in the developing intestine. Increased nonspecific transepithelial transport could also result in greater rates of enteric allergies, particularly against cow's milk proteins. It is clearly critical to determine the contribution of membrane trafficking to these clinical conditions.

REFERENCES

1. Sanderson IR, Walker WA. Uptake and transport of macromolecules by the intestine: possible role in clinical disorders. Gastroenterology 1993;104:622–39.
2. Kliegman RM, Walker WA, Yolken RH. Necrotizing enterocolitis: research agenda for a disease of unknown etiology and pathogenesis. Pediatr Res 1993;34:701–8.
3. Mukherjee S, Ghosh RN, Maxfield FR. Endocytosis. Physiol Rev 1997;7:759–803.
4. Schmid SL. Clathrin-coated vesicle formation and protein sorting: an integrated process. Annu Rev Biochem 1997;66:511–48.
5. Pearse BM, Bretscher MS. Membrane recycling by coated vesicles. Annu Rev Biochem 1981;50:85–101.
6. Pearse BMF. Receptors compete for adaptors found in plasma membrane coated pits. EMBO J 1988;7:3331–6.
7. Glickman JN, Conibear E, Pearse BMF. Specificity of binding of clathrin adaptors to signals on the mannose-6-phosphate/insulin-like growth factor II receptor. EMBO J 1989;8:1041–7.
8. Ohno H, Stewart J, Fournier MC, et al. Interaction of tyrosine-based sorting signals with clathrin associated proteins. Science 1995;269:1872–5.
9. Parton RG. Caveolae and caveolins. Curr Opin Cell Biol 1996;8:542–8.
10. Palade GE. Fine structure of blood capillaries. J Appl Physics 1953;24:1424.
11. Rothberg K, Heuser JE, Donzell WC, et al. Caveolin, a protein component of caveolae membrane coats. Cell 1992;68:673–82.
12. Schnitzer JE, Oh P, Pinney E, Allard J. Filipin-sensitive caveolae-mediated transport in endothelium: reduced transcytosis, scavenger endocytosis, and capillary permeability of select macromolecules. J Cell Biol 1994;27:1217–32.
13. Anderson RGW. Potocytosis of small molecules and ions by caveolae. Trends Cell Biol 1993;3:69–72.
14. Parton RG. Ultrastructural localization of gangliosides; GM1 is concentrated in caveolae. J Histochem Cytochem 1994;42:155–66.
15. Schnitzer JE, McIntosh DP, Dvorak AM, et al. Separation of caveolae from associated microdomains of GPI-anchored proteins. Science 1995;269:1435–9.
16. Dominguez P, Barros F, Lazo PS. The activation of adenylate cyclase from small intestinal epithelium by cholera toxin. Eur J Biochem 1985;146:533–8.
17. Parkinson DK, Ebel H, DiBona DR, Sharp GWG. Localization of the action of cholera toxin on adenyl cyclase in mucosal epithelial cells of rabbit intestine. J Clin Invest 1972;51:2292–8.
18. Holmgren J. Actions of cholera toxin and the prevention and treatment of cholera. Nature 1981;292:413–7.
19. Lencer WI, Delp C, Neutra MR, Madara JL. Mechanism of cholera toxin action on a polarized human intestinal epithelial cell line: role of vesicular traffic. J Cell Biol 1992;117:1197–209.
20. Kurzchalia TV, Dupree P, Parton RG, et al. VIP21, a 21KD membrane protein is an integral component of trans-Golgi network-derived transport vesicles. J Cell Biol 1992;118:1003–14.
21. Lamaze C, Schmid SL. The emergence of clathrin-independent pinocytic pathways. Curr Opin Cell Biol 1995;7:573–80.
22. Damke H, Baba T, Warnock DE, Schmid SL. Induction of mutant dynamin specifically blocks endocytic coated vesicle formation. J Cell Biol 1994;127:915–34.
23. Benedetti H, Raths S, Crausaz F, Riezman H. The END3 gene encodes a protein that is required for the internalization step of endocytosis and for actin cytoskeleton organization in yeast. Mol Biol Cell 1994;5:1023–37.
24. Radhakrishna H, Donaldson JG. ADP-ribosylation factor 6 regulates a novel plasma membrane recycling pathway. J Cell Biol 1997;139:49–61.
25. Levine JS, Allen RH, Alpers DH, Seetharam B. Immunocytochemical localization of the intrinsic factor-cobalamin receptor in dog-ileum: distribution of intracellular receptor during cell maturation. J Cell Biol 1984;98:1111–8.
26. Dix CJ, Hassan IF, Obray HY, et al. The transport of vitamin B12 through polarized monolayers of Caco-2 cells. Gastroenterology 1990;98:1272–9.
27. Dan N, Cutler DF. Transcytosis and processing of intrinsic factor-cobalamin in Caco-2 cells. J Biol Chem 1994;269:18849–55.
28. Gonnella PA, Siminoski K, Murphy RA, Neutra MR. Transepithelial transport of epidermal growth factor by absorptive cells of suckling rat ileum. J Clin Invest 1987;80:22–32.
29. Gonnella PA, Harmatz P, Walker WA. Prolactin is transported across the epithelium of the jejunum and ileum of the suckling rat. J Cell Physiol 1989;140:138–49.
30. Simonoski K, Gonnella P, Bernanke J, et al. Uptake and transepithelial transport of nerve growth factor in suckling rat ileum. J Cell Biol 1986;103:1979–90.
31. Gottlieb TA, Ivanov IE, Adesnik M, Sabatini DD. Actin microfilaments play a critical role in endocytosis at the apical but not the basolateral surface in polarized epithelial cells. J Cell Biol 1993;120:695–710.
32. Jackman MR, Shurety W, Ellis JA, Luzio JP. Inhibition of apical but not basolateral endocytosis of ricin and folate in Caco-2 cells by cytochalasin D. J Cell Sci 1994;107:2547–56.

33. Naim HY, Dodds DT, Brewer CB, Roth MG. Apical and basolateral coated pits of MDCK cells differ in their rates of maturation into coated vesicles, but not in the ability to distinguish between mutant hemagglutinin proteins with different internalization signals. J Cell Biol 1995;129: 1241–50.
34. Eker P, Holm PK, van Deurs B, Sandvig K. Selective regulation of apical endocytosis in polarized Madin-Darby canine kidney cells by mastoparan and cAMP. J Biol Chem 1994; 269:18607–15.
35. Bomsel M, Prydz K, Parton RG, et al. Endocytosis in filter-grown Madin-Darby Canine Kidney Cells. J Cell Biol 1989; 109:3243–58.
36. Parton RG, Prydz K, Bomsel M, et al. Meeting of the apical and basolateral endocytic pathways of the Madin-Darby canine kidney cells in late endosomes. J Cell Biol 1989;109: 3259–72.
37. Knight A, Hughson E, Hopkins CR, Cutler DF. Membrane protein trafficking through the common apical endosome compartment of polarized Caco-2 cells. Mol Biol Cell 1995; 6:597–610.
38. Hughson EJ, Hopkins CR. Endocytic pathways in polarized Caco-2 cells: identification of an endosomal compartment accessible from both apical and basolateral surfaces. J Cell Biol 1990;110:337–48.
39. Fujita M, Reinhart F, Neutra MR. Convergence of apical and basolateral endocytic pathways at the late endosome in intestinal absorptive cells of the suckling rat ileum. J Cell Sci 1990; 97:385–94.
40. Geuze HJ, Slot JW, Strous GJ, et al. Intracellular site of asialoglycoprotein receptor-ligand uncoupling: double-label immunoelectron microscopy during receptor-mediated endocytosis. Cell 1983;32:277–87.
41. Baenziger JU, Fiete D. Separation of two populations of endocytic vesicles involved in receptor-ligand sorting in rat hepatocytes. J Biol Chem 1986;261:7445–54.
42. Schmid SL, Fuchs R, Male P, Mellman I. Two distinct subpopulations of endosomes involved in membrane recycling and transport to lysosomes. Cell 1988;52:73–83.
43. Dunn KW, Maxfield FR. Delivery of ligands from sorting endosomes to late endosomes occurs by maturation of sorting endosomes. J Cell Biol 1992;117:301–10.
44. Bucci C, Parton RG, Mather IH, et al. The small GTPase rab5 functions as a regulatory factor in the early endocytic pathway. Cell 1992;70:715–28.
45. Bucci C, Wandinger-Ness A, Lutke A, et al. Rab5a is a common component of the apical and basolateral endocytic machinery in polarized epithelial cells. Proc Natl Acad Sci U S A 1994;91:5061–5.
46. Van der Sluijs P, Hull P, Webster P, et al. The small GTP-binding protein rab4 controls an early sorting event on the endocytic pathway. Cell 1992;70:729–40.
47. Wilson JM, Whitney JA, Neutra MR. Identification of an endosomal antigen specific to absorptive cells of suckling rat ileum. J Cell Biol 1987;105:691–703.
48. Dunn KW, McGraw TE, Maxfield FR. Iterative fractionation of recycling receptors from lysosomally destined ligands in an early sorting endosome. J Cell Biol 1989;109:3303–14.
49. Ghosh RN, Gelman DL, Maxfield FR. Quantitation of low-density lipoprotein and transferrin endocytic sorting in Hep2 cells using confocal microscopy. J Cell Sci 1994;107:2177–89.
50. Yamashiro DJ, Maxfield FR. Acidification of morphologically distinct endosomes in mutant and wild-type Chinese hamster ovary cells. J Cell Biol 1987;105:2723–33.
51. Linderman JJ, Lauffenburger DA. Analysis of intracellular receptor/ligand sorting in endosomes. J Theor Biol 1988; 132:203–45.
52. Stoorvogel W, Strous GJ, Geuze HJ, et al. Late endosomes derive from early endosomes by maturation. Cell 1991;65: 417–27.
53. Brown WJ, Goodhouse J, Farquhar MG. Mannose-6-phosphate receptors for lysosomal enzymes cycle between the Golgi complex and endosomes. J Cell Biol 1986;103:1235–47.
54. Kornfeld S, Mellman I. The biogenesis of lysosomes. Annu Rev Cell Biol 1989;5:483–525.
55. Lippincott-Schwartz J, Fambrough DM. Lysosomal membrane dynamics: structure and interorganellar movement of a major lysosomal membrane glycoprotein. J Cell Biol 1986; 102:1593–605.
56. Barriocanal JG, Bonifacino JS, Yuan L, Sandoval I. Biosynthesis, glycosylation, movement through the Golgi system, and transport to lysosomes by an N-linked carbohydrate-independent mechanism of three lysosomal integral membrane proteins. J Biol Chem 1986;261:16755–63.
57. Carlsson SR, Roth J, Piller F, Fukuda M. Isolation and characterization of human lysosomal membrane glycoproteins, h-lamp-1 and h-lamp-2. Major sialoglycoproteins carrying polylactosaminoglycan. J Biol Chem 1988;263:18911–9.
58. Lewis V, Green SA, Marsh M, et al. Glycoproteins of the lysosomal membrane. J Cell Biol 1985;100:1839–47.
59. Mayor S, Presley JF, Maxfield FR. Sorting of membrane components from endosomes and subsequent recycling to the cell surface occurs by a bulk flow process. J Cell Biol 1993; 121:1257–69.
60. Tooze J, Hollinshead M. Tubular early endosomal network in AtT20 and other cells. J Cell Biol 1991;115:635–54.
61. Yamashiro DJ, Tycko B, Fluss SR, Maxfield FR. Segregation of transferrin to a mildly acidic (pH 6.5) para-Golgi compartment in the recycling pathway. Cell 1984;37:789–800.
62. Barroso M, Sztul ES. Basolateral to apical transcytosis in polarized cells is indirect and involves BFA and trimeric G protein sensitive passage through the apical endosome. J Cell Biol 1994;124:83–100.
63. Apodaca G, Katz LA, Mostov KE. Receptor-mediated transcytosis of IgA in MDCK cells is via apical recycling endosomes. J Cell Biol 1994;125:67–86.
64. Nuoffer C, Balch WE. GTPases: multifunctional molecular switches regulating vesicular traffic. Annu Rev Biochem 1994;63:949–90.
65. DeCamilli P, Takei K, McPherson PS. The function of dynamin in endocytosis. Curr Opin Neurobiol 1995; 5:559–65.
66. Warnock DE, Schmid SL. Dynamin GTPase, a force-generating molecular switch. Bioessays 1996;18:885–93.
67. Tuma PL, Stachniak MC, Collins CA. Activation of dynamin GTPase by acidic phospholipids and endogenous rat brain vesicles. J Biol Chem 1993;268:17240–6.
68. Schpetner HS, Vallee RB. Dynamin is a GTPase stimulated to high levels of activity by microtubules. Nature 1992;355: 733–5.
69. Tuma PL, Collins CA. Dynamin forms polymeric complexes in the presence of lipid vesicles. Characterization of chemically cross-linked dynamin molecules. J Biol Chem 1995; 270:26707–14.
70. Lin HC, Gilman AG. Regulation of dynamin GTPase activity by G protein betagamma subunits and phosphatidylinositol 4,5 bisphosphate. J Biol Chem 1996;271:27979–82.
71. Gout I, Dhand R, Hiles ID, et al. The GTPase dynamin binds to and is activated by a subset of SH3 domains. Cell 1993; 75:25–36.
72. Herskovits JS, Shpetner HS, Burgess CC, Vallee RB. Microtubules and Src homology 3 domains stimulate the dynamin GTPase via its C-terminal domain. Proc Natl Acad Sci U S A 1993;90:11468–72.

73. Salim K, Bottomley MJ, Querfurth E, et al. Distinct specificity in the recognition of phosphoinositides by the pleckstrin homology domains of dynamin and Bruton's tyrosine kinase. EMBO J 1996;15:6241–50.
74. Warnock DE, Hinshaw JE, Schmid SL. Dynamin self-assembly stimulates its GTPase activity. J Biol Chem 1996;271:22310–4.
75. van der Bliek AM, Meyerowitz EM. Dynamin-like protein encoded by the *Drosophila* shibire gene associated with vesicular traffic. Nature 1991;351:411–4.
76. Takel K, McPherson PS, Schmid SL, De Camilli P. Tubular membrane invaginations coated by dynamin rings are induced by GTP-gamma S in nerve terminals. Nature 1995;374:186–90.
77. Clark SG, Shurland DL, Meyerowitz EM, et al. A dynamin GTPase mutation causes a rapid and reversible temperature-inducible locomotion defect in *C. elegans*. Proc Natl Acad Sci U S A 1997;94:10438–43.
78. Zerial M, Stenmark H. Rab GTPases in vesicular transport. Curr Opin Cell Biol 1993;5:613–20.
79. Gorvel JP, Chavrier P, Zerial M, Gruenberg J. Rab5 controls early endosome fusion in vitro. Cell 1991;64:915–25.
80. Stenmark H, Parton RG, Steele-Mortimer O, et al. Inhibition of rab5 GTPase activity stimulates membrane fusion in endocytosis. EMBO J 1994;13:1287–96.
81. Feng Y, Press B, Wandinger-Ness A. Rab7: an important regulator of late endocytic membrane traffic. J Cell Biol 1995;131:1435–52.
82. Ullrich O, Reinsch S, Urbe S, et al. Rab11 regulates recycling through the perinuclear recycling endosome. J Cell Biol 1996;135:913–24.
83. Goldenring JR, Smith J, Vaughan HD, et al. Rab11 is an apically located small GTP-binding protein in epithelial tissues. Am J Physiol 1996;270:G515–25.
84. Baldini G, Sherer PE, Lodish HF. Non-neuronal expression of rab3A: induction during adipogenesis and association with different intracellular membranes than rab3D. Proc Natl Acad Sci U S A 1995;92:4284–8.
85. Lütcke A, Jansson S, Parton RG, et al. Rab17, a novel small GTPase, is specific for epithelial cells and is induced during cell polarization. J Cell Biol 1993;121:553–64.
86. Goldenring JR, Shen KR, Vaughan HD, Modlin IM. Identification of a small GTP-binding protein, rab25, expressed in the gastrointestinal mucosa, kidney and lung. J Biol Chem 1993;268:18419–22.
87. Gekle M, Mildenberger S, Freudlinger R, et al. Albumin endocytosis in OK cells: dependence on actin and microtubules and regulation by protein kinases. Am J Physiol 1997;272:F668–77.
88. Bradbury NA, Bridges RJ. Endocytosis is regulated by protein kinase A, but not protein kinase C in a secretory epithelial cell line. Biochem Biophys Res Comm 1992;184:1173–80.
89. Bijlsma PB, Kiliaan AJ, Scholten G, et al. Carbachol, but not forskolin increases mucosal-to-serosal transport of intact protein in rat ileum in vitro. Am J Physiol 1996;271:G147–55.
90. Lukacs GL, Segal G, Kartner N, et al. Constitutive internalization of cystic fibrosis transmembrane conductance regulator occurs via clathrin-dependent endocytosis and is regulated by protein phosphorylation. Biochem J 1997;328:353–61.
91. Clark SL Jr. The ingestion of proteins and colloidal materials by columnar absorptive cells of the small intestine in rats and mice. J Biophys Biochem Cytol 1959;5:41–50.
92. Cornell R, Padykula HA. A cytological study of intestinal absorption in the suckling rat. Am J Anat 1969;125:291–361.
93. Abrahamson DR, Rodewald R. Evidence for the sorting of endocytic vesicle contents during the receptor-mediated transport of IgG across the newborn rat intestine. J Cell Biol 1981;91:270–80.
94. Rodewald R. Distribution of immunoglobulin G receptors in the small intestine of the young rat. J Cell Biol 1980;85:18–32.
95. Simister NE, Rees AR. Isolation and characterization of an Fc receptor from neonatal rat small intestine. Eur J Immunol 1985;15:733–8.
96. Rodewald R, Abrahamson DR. Receptor mediated transport of IgG across the intestinal epithelium of the neonatal rat. Ciba Foundation Symposium 92. London: Pitman Books; 1982. p. 209–32.
97. Cornell R, Walker WA, Isselbacher KJ. Small intestinal absorption of horseradish peroxidase. A cytochemical study. Lab Invest 1971;25:42–8.
98. Gebert A, Rothkotter H-J, Pabst R. M cells in Peyer's patches of the intestine. Int Rev Cytol 1996;167:91–159.
99. Neutra MR, Pringault E, Kraehenbuhl JP. Antigen sampling across epithelial barriers and induction of mucosal immune responses. Annu Rev Immunol 1996;14:275–300.
100. Moxey PC, Trier JS. Specialized cell types in the human fetal small intestine. Anat Rec 1978;191:269–86.
101. Geuze HJ, Slot JW, Strous GJAM, et al. Intracellular sorting during endocytosis: comparative immunoelectron microscopy of multiple receptors in rat liver. Cell 1984;37:195–204.
102. Casanova JE, Apodaca G, Mostov KE. An autonomous signal for basolateral sorting in the cytoplasmic domain of the polymeric immunoglobulin receptor. Cell 1991;66:65–75.
103. Breitfeld PP, Casanova JE, McKinnon WC, Mostov KE. Deletions in the cytoplasmic domain of the polymeric immunoglobulin receptor differentially affect endocytic rate and postendocytic traffic. J Biol Chem 1990;265:13750–7.
104. Casanova JE, Breitfeld PP, Ross SA, Mostov KE. Phosphorylation of the polymeric immunoglobulin receptor required for its efficient transcytosis. Science 1990;248;742–5.
105. Hirt RP, Hughes GJ, Frutiger S, et al. Transcytosis of the polymeric Ig receptor requires phosphorylation of serine 664 in the absence but not the presence of dimeric IgA. Cell 1993;74:245–55.
106. Cardone MH, Smith BL, Song W, et al. Phorbol myristate acetate-mediated stimulation of transcytosis and apical recycling in MDCK cells. J Cell Biol 1994;124:717–27.
107. Hansen SH, Casanova JE. Gsα stimulates transcytosis and apical secretion in MDCK cells through cAMP and protein kinase A. J Cell Biol 1994;126:677–87.
108. De Camilli P, Emr SD, McPherson PS, Novick P. Phosphoinositides as regulators in membrane traffic. Science 1996;271:1533–9.
109. Joly M, Kazlauskas A, Fay F, Corvera S. Phosphatidylinositol-3-kinase is required at a post-endocytic step in PDGF receptor trafficking. J Biol Chem 1995;270:13225–30.
110. Martys JL, Wjasow C, Gangi DM, et al. Wortmannin-sensitive trafficking pathways in chinese hamster ovary cells. Differential effects on endocytosis and lysosomal sorting. J Biol Chem 1996;271:10953–62.
111. Spiro DJ, Boll W, Kirchhausen T, Wessling-Resnick M. Wortmannin alters the transferrin receptor endocytic pathway in vivo and in vitro. Mol Biol Cell 1996;7:355–67.
112. Hansen SH, Olsson AM, Casanova JE. Wortmannin, an inhibitor of phosphoinositide-3-kinase, inhibits transcytosis in polarized epithelial cells. J Biol Chem 1995;270;28425–32.
113. Dunn JS. The fine structure of the absorptive epithelial cells of the developing small intestine of the rat. J Anat 1967;101:57–68.
114. Hayward AF. Changes in fine structure of developing intestinal epithelium associated with pinocytosis. J Anat 1967;102:57–70.
115. Colony PC, Neutra MR. Macromolecular transport in the fetal rat intestine. Dev Biol 1985;89:294–306.

116. Staley TE, Corley LD, Bush LJ, Jones EW. The ultrastucture of neonatal calf intestine and absorption of heterologous proteins. Anat Rec 1972;172:559–80.
117. Kraehenbuhl J-P, Gloor E, Blanc B. Resorption intestinale de la ferritine chez deux especes animales aux possibilities d'absorption proteique neonatale differentes. Z Zellforsh Mikrosk Anat 1967;76:170–86.
118. Colony Moxey P, Trier JS. Development of villus absorptive cells in the human fetal small intestine: a morphological and morphometric study. Anat Rec 1979;195:463–82.
119. Orlic D, Lev R. Fetal rat intestinal absorption of horseradish peroxidase from swallowed amniotic fluid. J Cell Biol 1973;56:106–19.
120. Lev R, Orlic D. Uptake of protein in swallowed amniotic fluid by monkey fetal intestine in utero. Gastroenterology 1973;65:60–8.
121. Gitlin D, Kumate J, Morales C, et al. The turnover of amniotic fluid protein in human conceptus. Am J Obstet Gynecol 1972;113:632–45.
122. Horibe N, Okamoto T, Itakura A, et al. Levels of hepatocyte growth factor in maternal serum and amniotic fluid. Am J Obstet Gynecol 1995;173:937–42.
123. Jenkin G, McFarlane JR, de Kretser DM. Implication of inhibin and related proteins in fetal development. Reprod Fertil Dev 1995;7:323–31.
124. Merimee TJ, Grant M, Tyson JE. Insulin-like growth factors in amniotic fluid. J Clin Endocrinol Metab 1984;59:752–5.
125. Laham N, Brennecke SP, Bendtzen K, Rice GE. Tumor necrosis factor alpha during human pregnancy and labour: maternal plasma and amniotic fluid concentrations and release from intrauterine tissues. Eur J Endocrinol 1994;131:607–14.
126. Wissig SL, Graney DO. Membrane modifications in the apical endocytic complex of ileal epithelial cells. J Cell Biol 1968;39:564–79.
127. Knutton S, Limbrick AR, Robertson JD. Regular structures in membranes: membranes in the endocytic complex of ileal epithelial cells. J Cell Biol 1974;62:679–94.
128. Trahair J, Wilson JM, Neutra MR. Endotubin: a marker antigen for the endocytic stage of intestinal development in rat, sheep, and human. J Pediatr Gastroenterol Nutr 1995;21:277–87.
129. Jakoi ER, Zampighi G, Roberston JD. Regular structures in unit membranes. II. Morphological and biochemical characterization of two water-soluble membrane proteins from the suckling rat ileum. J Cell Biol 1976;70:97–111.
130. Speelman BA, Allen K, Grounds TL, et al. Molecular characterization of an apical early endosomal glycoprotein from developing rat intestinal epithelial cells. J Biol Chem 1995;270:1583–8.
131. Allen K, Gokay KE, Thomas MA, et al. Biosynthesis of endotubin: an apical early endosomal glycoprotein from developing rat intestinal epithelial cells. Biochem J 1998. [In press]
132. Clark SL Jr. The ingestion of proteins and colloidal materials by columnar absorptive cells of the small intestine in rats and mice. J Biophys Biochem Cytol 1959;5:41–50.
133. Gonnella PA, Neutra MR. Membrane-bound and fluid-phase macromolecules enter separate prelysosomal compartments in absorptive cells of suckling rat ileum. J Cell Biol 1984;99:909–17.
134. Koldovsky O. Hormonally active peptides in human milk. Acta Paediatr Suppl 1994;402:89–93.
135. Murphy RA, Saide JD, Blanchard MH, Young M. Nerve growth factor in mouse serum and saliva: role of the submandibular gland. Proc Natl Acad Sci U S A 1977;74:2330–2.
136. Weaver LT, Freigberg E, Israel EJ, Walker WA. Epidermal growth factor in human amniotic fluid. Gastroenterology 1988;95:1436.
137. Thornburg W, Matrison L, Magun B, Koldovsky O. Gastrointestinal absorption of epidermal growth factor in suckling rats. Am J Physiol 1984;246:G80–5.
138. Wilson JM, Whitney JA, Neutra MR. Biogenesis of the apical endosome-lysosome complex during differentiation of absorptive epithelial cells in rat ileum. J Cell Sci 1991;100:133–43.
139. Israel EJ, Simister N, Freiberg E, et al. Immunoglobulin G binding sites on the human foetal intestine: a possible mechanism for the passive transfer of immunity from mother to infant. Immunology 1993;79:77–81.
140. Leissring JC, Anderson JW, Smith DW. Uptake of antibodies by the intestine of the newborn infant. Am J Dis Child 1962;103:160–5.
141. Menard D, Arsenault P, Pothier P. Biologic effects of epidermal growth factor in human fetal jejunum. Gastroenterology 1988;94:656–63.

CHAPTER 6

Cell Interactions through the Basement Membrane in Intestinal Development and Differentiation

Michèle Kedinger, PhD

Jean-Noel Freund, PhD

Jean-Francois Launay, PhD

Patricia Simon-Assmann, PhD

Intestinal morphogenesis, proximodistal regionalization, and maintenance of the steady state between cell proliferation and differentiation result from tightly controlled heterologous cell interactions. Various in vitro and in vivo cellular models have shown that this epithelial-mesenchymal crosstalk involves basement membrane molecules and is regulated by cytokines and hormonal factors. In this review, we will focus mainly on the current knowledge of the expression and role of basement membrane laminins in the gut and on the contribution of homeobox transcription factors in the permissive and inductive epitheliomesenchymal cell interactions, and in the laminin-induced epithelial cell response.

GENERAL CHARACTERISTICS OF THE ADULT AND DEVELOPING GUT

The intestinal wall consists of mucosa whose functional element, the simple epithelium, is mainly composed of absorptive, mucus, endocrine, and Paneth's cells. The structural support of the epithelial layer is provided by the mucosal connective tissue, the lamina propria, which contains various cellular elements, including fibroblasts, muscle fibers, nerve fibers, blood, and lymphatic vessels. The most external tissue layers of the gut form the continuous peripheral muscle coat.

Two Main Characteristics Displayed by the Adult Gut

First, the digestive epithelium is characterized by constant and vigorous cell renewal and differentiation, which lead to compartmentalizing into the crypts, composed of stem cells and proliferative cells, and the villi in the small intestine, composed of differentiating-differentiated cells. The crypts are monoclonal, and the different cell types that compose the epithelium derive from a single stem cell. For the enterocytes, at least, there is a clear onset of expression of most functional proteins at the crypt-villus (CV) junction. This peculiar organization results from a vertical migration of the intestinal epithelial cells from the crypts towards the villus tip, where cells are extruded into the lumen.[1-3] In the colon, the crypts/glands are deeper, and the villi are replaced by a flat surface epithelium (Figure 6–1A, B).

Second, the intestinal tube is characterized by a morphologic and functional proximodistal (PD) regionalization. Despite the same CV architecture along the three main portions of the small intestine—the duodenum, jejunum, and ileum—the height of the villi progressively decreases from the proximal to the distal segments. Similarly, although the crypt architecture is maintained throughout the colon, it can be subdivided into three anatomically distinct portions.

The functional regionalization along the gastrointestinal tract (exemplified in Figure 6–2) concerns every epithelial cell type. For instance, the digestive hydrolases, like sucrase or lactase, selectively expressed in the small intestinal absorptive cells, decrease along the PD axis. In addition, both enzymes exhibit developmental characteristics: their onset occurs proximodistally; in rodents, the first expression of sucrase occurs late, around weaning; and lactase, already present at birth, then decreases and, around weaning in rodents, is no more expressed in the distal ileum.[4] The intestinal fatty acid binding proteins (I-FABP) and the ileal lipid binding protein (I-LBP) have also been extensively studied, providing insight into the molecular regulatory processes involved in tissular and PD-specific expression.[1] Among other markers, pepsinogen and carbonic anhydrase, expressed respectively in gastric and colonic epithelial cells, have been used in studies of epithelial-mesenchymal interactions and of promoter activity.[5,6] The mucus or goblet cells increase in number with the distal progression along the small and large intestine. In parallel, various mucin genes are expressed specifically in the stomach, small intestine, or colon.[7] Associated with this cell lineage are also proteins of the trefoil factors family (TFF)[8] that are expressed differentially along the gastrointestinal tract: PS2 (TFF1, comprising one trefoil domain) and SP (TFF2, two domains) are expressed in a complementary manner in the gastric mucus cells; and ITF (TFF3, one domain) is associated with

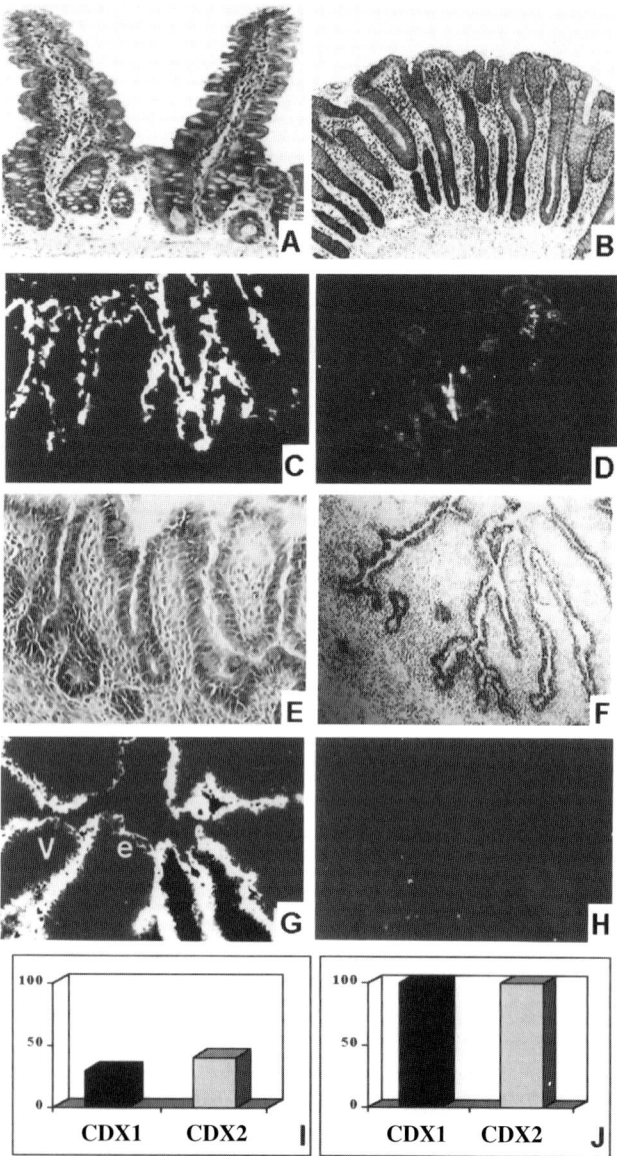

FIGURE 6–1. Experimental conditions leading to distinct patterns of intestinal morphogenesis and differentiation. A and B, Typical small intestine (A) and colon (B) structures. C and D, Immunocytochemical detection of sucrase on cryosections of associations composed of colon endoderm and small intestinal mesenchyme (C) and the corresponding control colon endoderm reassociated with its own mesenchyme (D) developed for 4 weeks under the skin of nude mice. E to H, Associations composed of small intestinal endoderms and F1G9 cells (E, G) or A1F1 cells (F, H) developed as intracoelomic grafts in chick embryos for 12 days. PAS staining (E, F) and immunocytochemical detection of lactase (G, H) on cryosections of the grafts. I and J, Semiquantitative analysis (arbitrary units) of CDX1 and CDX2 mRNA by RT-PCR, representative of the in vivo and experimental conditions illustrated, respectively, in A, C, E, G (small intestinal-type morphogenesis and differentiation) and in B, D, F, H (colon-type morphogenesis).

Monoclonal antirat sucrase and lactase antibodies have been kindly provided by A. Quaroni (Cornell University, Ithaca, NY). These experiments are published,[19,23,130] and the figure is taken from Kedinger M, Duluc I, Fritsch C, et al. Intestinal epithelial-mesenchymal cell interactions. Ann N Y Acad Sci 1998;859:1–17.

the mucus cells in the intestinal mucosa, except in the duodenal Brünner's gland cells that express SP. Interestingly, the glands surrounding the ulcerated intestinal mucosa in inflammatory bowel diseases display an ectopic PS2 and SP expression. Paneth's cells, which are confined to the crypt bottom, express various bacteriolytic enzymes, among which are defensin-related proteins, the crytdins (6 characterized so far in mice), which are found located in specific regions of the gut.[9] Finally, a variety of endocrine cells are scattered all over the gastrointestinal epithelium; the expression of various peptides also varies along the PD axis.[10]

Development of the Gut

The intestinal tube has a dual, endodermal and mesodermal, origin; it is formed from the association of the visceral endodermal and the splanchnic mesenchyme. These two embryonic anlagen differentiate, respectively, into the epithelial and the connective tissue-muscle layers. Gut development is characterized by morphogenetic processes—progressive outgrowth of the villi and, later on, downgrowth of the crypts in the stromal tissue—that are accompanied by a chronologic emergence of the different epithelial cell types: absorptive, mucus, endocrine, and, finally, Paneth's cells. The outer muscle layers and the mucosal and submucosal connective tissue form concurrently. The overall processes involved in the ontogenic maturation of the gastrointestinal tract are closely similar in most animal species; the temporal patterns, however, vary among them[11] (examples given in Figures 6–3 and 6–4.) Morphologic observations of the developing intestine emphasize the presence, at the basal surface of the deepest endodermal cell layer, of closely apposed elongated mesenchymal cells; later on, clumps of cuboidal mesenchymal cells concentrate at the apical edge of the growing villi.[12] In the adult organ, flat, elongated, subepithelial myofibroblasts underline the crypt compartment,[13] and a regular network of flat stellate fibroblastic cells has been described over the whole height of the villi.[14] An ultrastructurally recognizable basement membrane (BM) lies between the endodermal/epithelial and mesenchymal/fibroblastic cell layers from the fetal to the adult stages. Basement membranes are complex molecular structures composed mainly of collagens IV, laminins, proteoglycans, and nidogen (or entactin).

Experiments have shown that intestinal development, as well as the homeostasis in the adult organ, result from dynamic and reciprocal interactions between epithelial and mesenchymal (or mesenchyme-derived) cells. There is increasing evidence that this cellular crosstalk involves BM molecules, as well as various paracrine factors, acting on the cell behavior via membrane receptors (including integrins and tyrosine kinase receptors).

In this review we will (1) summarize the current knowledge and describe the latest experimental observations that emphasize the role of epithelial-mesenchymal cell interactions in gut development and homeostasis; (2) make an overview of the composition, cellular origin, and function of the intestinal basement membrane; and (3) discuss recent data suggesting that key transcription factors, i.e., homeodomain proteins, mediate the regulatory effects of BM molecules.

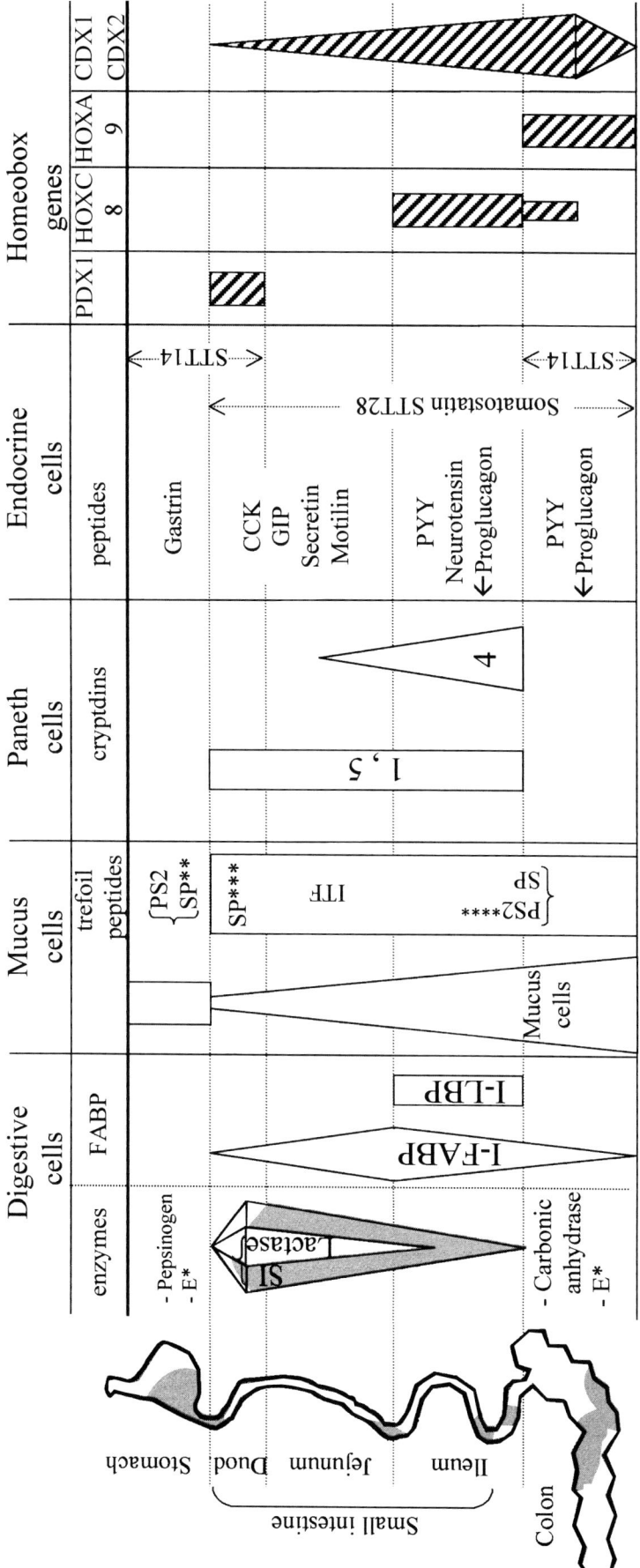

FIGURE 6–2. Nonexhaustive examples of proximodistal markers of various gastrointestinal epithelial cell lineages in the adult organ. Digestive cells: chief cells in the stomach; enterocytes in the small intestine; colonocytes in the colon. E = brushborder enzymes: sucrase-isomaltase (SI) and lactase; *= negative except in gastric intestinal metaplasia or differentiated colonic cancers; I-FABP = intestinal fatty acid binding protein; I-LBP = ileal lipid binding protein; CCK = cholecystokinin; GIP = gastric inhibitory polypeptide; PYY = peptide YY; ←proglucagon = peptides derived from the proglucagon gene; **= complementary expression in the stomach: PS2 (TFF1) in the surface mucus cells of the fundus and antrum, SP (TFF2) in the isthmus and glandular cells of both segments respectively; ***= confined in Brünner's gland cells; ****= induced in glands at the periphery of ulcers in inflamatory bowel disease. For corresponding references, see text.

RECIPROCAL EPITHELIAL-MESENCHYMAL CELL INTERACTIONS IN THE DEVELOPING AND ADULT GUT

The role of epithelial-mesenchymal cell interactions in the processes of morphogenesis and cytodifferentiation of the gastrointestinal tract during development and in the adult organ have been well documented using grafting models of interspecies and PD heterologous intestinal tissue associations developed in vivo in the coelom of chick embryos and/or under the kidney capsule or the skin in nude mice (see Figure 6–4).[11,15]

The basic conclusions of these studies have been reviewed formerly[11,16,17] and can be summarized as follows. (1) As a

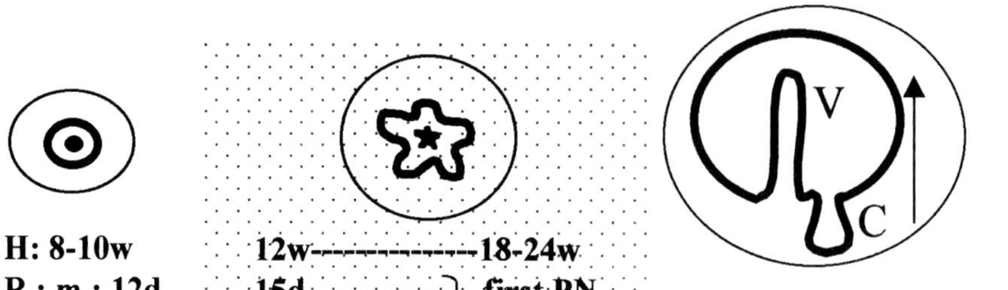

Stages	H: 8-10w R : m : 12d r : 14d	12w—18-24w 15d—} first PN 17d—} week	adult
Type IV collagen			
[α1(IV); α2 (IV)][152,153]	+ (R,H)	+ (R,H)	+ (R,H)
α5 (IV)[49]; α6 (IV)[155]	nd	α5;α6 + (H)	α5 - (H) ; α6 nd
[α3 (IV); α4 (IV)][49]	nd	- (H)	- (H)
Nidogen[152]	+ (R)	+ (R)	+ (R)
Perlecan[153,57]	+ (R,H)	+ (R,H)	+ (R,H)
Laminins			
β1γ1 (commun to LN1, 2, 10)[50,154]	+ (R,H)	+ (R,H)	+ (R,H)
LN1 α1	+ (R[50],H[70,156])	+ (R[50],H[70,156])	+ R: crypts[50] + H: villi[70,154]
LN2 α2	- (R,H)[70]	+ (R,H)[70]: crypt formation	+ (R,H)[70,154] : crypts
LN10 α5[60]	+ (R)	+ (R)	+ (R) : villi : increasing gradient
LN5 β3	+ (H[59]; R[pd])	+ (H[59]; R[pd])	+ (H[59,54];R[pd]) } villi : increasing gradient
LN5 γ2[59]	+ (H,R)	+ (H,R)	+ (H,R) } villi : increasing gradient
LN5 α3	+ (H)[59] - (R)[59]	+ (H)[59] - (R)[59]	+ (H)[59,54] } villi : increasing gradient + (R)[59] } villus tip

FIGURE 6–3. Expression of BM molecules in the subepithelial BM during intestinal development. The schematic representation of the gut in the upper part of the figure corresponds respectively to an undifferentiated stage, a morphogenetic phase, and the adult stage; the bold line depicts the BM at the interface between the endoderm-epithelium and the outer mesenchyme-mesenchyme derived layers.
Unless otherwise stated in the adult, BM molecules are found all over the CV BM.
Numbers in exponents correspond to references. See also corresponding reviews 35, 45–47.
R = rodent; H = human; w = weeks; d = days; PN = postnatal; C = crypt; V = villus; pd = personal data; nd = not done; m = mouse; r = rat.

general rule, the endodermal-mesenchymal cell interactions are reciprocal and permissive; the mesenchyme allows the formation of a specific morphogenesis (illustrated in Figure 6–4), and the endoderm directs the type of the epithelial cytodifferentiation. (2) The integrity of the tissues is not required: indeed, either endodermal or mesenchymal cell cultures associated with the intact counterpart are able to form intestinal structures when developed as grafts; similarly, bilayered endodermal-mesenchymal cocultures allow the endodermal cells to differentiate. (3) Heterologous cell interactions are maintained in the mature gut: postnatal crypt cells (the IEC-17 cell line[18]) require the association with fetal intestinal mesenchyme to differentiate into the various epithelial cell phenotypes; reciprocally, fibroblastic cell cultures raised from the postnatal lamina propria develop the typical lamina propria cells and form the external muscle coat when they are associated with fetal intestinal endoderm and grafted. (4) In addition to the permissive cell interactions, some inductive effects have been shown; they concern, on the one hand, the ability of the chick embryonic small intestinal mesenchyme to induce gastric endoderm to turn on an intestinal cytodifferentiation, and on the other hand, the ability of the intestinal endoderm to induce skin fibroblastic cell cultures to differentiate into intestinal smooth muscle cell layers.

Tissue Determinants of the Proximodistal Cytodifferentiation

Using some PD markers that have been listed above, we showed that developmental and positional information along the length of the small and large bowel is already acquired in

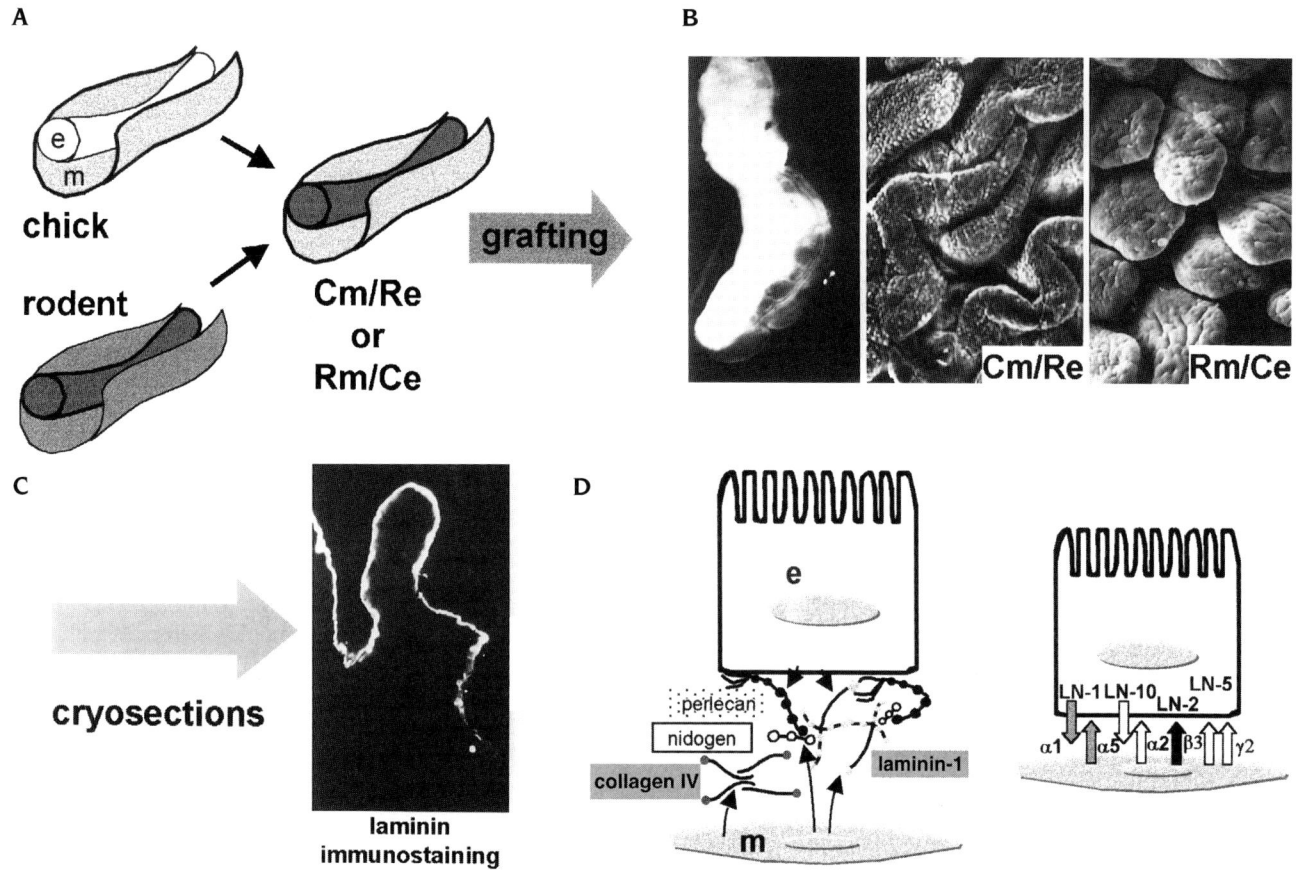

FIGURE 6–4. Epithelial-mesenchymal cooperation for the formation of the BM. A, The technique used consists of the construction of interspecies intestines by the dissociation (collagenase treatment and mechanical dissection) of the endoderm (e) from the mesenchyme (m) of chick (5 1/2 days) and rodent (12 days, mice; 14 days, rat) fetal intestines and cross-reassociation between chick mesenchyme and rodent endoderm (Cm/Re), or vice and versa (Rm/Ce). B, These hybrid associations are grafted in the coelom of 3-day chick embryos or in nude mice for various periods. The developed hybrid intestinal segments are individualized and vascularized; their luminal surface (scanning electron microscope) shows that the morphogenetic pattern corresponds to the species from which the mesenchyme is derived: zig-zag pattern in Cm/Re, and finger-like villi in Rm/Ce. C, Immunostaining with species-specific antibodies of the individual BM components (and laminin isoform chains) is performed on cryosections of the hybrid intestinal segment. The immunostaining illustrates the epithelial production and deposition in the subepithelial BM of laminin in a Cm/Re graft with an antibody-recognizing rodent antigens. D, Schematic representation of the epithelial or mesenchymal origin (*arrows*) of the main BM constituents (*left*) and laminin isoforms (*right*) resulting from the analysis of Cm/Re and Rm/Ce grafts developed for 13 to 17 days. The main binding sites among the BM components allowing the formation of a three-dimensional network are represented on the left panel.[35,51,56–60]

14-day rat fetal gut and is independent of luminal factors. The most significant example is given by the follow-up of lactase expression. Indeed, the mRNA and protein patterns, observed respectively in the 2- or 4-week grafts of fetal jejunum and ileum, recapitulate the normal pattern along the small intestine of neonates and adult animals and in particular the shut-off of lactase expression in the ileal segment that occurs at weaning.[19] The case of sucrase is also interesting as it is expressed in the xenografts precociously compared to its onset in situ, probably due to an effect of the hormonal status of the adult host. This precocious expression, visualized after 2 weeks of graft, displays a clear PD gradient: early turn-on of the sucrase gene in the proximal jejunum, where the protein is already detectable over the whole villus length; and late turn-on in the distal ileum, where sucrase is found only in the basal third of the villi.[19] The conclusion that position-specific information is acquired during fetal life was also made based on isografts of 15- to 16-day normal and transgenic (FABP/hGH) mice intestine.[20]

To analyze whether the positional information of functional marker expression displayed by the epithelial cells can be modulated by the mesenchyme, we analyzed grafted heterotopic associations composed of 14-day fetal endoderm and mesenchyme from proximal and distal small intestinal segments (e.g., jejunal mesenchyme combined with ileal endoderm, and vice versa). This study led to the conclusion that, at this developmental stage, the small-intestinal endoderm holds the cytodifferentiation information; indeed, each type of recombinant expressed an enzymatic pattern corresponding to the PD level from which the endoderm was originated, independently of the origin of the associated mesenchyme. The situation differs for the colon endoderm. Indeed, the ileal mesenchyme, and to a lesser extent the jejunal mesenchyme, was able to induce colonic endoderm to turn on a small intestinal-type enzymatic differentiation (Figure 6–1C, D),[19] indicating that the small intestinal mesenchyme can switch the endogenous cytodifferentiation program of the colonic endoderm. This observation is of special interest, as colon tumors also express small intestinal enzymes.[21] In contrast to the enterocytic transdifferentiation of the colonic absorptive cells, the endocrine cell lineage is not influenced by inductive actions of the mesenchyme. Indeed, endocrine cell types that are specific to the colon (those that express glucagon-like peptide and peptide YY; see Figure 6–2) are still found in tissular associations composed of small intestinal mesenchyme and colonic endoderm, and endocrine cells specific to the proximal part of the gut (cholecystokinine and gastric inhibitory polypeptide-positive cells) have not been found in these associations.[22] Another inductive action emanating from the mesenchyme has also been described at the molecular level in the chick embryonic stomach.[5] These authors took advantage of the specific expression of pepsinogen in the proventriculus (PV) (glandular stomach) but not in the gizzard (GZ) (muscular stomach). By using an in vitro model of cultured aggregates comprising mesenchymal cells and epithelial cells transiently transfected with a pepsinogen promoter-reporter gene construct, they demonstrated that the PV mesenchyme is able to induce pepsinogen expression in GZ epithelial cells as in PV cells; in contrast, GZ mesenchyme does not support expression in the PV epithelial cells.

Differential Properties of Individual Mesenchymal Cell Lines

To acquire a better knowledge of the phenotypic characteristics of the intestinal mesenchymal cells, we analyzed the properties of two morphologically distinct cell clones, A1F1 and F1G9—derived from primary cultures of postnatal rat ileal lamina propria—on associated epithelial cell.[23] It was particularly interesting to find that F1G9 cells induce the differentiation of intestinal endodermal cells in coculture and a CV morphogenesis in grafted associations, while the A1F1 cells stimulate proliferation rather than differentiation of the endodermal cells in vitro and induce a gland morphogenesis in vivo (see Figure 6–1E,F). The different inductive properties of these two mesenchymal cell lines can be correlated, although no causative link has been established, with the following observations: TGFβ1 induces F1G9, but not A1F1, cells to differentiate into myofibroblasts; and the F1G9 cell line produces more laminin than the A1F1 cells.[23] Moreover, human mesenchymal clonal cell lines derived from normal duodenal biopsies have been established and characterized. Interestingly, two of them (C9 and C11) display differences similar to those described for F1G9 and A1F1 with regard to their effect on epithelial cell behavior assessed on endodermal or CaCo-2 colonic cancer cells.[24] Further, the rat as well as the human mesenchymal cell lines analyzed exhibited different proliferative responses—inhibition or stimulation—to various cytokines. These data suggest that the lamina propria comprises various fibroblastic cell phenotypes that are differentially sensitive to cytokines, and that exhibit a different ability to support epithelial proliferation and differentiation. In addition, subepithelial fibroblasts have been shown to be involved in the inflammatory response.[13,25,26] Thus, based on these observations and on the variable properties of mesenchymal cells derived from the intestinal connective tissue, one may hypothesize that the epithelial-mesenchymal crosstalk is regulated, at least partly, by mesenchymal cells-lymphocytes interactions.[27–29] Indeed, an unbalanced cytokine rate may lead to changes in mesenchymal cell phenotypes or in the relative proportion of various mesenchymal cell types, which could, on the one hand, provoke impaired interactions with the epithelial cells and, as a consequence, tissue injury or, on the other hand, facilitate wound repair. These two situations may occur in chronic inflammatory bowel disease or in intestinal pathogenic infections.

INTESTINAL BASEMENT MEMBRANE

The BM is a specialization of the extracellular matrix (ECM). In the gut wall (without consideration of the vascular and nerve inputs), the ECM comprises the following:

1. The interstitial matrix, which is composed of a network of various types of collagens, noncollagenous glycoproteins, and proteoglycans, and which forms the core of the mucosal and submucosal connective tissue. Although a more detailed description is beyond the scope of this review, we will refer to some of these molecules on p. 94, because their expression is altered in intestinal bowel disease (IBD).

2. The muscular BM that surrounds individual smooth muscle cells in the outer muscular layers and in the muscularis mucosae.
3. The subepithelial BM, which will be focused on due to its location at the epithelial-mesenchymal-stromal interface. This specialized sheet-like extracellular matrix structure is recognizable ultrastructurally, between the endodermal-epithelial and the mesenchymal-fibroblastic cell layers, from the earliest fetal stages studied. This molecular structure is first regular and becomes interrupted during the phases of intense morphogenesis; in the adult organ, it is regular in the crypt region and becomes interrupted toward the apical third of the villi.[2]

Molecular Heterogeneity of the Developing to Adult Intestinal Subepithelial Basement Membrane

In general, the BMs are composed of various major molecules: type IV collagen, laminin, perlecan—a heparan sulfate proteoglycan—and nidogen/entactin. Details concerning the basic structures and main properties of these molecules can be found in comprehensive reviews.[30–32] We will focus on two main characteristics of these molecules as they are of fundamental importance for the understanding of the biologic role of the BMs and of the tissue- and stage-specific structure-function relationship.

First, the major BM molecules, type IV collagen and laminin, belong, in fact, to families of molecules. Collagen IV, like other collagens, is a triple helical-molecule composed of three α chains. The master molecule is formed by two $\alpha 1(IV)$ chains and one $\alpha 2(IV)$ chain encoded, respectively, by the COL4A1 and COL4A2 genes. In addition, two isoforms have been found: they are composed of $\alpha 3(IV)$ and $\alpha 4(IV)$ chains and of $\alpha 5(IV)$ and $\alpha 6(IV)$ chains, respectively.[33] The finding of collagen isoforms arose from studies of molecular defects of the renal glomerular basement membrane, i.e.: hereditary Alport's syndromes characterized by glomerulonephritis; diffuse esophageal leiomyomatosis, characterized by a benign proliferation of the smooth muscle cells; and Goodpasture's syndrome, an autoimmune disease characterized by glomerulonephritis and pulmonary hemorrhage. The family of laminins comprises cross- or T-shaped heterotrimeric proteins, composed of three chains named α (long arm chain), β, and γ (short arm chains).[30] The first laminin molecule identified in the intestinal BM corresponds to laminin-1; this molecule, first isolated from the Engelbreth-Holm-Swarm (EHS) tumor, is composed of three subunits, $\alpha 1$, $\beta 1$, $\gamma 1$, encoded by three distinct genes, LAMA1, LAMB1, and LAMC1. Thus far, 11 laminin variants have been described; their chain composition is summarized in Table 6–1A. They are expressed in a tissue- and developmental-specific manner, suggesting that they might generate functional diversity.[34,35] As with type IV collagens, laminin chain deficiencies have been associated with pathologic states: in particular, mutations in each gene encoding for the three constituent chains of laminin-5 ($\alpha 3$, $\beta 3$, $\gamma 2$) result in various types of junctional epidermolysis bullosa, characterized by skin blistering at the dermal-epidermal junction.[36,37] Mutations in the LAMA2 gene, encoding the $\alpha 2$ chain, are linked to a subtype of human muscular dystrophy,[38] which is also the major phenotype of $\alpha 2$-deficient mice (the mutant dy/dy mouse strain).[39]

Second, BM molecules, like ECM molecules in general, are characterized by complex modular structures with binding domains, allowing them, particularly in the case of laminin and collagen IV, to form networks by self-assembly and to bind several other components. For example, nidogen/entactin is able to link the laminin and collagen net-

TABLE 6–1
Constituent Chains of the Currently Known Laminin Isoforms and Integrins Binding to These Molecules

A											
Laminin	-1	-2	-3	-4	-5	-6	-7	-8	-9	-10	-11
Chains	$\alpha 1\beta 1\gamma 1$	$\alpha 2\beta 1\gamma 1$	$\alpha 1\beta 2\gamma 1$	$\alpha 2\beta 2\gamma 1$	$\alpha 3\beta 3\gamma 2$	$\alpha 3\beta 1\gamma 1$	$\alpha 3\beta 2\gamma 1$	$\alpha 4\beta 1\gamma 1$	$\alpha 4\beta 2\gamma 1$	$\alpha 5\beta 1\gamma 1$	$\alpha 5\beta 2\gamma 1$

B Laminins \ Integrins	$\alpha 1\beta 1$	$\alpha 2\beta 1$	$\alpha 3\beta 1$	$\alpha 6\beta 1$	$\alpha IIb\beta 3$	$\alpha 6\beta 4$	$\alpha 7\beta 1$	$\alpha 9\beta 1$	$\alpha v\beta 3$	$\alpha ?\beta 8$
Laminin-1	Y	Y	Y	Y	Y	Y	Y	Y	Y	Y
Laminin-2	N	N	Y	Y	Y	Y				
Laminin-3				Y						
Laminin-4	N	N				Y	Y			
Laminin-5		Y	Y	Y		Y				

Details can be found in[30,34] for the laminin isoforms and in [41,42,77] for the integrins. Y = yes; N = no.

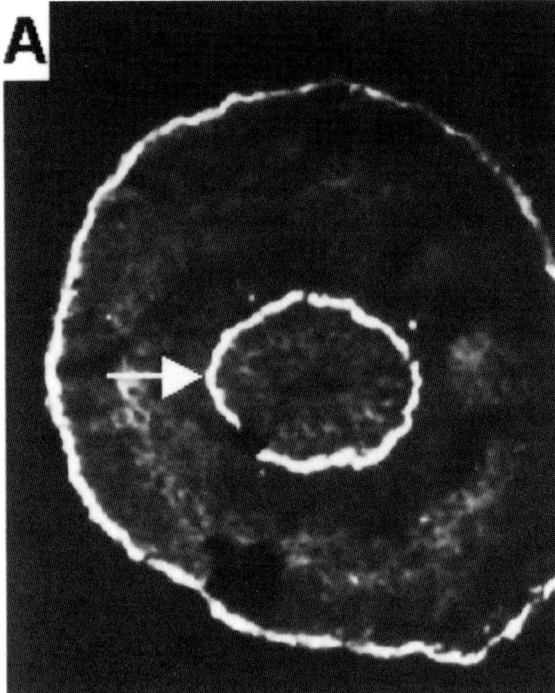 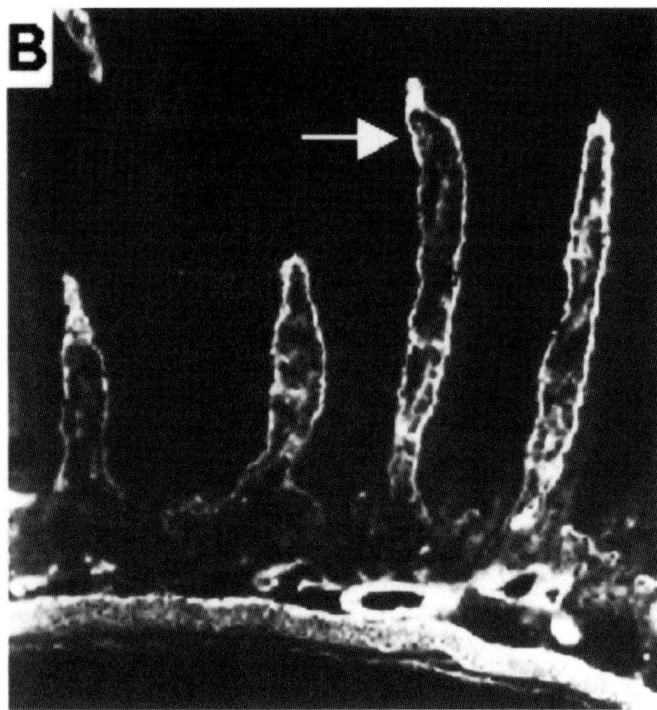

FIGURE 6–5. Immunostaining of LN-10 with anti-α5 antibodies (raised by L. Sorokin, Erlangen, Germany) in 12-day fetal (A) and adult (B) mouse intestines. Note that LN-10 is present at the endoderm-mesenchyme interface at early fetal stages and in the villus subepithelial BM in the mature organ[60] (*arrows*). Additionally, the α5 immunostaining is visible in the serosa, in the muscle layers, and surrounding blood vessels.

works and to form a ternary complex between laminin-1 and the protein core of proteoglycans.[32,40] Such intermolecular connections are schematized on Figure 6–4. Additionally, these molecules carry specific binding sites for cellular ECM receptors, the integrins, which consist of heterodimeric transmembrane proteins; the laminin-binding integrins are listed in Table 6–1B, and more details are available in reviews.[41,42] Furthermore, laminins containing α1 or α2 chains also bind to a component of a membrane receptor complex, the α-dystroglycan.[32,43] Knowledge about the function of the integrins has grown recently due to analysis of targeted mutations-deletions in mice;[44] however, there is still no indication of their role in intestinal development or adult steady-state. The expression pattern of the integrins in intestinal tissue has been reviewed by Beaulieu,[45,46] and will be referred to here only when necessary.

The precise composition of the BM and expression of integrins or other receptors vary among organs, and in the gut, do so as a function of the developmental stage and the CV position. The microheterogeneity of the BM is achieved by a time- and spatial-specific expression of the various isoforms of each family of molecules, leading to a precise three-dimensional organization that determines, through their receptors, the nature of the signals transmitted to the epithelial cells. Figure 6–3 summarizes the composition of the intestinal subepithelial BM at two developmental stages and along the CV axis in the mature organ. In addition to the main molecules referred to in Figure 6–3, decorin (a chondroitin sulfate proteoglycan), SPARC/BM40, and fibulins have been described in the gut BM.[32,46,47]

The three following points arise from these immunocytochemical studies in which the use of antibodies directed against individual BM-constituent chains allowed the researchers to focus specifically on the molecular composition of the subepithelial BM. The major references are quoted in Figure 6–3.

At the earliest stages of gut formation BM molecules, namely type IV collagen, nidogen, perlecan, and laminins 1, 5, and 10 (Figure 6–5), are already visible. No comprehensive studies have been done that analyze the chronologic deposition of these molecules in the primitive gut at embryonic stages preceding the association of the visceral endoderm with the splanchnic mesoderm. Our in vitro experimental models seem to indicate that, although individually both cell types produce some BM molecules (laminin-1 is known to be one of the earliest molecules produced by embryonic cells), they are not able to assemble them as a true BM before heterologous cell contacts have been achieved (see pp. 91, 92).

Simultaneously to the main morphogenetic phases, changes occur in the expression of collagen IV and laminin variants. First, collagen α5(IV) chain is expressed transiently, underlining the basolateral pole of the epithelial cells, around the 18th week in the human fetal intestine; the α6(IV) chain has also been found at the same gestational period in the human gut but has not been analyzed in the adult organ. In addition to this sporadic epithelial expression, these collagen IV chain molecules are mainly found to be associated with the intestinal smooth muscle.[48,49] Second, laminin-2, composed of an α2 chain associated with β1/γ1 chains, is expressed late during intestinal development. Its onset correlates to the formation of the crypts, where it is and remains restricted. In addition to these qualitative modifications of the BM, there are quantitative changes, as in the case of the laminin-α1 chain, which is synthesized in higher amounts (related to the β1-γ1 chains) during the phase of villus morphogenesis.[50]

The adult BM exhibits microheterogeneity and can be subdivided into a crypt and a villus BM; besides ubiquitous molecules (collagen α1/α2[IV], nidogen, perlecan), the crypt BM comprises laminin-2 whereas the villus BM contains both laminin-5 (Figure 6–6) and laminin-10 (see Figure 6–5), with an increasing gradient from the crypt mouth to the villus tip. In mouse intestine, laminin-1 is restricted to the crypts; in human, the immunocytochemical detection of this isoform using anti-α1 chain antibodies shows a villus localization but there is controversy regarding the specificity of the antihuman α1 antibodies that could crossreact with the α5 chain. Whether the difference between the two species is an artefact due to the tools used or whether it corresponds to a true difference is still not resolved.

Other ECM molecules, among them fibronectin, tenascin, and type VII collagen, are associated to the intestinal BM. The two former molecules exhibit an interesting complementary expression pattern in the adult intestine: fibronectin shows a decreasing gradient from the crypt BM to the villus tip, whereas tenascin increases towards the villus tip.[46,51] On the basis of in vitro analysis of the adhesion properties of intestinal epithelial cells to these molecules, this complementary expression pattern underlines a possible antiadhesive role of tenascin when epithelial cells move up to the villus tip.[52] This property is of interest, since tenascin is overexpressed in colitis. As far as type VII collagen is concerned, this molecule, composed of three α1(VII) chains, was thought to be exclusively expressed in squamous epithelia, where these anchoring fibrils connect the BMs to the underlying stroma.[53] A recent study describes an interesting expression pattern along the intestinal CV axis with changes along the anteroposterior axis: (1) negligible staining in the duodenum; (2) staining restricted to the lower part of the villus compartment in the jejunum; (3) prominent staining along the whole villus BM in the ileum; and (4) staining confined to the surface epithelium in the colon.[54,55] This molecule may form, together with laminin-5 and other constituents, the so-called hemidesmosome type II structures (see p. 92).

Epithelial-Mesenchymal Complementarity in the Formation of the Basement Membrane

In vitro experiments have demonstrated the importance of epithelial-mesenchymal contacts in both the formation of a BM and intestinal epithelial differentiation. To discover the physiological significance of the developmental and spatial microheterogeneities in the intestinal BM composition, we analyzed the cellular origin of individual BM components as a function of the developmental stage of the tissue, using interspecies chick-rodent embryonic epithelial-mesenchymal tissue recombinants. The hybrid intestines are developed as grafts in the chick embryo over varying periods of time, and the deposition of individual BM components in

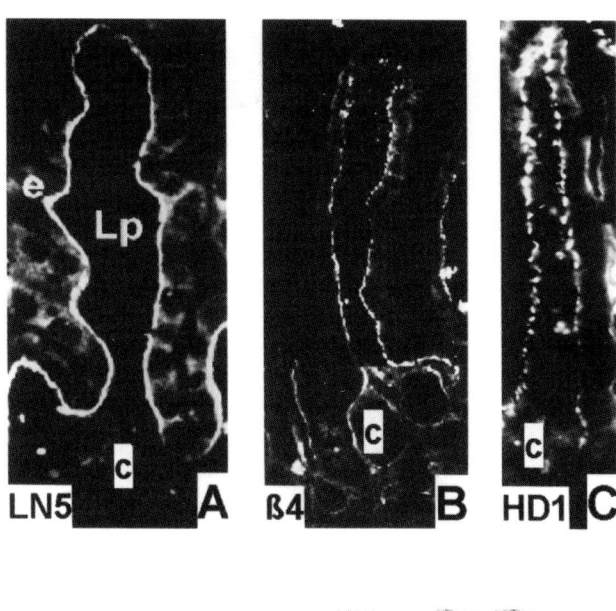

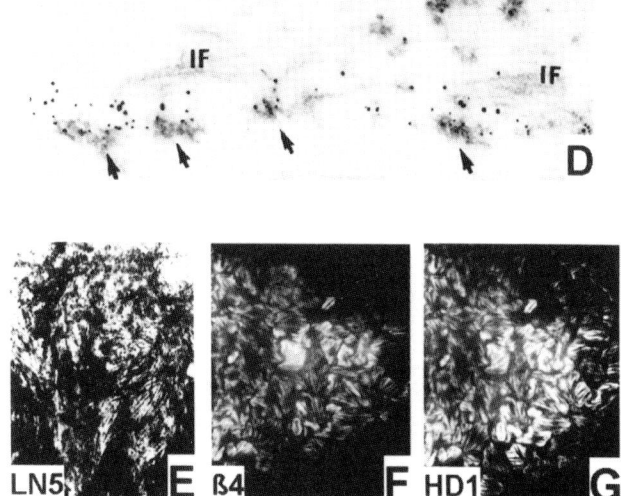

FIGURE 6–6. Type II hemidesmosomes are present in intestinal epithelial cells. Localization along the CV axis in the adult intestine (A to C) and at the basal surface of human colonic cancer HT29 cells (D to G) of laminin-5 and of α6β4 and HD1, constituents of type II hemidesmosomes. Pictures A to C show that the three components are colocalized in the subepithelial BM (LN-5) and at the basal pole (β4 integrin subunit, HD1) of the villus epithelial cells. Crypts (c) are almost devoid of LN-5 and HD1. e = epithelial cells; Lp = lamina propria. Picture D represents an ultrastructural immunolocalization of the β4 integrin subunit (5 nm gold particles) and of the plectin-like protein HD1 (10 nm gold particles). The latter is associated with the basal intermediate microfilaments (IF). The fixation-permeabilization steps that have been used allow the visualization of basal dense-type II HD structures (arrows). Pictures E to G correspond to immunocytochemical staining of LN-5 (E) deposited on the culture dish (after detachment of the cells from the substratum by EDTA treatment), and of β4 integrin subunit and HD1 (F, G: double staining) visualized at the ventral pole of the cells. Note that there is a clear colocalization of the two latter components and that LN-5 is deposited as basal patches similar to those depicted for β4 and HD1. These data can be found in vivo[59,70] and in vitro.[74–77]

the hybrid intestines is detected using species-specific antibodies. The experimental procedure and the main data obtained at the final developmental stage of the tissue recombinants are summarized in Figure 6–4 and reviewed in Simon-Assmann et al.[35,47]

Briefly, this technique allowed us to show that perlecan deposition is achieved by the epithelial compartment, while collagen type IV and nidogen are mostly mesenchymal products.[47,56,57] The production of the various laminin isoforms deposited at the epithelial-mesenchymal interface is complex: individual α, β, and γ chains are produced either by both cell types (α1, α5, β1, γ1, γ2) or exclusively by the mesenchymal ones (α2, β3).[35,58–60] Some of these data have been confirmed by in situ hybridization (laminin-β1 chain;[61] collagen IV;[62] laminin-α2 and laminin-α5 chains[60]). This latter technique alone, however, in contrast to the use of the interspecies recombinants, cannot prove that the molecules produced by the cell population in which the transcripts are found are, indeed, associated with the subepithelial BM.

Two major chronologic changes were revealed by observation of interspecific hybrids at various developmental stages: (1) the α1 chain of laminin-1 is produced by the epithelial cells during the whole development of the hybrids, and additionally by the mesenchymal cells only at advanced differentiated states;[58] (2) the α2 chain of laminin-5 is also of great interest since it presents a shift in its cellular expression; indeed, this chain is deposited by undifferentiated epithelial cells at early stages of development and by the mesenchymal cells at later stages parallel to the establishment of the adult pattern.[59]

Epithelial and mesenchymal cells, therefore, cooperate in the chronologic production of laminin isoforms: epithelial cells produce the laminin-1 and laminin-10 isoforms, and the mesenchymal cells produce laminin-2 and laminin-10 at any stage of differentiation. In addition, mesenchymal cells display a delayed expression/deposition of α1 and γ2 chains, which suggests that reciprocal inductive cell interaction processes leading to the mesenchymal differentiation are necessary for the expression of these specific BM molecules. Suggestion of requirement of a close tissue cooperation for the assembly of the BM is reinforced by the findings related to the formation of the laminin-nidogen-collagen IV complex (see above).[63]

The physiologic importance of the epithelial-mesenchymal cooperation for the establishment of the BM is also illustrated by the fact that glucocorticoids, which induce a precocious maturation of the fetal and postnatal intestines,[64,65] and retinoic acid, which is an intestinal morphogen that accelerates villus formation, crypt proliferation, and enterocytic differentiation,[66] may act through the mesenchymal compartment by increasing, in particular, laminin deposition.[66,67]

Understanding the Role of Basement Membrane Molecules in the Intestine

An increasing understanding of the role of BM molecules in general, and in the gut in particular, has been possible using a combination of in situ observations of developing and mature tissues (immunofluorescence, in situ hybridization; see p. 89); in situ examinations of tissues from animals or humans with gene deficiencies; and in vitro experiments using cultures of cells grown on various extracellular matrix substrates or on heterologous cells (cocultures). Combining the data obtained from these approaches is important because each has its limitation. For example, cells used in vitro are often immortalized or derived from tumors while the in vivo inhibitions of gene expression by homologous recombination can be either lethal or compensated by rescue pathways.

The role of the BM in the gastrointestinal system was first indicated when it was observed that early embryonic gastric or intestinal endodermal cells are not able to polarize/differentiate unless they are cocultured, associated with mesenchyme-derived cells, or seeded on ECM substrates.[2,51,68,69] A systematic study of the expression of differentiation markers and deposition of BM components in a coculture system led to the concept that heterologous cell contacts are necessary for the formation of the BM, and that BM formation precedes the onset of functional markers. The BM molecules whose function in intestinal cells has been most widely studied belong to the laminin family. Below are data and conclusions obtained for individual molecules.

Laminin-2 (α2β1γ1)

The restricted localization of this laminin isoform in the crypt BM indicated that it could play a role in crypt cell proliferation, in Paneth's cell differentiation, and/or in the maintenance of the stem cell microenvironment, allowing the emergence of the four intestinal cell lineages. Surprisingly, in dy/dy mice lacking the α2 chain (see p. 89), the crypt compartment, the villus height, or the various intestinal cell phenotypes were not altered.[70] Since α1 chains are also present in the mouse crypt BM, their presence may compensate for the lack of α2 chains. When cultured on laminin-2 coatings, human colonic cancer CaCo-2 cells, characterized by a high degree of differentiation,[71,72] exhibit an increased expression of two brush border enzymes, aminopeptidase and alkaline phosphatase; however, the typical intestinal enzymes sucrase and lactase were unchanged.[73] Thus, no clear conclusion about the role of laminin-2 in the gut can be drawn from these sporadic experiments.

Laminin-5 (α3β3γ2)

As mentioned earlier, this laminin isoform plays a crucial role in the dermal-epidermal integrity; in the squamous epithelia, laminin-5 forms the extracellular anchoring filaments of the hemidesmosomes (HDs), structures localized at the basal pole of the cells facing the BM. Typical HDs are composed of the transmembrane BPAG2-BP180 (Bullous Pemphigoid Antigen) and α6β4 integrin, and of intermediate filament-associated proteins HD1-plectin-IFAP300 and BPAG1-BP230, which form, respectively, the intracellular cytoplasmic and inner plaques that are linked to the intermediate filaments. Type VII collagen is also associated with these structures and constitutes the anchoring fibrils. In the simple intestinal epithelium, typical HDs have never been observed at the ultrastructural level. Nevertheless, a recent immunogold electron microscopic analysis of human HT29 colonic cancer cells clearly shows the presence of the cytoplasmic plaques of the HDs at the basal side of the cells (Figure 6–6D[74]). These structures in situ and in cell lines are composed of α6β4 integrin, HD1 protein, and laminin-5 but lack the two BPAG proteins;[59,70,74–77] they are called type II HDs. In HT29 cells, the three components are colocalized as patches at the ventral pole of the cells (Figure 6–6E to G). It is worth noting that in vivo the three constituents of type II HDs (α6β4, HD1, and laminin-5) are colocalized at the basal domain of the villus epithelial cells in the human intestine (Figure 6–6A to C). Leivo et al.[54] additionally showed that the onset of laminin-5 is immediately adjacent to the proliferative cells labelled with BrDU. Although type VII collagen exhibits important variations along the anteroposterior axis of the gut (see above), its distribution at least in the ileum fits with that of the other constituents of type II HDs.[54]

The dramatic consequences of mutations in the laminin-5 genes emphasize its functional importance in the skin (see p. 89); in some cases, intestinal disorders have been observed in these patients but the morphologic and functional natures of these defects in the gut have not been analyzed until now. Pyloric atresia can be associated with subtypes of junctional epidermolysis bullosa resulting from mutations in the α6 or β4 integrin subunits. The study of the intestines of α6 or β4 integrin subunits knockout mice[78–80]—that die shortly after birth—would be interesting at later stages by grafting the fetal intestines from the knockout animals.

The fact that intestinal type II HDs lack the BPAGs and that these structures are localized at the level of the villus enterocytes, where active migration occurs, suggests that they may participate in cell migration rather than function as anchoring devices as in the skin. The possible involvement of laminin-5 in intestinal epithelial cell migration has been documented in vitro using the polarized human colonic T84 cancer cells, which produce mainly laminin isoforms containing the α3 chain: laminins -5, -6, and -7.[81] Indeed, the restitution of T84 monolayers after mechanical wounding is blocked by antibodies directed against the laminin-α3 chain or against the corresponding receptors, the integrins α6β4 or α3β1.[81] In accordance with these results, HT29-FU cells,[82] seeded on a matrix enriched in LN-5, are induced to form threadlike extensions at the end of which a bright, colocalized staining of HD1 and the β4 integrin subunit can be seen.[74] Further, laminin-5 has been shown to be a primary target of the matrix metalloprotease-2, which cleaves the α2 chain, allowing a subsequent activation of cryptic sites on the α3 chain that trigger cell motility.[83] It would thus be of particular interest to know whether the truncated form of the γ2 chain is present in the developing intestine that undergoes intensive remodeling, and in the mature organ, where active cell migration occurs.

Correlations have, moreover, been reported between the expression of LN-5 and the size of tumors developed in nude mice by injections of various colonic cancer cell lines and/or their invasive properties. They are as follows: (1) Highly-producing LN5-α6β4-HT29 cells form larger tumors than CaCo-2 cells, which produce only low amounts of the LN5 γ2 chain and do not express the integrin α6β4 (personal data).[77] (2) CaCo-2 cells in which the synthesis of the laminin-5-γ2 chain and of the β4 integrin subunit are stimulated as a result of an overexpression of the CDX2 homeobox gene (see p. 95) develop significantly larger tumors than control cells.[84] (3) Targeted expression of α6β4 integrin in β4-deficient colon carcinoma cells increased the rate at which cells became invasive.[85] (4) The level of laminin-5α3 chain expressed in vitro by various clones of the human LoVo colonic cancer cell line correlates with the potential of the clones to develop metastasis.[86]

These observations are reinforced by the following findings. First, there is a preferential expression of the laminin-5-γ2 chain in invasive malignant colon cancer cells, with a high accumulation of the transcripts in cells localized at the front of migration.[87] Second, the LAMC2 (γ2) gene-promoter activity is significantly enhanced in HT29-MTX cells[88] under the influence of hepatocyte growth factor-scatter factor (HGF-SF),[89] which is known to be overexpressed in tumors,[90] and whose overexpression in transgenic mice induces tumorigenesis.[91] These data strongly indicate that laminin-5, associated with type II hemidesmosomes, is involved in cell migration along the villus axis and participates in tumor growth and invasion.

Laminin-1 (α1β1γ1)

Several lines of evidence indicating that laminin-1 is intimately involved in triggering differentiation of intestinal epithelial cells were provided by in vitro models. First, the addition of antilaminin-1 antibodies to intestinal endodermal/fibroblastic cocultures inhibits the onset of lactase, a typical differentiation marker of the intestinal epithelium.[67] Second, laminin-1, used as a substratum, significantly increases the expression of digestive enzymes such as lactase and sucrase in CaCo-2 cells.[73,92] Beaulieu's group also showed that there is a direct relationship between the apical expression of sucrase in these cells and their basal expression of laminin α1 chain,[73] and that the onset of sucrase expression is preceded by a transient expression of the α7Bβ1 integrin isoform, which is found in situ at the base of the villi and could be involved in the signaling pathway of laminin-1.[93] Third, correlations can be inferred among the capacity of the two human colonic cancer cell lines, HT29 and CaCo-2 cells, to produce laminin α1 chain, their degree of differentiation, and their ability to form a monolayer and a well organized BM when cultured on fibroblastic cells.[94,95]

Direct evidence of the role of laminin-1 in enterocytic differentiation has been provided in vitro using an antisense RNA strategy.[96] The inhibition of α1 chain expression in the CaCo-2 cells leads to (1) an incorrect secretion of the two other constituent chains of laminin, the β1 and γ1 chains; (2) the lack of BM formation in the coculture model, despite the production of other BM components—type IV collagen and nidogen—by the mesenchymal cells; and (3) alterations in the structural and functional polarity of the cells (poorly developed microvilli, absence of sucrase expression). However, in complementary experiments, the transfection of the full-length laminin α1 cDNA in α1-deficient HT29 cells promoted neither cell differentiation nor the formation of a BM in cocultures (De Arcangelis et al.,[96] and personal data). This could be linked to the peculiar repertoire of laminin isoforms and integrins in these cells, which may prevent the assembly of the ectopic α1 chains in a functional laminin-1 molecule, and/or the normal cell-cell and cell-matrix adhesion.

The prime importance of laminin-1 constituent chains is also suggested by in vivo observations. Indeed, disruption of the ubiquitously expressed LAMC1 gene encoding the γ1 chain leads to early embryonic lethality (Smith and Edgar, personal communication). Embryonic lethality due to multiple defects, among them an altered intestinal epithelial cell polarization, has been reported in *Drosophila* lacking the LAMA,[97–99] but no equivalent model has been obtained in mice. Due to the expected embryonic lethality of laminin-α1-deficient mice, we are developing a targeted disruption strategy in the intestine using the Cre-lox P system (Lefebvre et al., unpublished observations).

Laminin-1 thus appears to play a prime role in intestinal BM assembly and epithelial cell differentiation. Recent data that bring new insights to the understanding of the molecular mechanisms whereby extracellular matrix components trigger cell differentiation are detailed in p. 95.

Alterations of Basement Membrane Molecules in Intestinal Pathologies

The major alterations of the BMs are described in tumors, where a correlation between the degree of BM disruption and of the malignity has often been reported. Only a few intestinal pathologies have been found to be associated with defects in BM molecules.

A deficiency of laminin staining was observed in intestinal biopsies taken from children affected by a peculiar type of intractable diarrhea, called tufting enteropathy.[100] In this case, it has not been possible to determine whether the drop in laminin deposition at the subepithelial level was the primary defect of this disease, or whether it was secondary to an epithelial alteration. Patey et al.[101] recently showed that in tufting enteropathy, epithelial cells display an increased number of desmosomes, indicating an increased cell-cell adhesion which may cause alterations in the cell-matrix interactions.

A disruption of the BM heparan sulfate proteoglycan (perlecan) has been described in intestinal biopsies from patients affected by inflammatory bowel disease (IBD);[102] as these disruptions were found in the vicinity of tumor necrosis factor α (TNFα)-producing macrophages, they may result from a cytokine-dependent BM degradation. Conversely, other cytokines, transforming growth factor β (TGFβ) in particular, are also known to induce an overexpression of extracellular matrix molecules or of integrin receptors in various systems.[103] TGFβ1 is increased in IBDs[104] and may, among other changes (i.e., induction of fibrillar collagens leading to fibrosis), enhance the synthesis of tenascin, a phenomenon that has been reported in different types of colitis;[105] this abnormal expression of tenascin possibly competes with epithelial cell adhesion to fibronectin and induces cell shedding[52] (see p. 89), which could result from cell apoptosis following disruption of β1 integrin-matrix interactions.[106] Thus, in IBDs, changes in the composition of the intestinal BM or in the expression of integrins may, on one hand, result in a massive epithelial cell loss leading to ulcerations or, on the other hand, allow a subsequent re-epithelialization.[107]

Finally, an increased expression and deposition of laminin-1 and type IV collagen have been reported in the intestinal muscle layers in Hirschsprung's disease and in ls/ls mice, both being characterized by a deficient innervation of the distal gut. This defect could result from a precocious differentiation, induced by an overexpression of laminin-1, of the migrating neural crest cells that colonize the gut.[11,108]

BASEMENT MEMBRANE AND HOMEOBOX GENES INVOLVED IN CONTROL OF GENE EXPRESSION

The role of cell interactions, of BM components, and of some growth factors in intestinal development and homeostasis have been summarized. The transcriptional events that mediate these effects were poorly understood until recently. Here, we will focus on studies concerning the role of homeobox genes in the intestine and their regulation by extracellular matrix components and cell interactions.

Homeobox genes were identified in the mid-'80s in *Drosophila*, and later throughout the animal kingdom and in plants. This family of genes encodes nuclear transacting factors that bind DNA via a conserved basic helix-turn-helix domain, the so-called homeodomain.[109] They play a key role in the control of morphogenesis, in positional information, and in cell identity. They are regulated by morphogenetic agents such as retinoic acids, and by growth factors.[110] Among the targets of homeoproteins are the promoters of cell adhesion molecules and extracellular matrix components, providing a link between the control of gene expression and morphogenetic and differentiation events.[109,111] Consistent with their function during early development, homeobox genes are essentially expressed in the fetus; however, their expression is maintained at the adult stage in a small number of tissues including the intestine.

Homeobox Gene Expression in the Digestive Tract

Several homeobox genes are expressed in the digestive tract. During morphogenesis, they are expressed in cells of both mesenchymal and endodermal origin, and they become progressively restricted to the epithelial cell layer at the perinatal stage. As described at the beginning of this article, the gut, although not segmented, displays a morphologic and functional regionalization. According to a possible role of homeobox genes in defining the positional information and/or the cell identity, some of them exhibit differences in expression along the proximodistal axis of gut (Figure 6–2). For instance, PDX1, HOXC-8 (HOX3-1), and HOXA-9 (HOX1-7) transcripts are found, respectively, only in the duodenal, ileal, and colonic epithelium.[112,113] The only indication of the role of HOX genes in the gut concerns HOXA-4, expressed in the mesenchyme, and whose overexpression is associated with megacolon in transgenic mice.[114] In addition to its duodenal localization, PDX1 is expressed in the pancreas; it transactivates insulin and somatostatin. The primary role of PDX1 is indicated by the fact that knockout mice display defects in pancreatic and duodenal development. In the pancreas, PDX1 deficiency is linked to an early failure of exocrine and endocrine cells to proliferate and differentiate (absence of amylase and insulin positive cells) in response to mesenchymal signals;[115] in the rostral duodenum, the epithelial cells remain cuboidal, Brünner's gland cells do not differentiate, and there is a decrease in the number of endocrine cells (serotonin, secretin, and CCK). Interestingly, the inhibition by homologous recombination of other homeobox genes belonging to the PAX family, PAX-4 and PAX-6,[116–118] and of a transcription factor BETA2,[119] strongly suggests that these genes control the cytodifferentiation of cellular subsets from the pancreatic and intestinal endocrine cell lineage, respectively, PAX-4, those secreting insulin (β) or somatostatin (δ) cells; PAX-6, glucagon (α) cells; and BETA2, insulin (β) or secretin (S) cells. Whether the expression of these genes along the PD axis of the gut correlates with the occurrence of the various endocrine cell types (Figure 6–2) remains unanalyzed. Additional homeobox genes, namely CDX1 and CDX2 genes, display an increasing expression gradient along the intestinal PD axis; they are discussed below.

Intestinal Caudal-Related CDX1 and CDX2 Homeobox Genes

Two homeobox genes of the caudal family, CDX1[120] and CDX2[121]—the murine CDX2 gene is homologous to CDX3, originally identified in the hamster—have been extensively studied in recent years. In *Drosophila*, caudal participates in the determination of the embryonic anteroposterior axis; later it is restricted to posterior structures, in particular, the intestine of adult flies.[122] In mammals, CDX1 and CDX2 display a biphasic pattern. They are expressed in many tissues during early embryonic development and become restricted to the intestinal epithelium at the time of intestinal formation. For instance, CDX1 is transiently expressed in limb buds and along the central axis;[123] accordingly, CDX1 knockout mice show homeotic transformation of vertebrae, probably due to a CDX1-dependent shift of HOX gene expression domains.[124] CDX2 exhibits a transient expression in extraembryonic structures at day 3.5 post-coitum, as well as in the lateral splanchnic derivatives that provide the mesenchymal support of the digestive tract; accordingly, the homozygous null mutants do not survive the peri-implantation period.[125] The chicken CDX2 homologue, CDXA, shows a similar expression pattern.[126,127]

Once the expression of CDX1 and CDX2 is restricted to the intestinal tract, two peculiar features suggest they may be involved in the positional information and/or in the control of epithelial cell proliferation and differentiation. First, both genes exhibit an increasing gradient along the intestinal PD axis; this gradient is already established in the fetus and is maintained throughout adulthood.[112,121,128–130] Second, the CDX1 protein is predominantly expressed in the crypt compartment whereas the CDX2 protein is preferentially expressed in the differentiating compartment.[121,131] Consistent with this localization, CDX2 has been shown to be involved in the regulation of differentiation gene expression, such as sucrase and lactase.[132,133] The prime role of CDX1 and CDX2 in the intestinal epithelium is reiterated by the facts that CDX1 is turned on in small intestinal metaplasia of the esophagus and stomach,[131] and that heterozygous CDX2 knockout mice develop multiple colonic adenomas.[125] Consistently, CDX2 expression is decreased in human colon cancers and in chemically-induced colonic tumors in the rat.[134,135] A decline of CDX1 has also been reported in colonic tumors but without correlation between the degree of this decrease and the severity of dysplasia.[131,135,136] These observations and those arising from the experiments described below suggest that CDX1 may be a proto-oncogene whereas CDX2 is a new colonic tumor-suppressor gene.

The function of CDX1 and CDX2 was further investigated by cell transfection. In spontaneously differentiating colonic CaCo-2 TC7 cells,[72] CDX1-overexpression does not modify the rate of proliferation or differentiation; however, CDX1 inhibition by antisense RNA in these cells reduces cell proliferation,[84] and in nonintestinal cells CDX1 stimulates cell proliferation, suggesting a possible oncogenic effect of this homeobox gene.[137] Regarding CDX2, we failed to develop CaCo-2 TC7 cell clones expressing the antisense cDNA; cells displayed defects in adhesion to the substrate.[84] In contrast, CDX2 overexpression in undifferentiated IEC crypt cell lines, as well as in CaCo-2 TC7 cells, reduces cell proliferation and concomitantly stimulates cell polarization and differentiation[84,138] (personal data). In CaCo-2 cells, we observed pleiotropic effects in response to CDX2 overexpression[84] (Figure 6–7A). First, a clear stimulation of sucrase transcripts and activity was observed. Second, a modification of the overall cell adhesion properties was accompanied by (1) changes in laminin gene expression (decrease in laminin α1 mRNA and increase in laminin γ2 mRNA) and modifications of the integrin repertoire (decrease in integrin β1 subunit and increase in the β4 integrin subunit and its associated HD1 protein), visualized immunocytochemically by a shift from the α6β1 to the α6β4 integrin at the ventral domain of the cells;[139] (2) and increased expression of intercellular adhesion molecules or associated proteins (E-cadherin, APC). Third, CDX2 overexpression led to modifications in homeobox gene expression (increase in HOXA-9 and decrease in CDX1 transcripts). It is worth mentioning that the molecules stimulated by CDX2 are predominantly expressed in the differentiating enterocytes in vivo whereas those downregulated by CDX2 transfection are predominantly expressed in the crypt compartment (Figure 6–7B). These results suggest that CDX2 plays a key role in the control of the coordinated process of cell differentiation during the constant renewal of the intestinal epithelium. Further, CDX1 appears to be mainly involved in the control of cell proliferation although an effect on cell differentiation cannot be ruled out.

Regulation of the CDX1 and CDX2 Homeobox Genes by Epithelial-Mesenchymal Cell Interactions: In Vivo Models

The role attributed to the *Drosophila* caudal gene in defining the anteroposterior information, along with the function of the mammalian CDX1 and CDX2 homologues in intestinal cell proliferation and differentiation, prompted us to investigate whether these genes are involved in the mesenchymal-dependent regionalization of the gut. For this purpose, we took advantage of the grafting model in which fetal colonic

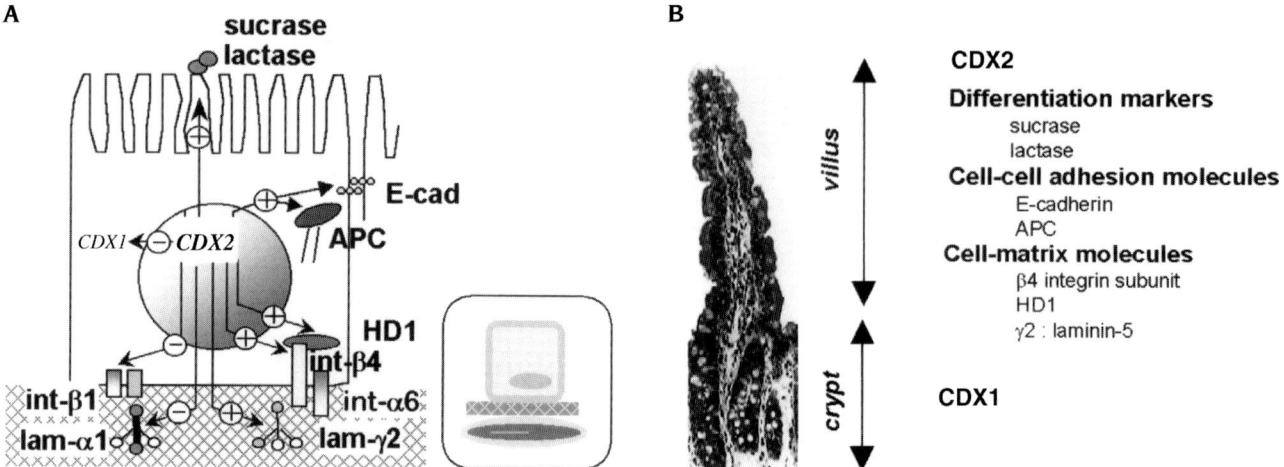

FIGURE 6–7. Schematic representation of the phenotypic changes induced in CaCo-2-TC7 cells transfected with the full-length CDX2 cDNA as in CaCo-2 cells cultured on laminin coatings or on stromal cells (*insert*). A, Data are published;[84] representation of the preferential expression along the CV axis in situ of CDX1 and CDX2 and of the markers that have been stimulated by CDX2 overexpression. B, Note that the β1 integrin subunit and the α1 laminin chain, which are both downregulated by CDX2, are found, respectively, over the whole CV axis and in the crypts in rodents (see text). + = increased expression; − = decreased.

endoderm differentiates either into small intestinal-type or colonic-type[19] (see p. 88). The results indicate that CDX1 and CDX2 expression are lower in the colonic epithelium that has undergone small intestinal-like heterodifferentiation under the influence of the small intestinal mesenchyme, compared to the colonic epithelium that differentiated normally in association with colonic mesenchyme[130] (see Figure 6–1). This is consistent with the fact that both homeobox genes exhibit a higher level of expression in the colon than in the small intestine in situ. Using a similar approach in chicken, Ishii et al.[127] have recently reported that in tissue recombinants composed of embryonic stomach endoderm and small-intestinal mesenchyme, the heterologous mesenchyme induces an intestinal transformation of the gastric endoderm and concomitantly the onset of CDXA expression, whose rostral limit normally lies at the boundary between the stomach and the duodenum. These data demonstrate that the caudal-related genes expressed in the digestive tract of mammals and birds are influenced by epithelial-mesenchymal cell interactions, and that these genes may actually participate in the positional information that dictates the epithelial differentiation along the small and large intestines.

To further document the effect of the mesenchyme on epithelial cell differentiation related to CDX1 and CDX2 expression, fetal endoderm was associated and grafted with the established F1G9 or A1F1 mesenchymal cell lines.[23] Again, the levels of CDX1 and CDX2 expression were lower in grafts exhibiting a typical small intestinal phenotype under the influence of the F1G9 cells than in glandular colonic-like grafts comprising the A1F1 mesenchymal cells[130] (see Figure 6–1). From these data, one can conclude that phenotypically different mesenchymal cell clones—that induce variable morphogenesis and proliferation-differentiation rates of the adjacent epithelium—are able to modify the epithelial expression of the CDX1 and CDX2 homeobox genes.

These results can be related to the findings[140,141] that the intestinal mesenchyme expresses several transcription factors, among which are those encoded by the HLX homeobox gene and by the winged helix transcription factor FKH6, which regulate the mitogenic signal of the visceral endoderm during development. Indeed, targeted disruption of the murine HLX or FKH6 genes is associated with a deficient gut elongation and looping for the former, and with expanded, branched crypts and lengthening of the villi with an overall altered architecture and cytodifferentiation for the latter. Thus, these two regulatory genes appear to control the epithelial cell proliferation and differentiation. According to Kaestner et al.,[141] BMP2 and BMP4 (bone morphogenetic proteins, members of the TGFβ family) could be the targets of FKH6, implicated in the signaling pathway from the mesenchyme to the epithelium. Correlated to this latter conclusion, it is worth noting that TGFβ produced by intestinal fibroblasts induces colon carcinoma T84 cells to form organized luminal structures composed of polarized cells.[142] Moreover, as mentioned on pp. 86 to 88, epithelial-mesenchymal cell interactions in the developing intestine are reciprocal; linked to this, Sonic hedgehog expressed by the endoderm activates regulatory genes, such as BMP4, HOX genes, and possibly others,[143,144] involved in intestinal mesoderm patterning and hindgut formation. Similarly, a chronologic homeobox gene expression is described in *Drosophila* in endoderm-mesenchyme-dependent gut formation.[1,145]

Crosstalk between the Basement Membrane and the CDX2 Homeobox Gene: In Vitro Approach

The findings that, first, CDX2 plays a key role in enterocytic cytodifferentiation and, second, that laminin-1 stimulates intestinal cell differentiation raised the hypothesis that

CDX2 was a good candidate as mediator of the effect of laminin-1. This idea is further supported by the fact that a major consequence of laminin-1 for cell differentiation concerns the stimulation of sucrase-isomaltase,[73,92,96] and that the CDX2 homeoprotein binds and transactivates the sucrase-isomaltase gene promoter.[132]

The analysis of CaCo-2 cells grown on laminin-1 coatings and, inversely, of CaCo-2 clones in which the endogenous production of laminin-1 is prevented by antisense RNA allowed us to establish a direct correlation between laminin-1, the level of CDX2 expression, and cell differentiation.[84] Further, the molecular changes induced in CaCo-2 cells by laminin-1 recapitulate those resulting from the overexpression of CDX2 by transfection, as assessed by the stimulation of APC and integrin β4 subunit, and by the decrease in CDX1 and integrin β1 subunit. In addition, the rise of CDX2 on laminin-1 coatings precedes the changes of APC, integrin β4 and β1, and CDX1 (Lorentz et al.[146] and personal data).

These data strongly suggest that the CDX2 homeobox gene is a mediator of the differentiating effect of laminin-1 on intestinal epithelial cells or, in other words, that CDX2 is controlled by laminin-1. They also provide substantial evidence in favor of a reciprocal control between BM molecules, their integrin receptors, and the CDX2 homeobox gene during intestinal cell differentiation (Figure 6–7). In this model, laminin-1 delivers a stimulatory signal to CDX2, most likely via integrin(s) containing a β1 subunit; consequently, CDX2 triggers cell differentiation and, in particular, it modifies the production of BM components and the integrin repertoire. Although it is difficult to extrapolate results obtained from cells cultured in vitro to the normal situation in vivo, the chronology of events proposed in this model is consistent with the distribution of the corresponding molecules along the CV axis.

The intracellular steps involved in signal transduction from the ECM to tissue-specific gene expression are far from being elucidated; the most extensively documented example concerns the control of mammary gland cells behavior, in which cell shape and laminin signalling via integrins lead to specific gene expression.[147] It has become obvious recently that phosphorylation cascades participate in these processes.[148] We do not yet have any evidence of the regulatory machinery involved in the control of CDX2 gene expression by laminin-1 in the intestinal epithelial cells. However, independently of the integrin signaling, we have demonstrated that the transcriptional activity of the CDX1 and CDX2 promoters is regulated by two different intracellular signaling pathways.[146] Indeed, ras activation stimulates the CDX1 promoter but inhibits the CDX2 promoter. The effect on CDX1 is mediated by the raf-dependent activation of MEK-1 (mitogen-activated-extracellular-related kinase) while the effect on CDX2 is mediated by PKC (protein kinase C) activation and by a modification of the balance between the Jun and Fos transcription factors. It is tempting to extrapolate from these results that extracellular molecules, i.e., BM components, acting via integrins on intracellular transduction pathways and finally on nuclear transcription factors, may influence the level of expression of CDX1 and CDX2, which represent key and specific regulatory genes of intestinal epithelial cell proliferation and differentiation. These results also have implications with regard to the altered expression of these homeobox genes in colonic cancers after oncogenic activation of ras.

CONCLUSION

Various recent discoveries have allowed us to determine the contribution of the crosstalk either between the embryonic tissue anlagen or between the different cellular partners of the intestinal mucosa (epithelial cells, [myo-]fibroblasts, mononuclear cells) in morphogenesis, proximodistal patterning, and regulation of proliferation versus cytodifferentiation during development and in the adult organ. The observation that the BM, which lies at the strategic epithelial-mesenchymal or stromal interface, is composed of molecules produced in an orderly and complementary manner by both tissue components enhances the significance of this heterologous cell crosstalk. Three points are potentially important in the understanding of the cellular and molecular control of the intestinal tissue homeostasis. First, the mesenchymal contribution in these processes has been emphasized by the demonstration of its implication in the deposition of major proteins of the subepithelial BM: type IV collagen, nidogen, and specific constituent chains of laminins. In addition, various soluble factors that control epithelial growth, motility, and morphogenesis are expressed in the gut by the mesenchymal cell compartment—in the vicinity of the epithelium—during the fetal and perinatal period: hepatic growth factor-scatter factor (HGF/SF), neuregulin (NGF), and keratinocyte growth factor (KGF). These factors function via tyrosine kinase receptors that are expressed exclusively or predominantly by epithelial cells.[149] Various human or rat mesenchymal cell lines established recently were shown to express variable amounts of HGF, TGFβ1, and epimorphin;[24,150] interestingly, these cell lines also display proliferative differentiation and adhesive inductive properties on epithelial cells.

Second, homeobox genes/transcription factors expressed either by the mesenchymal or the epithelial cells have been shown to be involved in the main cellular processes—proliferation, differentiation, and proximodistal cell identity—and to be controlled by epithelial-mesenchymal cell interactions via proteins of the TGFβ family, for example.

Third, one of these homeobox genes, CDX2, expressed specifically by the intestinal epithelial cells, is controlled by extracellular laminin-1. This observation is of major interest as this laminin isoform is essential for BM assembly and for epithelial cell differentiation. Interestingly, the experimental overexpression of CDX2 leads to pleiotrophic effects, modifying the expression of cell-cell and cell-matrix adhesion molecules, of differentiation markers, and of other homeobox genes, among them CDX1. Expression of both CDX1 and CDX2 is altered in colonic tumors, CDX2 knockout mice develop tumors, and both homeobox genes are targets of oncogenic signaling.

The challenges for the future are to further clarify the involvement of individual BM molecules via integrins in intestinal homeostasis and to understand the signaling pathways that link the outside of the cells to the nuclear factors and, more generally, those involved in the heterologous cell interactions. That knowledge should allow us to integrate the huge number of experimental observations and the morphofunctional characteristics of the gut, and finally to better understand some pathologic alterations that could lead to the elaboration of new therapies.

The authors would like to thank J. Stutzmann, who provided the ultrastructural picture presented on Figure 6. We would like also to acknowledge the colleagues who participated in the work presented in this review: A. De Arcangelis, C. Foltzer-Jourdainne, L. Fontao, C. Fritsch, O. Lefebvre, O. Lorentz, V. Orian-Rousseau, A. Waydelich, and M. Plateroti, as well as G. Evans (Sheffield, UK), D. Rubin (St. Louis, MO), and L. Sorokin (Erlangen, Germany), who are involved in collaborative programs. We are kindly indebted to C. Arnold and C. Leberquier for their expert technical assistance, and would like to thank I. Gillot and L. Mathern for their help in the finalization of the manuscript and figures.

The work presented in this review has been supported by the INSERM and by grants from the Association François Aupetit, Ferring Pharmaceuticals, Association pour la Recherche sur le Cancer, and Ligue Nationale-contre le Cancer.

REFERENCES

1. Hermiston ML, Simon T, Grossman MW, Gordon JI. Model systems for studying cell fate specification and differentiation in the gut epithelium. In: Johnson LR, editor. Physiology of the gastrointestinal tract. 3rd ed. New York: Raven Press; 1994. p. 521–69.
2. Kedinger M. Growth and development of intestinal mucosa. In: Campbell FC, editor. Small bowel enterocyte culture and transplantation. Austin: R.G. Landes Company; 1994. p. 1–31.
3. Potten CS, Booth C, Pritchard DM. The intestinal epithelial stem cell: the mucosal governor. Int J Exp Pathol 1997; 78:219–43.
4. Duluc I, Jost B, Freund JN. Multiple levels of control of the stage- and region-specific expression of rat intestinal lactase. J Cell Biol 1993;123:1577–86.
5. Fukuda K, Ishii Y, Saiga H, et al. Mesenchymal regulation of epithelial gene expression in developing avian stomach: 5′-flanking region of pepsinogen gene can mediate mesenchymal influence on its expression. Development 1994;120:3487–95.
6. Drummond F, Sowden J, Morrison K, Edwards YH. The caudal-type homeobox protein Cdx-2 binds to the colon promoter of the carbonic anhydrase 1 gene. Eur J Biochem 1996; 236:670–81.
7. van Klinken BJW, Dekker J, Büller HA, Einerhand AWC. Mucin gene structure and expression: protection vs adhesion. Am J Physiol 1995;269:G613–27.
8. Thim L. Trefoil peptides: from structure to function. Cell Mol Life Sci 1997;53:888–903.
9. Ouellette AJ, Selsted ME. Paneth cell defensins: endogenous peptide components of intestinal host defense. FASEB J 1996; 10:1280–9.
10. Desbuquois B. Gastrointestinal hormones. In: Beaulieu EE, Kelly PA, editors. Hormones from molecules to disease. Hermann Publishers in Arts and Science; 1990. p. 540–89.
11. Kedinger M, Newgreen D. The gut and enteric nervous system. In: Thorogood P, editor. Embryos, genes and birth defects. Chester, UK: John Wiley & Sons Ltd; 1997. p. 153–96.
12. Colony PC, Conforti JC. Morphogenesis in the fetal rat proximal colon: effects of cytochalasin D. Anat Rec 1993; 235:241–52.
13. Valentich JD, Powell DW. Intestinal subepithelial myofibroblasts and mucosal immunophysiology. Curr Opin Gastroenterol 1994;10:645–51.
14. Komuro T, Hashimoto Y. Three-dimensional structure of the rat intestinal wall (mucosa and submucosa). Arch Histol Cytol 1990;53:1–21.
15. Kedinger M, Fritsch C, Evans et al. Role of stromal-epithelial cell interactions and of basement membrane molecules in the onset and maintenance of epithelial integrity. In: Kagnoff MF, Kiyono H, editors. Essentials of mucosal immunology. San Diego: Academic Press; 1996. p. 111–23.
16. Haffen K, Kedinger M, Simon-Assmann P. Cell-contact dependent regulation of enterocytic differentiation. In: Lebenthal E, editor. Human gastrointestinal development. New-York: Raven Press; 1989. p. 19–40.
17. Yasugi S. Role of epithelial-mesenchymal interactions in differentiation of epithelium of vertebrate digestive organs. Dev Growth Differ 1993;35:1–9.
18. Quaroni A, Isselbacher KJ. Cytotoxic effects and metabolism of benzo-a-pyrene and 7,12-dimethylbenz-a-anthracene in duodenal and ileal epithelial cell cultures. J Natl Cancer Inst 1981;67:1353–62.
19. Duluc I, Freund J, Leberquier C, Kedinger M. Fetal endoderm primarily holds the temporal and positional information required for mammalian intestinal development. J Cell Biol 1994;126:211–21.
20. Rubin DC, Swietlicki E, Roth KA, Gordon JI. Use of fetal intestinal isografts from normal and transgenic mice to study the programming of positional information along the duodenal-to-colonic axis. J Biol Chem 1992;267:15122–33.
21. Czernichow B, Simon-Assmann P, Kedinger M, et al. Sucrase-isomaltase expression and enterocytic ultrastructure of human colorectal tumors. Int J Cancer 1989;44:238–44.
22. Ratineau C, Duluc I, Dumortier J, et al. Uncoupling of morphological and endocrine differentiation in the rat intestine during organogenesis [abstract]. American Gastroenterology Association; 1998 May 16–22; New Orleans, USA.
23. Fritsch C, Simon-Assmann P, Kedinger M, Evans GS. Cytokines modulate fibroblast phenotype and epithelial-stroma interactions in rat intestine. Gastroenterology 1997; 112:826–38.
24. Fritsch C, Orian-Rousseau V, Simon-Assmann P, et al. Characterization of three human stromal cell lines: interactions with colonic cancer cells and response to cytokines. Forthcoming.
25. Berschneider HM, Powell DW. Fibroblasts modulate intestinal secretory responses to inflammatory mediators. J Clin Invest 1992;89:484–9.
26. Mahida YR, Beltinger J, Makh S, et al. Adult human colonic subepithelial myofibroblasts express extracellular matrix proteins & cyclooxygenase-1 & -2. Am J Physiol 1998;273: G1341–8.
27. Griebel P, Hein WR, Dudler L, Ferrari G. Phenotype and function of stromal cells cloned from the ileal Peyer's patch of sheep. Stem Cells 1993; 11:130–43.
28. Hogaboam CM, Snider DP, Collins SM. Cytokine modulation of T-lymphocyte activation by intestinal smooth muscle cells. Gastroenterology 1997;112:1986–95.
29. Roberts AI, Nadler SC, Ebert EC. Mesenchymal cells stimulate human intestinal intraepithelial lymphocytes. Gastroenterology 1997;113:144–50.
30. Burgeson RE, Chiquet M, Deutzmann R, et al. A new nomenclature for the laminins. Matrix Biol 1994;14:209–11.
31. Yurchenco PD, O'Rear JJ. Basal lamina assembly. Curr Opin Cell Biol 1994;6:674–81.
32. Timpl R, Brown JC. Supramolecular assembly of basement membranes. Bioessays 1996;18:123–32.
33. Hudson BG, Reeders ST, Tryggvason K. Type IV collagen: structure, gene organization, and role in human diseases. J Biol Chem 1993;268:26033–6.

34. Miner JH, Patton BL, Lentz SI, et al. The laminin alpha chains: expression, developmental transitions, and chromosomal locations of alpha1-5, identification of heterotrimeric laminins 8-11, and cloning of a novel alpha3 isoform. J Cell Biol 1997;137:685–701.
35. Simon-Assmann P, Lefebvre O, Bellissent-Waydelich A, et al. The laminins: role of intestinal morphogenesis and differentiation. Ann N Y Acad Sci 1998;859:46–64.
36. Fine JD. International Symposium on Epidermolysis Bullosa - The William and Ida Friday Continuing Education Center, The University of North Carolina at Chapel Hill, April 25–26. J Invest Dermatol 1994;103:839–43.
37. Uitto J, Pulkkinen L. Molecular complexity of the cutaneous basement membrane zone. Mol Biol Rep 1996;23:35–46.
38. Tome FMS, Evangelista T, Leclerc A, et al. Congenital muscular dystrophy with merosin deficiency. C R Acad Sci III 1994;317:351–7.
39. Xu H, Christmas P, Wu XR, et al. Defective muscle basement membrane and lack of M-laminin in the dystrophic dy/dy mouse. Proc Natl Acad Sci U S A 1994;91:5572–6.
40. Aumailley M, Battaglia C, Mayer U, et al. Nidogen mediates the formation of ternary complexes of basement membrane components. Kidney Int 1993;43:7–12.
41. Delwel GO, Sonnenberg A. Laminin isoforms and their integrin receptors. In: Horton MA, editor. Adhesion receptors as therapeutic targets. London: CRC Press; 1996. p. 9–36.
42. Mercurio AM. Laminin receptors: achieving specificity through cooperation. Trends Cell Biol 1995;5:419–23.
43. Ekblom P. Receptors for laminins during epithelial morphogenesis. Curr Opin Cell Biol 1996;8:700–6.
44. Fässler R, Georges-Labouesse E, Hirsch E. Genetic analyses of integrin function in mice. Curr Opin Cell Biol 1996; 8:641–6.
45. Beaulieu JF. Recent work with migration/patterns of expression: cell-matrix interactions in human intestinal cell differentiation. In: Halter F, Winton D, Wright NA, editors. The gut as a model in cell and molecular biology. Proceedings of the Falk Symposium 94. Kluwer Academic Publishers; 1997. p. 165–79.
46. Beaulieu JF. Extracellular matrix components and integrins in relationship to human intestinal epithelial cell differentiation. Prog Histochem Cytochem 1997;31:1–77.
47. Simon-Assmann P, Kedinger M, De Arcangelis A, et al. Extracellular matrix components in intestinal development. Experientia 1995;51:883–900.
48. Zhou J, Mochizuki T, Smeets H, et al. Deletion of the paired alpha-5(IV) and alpha-6(IV) collagen genes in inherited smooth muscle tumors. Science 1993;261:1167–9.
49. Beaulieu JF, Vachon PH, Herring-Gillam FE, et al. Expression of the alpha-5(IV) collagen chain in the fetal human small intestine. Gastroenterology 1994;107:957–67.
50. Simo P, Simon-Assmann P, Bouziges F, et al. Changes in the expression of laminin during intestinal development. Development 1991;112:477–87.
51. Simon-Assmann P, Kedinger M. Heterotypic cellular cooperation in gut morphogenesis and differentiation. Semin Cell Biol 1993;4:221–30.
52. Probstmeier R, Martini R, Schachner M. Expression of J1/tenascin in the crypt-villus unit of adult mouse small intestine—implications for its role in epithelial cell shedding. Development 1990;109:313–21.
53. Gerecke DR, Gordon MK, Wagman DW, et al. Hemidesmosomes, anchoring filaments, and anchoring fibrils: components of a unique attachment complex. In: Yurchenco PD, Bird DE, Mecham RP, editors. Extracellular matrix assembly and structure. New York: Academic Press; 1994. p. 417–39.
54. Leivo I, Tani T, Laitinen L, et al. Anchoring complex components laminin-5 and type VII collagen in intestine: association with migrating and differentiating enterocytes. J Histochem Cytochem 1996;44:1267–77.
55. Lohi J, Leivo I, Tani T, et al. Laminins, tenascin and type VII collagen in colorectal mucosa. Histochem J 1996;28:431–40.
56. Simon-Assmann P, Bouziges F, Arnold C, et al. Epithelial-mesenchymal interactions in the production of basement membrane components in the gut. Development 1988;102: 339–47.
57. Simon-Assmann P, Bouziges F, Vigny M, Kedinger M. Origin and deposition of basement membrane heparan sulfate proteoglycan in the developing intestine. J Cell Biol 1989; 109:1837–48.
58. Simo P, Bouziges F, Lissitzky JC, et al. Dual and asynchronous deposition of laminin chains at the epithelial-mesenchymal interface in the gut. Gastroenterology 1992;102: 1835–45.
59. Orian-Rousseau V, Aberdam D, Fontao L, et al. Developmental expression of laminin-5 and HD1 in the intestine: epithelial to mesenchymal shift for the laminin gamma-2 chain subunit deposition. Dev Dyn 1996;206:12–23.
60. Lefebvre O, Kedinger M, Sorokin L, Simon-Assmann P. Developmental expression and cellular origin of the laminin alpha-2 and alpha-5 chains in the intestine. Forthcoming 1998.
61. Senior PV, Critchley DR, Beck F, et al. The localization of laminin mRNA and protein in the postimplantation embryo and placenta of the mouse: an in situ hybridization and immunocytochemical study. Development 1988;104:431–46.
62. Simon-Assmann P, Bouziges F, Freund JN, et al. Type IV collagen mRNA accumulates in the mesenchymal compartment at early stages of murine developing intestine. J Cell Biol 1990;110:849–57.
63. Dziadek M. Role of laminin-nidogen complexes in basement membrane formation during embryonic development. Experientia 1995;51:901–13.
64. Kedinger M, Simon-Assmann P, Bouziges F, et al. Mesenchyme-mediation of glucocorticoid effects on the expression of epithelial cell markers. Exp Clin Endocrinol (Life Sci Adv) 1989;8:119–35.
65. Henning SJ, Rubin DC, Shulman J. Ontogeny of the intestinal mucosa. In: Johnson, LR, editor. Physiology of the gastrointestinal tract. 3rd ed. New York: Raven Press; 1994. p. 571–610.
66. Plateroti M, Freund JN, Leberquier C, Kedinger M. Mesenchyme-mediated effects of retinoic acid during rat intestinal development. J Cell Sci 1997;110:1227–38.
67. Simo P, Simon-Assmann P, Arnold C, Kedinger M. Mesenchyme-mediated effect of dexamethasone on laminin in cocultures of embryonic gut epithelial cells and mesenchyme-derived cells. J Cell Sci 1992;101:161–71.
68. Kedinger M, Simon-Assmann P, Alexandre E, Haffen K. Importance of a fibroblastic support for in vitro differentiation of intestinal endodermal cells and for their response to glucocorticoids. Cell Differ 1987;20:171–82.
69. Takiguchi-Hayashi K, Yasugi S. Transfilter analysis of the inductive influence of proventricular mesenchyme on stomach epithelial differentiation of chick embryos. Roux' Arch Dev Biol 1990;198:400–66.
70. Simon-Assmann P, Duclos B, Orian-Rousseau V, et al. Differential expression of laminin isoforms and alpha 6-beta 4 integrin subunits in the developing human and mouse intestine. Dev Dyn 1994;201:71–85.
71. Pinto M, Robine-Léon S, Appay MD, et al. Enterocyte-like differentiation and polarization of the human colon carcinoma cell line Caco-2 in culture. Biol Cell 1983;47:323–30.

72. Chantret I, Rodolosse A, Barbat A, et al. Differential expression of sucrase-isomaltase in clones isolated from early and late passages of the cell line Caco-2: evidence for glucose-dependent negative regulation. J Cell Sci 1994;107:213–25.
73. Vachon PH, Beaulieu JF. Extracellular heterotrimeric laminin promotes differentiation in human enterocytes. Am J Physiol 1995;268:G857–67.
74. Fontao L, Stutzmann J, Launay JF. Triggering of type II hemidesmosome organization by actin assembly in a human colonic tumoral cell line. Exp Cell Res [In revision] 1998.
75. Simon-Assmann P, Leberquier C, Molto N, et al. Adhesive properties and integrin expression profiles of two colonic cancer populations differing by their spreading on laminin. J Cell Sci 1994;107:577–87.
76. Fontao L, Dirrig S, Owaribe K, et al. Polarized expression of HD1: relationship with the cytoskeleton in cultured human colonic carcinoma cells. Exp Cell Res 1997;231:319–27.
77. Orian-Rousseau V, Aberdam D, Rousselle P, et al. Human colonic cancer cells synthesize and adhere to laminin-5; their adhesion to laminin-5 involves multiple receptors among which integrin alpha-2 beta-1. J Cell Sci 1998 Jul;111:1993–2004.
78. Dowling J, Yu QC, Fuchs E. Beta-4 integrin is required for hemidesmosome formation, cell adhesion and cell survival. J Cell Biol 1996;134:559–72.
79. Georges-Labouesse E, Messadeq N, Yehia G, et al. Absence of the alpha-6 integrin leads to epidermolysis bullosa and neonatal death in mice. Nat Genet 1996;13:370–3.
80. Van der Neut R, Krimpenfort P, Calafat J, et al. Epithelial detachment due to absence of hemidesmosomes in integrin beta-4 null mice. Nat Genet 1996;13:366–9.
81. Lotz MM, Nusrat A, Madara JL, et al. Intestinal epithelial restitution. Involvement of specific laminin isoforms and integrin laminin receptors in wound closure of a transformed model epithelium. Am J Pathol 1997;150:747–60.
82. Lesuffleur T, Kornowski A, Luccioni C, et al. Adaptation to 5-fluorouracil of the heterogeneous human colon tumor cell line HT-29 results in the selection of cells committed to differentiation. Int J Cancer 1991;49:721–30.
83. Giannelli G, Falk-Marzillier J, Schiraldi O, et al. Induction of cell migration by matrix metalloprotease-2 cleavage of laminin-5. Science 1997;277:225–8.
84. Lorentz O, Duluc I, De Arcangelis A, et al. Key role of the Cdx2 homeobox gene in the extracellular matrix-mediated intestinal cell differentiation. J Cell Biol 1997;139:1553–65.
85. Rabinovitz I, Mercurio AM. The integrin alpha-6 beta-4 and the biology of carcinoma. Biochem Cell Biol 1996;74:811–21.
86. Dumortier J, Daemi N, Pourreyron C, et al. Selection of highly metastatic human colon carcinoma LoVo C5 variants obtained from metastastis in immunosuppressed newborn rat furthers expression of laminin-5. Fiftieth Annual Symposium on Fundamental Cancer Research: Molecular Determinants of Cancer Metastasis [abstract]. 1998 Oct; Houston, USA.
87. Pyke C, Sale S, Ralfkiaer E, et al. Laminin-5 is a marker of invading cancer cells in some human carcinomas and is coexpressed with the receptor for urokinase plasminogen activator in budding cancer cells in colon adenocarcinomas. Cancer Res 1995;15:4132–9.
88. Lesuffleur T, Barbat A, Dussaulx E, Zweibaum A. Growth adaptation to methotrexate of HT-29 human colon carcinoma cells is associated with their ability to differentiate into columnar absorptive and mucus-secreting cells. Cancer Res 1990;50:6334–43.
89. Olsen J, Fritsch C, Orian-Rousseau V, et al. Involvement of AP-1 proteins in the epithelial specific activation of the LAMC2 promoter by hepatocyte growth factor (scatter factor). Forthcoming 1998.
90. Di Renzo MF, Narsimham RP, Olivero M, et al. Expression of the Met/HGF receptor in normal and neoplastic human tissues. Oncogene 1991;6:1997–2003.
91. Takayama H, LaRochelle WJ, Sharp R, et al. Diverse tumorigenesis associated with aberrant development in mice overexpressing hepatocyte growth factor/scatter factor. Proc Natl Acad Sci U S A 1997;94:701–6.
92. Basson MD, Turowski G, Emenaker NJ. Regulation of human (Caco-2) intestinal epithelial cell differentiation by extracellular matrix proteins. Exp Cell Res 1996;225:301–5.
93. Basora N, Vachon PH, Herring-Gillam FE, et al. Relation between integrin alpha-7B beta-1 expression in human intestinal cells and enterocytic differentiation. Gastroenterology 1997;113:1510–21.
94. Bouziges F, Simo P, Simon-Assmann P, et al. Altered deposition of basement membrane molecules in cocultures of colonic cancer cells and fibroblasts. Int J Cancer 1991;48:101–8.
95. De Arcangelis A, Simo P, Lesuffleur T, et al. L'expression de la laminine est corrélée à la différenciation des cellules cancéreuses coliques humaines. Gastroentérol Clin Biol 1994;18:630–7.
96. De Arcangelis A, Neuville P, Boukamel R, et al. Inhibition of laminin alpha 1-chain expression leads to alteration of basement membrane assembly and cell differentiation. J Cell Biol 1996;133:417–30.
97. Henchcliffe C, Garcia-Alonso L, Tang J, Goodman CS. Genetic analysis of laminin A reveals diverse functions during morphogenesis in *Drosophila*. Development 1993;118:325–37.
98. Yarnitzky T, Volk T. Laminin is required for heart, somatic muscles, and gut development in the *Drosophila* embryo. Dev Biol 1995;169:609–18.
99. Garcia-Alonso L, Fetter RD, Goodman CS. Genetic analysis of laminin A in *Drosophila*: extracellular matrix containing laminin A is required for ocellar axon pathfinding. Development 1996;122:2611–21.
100. Goulet O, Kedinger M, Brousse M, et al. Intractable diarrhea of infancy with epithelial and basement membrane abnormalities. J Pediatr 1995;127:212–9.
101. Patey N, Scoazec JY, Cuenod-Jabri B, et al. Distribution of cell adhesion molecules in infants with intestinal epithelial dysplasia (tufting enteropathy). Gastroenterology 1997;113:833–43.
102. Murch SH, MacDonald TT, Walker-Smith JA, et al. Disruption of sulphated glycosaminoglycans in intestinal inflammation. Lancet 1993;341:711–4.
103. Postlethwaite AE, Kang AH. Fibroblasts and matrix proteins. In: Gallin JI, et al. editors. Inflammation: basic principles and clinical correlates. 2nd ed. New York: Raven Press; 1992;747–73.
104. Babyatsky MW, Rossiter G, Podolsky DK. Expression of transforming growth factors alpha and beta in colonic mucosa in inflammatory bowel disease. Gastroenterology 1996;110:975–84.
105. Riedl SE, Faissner A, Schlag P, et al. Altered content and distribution of tenascin in colitis, colon adenoma, and colorectal carcinoma. Gastroenterology 1992;103:400–6.
106. Sträter J, Wedding U, Barth TFE, et al. Rapid onset of apoptosis in vitro follows disruption of β1-integrin/matrix interactions in human colonic crypt cells. Gastroenterology 1996;110:1776–84.
107. Podolsky DK. Regulatory peptides and integration of the intestinal epithelium in mucosal responses. In: Kagnoff F, Kiyono H, editors. Essentials of mucosal immunology. San Diego: Academic Press; 1996. p. 101–10.
108. Rothman TP, Chen JX, Howard MJ, et al. Increased expression of laminin-1 and collagen (IV) subunits in the aganglionic bowel of ls/ls, but not c-ret-/- mice. Develop Biol 1996;178:498–513.

109. Botas J. Control of morphogenesis and differentiation by HOM/Hox genes. Curr Opin Cell Biol 1993;5:1015–22.
110. McGinnis W, Krumlauf R. Homeobox genes and axial patterning. Cell 1992;68:283–302.
111. Edelman GM, Jones JS. Outside and downstream of the homeobox. J Biol Chem 1993;268:20683–6.
112. James R, Kazenwadel J. Homeobox gene expression in the intestinal epithelium of adult mice. J Biol Chem 1991; 266:3246–51.
113. Walters JR, Howard A, Rumble HE, et al. Differences in expression of homeobox transcription factors in proximal and distal human small intestine. Gastroenterology 1997;113:472–7.
114. Tennyson VM, Gershon MD, Sherman DL, et al. Structural abnormalities associated with congenital megacolon in transgenic mice that overexpress the Hoxa-4 gene. Dev Dyn 1993; 198:28–53.
115. Offield M, Jetton TL, Labosky PA, et al. PDX-1 is required for pancreatic outgrowth and differentiation of the rostral duodenum. Development 1996;122:983–95.
116. Mansouri A, Hallonet M, Gruss P. Pax genes and their roles in cell differentiation and development. Curr Opin Cell Biol 1996;8:851–7.
117. St-Onge L, Sosa-Pineda B, Chowdhury K, et al. Pax6 is required for differentiation of glucagon-producing alpha-cells in mouse pancreas. Nature 1997;387:406–9.
118. Sosa-Pineda B, Chowdhury K, Torres M, et al. The Pax-4 gene is essential for differentiation of insulin-producing beta cells in the mammalian pancreas. Nature 1997;386:399–402.
119. Mutoh H, Fung BP, Naya FJ, et al. The basic helix-loop-helix transcription factor BETA2/NeuroD is expressed in mammalian enteroendocrine cells and activates secretion gene expression. Proc Natl Acad Sci U S A 1998;94:3560–4.
120. Duprey P, Chowdhury K, Dressler GR, et al. A mouse gene homologous to the *Drosophila* gene caudal is expressed in epithelial cells from the embryonic intestine. Genes Dev 1988;2:1647–54.
121. James R, Erler T, Kazenwadel J. Structure of the murine homeobox gene cdx-2. Expression in embryonic and adult intestinal epithelium. J Biol Chem 1994;269:15229–37.
122. Macdonald PM, Struhl G. A molecular gradient in early *Drosophila* embryos and its role in specifying the body pattern. Nature 1986;324:537–45.
123. Meyer BL, Gruss P. Mouse Cdx1 expression during gastrulation. Development 1998;117:191–203.
124. Subramanian V, Meyer BI, Gruss P. Disruption of the murine homeobox gene Cdx1 affects axial skeletal identities by altering the mesodermal expression domains of Hox genes. Cell 1995;83:641–53.
125. Chawengsaksophak K, James R, Hammond VE, et al. Homeosis and intestinal tumours in Cdx2 mutant mice. Nature 1997;385:84–7.
126. Frumkin A, Pillemer G, Haffner R, et al. A role for CdxA in gut closure and intestinal epithelia differentiation. Development 1994;120:253–63.
127. Ishii Y, Fukuda K, Saiga H, et al. Early specification of intestinal epithelium in the chicken embryo: a study on the localization and regulation of CdxA expression. Dev Growth Differ 1997;39:643–53.
128. Freund JN, Boukamel R, Benazzouz A. Gradient expression of Cdx along the rat intestine throughout postnatal development. FEBS Lett 1992;314:163–6.
129. Hu Y, Kazenwadel J, James R. Isolation and characterization of the murine homeobox gene cdx-1. Regulation of expression in intestinal epithelial cells. J Biol Chem 1993;268:27214–25.
130. Duluc I, Lorentz O, Fritsch C, et al. Changing intestinal connective tissue interactions alters homeobox gene expression in epithelial cells. J Cell Sci 1997;110:1317–24.
131. Silberg DG, Furth EE, Taylor JK, et al. CDX1 protein expression in normal, metaplastic, and neoplastic human alimentary tract epithelium. Gastroenterology 1997;113:478–86.
132. Suh E, Chen L, Taylor J, Traber PG. A homeodomain protein related to caudal regulates intestine-specific gene transcription. Mol Cell Biol 1994;14:7340–51.
133. Troelsen JT, Mitchelmore C, Spodsberg N, et al. Regulation of lactase-phlorizin hydrolase gene expression by the caudal-related homoeodomain protein Cdx-2. Biochem J 1997; 322: 833–8.
134. Ee HC, Erler T, Bhathal PS, et al. Cdx-2 homeodomain protein expression in human and rat colorectal adenoma and carcinoma. Am J Pathol 1995;147:586–92.
135. Mallo GV, Rechreche H, Frigerio JM, et al. Molecular cloning, sequencing and expression of the mRNA encoding human Cdx1 and Cdx2 homeobox. Down-regulation of Cdx1 and Cdx2 mRNA expression during colorectal carcinogenesis. Int J Cancer 1997;74:35–44.
136. Vider BZ, Zimber A, Hirsch D, et al. Human colorectal carcinogenesis is associated with deregulation of homeobox gene expression. Biochem Biophys Res Commun 1997;232:742–8.
137. Maulbecker CC, Gruss P. The oncogenic potential of deregulated homeobox genes. Cell Growth Differ 1993;4:431–41.
138. Suh E, Traber PG. An intestine-specific homeobox gene regulates proliferation and differentiation. Mol Cell Biol 1996; 16:619–25.
139. Kedinger M. Cellular and molecular partners involved in gut morphogenesis and differentiation. The Royal Society of Philosophical Transactions Biological Sciences 1998;353: 847–56.
140. Hentsch B, Lyons I, Li R, et al. Hlx homeobox gene is essential for an inductive tissue interaction that drives expansion of embryonic liver and gut. Genes Dev 1996;10:70–9.
141. Kaestner KH, Silberg DG, Traber PG, Schutz G. The mesenchymal winged helix transcription factor Fkh6 is required for the control of gastrointestinal proliferation and differentiation. Genes Dev 1997;11:1583–95.
142. Halttunen T, Marttinen A, Rantala I, et al. Fibroblasts and transforming growth factor beta induce organization and differentiation of T84 human epithelial cells. Gastroenterology 1996;111:1252–62.
143. Roberts DJ, Johnson RL, Burke AC, et al. Sonic hedgehog is an endodermal signal inducing Bmp-4 and Hox genes during induction and regionalization of the chick hindgut. Development 1995;121:3163–74.
144. Pabst O, Schneider A, Brand T, Arnold HH. The mouse Nkx2-3 homeodomain gene is expressed in gut mesenchyme during pre- and postnatal mouse development. Dev Dyn 1997; 209:29–35.
145. Shaw-Smith C, Wright NA. Aspects of gut development. Proc Nutr Soc 1996;55:519–27.
146. Lorentz O, Cadoret A, Duluc I, et al. Oncogenic ras downregulates the colon tumour-suppressor Cdx2 homeobox gene. Oncogene 1999;18:87–92.
147. Roskelley CD, Srebrow A, Bissel MJ. A hierarchy of ECM-mediated signalling regulates tissue-specific gene expression. Curr Opin Cell Biol 1995 Oct;7:736–47.
148. Lafrenie RM, Yamada KM. Integrin-dependent signal transduction. J Cell Biochem 1996;61:543–53.
149. Birchmeier C, Meyer D, Riethmacher D. Factors controlling growth, motility, and morphogenesis of normal and malignant epithelial cells. Int Rev Cytol 1995;160:221–66.
150. Plateroti M, Rubin D, Duluc I, et al. Subepithelial fibroblast cell lines from different levels of the gut axis display regional characteristics. Am J Physiol 1998;274:6945–54.
151. Kedinger M, Duluc I, Fritsch C, et al. Intestinal epithelial-mesenchymal cell interactions. Ann N Y Acad Sci 1998;859:1–17.

152. Simon-Assmann P, Kedinger M, Haffen K. Immunocytochemical localization of extracellular matrix proteins in relation to rat intestinal morphogenesis. Differentiation 1986;32:59–66.
153. Beaulieu JF, Vachon PH, Chartrand A. Immunolocalization of extracellular matrix components during organogenesis in the human small intestine. Anat Embryol (Berlin) 1991;183:363–9.
154. Beaulieu JF, Vachon PH. Reciprocal expression of laminin A-chain isoforms along the crypt-villus axis in the human small intestine. Gastroenterology 1994;106:829–39.
155. Peissel B, Geng L, Kalluri R, et al. Comparative distribution of the alpha-1(IV) and alpha-6(IV) collagen chains in normal human adult and fetal tissues and in kidneys from X-linked alport syndrome patients. J Clin Invest 1995;96:1948–57.
156. Perreault N, Vachon PH, Beaulieu JF. Appearance and distribution of laminin A chain isoforms and integrin alpha-2, alpha-3, alpha-6, beta-1, and beta-4 subunits in the developing human small intestinal mucosa. Anat Rec 1995;242:242–50.

CHAPTER 7

Development of Brushborder Enzyme Activity

Peter G. Traber, MD

The intestinal mucosa is lined by a simple columnar epithelium that performs a wide array of functions. In the absence of disease or surgical intervention, the epithelium maintains a highly ordered functional organization. The epithelium of the small intestine and colon is composed of four epithelial cells: phenotypes, including absorptive enterocytes; mucus-secreting goblet cells; a variety of enteroendocrine cells; and Paneth's cells. The predominant cell type is the absorptive enterocyte, which presents an apical membrane to the luminal environment. The interface between the apical membrane of enterocytes and the luminal contents of the intestine is where much of the function of the intestine occurs. The apical membrane is structured in a well-ordered lawn of microvilli that provides a vast surface area for interaction with the luminal contents. The light microscopic appearance of apical microvilli is that of an indistinct brush covering the apical surface of enterocytes, leading to the term "brushborder." The plasma membrane of the enterocyte brushborder contains integral membrane proteins that have a variety of functions, including enzyme activity and molecular transport. Many brushborder proteins have enzymatic domains that are presented to the extracellular milieu to perform important digestive enzymatic functions. These ectoenzymes perform hydrolysis of complex nutrients to simpler forms that may be absorbed by brushborder transport processes. These hydrolases are responsible for enzymatic breakdown of carbohydrates and peptides. This fundamental role in nutrient absorption has made the brushborder hydrolases a primary focus of research in the development of intestinal function.

The function, synthesis, and regulation of intestinal brushborder carbohydrases have been studied intensively. An understanding of the regulation of expression and function of carbohydrases has provided much information about intestinal epithelial cell gene expression and the processes of differentiation and development. Although many carbohydrases and other brushborder hydrolytic enzymes have been studied, this chapter will concentrate on the two best characterized with regard to molecular mechanisms, sucrase-isomaltase (SI) and lactase-phlorizin hydrolase (LPH). An understanding of the synthesis of these brushborder enzymes provides a window to molecular mechanisms directing intestinal epithelial differentiation and development. Although it is certain that other brushborder enzymes are regulated in diverse ways, the mechanisms of other enzymes are not as well characterized as those of SI and LPH. Comparing information on these two genes provides hypotheses and direction for a deeper understanding of the mechanisms that regulate carbohydrase expression.

In the final analysis, a complete understanding of human developmental physiology is the ultimate goal of investigators in the field. However, a discussion of brushborder enzyme development requires an understanding of a variety of mammalian species with different gestational durations. Humans are long gestational animals whose young are born with mature intestinal carbohydrase activities. In contrast, shorter gestational animals, such as rodents, do not complete the developmental process of carbohydrase expression until after birth. This difference between rodents and humans makes the correlation of certain molecular mechanisms more difficult. However, rodent models of intestinal development are of critical importance to elucidate the molecular mechanisms underlying carbohydrase expression. Therefore, the developmental patterns and mechanisms for carbohydrase expression in humans will be compared to and contrasted with those in rodents. In particular, the ability to genetically manipulate mice has made this model of prime importance in understanding the mechanisms of intestinal development and carbohydrase expression.

REGULATION OF GENE EXPRESSION AND PROTEIN FUNCTION DURING DEVELOPMENT

The development of organ systems is characterized by a continuous series of transitions in cellular phenotypes. These transitions are directed by interactions between cells of the same general type as well as between cells in different embryonic layers.[1] Cellular changes depend on signaling events that involve soluble and membrane-bound mediators from multiple cell types. These signals act on cells whose response may vary at different times during development. In the developing gut, the interaction between mesoderm and endoderm is crucial for defining cellular phenotypes during the developmental process.[2-8] These interactions occur via secreted proteins, direct cell-cell interactions, and the interaction of cell-surface molecules with extracellular matrix. The constituents of extracellular matrix are synthesized by both endoderm- and mesoderm-derived cells.[7,8]

At any point during development, the cellular phenotype is defined by the expression of specific sets of genes in individual cells. The sets of genes expressed in intestinal epithelial cells can be described as "transcriptomes," a term recently coined to refer to the entire set of genes transcribed in a given cell.[9] Transcriptomes in intestinal epithelial cells shift in well-orchestrated patterns during development, differentiation, and adaptive processes of the intestinal mucosa. Therefore, the mechanisms that regulate shifts in the epithelial cell transcriptome form the foundation for understanding developmental events.

Our current understanding of the complete transcriptome of intestinal epithelial cells is limited. Only a handful of genes have been fully characterized, and even fewer have been examined in detail during developmental transitions. It is very likely that, as larger sets of genes are described and their regulation explored, many types of complex patterns will be identified. However, we are currently limited to viewing this process through the window of several well-characterized genes: another reason this review concentrates on the two best-characterized brushborder enzymes, SI and LPH.

The predominant point of gene regulation during development is transcription. Although other mechanisms are important in a variety of organisms, transcriptional initiation remains the most crucial step in developmental processes in most mammalian cells and organs. Transcriptional initiation is an intricate biochemical process that involves the interaction of core nuclear machinery with cell-specific DNA binding proteins. The core nuclear machinery is called the basal transcription apparatus and is comprised of a large nuclear complex of proteins that interact with DNA elements immediately upstream of the transcriptional initiation site. The formation of the transcriptional initiation complex is catalyzed by protein interactions involving nuclear transcription factors that bind to DNA elements located on the same DNA strand as the structural gene. These DNA elements may act immediately upstream of the transcriptional initiation site, in which case they are called promoter elements, or distant from the transcriptional initiation site. Promoter regions contain DNA elements that interact with multiple proteins, including a combination of ubiquitous, cell-restricted, or cell-specific transcription factors. Regulatory regions located distant from the transcriptional initiation site may contain multiple DNA elements, including enhancers of transcriptional activation and silencers that can repress transcription. In addition to DNA-binding proteins that interact with proximal and distal elements, there are coadaptor proteins that serve to link the specific DNA-binding proteins to portions of the basal transcriptional apparatus. The coordinated assembly of a complex of many proteins at the transcriptional initiation site of a gene leads to modification of chromosome structure and initiation of RNA synthesis via the RNA polymerase II molecular complex. The biochemical interactions between all these proteins are modulated by a variety of protein modifications, including phosphorylation and acetylation. These protein modifications are, in turn, regulated by complex cellular signaling pathways. Therefore, regulation of gene expression is modulated by many processes that extend beyond simple expression of transcription proteins. Other important issues include the cellular localization of transcription proteins, post-translational modifications of DNA binding proteins and coadaptors, the presence or absence of intracellular ligands, and the physical state of chromatin domains.

Following synthesis of the primary RNA transcript, intron-encoded RNA is removed by splicosomes, a process regulated in a number of cells and which may result in multiple RNA sequences from a single primary transcript. This process of differential splicing has been demonstrated for many genes. A number of distinct protein products may result from transcription of a single gene. The two disaccharidase molecules discussed in this chapter are not regulated at the level of primary transcript splicing. However, there will almost certainly be important intestinal genes regulated by this process during development. These are likely to be regulatory molecules, since these proteins often have a modular domain structure, providing the opportunity to include or exclude a particular functional domain. In contrast, the functions of brushborder enzymes and transport proteins are more likely to depend on inclusion of all of the exons in the structural gene.

Additional nuclear processing involves the addition of a polyadenylated tail before the mature mRNA is transported from the nucleus to the cytoplasm. After transport of the mRNA out of the nucleus, there is compartmentalization of mRNA within the cytoplasm, and various mRNAs are targeted to different cellular locations. This has been shown in enterocytes for both SI and LPH mRNAs using in situ hybridization.[10,11] Sucrase-isomaltase and LPH mRNAs are localized immediately subjacent to the brushborder membrane, suggesting that localization of mRNAs may be linked to the final destination of the protein. The targeting mechanisms for mRNAs, the translational processes at their destination, and the functional significance of this finding will require additional study. If RNA targeting becomes an important regulatory mechanism, there is potential for this mechanism to be involved in development.

Brushborder proteins undergo extensive processing that may include cleavage of the primary peptide, glycosylation, and addition of lipids. These post-translational processing events may have profound effects on the trafficking of brushborder enzymes, as well as the ultimate function of the protein. Sucrase-isomaltase and LPH undergo extensive post-translational processing. There is some evidence that this processing is involved in certain aspects of regional and developmental enzyme function.

Brushborder membrane proteins undergo additional alterations once they are inserted in the apical membrane. These alterations are caused by exposure to enzymatic activities in the lumen of the bowel. Although basolateral membrane proteins may also be altered once they are inserted into the plasma membrane, brushborder enzymes are unique in their modification by digestive enzymes. Sucrase-isomaltase is the classic example of such a modification. Once the SI protein is inserted into the brushborder membrane, the ectodomain that contains both sucrase and isomaltase subunits is cleaved between those subunits by luminal proteases. The isomaltase and sucrase subunits of SI remain associated by noncovalent bonding. Therefore, it is important to consider changes in functional activity of brushborder enzymes as a result of intraluminal modifications.

In summary, the emergence of a functional brushborder enzyme depends on a complex series of events from nucleus to apical membrane. All the steps involved in this process are potential regulatory points during differentiation and development. It is likely that cells and organs use the entire complement of potential regulatory points in modifying phenotypes during development. However, the most important and fundamental regulatory step in developmental processes is transcriptional initiation. In the most fundamental sense, the network of interacting nuclear proteins in a given cell determines the transcriptome and thus the cellular phenotype.

DEVELOPMENTAL REGULATION OF SUCRASE-ISOMALTASE

Sucrase-isomaltase is a bifunctional disaccharidase with two active sites comprising 100%, 90%, and 80% of the sucrase, isomaltase, and maltase activity, respectively, in the intestine.[12] The human SI mRNA contains 5481 bases encoding a 1827 amino acid polypeptide that correlates with the measured molecular weight of the nonglycosylated human SI protein of 185 kDa.[13,14] The primary structure of SI predicts a five-domain model of the molecule, including a short intracytoplasmic aminoterminus, a single membrane-spanning anchor, and an extracellular glycosylated stalk that is linked to the isomaltase and sucrase subunits in series.[15–17] Following intraluminal digestion, the carboxyterminal sucrase subunit is linked to the isomaltase subunit by noncovalent, ionic bonding.

Sucrase-isomaltase gene regulation has been studied using a combination of model systems, including cell lines and animals. The use of cell lines can provide important information on mechanisms but the conclusions from these studies must be confirmed in the intact animal. Moreover, processes in cancer cell lines may be reflective of various stages in development rather than the adult state. In the following sections, the patterns of expression in the adult and developing intestine will be presented, followed by a description of what is known about the processes that lead to a functional SI protein.

Spatial and Regional Expression of Sucrase-Isomaltase in the Fully Developed Intestine

The adult pattern of SI gene expression provides the foundation for understanding how this pattern develops during fetal life. Since the patterns of adult SI expression are quite similar in human and mouse, the species will be discussed together.

The expression of many genes in the intestine has complex spatial patterns along the vertical (crypt-to-villus) (CV) and horizontal (proximal-to-distal) axes of the gut.[18] Sections of frozen tissue taken sequentially from villus to crypt cells have been used to measure enzymatic activity along the CV axis. These studies showed there was little sucrase enzyme activity in crypts, maximal activity in lower and midvillus, and decreased levels in villus tip cells.[19]

Immunohistochemistry for SI protein showed that this pattern of enzyme activity is consistent with SI protein localization.[20] In mouse intestine, SI protein in the intestinal mucosa is not detectable in crypt cells, but is expressed from the CV junction to the villus tip, with a minimal decrease in intensity at the tips.[21] The slight decrease in protein immunoreactivity at the villus tips may be the cause of the decrease in enzymatic activity, although loss of the sucrase subunit in more mature enterocytes exposed to the intestinal lumen may also be involved. This pattern of SI expression is generally accepted, although there are data using monoclonal antibodies that show that SI protein is expressed to some degree in human small intestinal crypts in a form that is processed differently than in villus cells[22] (discussed below).

In situ RNA hybridization performed in rat,[23] mouse,[21] and human[11,24] small intestine shows that SI mRNA is not detectable in crypt cells. It remains possible that there are low levels of SI mRNA in crypt cells, but the relative amount compared to villus cells is vanishingly small. Sucrase-isomaltase mRNA is first detected in significant amounts in the upper region of the crypt near the CV junction. Within only a few cell positions, the levels of SI mRNA are maximal and remain at a similar level approximately two-thirds of the way up the villus, followed by decreasing levels at the villus tip. These data suggest that the major mechanism for regulating the expression of the SI protein along the CV axis is the steady state level of SI mRNA. However, post-transcriptional and post-translational regulation likely play a role in the expression of functional SI protein[22] and in colon carcinoma cell lines that can undergo partial enterocytic differentiation.[25]

The regulation of SI mRNA levels along the CV axis may occur as a result of changes in mRNA synthesis or in the rates of mRNA degradation. As discussed below, experiments in transgenic mice provide some important insights into the level of regulation of SI mRNA. These data suggest that the complex patterns of SI mRNA expression along the CV axis may result primarily from events associated with transcriptional regulation of the gene.

There are many functional differences between the jejunum and the ileum that reflect differences in gene expression of different genes along the proximal-distal axis of the intestine. In the human small intestine, SI enzyme activity is greatest in the proximal small intestine and decreases in the more distal portions of the bowel.[26] Similarly, in rat small intestine SI activity is four- to fivefold greater in the jejunum than in the ileum.[27] Interestingly, in the rat and mouse sucrase mRNA appears similar between the two regions.[21,28] There are minor differences in the pattern of Golgi's glycosylation between the two regions, but these do not seem to affect the resultant protein.[27,28] The major difference in regulation between jejunum and ileum appears to be at the level of mRNA translation.[28]

The opposite end of the spectrum from development is aging. A number of studies have been conducted in aged rodents with respect to the expression of SI. The total sucrase activity in 24-month-old rats is 38% lower than the levels in 3-month-old animals,[29] whereas SI mRNA levels are the same. Thus, post-transcriptional mechanisms appear to alter the function of the protein in aged animals. Additional insight into the mechanism of this effect of aging was suggested by studies in a senescence-accelerated strain of mouse.[30] These investigators found that sucrase activity was decreased but isomaltase activity was maintained, and that pancreatic duct ligation resulted in a marked increase in sucrase activity. Taken together, these results suggest that there may be enhanced sensitivity of the sucrase subunit in the senescent mice to pancreatic proteases.

Expression of Sucrase-Isomaltase in the Developing Intestine and Colon

Expression of Sucrase-Isomaltase in Development of the Small Intestine

Sucrase-isomaltase has served as a model to examine developmental processes in the intestine because its expression mirrors many of the developmental transitions that occur in the establishment of the adult intestine.[31–35]

Human small intestinal development. The endoderm of the human small intestine remains an undifferentiated stratified epithelium until approximately week 9 of development (Figure 7–1) (for review see[1]). Between weeks 9 and 10 the stratified endoderm changes morphology to a single layer of columnar epithelial cells with nascent villi protruding into the gut lumen. At the same time three of the primary phenotypes are established, including enterocytes, enteroendocrine cells, and goblet cells. Several days later Paneth's cells appear. These developmental events begin in the most proximal regions of the gut and proceed in an orderly progression toward more distal regions of the small intestine. At approximately 11 to 12 weeks crypts begin to develop from the intervillus cells and villi length, until, by week 16, the CV structure of the small intestine is well established. Cellular proliferation is randomly distributed in the endoderm, but is rapidly localized to intervillus cells and then crypts after the endoderm-intestinal transition.

In the human small intestine, SI activity and protein appear to be first expressed just after the endoderm-intestinal transition (see Figure 7–1). Expression reaches substantial levels between gestational weeks 10 and 22, after which there is a gradual increase in levels to just prior to birth, when there is a marked increase.[26,31] The increase in SI activity is paralleled by an increase in the level of mRNA, suggesting that this is the major level of developmental regulation in the human fetal small intestine.[31,36] After birth there is a rapid decline in levels, such that comparable levels to those found early in gestation are reached between 2 and 11 months of age.[26] In children, expression of SI mRNA also correlates with protein and enzymatic activity, and there are no significant changes in expression between ages 1 to 18 years.[37]

Rodent small intestinal development. In rats, mice, and rabbits the maturation of the small intestine is completed in the neonatal period.[32] In the mouse intestine, the endoderm remains as an undifferentiated stratified epithelium until late in intrauterine development. Between embryonic day's 14 and 15 the endoderm is transformed into an intestinal-type columnar epithelium in a similar way as described for the human small intestine (Figure 7–2). The same processes of cell lineage allocation and development of villi and crypts occur in the mouse small intestine. The major difference is that much of this occurs after birth. In the third week of life there is a dramatic change in the pattern of gene expression in the intestinal

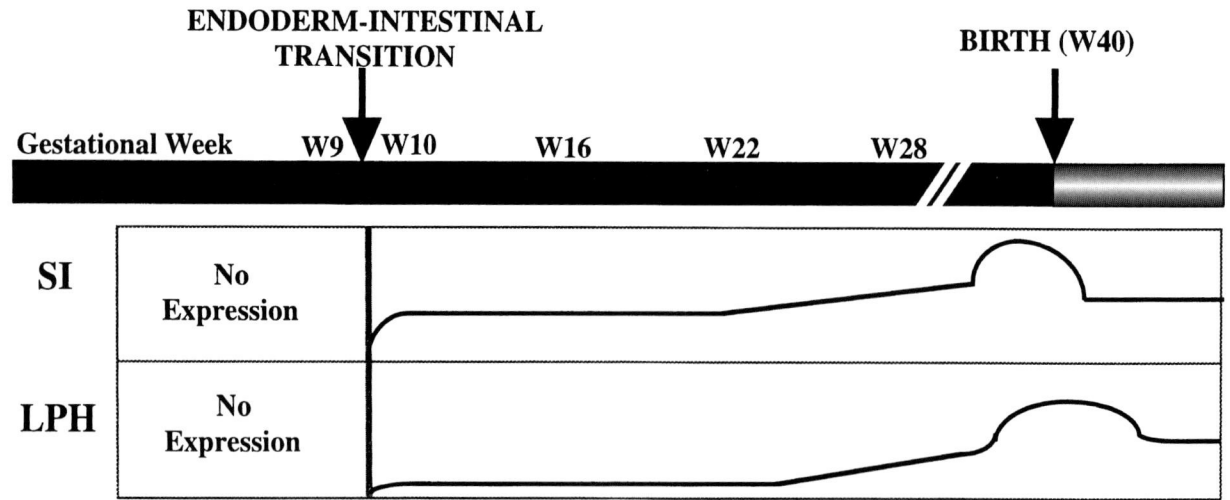

FIGURE 7–1. Regulation of gene expression during development of the human small intestine. The bar at the top of the figure represents the gestational time line for human fetal development. The transition from a stratified, undifferentiated endoderm to a columnar intestinal-type epithelium occurs in the fetal period between gestational weeks 9 and 10. This represents the initial time when sucrase-isomaltase (SI) and lactase-phlorizin hydrolase (LPH) are first expressed. The patterns of expression of both SI and LPH represent enzymatic activity for the two enzymes; expression of mRNAs is discussed in the text. The pattern of expression shown in the figure is a stylized representation of data reported in the literature. The smooth transitions of the expression curves throughout human development do not imply that there are data for each of these gestational time points.

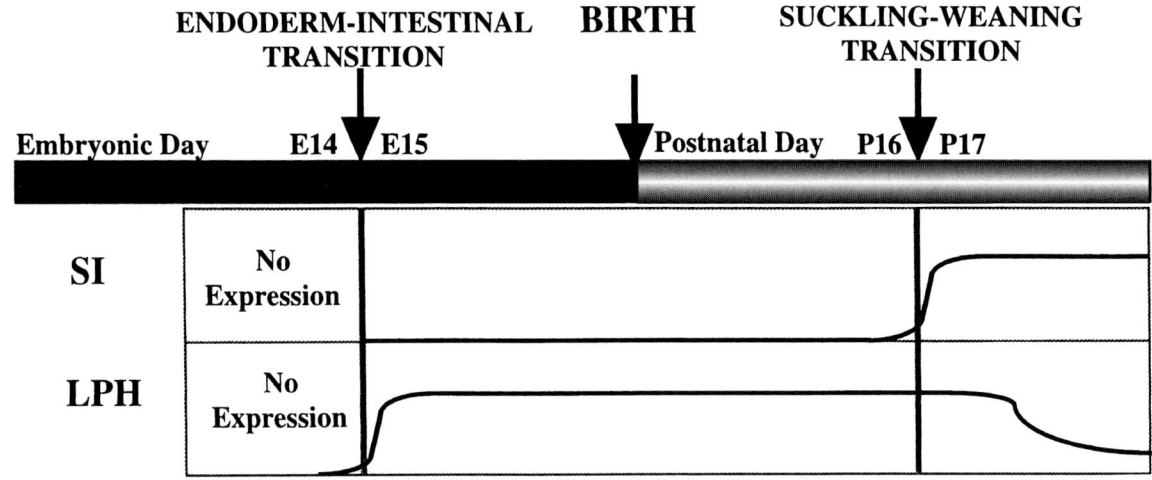

FIGURE 7–2. Regulation of gene expression during development of rodent small intestine. The developmental time line in this figure underscores the fact that intestinal development and regulation of SI and LPH gene expression occurs in both prenatal and postnatal time periods. Since the total gestational time in mice is approximately 20 days, the endoderm-intestinal transition between embryonic days 14 and 15 occurs relatively late in development. Developmental processes in the small intestine continue through the suckling-weaning transition in the third week of life, after which the intestinal epithelium has a mature phenotype. The patterns of expression of SI and LPH represent enzyme activities as reported in multiple studies in the literature. Sucrase-isomaltase activity is not detectable in the small intestine of suckling rodents although small amounts of SI mRNA are detectable, as indicated in the text.

epithelium coincident with the switch from a diet of milk to more solid food. This event occurs over a period of several days in a mouse, but the most dramatic transition for SI gene expression occurs between postnatal days 16 and 17. Near the end of the fourth week of life the mouse small intestine has attained its adult architecture, which is maintained throughout life.

It has been shown in many studies that there is no SI enzymatic activity in the small intestine from birth until the time of weaning.[38,39] At weaning there is a dramatic induction of SI activity that rapidly establishes the adult levels. There is evidence to suggest that although enzymatic activity seems to appear suddenly at the suckling-weaning transition, the activation of the SI gene occurs in two stages.[35] Sucrase-isomaltase mRNA is first detectable in the mouse small intestine at very low levels in the mouse fetus, coincident with the endoderm-intestinal transition.[35] These levels are quite low and only demonstrated using the reverse transcriptase polymerase chain reaction (RT-PCR).[35] Low levels of SI mRNA are maintained for the first 16 days of postnatal life, again only detectable by sensitive methods of mRNA measurement.[35] During this entire time of low-level SI mRNA expression, SI protein and enzymatic activity are not detectable using available methods of measurement. At the time of the suckling-weaning transition there is a dramatic induction of both SI mRNA and protein.[35] The expression of SI mRNA and protein is first detected in cells located at the CV junction, suggesting that changes in the cells are programmed in the crypt compartment. As the enterocytes migrate toward the villus tip the entire villus becomes populated by cells expressing SI, a process essentially complete between 21 and 23 days following birth. The process of SI expression at the suckling-weaning transition begins in the most proximal portions of the intestine and proceeds to distal segments in an orderly progression. Thus, this proximal-to-distal patterning is maintained in both early and late developmental events. Thereafter, the expression of SI in the mouse small intestine remains essentially unchanged. Transgenic mouse experiments, described below, show that transcriptional regulation is primarily responsible for developmental patterns of SI expression. These two stages of SI mRNA expression, before and after weaning, suggest that the epithelial cells become competent to transcribe the SI gene in late fetal development; but there are missing factors that trigger full expression of the gene at weaning.

The dramatic induction of SI in rodent intestine appears to be a genetically programmed event that is not significantly affected by the type of food ingested.[32–34,40] Stress in unweaned pups or administration of corticosteroids and/or thyroid hormone results in premature induction of SI before the normal time of weaning.[32–34,40] It appears that the normal induction of SI at the suckling-weaning transition and the precocious induction by corticosteroids occur through separate molecular pathways.[35,41] Corticosteroids do not have an effect on the expression of human SI in utero as assessed in organ culture.[31] Although one time it was felt that thyroid hormone may simply increase the migration of enterocytes, there is now evidence that the increase in SI expression in response to a combination of corticosteroids and thyroxine is due to greater expression of SI per cell.[42] In addition to corticosteroids and thyroxine, there is evidence that insulin can regulate the developmental expression of SI. Low doses of insulin can induce precocious expression of SI activity and mRNA, an effect that can be reversed by antibodies to the insulin receptor.[43]

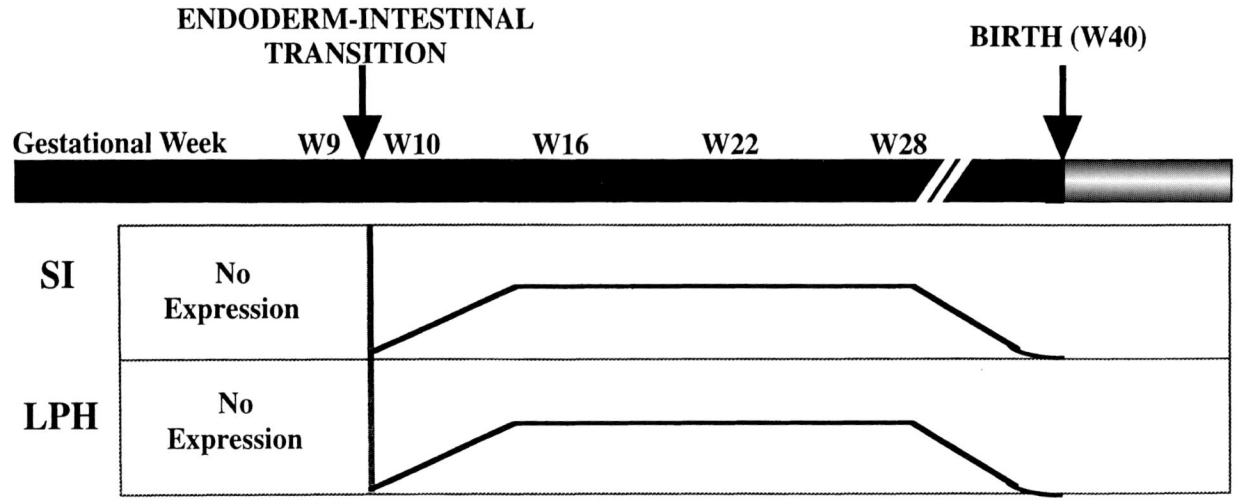

FIGURE 7-3. Regulation of gene expression during development of human colon. The bar at the top of the figure represents the gestational time line for human fetal development. The transition from a stratified, undifferentiated endoderm to a columnar epithelium occurs in the fetal period between gestational weeks 9 and 10, somewhat delayed after the same transition in the small intestine. The patterns of expression of both SI and LPH represent enzymatic activity for the two enzymes. The pattern of expression shown in the figure is a stylized representation of data reported in the literature. The smooth transitions of the expression curves throughout human development do not imply that there are data for each of these gestational time points.

Expression of Sucrose-Isomaltase during Development of the Colon

Sucrose-isomaltase is expressed transiently in the colon of both humans and rodents.[35,44-48] This finding is important for two issues in intestinal biology. First, the mechanisms of this colonic expression will provide insight into differences in regulatory mechanisms of gene expression in the small intestine and colon. Second, an understanding of these mechanisms may provide a window to the regulation of gene expression in colorectal cancer cells because the majority of colorectal cancers express SI.

Human colonic development. There are many similarities between the developmental events in the small intestine and colon in humans. At the beginning of the embryonic period (4 weeks) the colon consists of a tube of stratified endoderm surrounded by mesodermal tissue.[49] Between 7 and 8 weeks three longitudinal ridges arise in the epithelium, and by 9 weeks mesenchyme has moved to indent the underside of the ridges to form folds in the epithelium that continue to develop into true villiform protrusions by week 10. Between weeks 10 and 11 is the first appearance of glands as protuberances into the mesenchyme between the folds and villi. The villi continue to form until the lumen is nearly filled with villi by week 16, at which time the architectures of the fetal colon and small intestine are similar. The glands continue to develop during the fetal period by splitting of existing glands from the bottom up. The earliest appearance of goblet cells is between weeks 9 and 10, although appreciable numbers are not seen until week 12.[50] Unlike the small intestine, the colonic goblet cells rapidly become the predominant epithelial cell lining the fetal colon.[50] Enteroendocrine cells are also first identified between weeks 9 and 10, with numbers increasing up to week 20.[51] The fetal colonic villi gradually regress over the remainder of gestation such that the newborn human has the typical adult pattern of crypts and surface epithelium without a villus structure.

Sucrose-isomaltase is expressed in the fetal colon beginning at approximately gestational week 11 and reaches a plateau in week 14 that is maintained until week 28 (Figure 7-3).[47] After week 28 there is a gradual loss of SI expression, with total absence of SI in the newborn colon.[45,47] The level of expression of SI in the fetal colon is substantial, with some studies indicating that it may be as high as the small intestine at similar times of development. Studies using the RT-PCR suggest that there is no expression of SI mRNA in the adult human colon,[52] although there is controversy about this issue.[52-56] Importantly, SI is expressed in neoplastic tissue from the colon, including adenomas and adenocarcinomas.[52-55,57] This may represent a reversion to a fetal type of regulation of the SI gene.

Rodent colonic development. The histologic morphology of the rodent colon during development is similar to that of the human colon, with the same timing differences that pertain to small intestinal development (Figure 7-4). In the first 2 postnatal weeks the colonic epithelium has a villus structure reminiscent of the small intestine.[48,58-62] This villus structure rapidly regresses such that after weaning is completed the colonic villi have disappeared. Sucrose-isomaltase protein and enzymatic activity are not measurable in the developing colon.[48] However, SI protein is detectable by immunohistochemistry in neonatal rat colon after exposure to exogenously administered corticosteroids.[48] In contrast to the protein, SI mRNA is detected in the neonatal mouse colon when measured using sensitive methods.[35] Low levels of SI mRNA are expressed in the mouse colon at birth, peak between 8 and 10 days and then

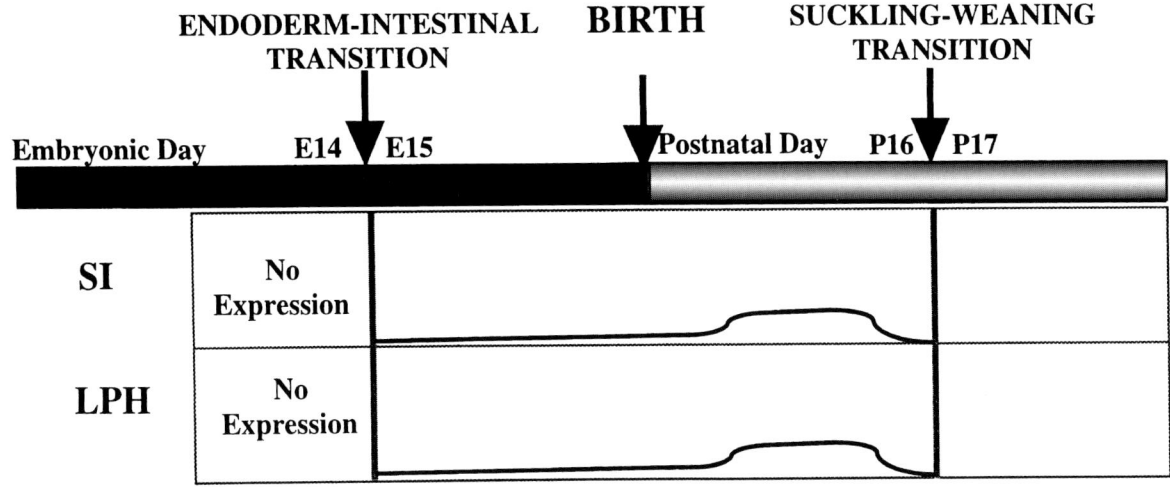

FIGURE 7–4. Regulation of gene expression during development of rodent colon. The developmental time line in this figure demonstrates that colonic development occurs in both prenatal and postnatal time periods. Developmental processes in the colon, as in the small intestine, continue through the suckling-weaning transition in the third week of life. The patterns of expression of SI and LPH in the neonatal colon represent enzyme activities as reported in the literature.

regress after postnatal day 16.[35] The level of SI expression in the mouse colon at the peak of expression is greater than comparable levels in the small intestine at the same time during postnatal development.[35] However, the levels of SI mRNA in the colon are many fold less than the expression in the adult small intestine.

These results suggest that the cellular machinery is present in developing colonocytes to express SI and that this expression is linked in time with the appearance of a small intestinal morphology. The loss of expression in adult colon may be due to loss of this cellular machinery. However, since there is re-expression in colorectal cancer cells, the more likely explanation is that there are factors that actively repress SI expression in the adult colon, and that these factors may be lost in cancer cells.

Regulation of Sucrose-Isomaltase Synthesis

Although enzymatic activity of SI may be modulated by post-transcriptional mechanisms that involve either translation or processing, the most important level of regulation of SI expression is focused on transcriptional initiation. This discussion will emphasize transcription as a developmental regulatory mechanism as elucidated from experiments in experimental animals and cell lines.

Transcriptional Regulation of the Sucrase-Isomaltase Gene

There appears to be only a single SI gene in multiple species.[23,63,64] The DNA region upstream of the transcriptional start site has been sequenced and analyzed in human,[14,63] mouse,[64] and rat,[65] demonstrating a high degree of homology within the immediate 200 nucleotides upstream of the start site. As has been demonstrated for many eukaryotic genes, this immediate upstream promoter region of the SI gene has been shown to be critical for transcriptional initiation.[21,35,63,64,66,67] The promoter structure contains a TATA box located 27 nucleotides upstream of the defined start of transcription, correlating with the appropriate distance for the binding of TATA-binding protein (TBP) and the initiation complex.[64] A number of DNA regulatory elements have been characterized immediately upstream of the TATA box and extending to approximately 180 nucleotides upstream of the transcriptional initiation site. The functions of these elements and their cognate DNA binding proteins will be described in detail.

Transcriptional regulation of the sucrase-isomaltase gene in transgenic mice. Developmental expression of genes in a complex organ system such as the intestine requires in vivo analysis of regulation. Characterization of transcriptional regulation using in vitro systems or cell lines would be incomplete without correlative studies on the regulation in intact tissues. For this purpose, the use of transgenic animals that link gene regulatory regions to reporter genes has been most instructive. Developmental patterns of expression of transgenes made using both human and mouse SI genes have been examined in transgenic mice.[21,35,67]

Initial studies involved the generation of transgenic mouse lines with a construct containing nucleotides −3424 to +54 of the human SI gene linked to the human growth hormone structural gene as a reporter.[21] Transgene expression was limited to the small intestine and, to a much lesser degree, the colon but the pattern of expression was different than the endogenous gene. In both the small intestine and colon, expression of the transgene was found to be in the distal portions of the intestinal tract, including the distal jejunum, ileum, and distal colon. Expression of the transgene was found in enterocytic cells of the ileum, as well as enteroendocrine cells in the ileum and colon. Since SI is ordinarily expressed only in the enterocyte lineage, enteroendocrine cells represented ectopic expression. Thus, experiments with this transgenic construct revealed that the regulatory region used contained elements necessary for intestine-specific transcription, but additional elements are necessary to recapitulate the expression pattern of the endogenous gene.

Because of potential differences between the human and mouse genes, additional transgenic mice were made using the mouse SI gene.[35,67] These transgenes have provided a more complete view of transcriptional regulation during development. Two transgene constructs have been examined in detail, one that linked nucleotides −201 to +54 of the mouse SI gene to the human growth hormone reporter gene (short construct) and a second linking nucleotides −8500 to +54 of the mouse SI gene to the same reporter (long construct). The short construct represents a highly evolutionarily conserved region of the SI gene. This conserved promoter region of the SI gene was capable of directing transgene expression specifically to small intestinal tissues in multiple founder lines.[35] Expression of the transgene was found in all portions of the small intestine and in much lower levels in the cecum and proximal colon.[35] Several founder lines either lacked expression of the transgene or had very minimal expression in a scattered distribution. These data indicated that the insertion site of the transgene in the mouse genome had an effect on the ability of the transgene to be expressed. Immunohistochemical staining for human growth hormone revealed that the short transgene was expressed predominantly in enterocytes of the small intestine, with prominent expression in a number of enteroendocrine cells. Expression in goblet and Paneth's cells was rarely identified in several transgenic lines. Similar to the expression of the endogenous SI gene, there was a marked differential in expression of the transgene between the crypt and villus compartments, with initiation of transgene expression in enterocytes at the CV junction. The expression of the transgene mRNA in the colon was very low, and in only one of six founder lines was there detection of immunostaining of the proximal colon in scattered enteroendocrine cells.

Developmental expression of the short transgene revealed the first onset of expression at embryonic day 16.5 in enteroendocrine cells.[35] Recall, from the developmental expression of the endogenous gene, that this is the first time that expression can be detected at very low levels. However, at no time during development is there evidence that the endogenous SI gene is expressed in enteroendocrine cells. Thus, this cellular pattern of expression of the transgene represents ectopic expression, but does indicate that this is the time at which intestinal epithelial cells become competent to transcribe the gene. Since in situ techniques are unable to identify the low-level expression of the endogenous gene, it is unreasonable to expect the transgene to be expressed at levels sufficient to be identified in enterocytes at this early stage in development. Enteroendocrine cell expression continued through the early postnatal period and into adulthood. Enterocyte expression, the site of endogenous SI expression, was initiated by postnatal day 16 at the CV junction. In subsequent postnatal days, transgene expression was extended throughout the villus by migration of the cells. Therefore, the short evolutionarily conserved promoter was able to recapitulate to a remarkable degree the developmental patterns of SI gene expression.

Evaluation of the long transgenic construct revealed added complexity.[67] In these transgenic animals, there was high-level expression of the transgene in all founder lines in a copy number-dependent fashion. These results suggest that in contrast to the short construct, the expression of this transgene was not dependent on the site of insertion in the genome and directed expression dependent on the number of copies of the transgene. This leads to the conclusion that the added DNA in the long construct may contain regulatory regions that insulate the promoter region from the effects of surrounding chromatin.[67] A second interesting finding from the long construct was that all four cell lineages in the small intestine expressed the transgene. Similar to the short construct, there was an increase in expression in enterocytes as they moved from the crypt compartment onto the villus; but there was also high-level expression in enteroendocrine and goblet cells in both crypt and villus compartments and in Paneth's cells in the base of crypts.[67] The expression of the transgene in the colon was restricted to the proximal colon predominately in enteroendocrine cells, although a few colonocytes also stained.

Developmental expression of the long transgene construct in different cell lineages revealed an interesting temporal pattern. Enterocyte expression was very similar to the short construct, with no expression until the suckling-weaning transition, after which there was high-level expression in villus-associated enterocytes. Unlike the short construct, there was easily identifiable transgene expression in crypt enterocytes, although the difference between crypt and villus remained dramatic. Enteroendocrine cell expression was first noted in fetal life after the endoderm-intestinal transition and was maintained throughout postnatal life, although there was a progressive increase in the number of enteroendocrine cells that expressed the transgene. After the onset of transgene expression in enterocytes at the suckling-weaning transition there was progressive expression in subsequent days in goblet and Paneth's cells. Thus, by postnatal day 30 there was high-level expression in all the epithelial cells in the small intestine.

Because it has been recognized for many years that corticosteroids are capable of mediating precocious induction of intestinal maturation, we examined whether the treatment of suckling animals with dexamethasone was able to induce transgene expression. Although dexamethasone was able to induce the SI protein, as previously reported, there was no induction of human growth hormone protein expression in enterocytes using the transgenic animals containing either the long or short constructs.[35] These results indicate that regulatory elements that mediate the induction of SI expression by corticosteroids must lie outside the region of the SI gene bounded by nucleotides −8500 to +54 of the mouse SI gene.

A summary of the results of transgenic experiments using the SI gene suggests that a complex array of regulatory elements are necessary to direct the patterns of SI gene transcription. The evolutionarily conserved promoter region is able to direct intestine-specific and developmental expression to a remarkable degree. The promoter directs expression to enterocytes in the proper developmental and spatial patterns in the small intestinal epithelium. However, ectopic expression in enteroendocrine cells reveals that additional elements are required for regulation. Results of experiments with the long promoter construct suggest that the region

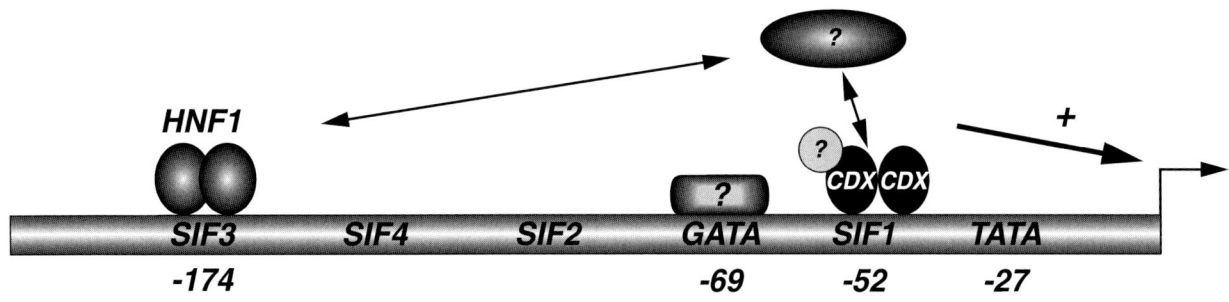

FIGURE 7–5. Evolutionarily conserved SI gene promoter. This figure depicts the DNA regulatory elements and their cognate DNA binding proteins that have been thus far described in the SI promoter. SIF stands for sucrase isomaltase footprint. The SIF1 element has been shown to contain two binding sites for caudal-related homeobox proteins, or CDX. The SIF3 site has been shown to interact with hepatocyte nuclear factor 1 proteins, HNF1α and HNF1β. Sucrase-isomaltase footprint 2 and SIF4 remain as potential regulatory elements, although differences between mouse and human promoters make them of questionable significance, as discussed. The GATA site is a potential regulatory element that may interact with GATA-type zinc-finger transcription factors. The small circle with a question mark attached to the CDX protein indicates the possibility that post-translational processing of CDX proteins may modify their function. The elongated circle with a question mark represents potential cofactors that may mediate protein-protein interaction between DNA-binding proteins or the basal transcriptional apparatus.

between −8500 and −201 nucleotides may contain several regulatory elements. One element may be an insulator that protects the promoter region from chromatin effects. It is also possible that there are enhancer elements for the expression of the transgene in Paneth's cells and goblet cells, since there was little expression in these cells with the short construct. However, it is also possible that the expression in these cell lineages is related to overall enhancement of the ability of the promoter to drive expression because of the insulator function. This issue cannot be resolved from the current data.

The fact that the long construct directs high-level expression in all four cell lineages in the small intestine suggests that elements located outside the region from −8500 to +54 are required to silence transcription in nonenterocytic cells. Such a silencing mechanism has increasingly been described in the regulation of gene expression, including other intestinal genes.[68] Finally, the well-described mechanism of precocious induction of SI is also regulated by elements located outside the region bounded by these transgenic experiments. In sum, the evolutionarily conserved promoter is critically important for developmental and differentiation-dependent expression of the SI gene. Additional elements located outside the promoter are necessary for modulation of expression in various cell lineages, as well as the response to corticosteroids.

Regulatory elements and cognate DNA-binding proteins in the sucrase-isomaltase promoter. The transgenic mouse experiments showed that the first 200 nucleotides upstream of the transcriptional start site were critical for regulation of developmental expression of the SI gene. Therefore, a careful analysis of the DNA regulatory elements and DNA-binding proteins has focused on this region. The nucleotide sequence of the human, mouse, and rat sequences show a high degree of identity between the three species. Several regions show identical nucleotides over long stretches of DNA that make these regions likely regulatory elements.

Initially, an unbiased approach to defining regulatory elements was taken by examining the promoter for regions that interacted with nuclear proteins.[64] Nuclear proteins were isolated from the CaCo-2 cell line which have many characteristics of enterocytes, including expression of the SI gene. Nonintestinal cell lines were used for comparative purposes. DNase I footprinting analysis showed that there were three regions that interacted with nuclear extracts from CaCo-2 cells, only one of which was unique to the intestinal line.[64] These three elements were named SIF1, SIF2, and SIF3 for sucrase-isomaltase footprint (Figure 7–5). Both the mouse and the human promoters were used in this analysis and gave similar results. Transfection experiments with deletional reporter gene constructs showed that each of the elements was important for transcriptional induction of the SI gene in CaCo-2 cells. The promoter was not active in nonintestinal cell lines.[64]

The SIF1 site has received the most attention since it binds to proteins expressed in nuclei of both intestinal cell lines and intestinal epithelial cells.[64] A variety of experiments showed that this element contained two adjacent binding sites for a similar protein.[64,69] A mouse intestinal cDNA expression library was screened using this element as a probe to identify the nuclear proteins that interact with this site.[69] This approach was successful in identifying a specific DNA-binding protein that was able to bind to the SIF1 site and transactivate the SI gene promoter. This protein was a caudal-related homeodomain protein (CDX2) that turned out to be a member of a three-gene subfamily of homeobox genes in the mouse. Antibodies raised to recognize CDX2 were used to show that the predominant SIF1-interacting protein in nuclear extract from intestinal cell lines was CDX2. Recently, the HOXC11 protein has been shown to interact with the SIF1 element.[70] This finding will be discussed in more detail.

The SIF3 site, and to a lesser extent the SIF2 site, were shown to interact with hepatocyte nuclear factor 1 (HNF1).[66] Hepatocyte nuclear factor 1α and HNF1β, the two known members of the HNF1 family, are diverged homeodomain proteins that form homo- and heterodimers on DNA and activate transcription. Both HNF1α and HNF1β interact specifically with SIF2 and SIF3, whereas only HNF1α is able to activate transcription of the SI promoter to a significant degree. The relative function of HNF1 proteins on the SIF2 and SIF3 elements has not been elucidated.

There are several other sites in the SI gene promoter that have potential regulatory significance. Immediately upstream of the SIF1 element is a sequence that was shown to interact with GATA zinc-finger transcription factors (TGATAG).[71] There are at least three GATA proteins expressed in the small intestinal epithelium,[72] but the functional significance of this site remains unclear. Although there may be an important functional significance to this site, an understanding of the GATA element function and which proteins actually interact with the site will require additional investigation. Transfection experiments showed a marked decrease in transcriptional activation when nucleotides −94 to −66 were deleted from the SI promoter, which could be secondary to either the SIF2 or GATA binding elements.[64]

Another potential regulatory site is an inverted repeat with the sequence TTTATGTAAA that was described as SIF4 in a preliminary communication.[73] The SIF4 site was used to screen a mouse liver cDNA expression library and was found to interact with the mouse homolog of human E4BP4, a basic leucine zipper protein that has been shown to act as a transcriptional repressor.[74] This work was not followed up because the mouse E4BP4 did not affect transcription of the SI promoter in transfection experiments, and mutation of the SIF4 site did not affect transcription of the promoter in CaCo-2 cells. However, this site has not formally been excluded as a regulatory region.

Hepatocyte nuclear factor 6 is a liver-enriched nuclear protein that interacts with a specific nucleotide sequence in the HNF3 beta gene[75]; HNF6 is a cut-homeodomain transcription factor that can activate target genes and is expressed in liver, pancreas, and intestinal epithelium.[75,76] There is consensus HNF6 binding element located between the TATA box and the SIF1 element in both the mouse and human SI gene promoter.[75] The potential functional significance of this site has not been explored.

In summary, the SI promoter appears to have a limited number of regulatory elements important for regulation of gene transcription. The most important functional elements that have been characterized thus far are SIF1, SIF3, and the region between −94 and −66 (which contains both SIF2 and GATA elements). Although it is clear that SIF1 interacts with CDX proteins, it remains possible that other transcription factors bind to this element. Moreover, it is formally possible that other sequences in the promoter are important for regulation but have eluded the experimental systems and methods used thus far. How these elements and their DNA-binding proteins may act during development to direct intestinal gene expression will be discussed below.

Function of CDX proteins. The CDX proteins appear to be major regulators of the SI gene promoter via interaction with the SIF1 DNA element. Thus a more complete description of the function of these proteins is important for understanding their potential function in the regulation of SI gene transcription. Caudal (cad) was first described in *Drosophila melanogaster*, and the first caudal-related gene in another organism was CDX1, cloned from mouse embryo cDNA library using cad as a probe.[77] The CDX genes have now been cloned from many organisms, including a family of three genes in mouse (CDX1,[77] CDX2,[69,78,79] and CDX4[80]) and two in human (CDX1[81,82] and CDX2[82,83]).

The pattern of expression of the CDX genes in mice provides insight into possible functional roles. CDX4 is expressed exclusively in posterior structures of early embryos,[80] and not later in development. CDX1 is expressed just after gastrulation in mouse embryogenesis in posterior structures, and expression throughout the embryo appears to be extinguished by approximately embryonic day 12.[84] The CDX1 mRNA is then re-expressed in the gut endoderm at approximately post coital day 14,[77] immediately before the endoderm-intestinal transition. The CDX1 protein becomes preferentially localized to the crypt compartment of the small intestine and colon.[85] CDX2 is first expressed in preimplantation embryos in placental precursor cells, and then at the time of gastrulation it is expressed in posterior structures.[86] Expression continues in the gut endoderm after turning of the embryo and continues to be expressed throughout life.[86] In the adult intestinal tract there is some evidence of an increasing gradient of both CDX1 and CDX2 mRNAs toward the distal portions of the bowel.[78,87] However, the patterns of expression require more careful analysis of both mRNA and protein before firm conclusions can be made.

CDX1 and CDX2 bind to specific sequences of DNA via their homeodomain. CDX2 was first shown to interact with an AT-rich sequence in the SI promoter but since then has been shown to interact with elements in a number of other promoters of genes expressed in the intestine, including lactase-phlorizin hydrolase,[88] intestinal phospholipase A/lysophospholipase (IPAL),[89] calbindin D9K,[90] carbonic anhydrase,[91] and glucagon.[92–94] Studies with the IPAL promoter showed that both CDX1 and CDX2 were capable of activating transcription in a DNA-binding dependent fashion and that CDX proteins could activate transcription from a single binding site in the promoter.[89] Only minimal information is available regarding the functional domains of CDX proteins. The activation domain for both proteins was shown to be in the aminoterminal end of the protein.[95] Nothing is currently known about how the activation domain functions, the function of the domain that is carboxyterminal to the homeodomain, or what protein modifications, such as phosphorylation or acetylation, may occur in these proteins.

Null mutants in mice have been created for both CDX1 and CDX2. The CDX1 null mice are live born and survive until adulthood, although there is an anterior homeotic shift in vertebral structures, indicating that expression of CDX1 in the early embryo is important for patterning of the axial skeleton.[96] Although a detailed report on the small intestine and colon was not provided, the intestinal tract was grossly intact and must have been functional, since the animals survived. The CDX2 null mice are not viable and die in utero before implantation.[97] Interestingly, the axial skeleton of CDX2 (+/−) mice had an anterior homeotic shift nearly identical to that reported for the CDX1 null mice.[97] The small intestine and colon developed normally in the CDX2(+/−) mice, but several weeks after birth they developed colonic tumors with evidence of squamous metaplasia. Of great interest, the expression of CDX2 proteins was completely lost in the tumor cells, whereas it was expressed in the normal colonocytes. The investigators showed that the normal CDX2 allele was not lost in the tumors, suggesting that there were either point mutations that could not be identified by restriction fragment length polymorphism (RFLP) analysis or, more likely, an epigenetic event that extinguished expression of CDX2. These results show that continued expression of CDX2 is necessary to maintain the normal intestinal phenotype.

Several studies in intestinal cell lines have demonstrated the importance of CDX proteins on the regulation of differentiation and proliferation.[98–101] In summary, both CDX1 and CDX2 are expressed in the intestinal epithelium and have a demonstrated role in regulation of the intestinal cell phenotype, as demonstrated by studies in the whole animal or cell lines.

Translation and Processing of the Sucrase-Isomaltase Messenger Ribonucleic Acid

Following synthesis and processing, the mature mRNA for SI is translated in the cytoplasm to yield a single protein.[13,16] As mentioned, the mRNA for SI is localized in a sub-brushborder compartment of the enterocyte near the site of insertion into the apical membrane.[10,11] It is unknown whether this localization plays a role in developmental expression or regulation of SI protein in different regions of the intestine or in response to physiologic stimuli.

The N-terminus forms a short membrane anchor that remains embedded in the endoplasmic reticulum (ER)[16,102] and may be phosphorylated under certain conditions.[103] Protein N-glycosylation, with the addition of a branched oligosaccharide to an asparagine residue, occurs during translation of the SI protein in the ER. Because this oligosaccharide contains nine mannose molecules, the SI protein with this modification has been called the high-mannose form. The high-mannose form is modified in the Golgi by removal of mannose residues and the addition of other sugars. O-glycosylation occurs at the hydroxyl group of serine and threonine residues in Golgi's apparatus. The fully glycosylated SI molecule has a molecular weight of 245 kDa, and it has been shown that both N- and O-glycosylation occurs equally on the isomaltase and sucrase subunits.[13] These data are for the human protein, and although other species show essentially the same pattern of synthesis, there are slight differences in the molecular weights of the forms.[102,104–106]

The fully glycosylated SI molecule is transported uncleaved to the apical membrane of the enterocyte via direct transport in vesicles from Golgi's apparatus.[20] The cleavage of the molecule to the two subunits occurs by an enzymatic step in the lumen of the intestine.[12,16] The cleavage of the molecules into the two subunits (145 kDa for isomaltase and 130 kDa for sucrase) occurs by tryptic digestion in the lumen of the human intestine.[13] The two subunits remain associated by hydrostatic bonds. The degradation of SI in the lumen of the intestine is mediated by pancreatic proteases.[107,108]

Understanding of the processing and transport of the SI molecule has been instrumental in elucidating the site of the defect in inherited SI deficiency in humans. The enzymatic deficiency in these individuals appears related to a number of different defects in glycosylation, intracellular transport, and possibly altered catalytic activity.[109] The two situations in which translational or post-translational mechanisms have been implicated in regulation are in aging[29] and in the regional distribution of protein in the rat.[27,28] As described above, in aged rats there appears to be an increased sensitivity to the degradation of the sucrase subunit by pancreatic proteases. The underlying mechanisms of this are unexplored, but could be related to changes in folding during translation or in the post-translational modification by glycosylation. Either of these changes may alter the three-dimensional structure of the final protein, providing easier access for proteases. The mechanisms of the differences in the translation of SI mRNA between the proximal and distal small intestine in rats have not been elucidated.

Another area of post-transcriptional regulation has been suggested. Monoclonal antibodies have been described that recognize different forms of the SI molecule.[22] Immunoblot analysis of these antibodies was able to immunoprecipitate SI, and in immunoblots recognized different portions of the SI molecule.[22] When these antibodies were used in immunohistochemical staining of human small intestine, there were three patterns of staining: (1) intense staining of the brushborder of enterocytes located on the villus with no staining of crypt cells; (2) intense staining of villus enterocytes with weak staining of the apical membrane of crypt cells; and (3) weak staining of apical membranes of both crypt and villus enterocytes.[22] These results suggested to the authors that the primary difference in the expression of SI activity between crypt and villus enterocytes was at the level of post-translational processing with different glycosylated forms. This level of regulation would be a novel mechanism and quite interesting for intestinal gene regulation. However, it is clear from studies in multiple species, including human,[11,24] that the primary level of regulation of SI gene expression along the CV axis is the steady state amount of SI mRNA. There may, however, be a role for the type of regulation suggested by these authors over short segments of the CV axis. Moreover, the in situ hybridization experiments do not rule out the possibility that there are small amounts of protein in crypt enterocytes. The overall importance of these findings remains unclear.

Working Model of Sucrase-Isomaltase Regulation during Intestinal Development

Transcriptional initiation appears to be the most important level of regulation for the SI gene during development. The findings in transgenic mice place the focus for a model of developmental SI gene transcription on the evolutionarily conserved promoter. The CDX and HNF1 transcription factors that interact with DNA regulatory elements are likely to be central participants in the regulation of developmental SI gene transcription. However, it is clear from the patterns of expression of CDX and HNF1 that the presence of these factors alone is insufficient to regulate the developmental patterns of expression directed by the SI promoter. As shown in Figure 7–6, the patterns of expression of the endogenous SI gene and the short transgene in enterocytes do not correspond to the expression of CDX1, CDX2, HNF1α, or HNF1β. It should be noted, however, that confirmation of the importance of the DNA regulatory elements and their putative cognate DNA-binding proteins for SI gene transcription will require more specific experiments, including point mutations in promoter transgenic constructs, and creative ways to manipulate the expression of the individual transcription factors, alone and in combination.

Given that it is unlikely that the known transcription factors are able to regulate SI gene transcription by the fact that they are expressed alone, what are the other potential mechanisms that allow the evolutionarily conserved SI promoter to direct developmental expression? First, there may be other nuclear proteins that interact with the currently described DNA elements. In this regard, data have been presented that HOXC11 binds to the SIF1 element and is able to activate transcription.[70] Additionally, other homeodomain proteins may be able to bind to SIF1.[96] It has also been reported that different rat intestinal nuclear proteins bind the SIF1 element depending on the developmental times of isolation.[65] Nuclear proteins isolated from the suckling rat intestine formed a high mobility complex with SIF1 whereas the weaned intestinal nuclear extract showed a slower mobility complex that was not confirmed to be CDX2.[65] It should be noted that these results differ from preliminary

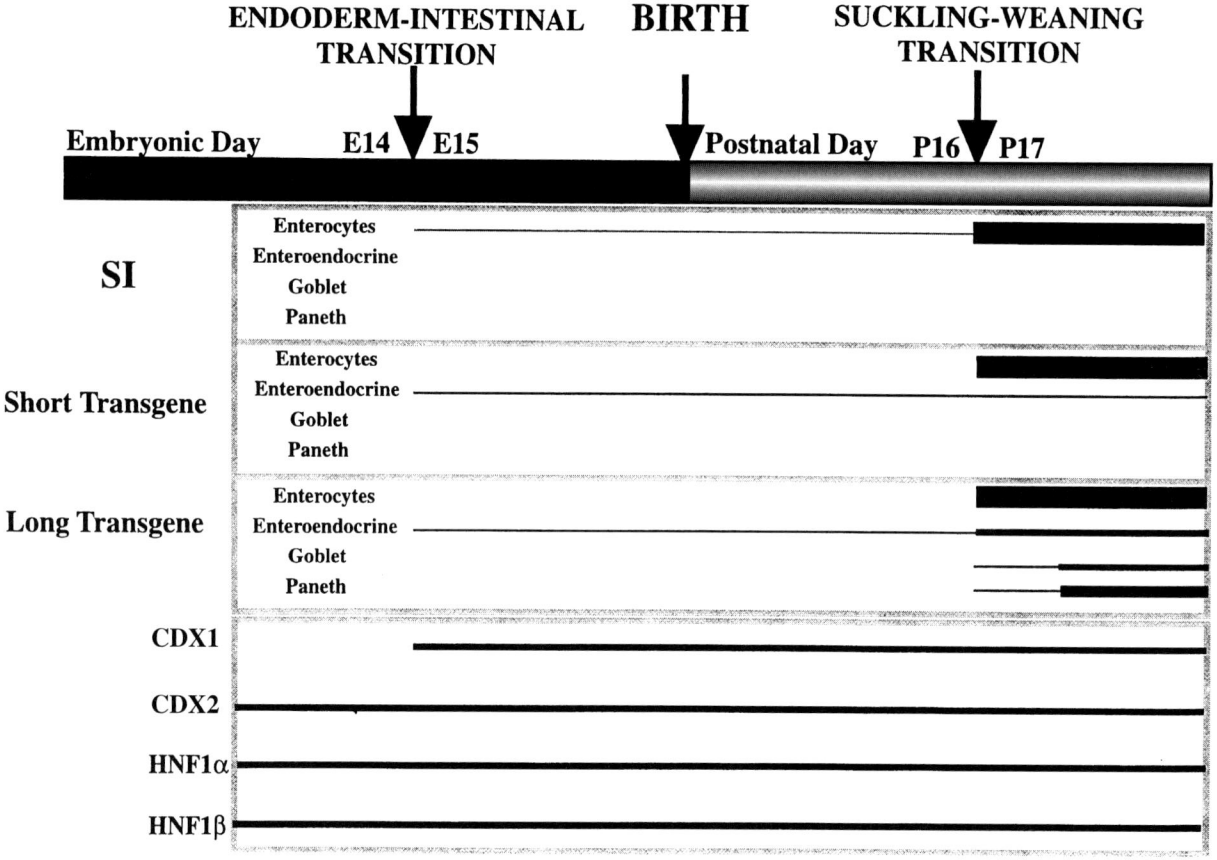

FIGURE 7–6. Regulation of SI gene expression during development of mouse small intestine. This figure depicts the expression of the endogenous SI gene, as well as transgenic constructs placed on the developmental time line in mice. These expression data represent a combination of SI mRNA and protein data. The endogenous SI gene is expressed in enterocytes at low levels beginning at the endoderm-intestinal transition. At the suckling-weaning transition, there is marked induction of the endogenous gene, resulting in adult levels by the fourth week of life. Expression of the endogenous gene is not detected in enteroendocrine, goblet, or Paneth's cells at any time during intestinal development. The short transgenic construct includes nucleotides –201 to +54 of the mouse SI gene linked to a reporter gene. This short transgene directs expression of the reporter gene in enterocytes that recapitulates the pattern of the endogenous gene to a remarkable degree, as described in the text. There is ectopic expression of this short transgene construct in enteroendocrine cells, beginning after the endoderm intestinal transition. Highly variable and rare expression is noted in goblet cells and Paneth's cells. The long transgene construct includes nucleotides –8500 to +54 of the mouse SI gene and promotes expression in enterocytes in a pattern similar to that of the short transgene, although the levels are increased, as described. A similar pattern of enteroendocrine cell expression is also seen, although there is an increase after the suckling-weaning transition. Moreover, following the suckling-weaning transition expression is noted in both goblet cells and Paneth's cells that is maximal after the fourth week of life. The bottom of this figure demonstrates the patterns of expression of the caudal-related homeobox genes CDX1 and CDX2 and the hepatocyte nuclear factor 1, HNF1α and HNF1β. Relative levels of these genes are not depicted, but rather their onset of expression. Each of these transcription factors has been implicated in the regulation of the promoter used in the short transgene construct. The lack of concordant expression patterns for these transcription factors and the transgene constructs is discussed in the text.

experiments in the mouse small intestine, where CDX1 and CDX2 were found to bind to the SIF1 element in both suckling and weaned intestine.[110] Therefore, various DNA-binding proteins may compete for binding with the SIF1 element during intestinal development and thereby regulate activity of the SI promoter. This possibility requires additional study. The same situation could involve the SIF3 site, although there are no candidates currently.

A second possibility is that there are undiscovered DNA-binding proteins that interact with other elements in the SI promoter. As described, these sites may include SIF4 or the GATA site. A third possible scenario for promoter regulation is modification of CDX or HNF1 proteins that alters their interaction with DNA or affects their ability to activate transcription. It has been reported that there is an increase in SIF1 binding upon differentiation of CaCo-2 cells, thus correlating with SI expression.[111] Although an increase in expression of the binding proteins is a possible explanation for these findings, an increase in binding affinity for the site is also possible.

Finally, the mediation of transcriptional activation by CDX and HNF1, as well as any other factors described subsequently, may depend on interactions with other proteins that link the transcription factors to the basal apparatus. This interaction may be direct with the basal apparatus or indirect via coadaptor proteins. It is likely that each of these possibilities is involved in regulation. As the model is refined through additional experimentation, a network of interacting proteins will be required to assemble on the promoter to initiate SI gene transcription, and developmental transitions will be mediated by addition or subtraction of individual proteins or modification of those proteins as a result of signaling events.

DEVELOPMENTAL REGULATION OF LACTASE-PHLORIZIN HYDROLASE

The major carbohydrate in milk is the disaccharide lactose, which is produced exclusively in the mammary glands of mammals by lactose synthase. Brushborder lactase is the only enzyme that cleaves lactose into glucose and galactose and is therefore essential for the survival of mammals early in life.[112] Lactase has other enzymatic activities, including phlorizin hydrolase, glycosylceramidase, and β-galactosidase activity.[113] The human LPH cDNA encodes for a single polypeptide chain containing 1972 amino acids,[114] and the structural gene is approximately 55 kb long with 17 exons.[115,116] An understanding of LPH regulation has been a goal for many investigators because its expression declines in the majority of humans, resulting in varying degrees of lactose intolerance in adults.

Spatial and Regional Expression of Lactase-Phlorizin Hydrolase in the Fully Developed Intestine

Unlike SI, the expression of LPH in the adult intestinal epithelium is not the norm in most mammalian species. Lactase-phlorizin hydrolase is a crucial intestinal enzyme in neonatal life when the immature animal depends on mother's milk for nourishment. After the transition is made to solid food, LPH activity markedly diminishes or disappears in most species, including the majority of the human population. Persistence of LPH expression in some human populations appears to be the exception in nature. For these reasons, the patterns of expression of LPH are appropriately discussed in the context of intestinal development. Thus, the next section will describe developmental expression of LPH as well as persistent expression in adult humans.

Developmental Expression of Lactase-Phlorizin Hydrolase

The developmental expression of LPH is as complex as that of SI and has been studied extensively.[16,34,40,113] In many respects there is a reciprocal relationship between the developmental expression of LPH and SI. Thus, a comparison of the regulatory mechanisms of these two brushborder enzymes will likely reveal important paradigms for intestinal gene regulation. The discussion of SI regulation in the previous sections allows this section on LPH to be more concise, and the reader is referred to the SI sections for more detailed description of general developmental changes.

Expression of Lactase-Phlorizin Hydrolase in Development of the Small Intestine

Human small intestinal development. Lactase-phlorizin hydrolase is expressed in human fetal small intestine at a time in gestation just after the onset of expression of SI[31,44] (see Figure 7–1). The expression of LPH remains relatively low in the fetal intestine until approximately 24 weeks, after which there is a gradual increase until late in gestation, when there is a marked increase in activity at approximately 32 weeks of gestation.[26,117] This increased activity remains through birth and early infancy, with decreases to lower levels in the first year of life.[26,117] Expression of LPH is then maintained at these levels during childhood. The expression of LPH mRNA during human intestinal development correlates well with the level of enzyme activity, suggesting that steady state mRNA is the major level of regulatory control.[117] There is some evidence that the increase in LPH late in gestation is related to corticosteroids.[26,117] In organ culture LPH activity, but not mRNA, was induced by corticosteroids, suggesting a posttranscriptional level of regulatory control.[117]

Lactase-phlorizin hydrolase mRNA and protein in the mature human intestinal epithelium has a complex pattern of expression along the CV axis.[11] There is very little expression of the mRNA or protein in crypt cells. At the CV junction high levels of LPH mRNA appear, which are maintained at similar levels in cells out in the villus tips.[11] This pattern differs from SI mRNA, which is decreased in the villus tips,[11,24] and also from the pattern of LPH expression in rat intestine (see below). As for SI, the LPH mRNA is localized in a cellular compartment just under the brushborder membrane.[11] The LPH protein is found in the brushborder membrane out to the villus tip.[11]

Sometime during childhood or adolescence, LPH activity declines to between 5% and 10% of childhood levels in the majority of the worldwide population.[16,118] The age at which the enzyme disappears is variable, depending on the heritage of the individual. In selected human populations, such as those in northern Europe where dairy cattle have been developed as a continuing source of milk products, there is persistence of intestinal LPH activity throughout adulthood.[16,34,40,113] The hypolactasia phenotype is inherited as an autosomal recessive trait, and there is evidence that in heterozygous individuals there are intermediate levels of LPH activity.[16] The persistence of LPH activity is an autosomal dominant trait. As stated, nearly all other species of mammals lose LPH activity following weaning.[16,34,40,113]

The underlying mechanisms of hypolactasia in adult humans have been a focus of research for many years.[113,115,119–122] At times there have been divergent views in the literature on the pathophysiology and mechanisms of adult hypolactasia. This is because the disorder is heterogeneous with a number of underlying mechanisms. The coding sequence of the LPH gene predicts the same primary protein in subjects who have persistence and loss of lactase activity.[115] Evaluation of polymorphisms in the LPH gene reveals that the persistence or nonpersistence of LPH is controlled by DNA elements located on the same strand of DNA as the structural gene.[120,123] There is a strong correlation between LPH mRNA and prolactase levels in biopsies from individuals with persistence and nonpersistence of LPH.[121] However, there is less correlation between LPH mRNA and lactase activity. Analysis of data from a large group of individuals shows that there are likely both transcriptional and post-transcriptional mechanisms involved in the development of hypolactasia.

Studies of LPH mRNA and protein in patients with hypolactasia reveal a remarkable degree of heterogeneity in expression within the enterocyte population.[124,125] Lactase-phlorizin hydrolase mRNA in patients with hypolactasia is expressed in approximately half of the enterocytes in the small intestinal mucosa, distributed in an essentially random fashion.[125] Some, but not all, of the enterocytes that express LPH mRNA also express LPH protein and enzymatic activity.

Some infants are born with a severe deficiency of LPH that is inherited as an autosomal recessive trait. It has recently been shown that the genetic locus for this deficiency is near the LPH gene, but is separate.[126]

Rodent small intestinal development. Expression of LPH mRNA and protein is first detected just after the endoderm-intestinal transition during rodent development[127] (see Figure 7–2). In situ hybridization and immunohistochemistry of small intestine from fetal and neonatal rats reveal a complex pattern of expression of LPH mRNA.[127] Prior to birth, LPH mRNA and protein are expressed in all villus-associated enterocytes.[127] Immediately after birth, LPH mRNA is restricted to enterocytes located at the base of villi, in a fashion similar to the pattern of expression of SI mRNA in adult intestine. The protein, however, persists throughout all villus enterocytes.[127] As described, the pattern of expression of the LPH mRNA in human small intestinal epithelium differs from that of the rat.[11] However, similar to the human enterocyte, LPH mRNA is localized within the cell to the subvillus cytoplasm in the rat.[10]

In addition to the timing of expression during development along the CV axis, there are important changes in expression along the horizontal axis of the gut.[112,128–133] Expression of LPH is first detected in the proximal small intestine, which rapidly spreads distally until expression is found along the entire length of the intestine. During the postnatal life there are shifts in the patterns of expression along the length of the intestine, with decreased expression in the duodenum and the terminal ileum and distal jejunum.[128,134] Thus, the highest level of expression of LPH is in the middle portion of the jejunum.[128,134]

The expression of LPH remains high in the small intestine until after weaning, when there is a decline in activity. In fact, LPH activity declines at the same time that SI activity increases in the small intestine.[16,32,33] Similar to many of the changes that occur at the suckling-weaning transition, the decline in LPH activity is hastened by pharmacologic treatment with corticosteroids in parallel with the induction of SI. There have been many studies on the mechanisms for the postweaning decline in LPH activity in many animal species.[112,129–133,135–139] As in the human small intestine, there appear to be several mechanisms in rodents that lead to the decrease in LPH after weaning, but controversy remains about what is the predominant level of regulation. These controversies may be due in part to the fact that regulation is different along the length of the intestinal tract, a variable that was not taken careful note of in all studies.

Taken together, the results of a number of studies suggest that the primary reason for a decline in LPH activity in the proximal duodenum and ileum after weaning is a decrease in LPH mRNA levels.[128,131,133] Nuclear run-on experiments, using nuclei isolated from the entire length of intestine, showed that the decline in LPH mRNA is, at least in part, due to decreased transcription of the LPH gene.[128] The measurement of primary transcripts of the LPH mRNA suggested that the decrease in both proximal and distal intestine was due to decreased transcription.[128] Likewise, another study has shown a decrease in LPH gene transcription in the proximal duodenum.[133] However, there is evidence that the mechanisms of decreased LPH mRNA are different in the two regions of the intestine.[133] This study showed that nuclear transcription of the LPH gene is maintained in the ileum, although there is decreased ileal LPH mRNA.[133] Therefore, the decrease in expression in the proximal duodenum is likely due to decreased gene transcription, whereas the mechanism of the decrease in the ileum is unclear and may be due to decreased transcription or increased degradation of LPH mRNA in the face of continued gene transcription. In the middle regions of the intestine the expression of LPH mRNA and the amount of polysome-bound RNA are maintained, but there is a decrease in lactase activity, suggesting a post-translational mechanism.[133]

A number of studies have clearly shown that post-translational mechanisms are involved in the postweaning decline in LPH activity.[129,131–133,135–139] These mechanisms are particularly important for modulating the expression of functional LPH protein along the length of the intestine. Therefore, there are multiple regulatory mechanisms active in different regions of the intestinal tract.

Expression of Lactase-Phlorizin Hydrolase in Development of the Colon

Similar to SI, LPH is expressed during development of both the rodent and human colon (see Figures 7–3 and 7–4). The pattern of expression in the human colon is similar to SI and is not expressed in the neonatal colon. Moreover, as for SI, some colorectal cancer cell lines express LPH and thus simulate the fetal colonic phenotype. Lactase-phlorizin hydrolase is expressed in the neonatal rat colon[45,140] in the same manner as SI. Expression in the perinatal rat colon reaches a peak between 2 and 6 days after birth and then decreases to undetectable levels in the third week of life.[48]

Synthesis of Lactase-Phlorizin Hydrolase

Transcriptional Regulation of the Lactase-Phlorizin Hydrolase Gene

Similar to the SI gene, evidence has accumulated that transcriptional initiation is the primary level of regulation in the developmental expression of LPH. Various lengths of the 5'-flanking regions of the human,[115] pig,[141] and rat[142,143] LPH genes have been characterized. The LPH promoter is well conserved across species within the first 150 nucleotides from the start of transcription.[141]

Transcriptional regulation of the lactase-phlorizin hydrolase gene in transgenic mice. Transgenic mouse experiments have been employed to determine whether the 5'-flanking region of the LPH gene is able to direct developmental expression. Nucleotides −2038 to +15 of the rat LPH gene linked to a reporter gene were studied in transgenic mice.[143] This construct was expressed in the small intestine in only one of six founder lines, with two of the other lines expressing at low levels in kidney and three lines with no expression. These results suggest that this regulatory region is highly sensitive to the site of insertion in the mouse chromosomal DNA. The horizontal pattern of expression of the transgene differed from the endogenous LPH gene. Lactase-phlorizin hydrolase mRNA in the adult mouse small intestine is expressed at highest levels in the geometric middle of the small intestine, with lower levels in the more proximal and distal parts of the intestine. In contrast, the transgene was expressed at high levels in the proximal intestine, lower levels in scattered cells in the midintestine, and was not expressed in the distal intestine. The transgene was expressed appropriately along the CV axis, with no expression in crypt cells and high-level expression in enterocytes located on the villus. There was no expression in goblet, enteroendocrine, or Paneth's cells.[143] Developmental expression of this transgene showed surprising results. The transgene expression increased dramatically in the proximal small intestine after the second week of life, whereas the endogenous LPH mRNA decreased after weaning to very low levels. Thus, the pattern of expression of the LPH transgene was the opposite of what would have been expected.

In another transgenic study, nucleotides −994 to −17 of the pig LPH gene linked to a reporter gene were shown to direct expression specifically to the small intestine.[144] Two transgenic lines were shown to have this pattern of expression. In situ hybridization showed that the transgene mRNA was expressed predominantly in villus-associated enterocytes. Additionally, expression was limited to differentiated enterocytes located on the villus, and there was a postweaning decrease in expression. Interestingly, the transgene was predominantly expressed in the proximal small intestine, whereas the endogenous LPH mRNA was in the midintestine, similar to the results of the rat LPH transgenic experiments described. During development the transgene mRNA decreased in parallel with the LPH mRNA after weaning.[144]

Clearly the immediate upstream region of the LPH gene is able to direct intestinal expression with correct patterns along the CV axis. It appears that there are elements missing from both transgenic constructs reported that are responsible for directing the correct pattern of expression along the horizontal axis of the intestine, since both transgenes were expressed more proximally in the small intestine than the endogenous LPH gene. The discrepancy between the two studies with respect to the developmental pattern of expression is puzzling. This may be due to different locations for the element responsible for the downregulation of the LPH gene after weaning in the rat and pig LPH genes, although it may be related to ectopic expression in a single transgenic line. More refined studies will be required to narrow the regulatory region to determine whether the evolutionarily conserved region of the promoter is able to direct expression, as is the case with SI.

Regulatory Elements and Cognate DNA-Binding Proteins in the Lactase-Phlorizin Hydrolase Promoter

Studies in intestinal cell lines have identified functional DNA elements in the LPH promoter that interact with nuclear transcripton factors.[88,141,145,146] A cis-acting element called CE-LPH1 was identified immediately upstream of the TATA box that was shown to be critical for LPH gene transcription in transfection experiments.[88,141,147] Interestingly, it has been shown that CDX proteins bind to one region of this element and activate transcription.[88] A single CDX2 molecule binds to the LPH promoter, whereas the SI promoter binds two CDX molecules at two closely linked sites.[88] However, it has been found in a number of studies that there are likely other proteins that bind to CE-LPH1.[88,146]

Recently, a new transcription factor has been implicated in the regulation of LPH.[70] HOXC11 was found to bind to the CE-LPH1 site and activate transcription.[70] These findings show that other homeodomain transcription factors may regulate gene transcription through elements that also bind CDX proteins. However, it appears unlikely that expression of HOXC11 alone regulates LPH developmental expression, since it is expressed early in intestinal development before the expression of LPH.[70]

A member of the GATA-type zinc-finger transcription factor family, GATA6 has been shown to interact with the human LPH promoter and activate transcription.[145] Hepatocyte nuclear factor 1 proteins have also been shown to interact with and activate transcription of the LPH gene.[70] Therefore, it is quite striking that transcription factors similar to those that regulate the SI gene promoter may also be involved in the regulation of LPH.

Further characterization of the elements and DNA-binding proteins that regulate LPH would be facilitated by narrowing the regulatory region through transgenic mouse experiments.

Translation and Processing of the Lactase-Phlorizin Hydrolase Messenger Ribonucleic Acid

Biochemical experiments using both native LPH protein and cDNA-derived protein from transfected cells have provided a clear picture of the processing and structure of the mature enzyme. Lactase-phlorizin hydrolase is anchored to the apical membrane and has two active sites on the luminal side of the membrane. The carboxyterminal end of the LPH polypeptide is embedded in the plasma membrane, leaving the aminoterminal end in the lumen. The two active sites are located on the same peptide, which is not cleaved, in contrast to SI. The 19 N-terminal amino acids of the propeptide are cleaved in the ER, leaving the N-terminal end of the molecule free in the interior of the ER. Following synthesis of the polypeptide, the carboxyterminal end remains embedded in the membrane, serving as an anchor. This anchor consists of a cytoplasmic domain containing 26 amino acids and a membrane-spanning region containing 19 hydrophobic amino acids.[114] Correct folding of pro-LPH in the ER depends on intramolecular disulfide bonds.[148] The active sites have been identified with the lactase site at Glu^{1271} and the phlorizin hydrolyase site at Glu^{1747}.[149]

A single polypeptide precursor of approximately 210 kDa is synthesized from a single mRNA in humans,[150] and glycosylation results in a 215-kDa high-mannose form and a 225-kDa complex glycosylated form. The mature enzyme in the brushborder represents a cleavage product of the glycosylated precursor molecule.[16,113,151,152] The first cleavage occurs intracellularly at a dibasic residue (Arg_{734}-Leu_{735}), resulting in a 160-kDa intermediate form of LPH.[153,154] Although the cleaved polypeptide has structural similarities with the mature enzyme, the cleaved product is devoid of enzymatic activity.[155] Thus, the human enzyme is cleaved prior to the appearance of the protein on the plasma membrane[150] in a post-Golgi's compartment[156] following complex glycosylation.[151,157] The human LPH enzyme is cleaved at a second site by extracellular trypsin (Arg_{868}-Ala_{869}) once it is in the brushborder membrane to yield the mature 145-kDa form.[153] In contrast to human LPH, the cleavage of the rat enzyme appears to occur on the plasma membrane in several steps.[113,158,159]

It is clear that post-transcriptional mechanisms are important for certain aspects of LPH regulation.[131,136,137,139] However, the precise mechanism of this regulation is not yet well-defined. There are changes in the molecular forms of LPH, some of which are enzymatically inactive.[131,136,137]

Working Model of Lactase-Phlorizin Hydrolase Regulation during Intestinal Development

Much evidence points to transcriptional activation as an important mechanism for LPH regulation, including at the endoderm-intestinal transition, along the CV axis, and in the decrease in expression at weaning. Post-translational regulation plays an important role in restricting the functional expression of the protein along the horizontal intestinal axis and in the postweaning decline in activity. The relative roles of transcription and translation remain controversial.

The 5'-flanking region of the LPH gene appears to have important regulatory elements able to direct developmental patterns of LPH expression. However, the region has not been narrowed sufficiently to accurately define the individual elements. It is quite intriguing that similar transcription factors may be involved in the regulation of both SI and LPH. However, two lines of evidence suggest that there must be other proteins involved in transcriptional regulation. First, the patterns of expression of LPH and SI differ. In fact, their patterns of expression are mirror images in many respects. Lactase-phlorizin hydrolase is expressed at high levels after the endoderm-intestinal transition and decreases to low levels after weaning. In contrast, SI mRNA is only detectable until weaning, when there is a large increase in expression. Second, the transcription factors thus far identified as involved in LPH transcription do not have a pattern of developmental expression that completely explains the pattern of LPH expression.

There are many potential mechanisms for the transcriptional regulation of LPH during development, as discussed for SI. There may be other important DNA binding proteins and coadaptor proteins involved in LPH gene transcription.

INTEGRATED MODELS OF DEVELOPMENTAL EXPRESSION

The mechanisms of SI and LPH expression in the developing intestinal epithelium are complex. There are a number of similarities, but also significant differences in the patterns of expression and mechanisms between these two disaccharidases. Should the number of mechanisms and regulatory proteins involved in developmental gene expression in the intestine continue to increase with each newly characterized gene, the degree of complexity will greatly expand. However, even in the two genes described in this chapter there are enough similarities to suggest that there may be unified themes across large numbers of genes. First, transcription is a primary level of regulation, particularly at the endoderm-intestinal transition. At latter stages of development other levels of regulation are involved, although transcription remains predominant. Second, the molecular mechanisms that initiate transcription of the two genes seem to have a number of striking similarities. Two major transcription factor families, CDX and HNF1, are prominently involved in the regulation of both genes. In addition, we recently showed that another brushborder enzyme expressed in a similar pattern as SI also is regulated by both CDX and HNF1 proteins.[89] Therefore, there may be a relatively restricted set of transcriptional proteins that will act to coordinate expression of a large number of intestinal genes. How this is accomplished will be discovered in the interactions between these proteins and the various arrangements of DNA regulatory elements in different promoters.

An added benefit of understanding transcriptional regulation of intestinal genes during development relates to the discovery of generalized mechanisms involved in developmental processes. Once the mechanisms of transcriptional initiation of phenotypic genes have been described, the transcriptional regulatory proteins involved in this process can be identified. These transcription proteins often have broadbased regulatory effects during development beyond the regulation of the specific gene for which its function was originally characterized. An example of this benefit is the broadbased effect of CDX proteins on cellular proliferation and differentiation.

REFERENCES

1. Traber PG, Wu GD. Intestinal development and differentiation. In: Rustgi AK, editor. Gastrointestinal cancers: biology, diagnosis, and therapy. Philadelphia: Lippencott-Raven Publications; 1995. p. 21–43.
2. Birchmeier C, Birchmeier W. Molecular aspects of mesenchymal-epithelial interactions. Ann Rev Cell Biol 1993;9:511–40.
3. Carroll KM, Wong TT, Drabik DL, Chang EB. Differentiation of rat small intestinal epithelial cells by extracellular matrix. Am J Physiol 1988;254:G355–60.
4. Haffen K, Kedinger M, Simon-Assmann P. Mesenchyme-dependent differentiation of epithelial progenitor cells in the gut. J Pediatr Gastroenterol Nutr 1987;6:14–23.
5. Duluc I, Freund J-N, Leberquier C, Kedinger M. Fetal endoderm primarily holds the temporal and positional information required for mammalian intestinal development. J Cell Biol 1994;126:211–21.
6. Louvard D, Kedinger M, Hauri HP. The differentiating intestinal epithelial cell: establishment and maintenance of functions through interactions between cellular structures. Ann Rev Cell Biol 1992;8:157–95.
7. Beaulieu J-F. Extracellular matrix components and integrins in relationship to human intestinal epithelial cell differentiation. Prog Histochem Cytochem 1997;31:1–78.
8. Simon-Assmann P, Kedinger M, DeArchangelis A, et al. Extracellular matrix components in intestinal development. Experientia 1995;51:883–900.
9. Zang L, Zhou W, Veculsecu VE, et al. Gene expression profiles in normal and cancer cells. Science 1997;276:1268–72.
10. Rings EHHM, Buller HA, deBoer PAJ, et al. Messenger RNA sorting in enterocytes: co-localization with encoded proteins. FEBS Lett 1992;300:183–7.
11. Barth JA, Li W, Krasinski SD, et al. Asymmetrical localization of mRNAs in enterocytes of human jejunum. J Histochem Cytochem 1998;46:335–43.
12. Brunner J, Wacker H, Semenza G. Sucrase-isomaltase of the small-intestinal brush border membrane: assembly and biosynthesis. Methods Enzymol 1983;96:386–406.
13. Naim HY, Sterchi EE, Lentze MJ. Biosynthesis of the human sucrase-isomaltase complex. J Biol Chem 1988;267:7242–53.
14. Chantret I, Lacasa M, Chevalier G, et al. Sequence of the complete cDNA and the 5′ structure of the human sucrase-isomaltase gene. Biochem J 1992;285:915–23.
15. Semenza G. Anchoring and biosynthesis of stalked brush border membrane proteins: glucosidases and peptidases of enterocytes and renal tubuli. Ann Rev Cell Biol 1986;2:255–313.
16. Semenza G, Auricchio S. Small-intestinal disaccharidases. In: Scriver CR, Beaudet AL, Sey WS, Valle D, editors. The metabolic basis of inherited disease. 4th ed. New York: McGraw-Hill; 1989. p. 2975–97.
17. Hunziker W, Spiess M, Semenza G, Lodish HF. The sucrase-isomaltase complex: primary structure, membrane-orientation, and evolution of a stalked, intrinsic brush border protein. Cell 1986;46:227–34.
18. Gordon JI. Intestinal epithelial differentiation: new insights from chimeric and transgenic mice. J Cell Biol 1989;108:1187–94.
19. Dahlqvist A, Nordstrom C. The distribution of disaccharidase activities in the villi and crypts of the small-intestinal mucosa. Biochim Biophys Acta 1966;113:624–6.
20. Lorenzsonn V, Korsmo H, Olsen WA. Localization of sucrase-isomaltase in the rat enterocyte. Gastroenterology 1987;92:98–105.
21. Markowitz AJ, Wu GD, Birkenmeier EH, Traber PG. The human sucrase-isomaltase gene directs complex patterns of gene expression in transgenic mice. Am J Physiol 1993;265:G526–39.
22. Beaulieu JF, Nichols B, Quaroni A. Posttranslational regulation of sucrase-isomaltase expression in intestinal crypt and villus cells. J Biol Chem 1989;264:20000–11.
23. Traber PG. Regulation of sucrase-isomaltase gene expression along the crypt-villus axis of rat small intestine. Biochem Biophys Res Commun 1990;173:765–73.
24. Traber PG, Yu L, Wu G, Judge T. Sucrase-isomaltase gene expression along the crypt-villus axis of human small intestine is regulated at the level of mRNA abundance. Am J Physiol 1992;262:G123–30.
25. Trugnan G, Rousset M, Chantret I, et al. The posttranslational processing of sucrase-isomaltase in HT-29 cells is a function of their state of enterocytic differentiation. J Cell Biol 1987;104:1199–205.
26. Grand RJ, Watkins JB, Torti RM. Develpment of the human gastrointestinal tract. A review. Gastroenterology 1976;70:790–810.
27. Hoffman LR, Chang EB. Regional expression and regulation of intestinal sucrase-isomaltase. J Nutr Biochem 1993;4:130–41.
28. Hoffman LR, Chang EB. Determinants of regional sucrase-isomaltase expression in adult rat small intestine. J Biol Chem 1991;266:21815–20.
29. Lee MF, Russell RM, Montgomery RK, Krasinski SD. Total intestinal lactase and sucrase activities are reduced in aged rats. J Nutr 1997;127:1382–7.
30. Takenoshita M, Yabune M, Katsura H, et al. Low sucrase activity in the small intestine of a senescence-accelerated strain of mouse, SAMP1. Biosci Biotechnol Biochem 1998;62:965–9.
31. Auricchio S, Sebastio G. Development of disaccharidases. In: Lebenthal E, editor. Human gastrointestinal development. New York: Raven Press; 1989. p. 451–70.
32. Henning SJ. Ontogeny of enzymes in the small intestine. Annu Rev Physiol 1985;47:231–45.
33. Henning SJ. Functional development of the gastrointestinal tract. In: Johnson LR, editor. Physiology of the gastrointestinal tract. 2nd ed. New York: Raven Press; 1987. p. 285–300.
34. Galand G. Brush-border membrane sucrase-isomaltase, maltase-glucoamylase and trehalase in mammals. Comp Biochem Physiol 1989;94B:1–11.
35. Tung J, Markowitz AJ, Silberg DG, Traber PG. Developmental expression of SI in transgenic mice is regulated by an evolutionarily conserved promoter. Am J Physiol 1997;273:G83–92.
36. Sebastio G, Hunziker W, O'Neill B, et al. The biosynthesis of intestinal sucrase-isomaltase in human embryo is most likely controlled at the level of transcription. Biochem Biophys Res Commun 1987;149:830–9.
37. Van Beers EH, Rings EH, Taminiau JA, et al. Regulation of lactase and sucrase-isomaltase gene expression in the duodenum during childhood. J Pediatr Gastroenterol Nutr 1998;27:37–46.
38. Leeper LL, Henning SJ. Development and tissue distribution of sucrase-isomaltase mRNA in rats. Am J Physiol 1990;258:G52–8.
39. Sebastio G, Hunziker W, Ballabio A, et al. On the primary site of control in the spontaneous development of small-intestinal sucrase-isomaltase after birth. FEBS Lett 1986;208:460–5.

40. Kodolvsky O. Developmental, dietary and hormonal control of intestinal disaccharidases in mammals (including man). In: Randle PJ, Steiner DF, Whelan WJ, editors. Carbohydrate metabolism and its disorders. London: Academic Press; 1981. p. 481–522.
41. Nanthakumar NN, Henning SJ. Distinguishing normal and glucocorticoid-induced maturation of intestine using bromodeoxyuridine. Am J Physiol 1995;268:G139–45.
42. Leeper LL, McDonald MC, Heath JP, Henning SJ. Sucrase-isomaltse ontogeny: synergism between glucocorticoids and thyroxine reflects increased mRNA and no change in cell migration. Biochem Biophys Res Commun 1998;246:765–70.
43. Buts JP, Duranton B, DeKeyser N, et al. Premature stimulation of rat sucrase-isomaltase (SI) by exogenous insulin and the analog B-Asp10 is regulated by a receptor-mediated signal triggering SI gene transcription. Pediatr Res 1998;43:585–91.
44. Menard D. Growth-promoting factors and the development of the human gut. In: Lebenthal E, editor. Human gastrointestinal development. New York: Raven Press; 1989. p. 123–50.
45. Potter GD. Development of colonic function. In: Lebenthal E, editor. Human gastrointestinal development. New York: Raven Press; 1989. p. 545–59.
46. Zweibaum A, Triadou N, Kedinger M, et al. Sucrase-isomaltase: a marker of foetal and malignant epithelial cells of the human colon. Int J Cancer 1983;32:407–12.
47. Lacroix B, Kedinger M, Simon-Assmann P, et al. Developmental pattern of brush border enzymes in the human fetal colon. Correlation with some morphogenetic events. Early Hum Dev 1984;9:95–103.
48. Foltzer-Jourdainne C, Kedinger M, Raul F. Perinatal expression of brush-border hydrolases in rat colon: hormonal and tissue regulation. Am J Physiol 1989;257:G496–503.
49. Johnson FP. The development of the mucous membrane of the large intestine and vermiform process in the human embryo. Am J Anat 1913;14:187–233.
50. Lev R, Orlie D. Histochemical and radioautographic studies of normal human fetal colon. Histochemistry 1974;39:301–11.
51. Lehy T, Cristina ML. Ontogeny and distribution of certain endocrine cells in the human fetal large intestine. Cell Tissue Res 1979;203:415–26.
52. Wiltz O, O'Hara CJ, Steele GD, Mercurio AM. Expression of enzymatically active sucrase-isomaltase is a ubiquitous property of colon adenocarcinomas. Gastroenterology 1991;100:1266–78.
53. Real RX, Xu M, Vila MR, DeBolos C. Intestinal brush-border-associated enzymes: co-ordinated expression in colorectal cancer. Int J Cancer 1992;51:173–81.
54. Czernichow B, Simon-Assmann P, Kedinger M, et al. Sucrase-isomaltase expression and enterocytic ultrastructure of human colorectal tumors. Int J Cancer 1989;44:238–44.
55. Beaulieu JF, Weiser MM, Herrera L, Quaroni A. Detection and characterization of sucrase-isomaltase in adult human colon and in colonic polyps. Gastroenterology 1990;98:1467–77.
56. Tapscott SJ, Lassar AB, David RL, Weintraub H. 5-bromo-2'-deoxyuridine blocks myogenesis by extinguishing expression of myoD1. Science 1989;245:532–6.
57. Gorvel JP, Ferrero A, Chambraud L, et al. Expression of sucrase-isomaltase and dipeptidylpeptidase IV in human small intestine and colon. Gastroenterology 1991;101:618–25.
58. Colony PC, Kois JM, Peiffer LP. Structural and enzymatic changes during colonic maturation in the fetal and suckling rat. Gastroenterology 1989;97:338–47.
59. Sato M, Ahnen DJ. Regional variability of colonocyte growth and differentiation in the rat. Anat Rec 1992;233:409–14.
60. Williams L, Bell L. Asynchronous development of the rat colon. Anat Embryol (Berlin) 1991;183:573–8.
61. Brackett KA, Townsend SF. Organogenesis of the colon in rats. J Morphol 1980;163:191–201.
62. Helander HF. Morphological studies on the development of the rat colonic mucosa. Acta Anat (Basel) 1973;85:153–76.
63. Wu GD, Wang W, Traber PG. Isolation and characterization of the human sucrase-isomaltase gene and demonstration of intestine-specific transcriptional elements. J Biol Chem 1992;267:7863–70.
64. Traber PG, Wu GD, Wang W. Novel DNA-binding proteins regulate intestine-specific transcription of the sucrase-isomaltase gene. Mol Cell Biol 1992;12:3614–27.
65. Hecht A, Torbey CF, Korsmo HA, Olsen WA. Regulation of sucrase and lactase in developing rats: role of nuclear factors that bind to two gene regulatory elements. Gastroenterology 1997;112:803–12.
66. Wu GD, Chen L, Forslund K, Traber PG. Hepatocyte nuclear factor 1α (HNF-1α) and HNF-1β regulate transcription via two elements in an intestine-specific promoter. J Biol Chem 1994;269:17080–5.
67. Markowitz AJ, Wu GD, Bader A, et al. Regulation of lineage-specific transcription of the sucrase-isomaltase gene in transgenic mice and cell lines. Am J Physiol 1995;269:G925–39.
68. Simon TC, Roth KA, Gordon JI. Use of transgenic mice to map cis-acting elements in the liver fatty acid-binding protein gene (Fabpl) that regulate its cell lineage-specific differentiation-dependent and spatial patterns of expression in the gut epithelium and in the liver acinus. J Biol Chem 1993;268:18345–58.
69. Suh E-R, Chen L, Taylor J, Traber PG. A homeodomain protein related to caudal regulates intestine-specific gene transcription. Mol Cell Biol 1994;14:7340–51.
70. Mitchelmore C, Troelsen JT, Sjostrom H, Noren O. The HOXC11 homeodomain protein itneracts with the lactase-phlorizin hydrolase promoter and stimulates HNF 1 alpha-dependent transcription. J Biol Chem 1998;273:13297–306.
71. Silberg DG, Lon S, Morrisey E, et al. A conserved DNA element conforming to the GATA consensus is required for sucrase-isomaltase gene transcription. Gastroenterology 1997;112:A405.
72. Laverriere AC, MacNeill C, Mueller C, et al. GATA-4/5/6, a subfamily of three transcription factors transcribed in developing heart and gut. J Biol Chem 1994;269:23177–84.
73. Wu GD, Markowitz AJ, Birkenmeier E, Traber PG. A negative transcriptional regulatory element is involved in enterocyte and enteroendocrine cell lineage determination. Clin Res 1992;40.
74. Cowell IG, Skinner A, Hurst HC. Transcriptional repression by a novel member of the bZIP family of transcription factors. Mol Cell Biol 1992;12:3070–7.
75. Samadani U, Costa RH. The transcriptional activator hepatocyte nuclear factor 6 regulates liver gene expression. Mol Cell Biol 1996;16:6273–84.
76. Rausa F, Samadani U, Ye H, et al. The cut-homeodomain transcriptional activator HNF-6 is coexpressed with its target gene HNF-3 beta in the developing murine liver and pancreas. Dev Biol 1997;192:228–46.
77. Duprey P, Chowdhury K, Dressler GR, et al. A mouse gene homologous to the Drosophila gene caudal is expressed in epithelial cells from the embryonic intestine. Genes Dev 1988;2:1647–54.
78. James R, Kazenwadel J. Homeobox gene expression in intestinal epithelium of adult mice. J Biol Chem 1991;266:3246–51.
79. James R, Erler T, Kazenwadel J. Structure of the murine homeobox gene cdx-2: expression in embryonic and adult intestinal epithelium. J Biol Chem 1994;269:15229–37.

80. Gamer LW, Wright CVE. Murine Cdx-4 bears striking similarities to the *Drosophila* caudal gene in its homeodomain sequence and early expression pattern. Mech Dev 1993;43:71–81.
81. Bonner CA, Loftus SK, Wasmuth JJ. Isolation, characterization, and precise physical localization of human CDX1, a caudal–type homeobox gene. Genomics 1995;28:206–11.
82. Mallo GV, Rechreche H, Frigerio J-M, et al. Molecular cloning, sequencing, and expression of the mRNA encoding human CDX1 and CDX2 homeobox, down-regulation of CDX1 and CDX2 mRNA expression during colorectal carcinogenesis. Int J Cancer 1997;74:35–44.
83. Drummond F, Putt W, Fox M, Edwards YH. Cloning and chromosomal assignment of the human CDX2 gene. Ann Hum Genet 1997;61:393–400.
84. Meyer BI, Gruss P. Mouse cdx-1 expression during gastrulation. Development 1993;117:191–203.
85. Silberg DG, Furth EE, Taylor JK, et al. Cdx1 protein expression in normal, metaplastic and neoplastic human alimentary tract epithelium. Gastroenterology 1997;113:478–86.
86. Beck F, Erler T, Russell A, James R. Expression of Cdx-2 in the mouse embryo and placenta: possible role in patterning of the extra-embryonic membranes. Dev Dyn 1995;204:219–27.
87. Freund J-N, Boukamel R, Benazzouz A. Gradient expression of cdx along the rat intestine throughout postnatal development. FEBS Lett 1992;314:163–6.
88. Troelsen JT, Mitchelmore C, Spodsberg N, et al. Regulation of lactase-phlorizin hydrolase gene expression by the caudal-related homeodomain protein Cdx-2. Biochem J 1997;322:833–8.
89. Taylor JK, Boll W, Levy T, et al. Comparison of intestinal phospholipase A/lysophospholipase and sucrase-isomaltase genes suggests a common structure for enterocyte-specific promoters. DNA Cell Biol 1997;16:1419–28.
90. Lambert M, Colnot S, Suh ER, et al. cis-Acting elements and transcription factors involved in the intestinal specific expression of the rat calbindin-D9k gene: binding of the intestine-specific transcription factor Cdx-2 to the TATA box. Eur J Biochem 1996;236:778–88.
91. Drummond F, Sowden J, Morrison K, Edwards YH. The caudal-type homeobox protein Cdx-2 binds to the colon promoter of the carbonic anhydrase 1 gene. Eur J Biochem 1996;236:670–81.
92. Jin T, Drucker DJ. Activation of proglucagon gene transcription through a novel promoter element by the caudal-related homeodomain protein cdx-2/3. Mol Cell Biol 1996;16:19–28.
93. Jin RR, Trinh DKY, Wang F, Drucker DJ. The caudal homeobox protein cdx-2/3 activates endogenous proglucagon gene expression in InR1-G9 islet cells. Mol Endocrinol 1997;11:203–9.
94. Laser B, Meda P, Constant I, Philippe J. The caudal-related homeodomain protein Cdx-2/3 regulates glucagon gene expression in islet cells. J Biol Chem 1996;271:28984–94.
95. Taylor JK, Levy T, Suh ER, Traber PG. Activation of enhancer elements by the homeobox gene Cdx2 is cell line specific. Nucleic Acids Res 1997;25:2293–300.
96. Subramanian V, Meyer BI, Gruss P. Disruption of the murine homeobox gene Cdx1 affects axial skeletal identities by altering the mesodermal expression domains of Hox genes. Cell 1995;83:641–53.
97. Chawengsaksophak K, James R, Hammond VE, et al. Homeosis and intestinal tumors in Cdx2 mutant mice. Nature 1997;386:84–7.
98. Suh E-R, Traber PG. An intestine-specific homeobox gene regulates proliferation and differentiation. Mol Cell Biol 1996;16:619–25.
99. Duluc I, Lorentz O, Fritsch C, et al. Changing intestinal connective tissue interactions alters homeobox gene expression in epithelial cells. J Cell Sci 1997;110:1317–24.
100. Lorentz O, Duluc I, DeArcangelis A, et al. Key role of the Cdx2 homeobox gene in extracellular matrix-mediated intestinal cell differentiation. J Cell Biol 1997;139:1553–65.
101. Mallo GV, Soubeyran P, Lissitzky J-C, et al. Expression of Cdx1 and Cdx2 homeotic genes leads to reduced malignancy in colon cancer-derived cells. J Biol Chem 1998;273:14030–6.
102. Spiess M, Brunner J, Semenza G. Hydrophobic labeling, isolation, and partial characterization of the NH_2-terminal membranous segment of sucrase-isomaltase complex. J Biol Chem 1982;257:2370–7.
103. Keller P, Semenza G, Shaltiel S. Phosphorylation of the N-terminal intracellular tail of sucrase-isomaltase by cAMP-dependent protein kinase. Eur J Biochem 1995;233:963–8.
104. Ghersa P, Huber P, Semenza G, Wacker H. Cell-free synthesis, membrane integration, and glyucosylation of prp-sucrase-isomaltase. J Biol Chem 1986;261:7969–74.
105. Shapiro GL, Bulow SD, Conklin KA, et al. Postinsertional processing of sucrase-α dextrinase precursor to authentic subunits: mutliple step cleavage by trypsin. Am J Physiol 1991;261:G847–57.
106. Alpers DH, Helms D, Seetharam S, et al. In vitro translation of intestinal sucrase-isomaltase and glucoamylase. Biochem Biophys Res Commun 1986;134:37–43.
107. Alpers DH, Tedesco FJ. The possible role of pancreatic proteases in the turnover of intestinal brush border proteins. Biochim Biophys Acta 1975;401:28–40.
108. Kwong WKL, Seetharam B, Alpers DH. Effect of exocrine pancreatic insufficiency on small intestine in the mouse. Gastroenterology 1978;74:1277–82.
109. Fransen JAM, Hauri H-P, Ginsel LA, Naim HY. Naturally occurring mutations in intestinal sucrase-isomaltase provide evidence for the existence of an intracellular sorting signal in the isomaltase subunit. J Cell Biol 1991;115:45–57.
110. Zhu Y, Rosenberg E, Silberg DG, Traber PG. Characterization of nuclear proteins that interact with the sucrase-isomaltase promoter during development. Gastroenterology 1997;112:A917.
111. Olsen WA, Lloyd M, Korsmo H, He H-Z. Regulation of sucrase and lactase in Caco-2 cells: relationship to nuclear factors SIF-1 and NF-LPH-1. Am J Physiol 1996;271:G707–13.
112. Rings EHHM, VanBeers EH, Drasinski SD, et al. Lactase-origin, gene-expression, localization, and function. Nutr Res 1994;14:775–97.
113. Montgomery RK, Buller HA, Rings EHHM, Grand RJ. Lactose intolerance and the genetic regulation of intestinal lactase-phlorizin hydrolase. FASEB J 1991;5:2824–32.
114. Mantei N, Villa M, Enziler T, et al. Complete primary structure of human and rabbit lactase-phlorizin hydrolase: implications for biosynthesis, membrane anchoring and evolution of the enzyme. EMBO J 1988;7:2705–13.
115. Boll W, Wagner P, Mantei N. Structure of the chromosomal gene and cDNAs coding for lactase-phlorizin hydrolase in humans with adult-type hypolactasia or persistence of lactase. Am J Hum Genet 1991;48:889–902.
116. Kruse TA, Bolund L, Byskov A, et al. Mapping of the human lactase-phlorizin hydrolase gene to chromosome 2. Cytogenet Cell Genet 1989;51:1026.
117. Villa M, Menard D, Semenza G, Mantei N. The expression of lactase enzymatic activity and mRNA in human fetal jejunum. FEBS Lett 1992;301:202–6.
118. Buller HA, Grand RJ. Lactose intolerance. Annu Rev Med 1990 41:141–8.
119. Sterchi EE, Mills PR, Fransen JAM, et al. Biogenesis of intestinal lactase-phlorizin hydrolase in adults with lactose intolerance. J Clin Invest 1990;86:1329–37.

120. Wang Y, Harvey CB, Proatt WS, et al. The lactase persistence/non-persistence polymorphism is controlled by a cis-acting element. Hum Mol Genet 1995;4:657–62.
121. Rossi M, Maiuri L, Tusco MI, et al. Lactase persistence versus decline in human adults: multifactorial events are involved in down-regulation after weaning. Gastroenterology 1997;112:1506–14.
122. Witte J, Lloyd M, Lorenzsonn V, et al. The biosynthetic basis of adult lactase deficiency. J Clin Invest 1990;86:1338–42.
123. Harvey CB, Pratt WS, Islam I, et al. DNA polymorphisms in the lactase gene. Eur J Hum Genet 1995;3:27–41.
124. Maiuri L, Raia V, Potter J, et al. Mosaic pattern of lactase expression by villous enterocytes in human adult-type hypolactasia. Gastroenterology 1991;100:359–69.
125. Maiuri L, Rossi M, Raia V, et al. Mosaic regulation of lactase in human adult-type hypolactasia. Gastroenterology 1994;107:54–60.
126. Jarvela I, Enattah NS, Kokkonen J, et al. Assignment of the locus for congenital lactase deficiency to 2q21, in the vicinity of but separate from the lactase-phlorizin hydrolase gene. Am J Hum Genet 1998;63:1078–85.
127. Rings EHHM, DeBoar PAJ, Moorman AFM, et al. Lactase gene expression during early development of rat small intestine. Gastroenterology 1992;103:1154–61.
128. Krasinski S, Estrada G, Yeh K-Y, et al. Transcriptional regulation of intestinal hydrolase biosynthesis during postnatal development in rats. Am J Physiol 1994;267:G584–94.
129. Freund J-N, Duluc I, Raul F. Lactase expression is controlled differently in the jejunum and ileum during development in rats. Gastroenterology 1991;100:388–94.
130. Freund J-N, Torp N, Duluc I, et al. Comparative expression of the mRNA for three intestinal hydrolases during postnatal development in the rat. Cell Mol Biol 1990;36:729–36.
131. Rossi M, Maiuri L, Russomanno C, Auricchio S. In vitro biosynthesis of lactase in preweaning and adult rabbit. FEBS Lett 1992;313:260–4.
132. Keller P, Zwicker E, Mantei N, Semenza G. The levels of lactase and of sucrase-isomaltase along the rabbit small intestine are regulated both at the mRNA level and post-translationally. FEBS Lett 1992;313:265–9.
133. Duluc I, Jost B, Freund J-N. Multiple levels of control of the stage- and region-specific expression of rat intestinal lactase. J Cell Biol 1993;123:1577–86.
134. Rings EHHM, Krasinski SD, VanBeers EH, et al. Restriction of lactase gene-expression along the proximal-to-distal axis of rat small intestine occurs during postnatal development. Gastroenterology 1994;106:1223–32.
135. Rossi M, Maiuri L, Salvati VM, et al. In vitro biosynthesis of lactase in suckling and adult rabbits: regulatory mechanisms involved in the decline of the lactase activity. FEBS Lett 1993;329:106–10.
136. Castillo RO, Reisenauer AM, Kwong LK, et al. Intestinal lactase in the neonatal rat. J Biol Chem 1990;265:15889–93.
137. Quan R, Santiago NA, Tsuboi KK, Gray GM. Intestinal lactase. J Biol Chem 1990;265:15882–8.
138. Buller HA, Kothe MJC, Goldman DA, et al. Coordinate expression of lactate-phlorizin hydrolase mRNA and enzyme levels in rat intestine during development. J Biol Chem 1990;265:6978–83.
139. Nudell DM, Santiago NA, Zhu J-S, et al. Intestinal lactase: maturational excess expression of mRNA over enzyme protein. Am J Physiol 1993;265:G1108–15.
140. Buller HA, Rings EHHM, Montgomery RK, et al. Suckling rat colon synthesizes and processes active lactase-phlorizin hydrolase immunologically identical to that from jejunum. Pediatr Res 1989;26:232–6.
141. Troelsen JT, Olsen J, Noren O, Sjostrom H. A novel intestinal trans-factor (NF-LPH 1) interacts with the lactase-phlorizin hydrolase promoter and co-varies with the enzymatic activity. J Biol Chem 1992;267:20407–11.
142. Verhave M, Krasinski S, Mass S, et al. Identification of positive and negative transcriptional regulatory regions in the rat lactase-phlorizin hydroxylase gene. Gastroenterology 1993;104:A287.
143. Krasinski SD, Upchurch BH, Irons SJ, et al. Rat lactase-phlorizin hydrolase/human growth hormone transgene is expressed on small intestinal villi in transgenic mice. Gastroenterology 1997;113:844–55.
144. Troelsen JT, Mehlum A, Olsen J, et al. 1 kb of the lactase-phlorizin hydrolase promoter directs post-weaning decline and small intestinal-specific expression in transgenic mice. FEBS Lett 1994;342:291–6.
145. FitzGerald K, Bazar L, Avigan MI. GATA-6 stimulates a cell line-specific activation element in the human lactase promoter. Am J Physiol 1998;274:G314–24.
146. Boukamel R, Freund J-N. The cis-element CE-LPH 1 of the rat intestinal lactase gene promoter interacts in vitro with several nuclear factors present in endodermal tissues. FEBS Lett 1994;353:108–12.
147. Troelsen JT, Olsen J, Mitchelmore C, et al. Two intestinal specific nuclear factors binding to the lactase-phlorizin hydrolase and sucrase-isomaltase promoters are functionally related to oligomeric molecules. FEBS Lett 1994;342:297–301.
148. Jacob R, Bulleid N, Naim HY. Folding of human intestinal lactase-phlorizin hydrolase. Am Soc Biochem Mol Biol 1995;270:18678–84.
149. Wacker H, Keller P, Falchetto R, et al. Location of the two catalytic sites in intestinal lactase-phlorizin hydrolase. J Biol Chem 1992;267:18744–55.
150. Naim HY, Sterchi EE, Lentze MJ. Biosynthesis and maturation of lactase-phlorizin hydrolase in the human small intestinal epithelial cells. Biochem J 1987;241:427–34.
151. Naim HY, Lentze MJ. Impact of 0-glycosylation on the function of human intestinal lactase-phlorizin hydrolase. J Biol Chem 1992;267:25494–504.
152. Danielsen EM, Skovbjerg H, Noren O, Sjostrom H. Biosynthesis of intestinal microvillar proteins: intracellular processing of lactase-phlorizin hydrolase. Biochem Biophys Res Commun 1984;122:82–90.
153. Wuthrich M, Grunberg J, Hahn D, et al. Proteolytic processing of human lactase-phlorizin hydrolase is a two-step event: identification of the cleavage sites. Arch Biochem Biophys 1996;336:27–34.
154. Jacob R, Naim HY. Analysis of the putative cleavage site in human lactase-phlorizin hydrolase. Biochem Soc Trans 1995;23:305S.
155. Naim HY. The pro-region of human intestinal lactase-phlorizin hydrolase is enzymatically inactive towards lactose. Biol Chem 1995;376:255–8.
156. Lottaz D, Oberholzer T, Bahler P, et al. Maturation of human lactase-phlorizin hydrolase. Proteolytic cleavage of precursor occurs after passage through the Golgi complex. FEBS Lett 1992;313:270–6.
157. Naim HY. Processing of human pro-lactase-phlorizin hydrolase at reduced temperatures: cleavage is preceded by complex glycosylation. Biochem J 1992;285:13–6.
158. Buller HA, Montgomery RK, Sasak WV, Grand RJ. Biosynthesis, glycosylation, and intracellular transport of intestinal lactase-phlorizin hydrolase in rats. J Biol Chem 1987;262:1–6.
159. Yeh K, Yeh M, Pan P, Holt PR. Post-translational cleavage of rat intestinal lactase occurs at the luminal side of the brush border membrane. Gastroenterology 1991;101:312–8.

CHAPTER 8

Ontogeny of Nutrient Transporters

Ronaldo P. Ferraris, PhD

Randal K. Buddington, PhD

Elmer S. David, MD

Ontogenetic development has been studied for a variety of functions of the gastrointestinal tract, the most notable being intestinal brushborder hydrolases, digestive enzymes, and gastric acid secretion.[1] Except for intestinal transport of macromolecules, which is important for developing immunity in neonates, little information is available regarding the development of intestinal nutrient transport systems. Even less information can be found on the various mechanisms regulating their development. While the effects of diet and hormones on development of the enzymes sucrase and lactase have been studied since the 1960s,[1,2] their effects on intestinal nutrient transporters have been studied only recently.[3–5] This neglect has arisen mainly because intestinal absorptive capacity, especially in adults, has for many years been thought of as several orders of magnitude greater than possible dietary nutrient loads,[6] and because parenteral nutrition has been the preferred intervention for sustenance of prematurely born infants and neonates with gastrointestinal problems.[7]

Our laboratories have since shown that, in many cases, the small intestine possesses little or no excess capacity for nutrient absorption,[8] especially in developing animals.[3] Total parenteral nutrition was introduced to clinical medicine in the early 1970s[7] and was credited for substantial reductions in premature infant mortality and morbidity. Prolonged parenteral nutrition and prolonged absence of luminal nutrients in the gut, however, have been demonstrated to lead to numerous complications, including cholestatic jaundice, electrolyte imbalance, and metabolic bone disease, and are risk factors for delayed growth, nosocomial infections, and chronic lung disease.[9] These complications have fueled a recent surge of interest in enteral feeding,[10] which has been shown to lead to faster weight gain and faster gastrointestinal growth and maturation in premature infants.[11] The decision to enterally feed a premature infant, however, must take into account the developmental limitations in nutrient absorption as well as the potential for enhancing absorptive processes.[12] An increased understanding of these developmental limitations to absorption is important to the nutrition of the premature infant, whose gastrointestinal tract cannot process food at volumes and concentrations provided to term infants. For example, in prematurely born humans, digestion and absorption rates of glucose polymers are slow and increase with postnatal age.[13]

SIGNIFICANCE AND RELEVANCE

The clinical significance of this chapter is closely linked to the nutrition of neonates, especially that of premature infants. Studies of ontogeny of nutrient transporters, however, also have a much broader relevance that encompasses clinically related applications. The vertebrate gut undergoes two major developmental transitions associated with changing functional demands. The first is an abrupt transition from yolk or placental nutrition to nutrition derived solely from nutrients absorbed by the small intestine. The second is a gradual change in diet composition as vertebrates undergo weaning or metamorphosis. These nutritional and dietary transitions occur in parallel with changes in expression of transporter genes. Why are certain transporters expressed at certain times and not at others? Why do intestinal cells undergoing development express certain transporters and not others? This chapter also addresses these important questions.

SCOPE AND LIMITATIONS

This chapter will focus on the ontogeny of sugar, amino acid, peptide and bile acid transporters in the small intestine, and on the ontogeny of regulatory mechanisms modulating their activity. Ontogeny of transporters for vitamins and minerals will only be mentioned very briefly, mainly to highlight the facts that very few intestinal developmental studies have been done on these micronutrients, and that mechanisms of their transport are less known. Placental nutrient transporters will be excluded from this review, and, with few exceptions, so will results derived from intestinal cell cultures. Placental nutrient transporters are, however, important to fetal nutrition, as is shown by dramatic increases in transporter number during fetal development.[14]

Our review begins by briefly describing the different transport systems emphasized in this chapter, the various methods for measuring nutrient absorption, and, finally, the various procedures for normalizing absorption rates. We briefly describe the mechanistic bases for developmental changes in absorption. We then summarize the various patterns of prenatal and postnatal development of transporters of sugars, amino acids, peptides, and bile acids. We also explain how these changes in patterns of transport are related to age and to body weight. We then discuss whether these patterns are hardwired or inducible, the various dietary and hormonal signals regulating both hardwired and inducible transporters, and the cellular and molecular mechanisms underlying changes in transport patterns. Finally, we provide examples of clinical correlates of derangements in nutrient transport, and end with a list of promising directions for future work.

In humans, development of intestinal nutrient transporters is relatively well known for the first trimester of gestation, but very little is known for the third trimester. Nevertheless, development of intestinal transporters has been studied in a wide variety of animal models, including mice, rats, pigs, sheep, dogs, cats, mink, guinea pigs, rabbits, birds, frogs, and fish. Following the pattern found for studies of intestinal hydrolases, the majority of developmental studies of nutrient transport has used rats and mice as animal models not only because these rodents are, like humans, omnivores, but also because rodents are altricial, i.e., born premature, and many postnatal maturational changes in rat small intestine occur prenatally in humans, making neonatal rodents appropriate models of preterm infants.[15,16] There has also been a surge of studies using pig small intestine, again because of its similarity to the human small intestine and the pig's omnivorous habits.[17] Nevertheless, to limit the discussion to mice, rats, and pigs would neglect information from development of other feeding strategies that may be vital for increasing our understanding of human intestinal development; hence, we will use a broad, comparative approach in our discussion of ontogeny of nutrient transporters.

TRANSPORT SYSTEMS

The small intestine is lined by epithelial cells attached to each other by junctional complexes, consisting of: the tight junction; the belt desmosome, or zonula adherens; and the spot desmosome, or macula adherens.[18] Intestinal transport of nutrients, therefore, occurs by two pathways, one going through the cells and another through the junctional complexes (Figure 8–1). For the transcellular pathway, nutrients are initially transported across the apical or brushborder membrane by carriers, diffuse through the cytosol, then cross the basolateral membrane by another set of carriers. Carrier-mediated transport in either membrane may be active or passive. Passage through the paracellular pathway occurs by passive mechanisms only, but one of these mechanisms, solvent drag, is thought to be indirectly dependent on the activity of Na-dependent transporters.

The relative contributions of transcellular versus paracellular transport to nutrient absorption are the subject of much debate and are beyond the scope of this review. Readers are referred to Ferraris et al.,[19] Toloza et al.,[20] Diamond,[21] Ferraris and Diamond,[8] and Pappenheimer[22–24] for discussions. We consider the transcellular pathway to be the predominant mode of nutrient transport at the physiological concentrations that exist in the small intestine. Ontogenetic changes in levels of nutrient transporters that match changes in diet composition and in metabolic requirements of many animals are but one of the major reasons for the importance of the transcellular pathway to total intestinal nutrient transport.

The number of studies describing ontogenetic changes in transport systems in the brushborder is much larger than for those of the basolateral membrane. Since regulatory changes in the basolateral membrane match those in the brushborder and are undoubtedly important during development, we will also describe what is known for ontogeny of transporters in the basolateral membrane. Although we will emphasize changes in specific transport systems, we will also mention ontogenetic changes in major nonspecific mechanisms that indirectly affect transport, such as changes in surface area, electrochemical gradient for Na, membrane permeability, and ratio of transporting to nontransporting cells. The process of "intestinal closure," or changes in permeability of the neonatal gut to immunologically recognizable proteins, is discussed in detail elsewhere.

Sugars

The final products of carbohydrate digestion are glucose, galactose, and fructose. Glucose and galactose are absorbed by the Na-dependent glucose transporter SGLT1 in the brushborder membrane (Figure 8–1).[25] Fructose is transported across the brushborder membrane by GLUT5, a member of the large family of Na-independent, facilitative glucose transporters.[26] GLUT5 is also expressed in lesser amounts in adipose, muscle, and kidney tissues.[27] Glucose, galactose and fructose are subsequently and passively transported across the basolateral membrane by GLUT2.[28] GLUT2 is also expressed in the liver and pancreas, and acts as a high-capacity transport system to allow large fluxes of glucose. The amino acid sequences of the mammalian facilitative glucose transporters vary significantly. There is 39 to 65% sequence identity and 50 to 76% sequence similarity between isoforms; 26% of the residues are invariant in all 5 proteins, and another 13% represent conservative amino acid replacements.[29] The three intestinal sugar transporters, SGLT1, GLUT5, and GLUT2, have each been cloned, and there is an increasing number of studies on the cellular and molecular transport mechanisms underlying intestinal sugar transport and its regulation. A discussion of these mechanisms, as well as of the large number of transport systems covered in this chapter, is beyond the scope of this review. Readers may consult other recent reviews.[30–32]

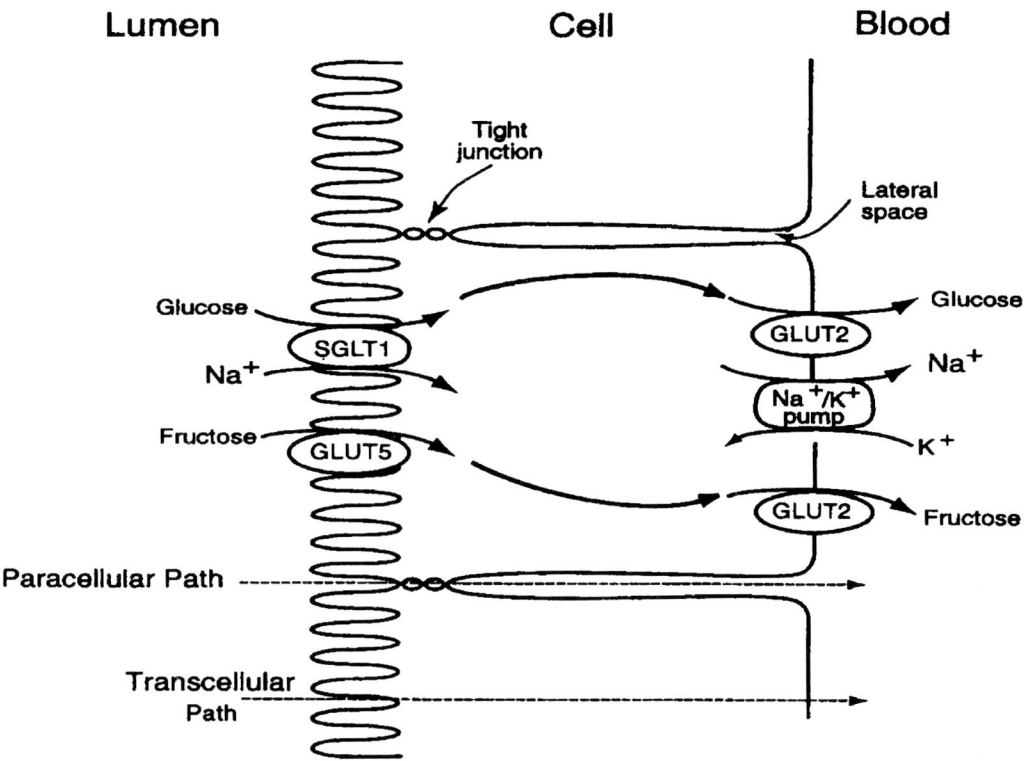

FIGURE 8–1. Transcellular absorption of monosaccharides involves three transporters. Glucose and galactose are cotransported with Na+ from the intestinal lumen across the brushborder or apical membrane into the cytosol by SGLT1, the Na+-dependent glucose transporter. Fructose is transported across the brushborder membrane by GLUT5, an Na+-independent transporter belonging to the family of facilitated GLUT transporters. Glucose, galactose, and fructose are transported across the basolateral membrane by GLUT2. (From Ferraris RP, Diamond JM. Regulation of intestinal sugar transport. Physiol Rev 1997;77:257–302. Reprinted with permission from the American Physiological Society.)

Amino Acids

Amino acid transport across either brushborder or basolateral membranes is a complicated subject, because of the large number of amino acids and a similarly large number of transport systems with overlapping substrate specificities. Moreover, some of these transport systems use the electrochemical gradient for Na, while others use those for Cl and K as well.[33,34] Hopfer[35] and Ganapathy et al.[36] mention at least 8 amino acid transporters in the brushborder of the small intestine (Table 8–1).

Whenever amino acid transport is mentioned in this review, it reflects the overall transport of that specific amino acid via all transporters recognizing that amino acid as a substrate. In sharp contrast, brushborder glucose transport reflects mainly the activity of SGLT1, and brushborder fructose transport that of GLUT5. The various transporters used by a single amino acid may differ in development, confounding the interpretation of appearance of transport activity and appearance of transporters. A notable exception is the transport of proline and other imino acids transported only by the IMINO transport system. Two of these amino acid transport systems have been cloned.[34,36] CAT1 not only shows properties similar to the amino acid transport system y^+ when CAT1 is expressed in *Xenopus* oocytes, but it is also found in tissues expressing significant y^+ transporter activity.[34] Other isoforms, CAT2A and CAT2B, were subsequently cloned. The X^-_{AG} transport system in the brushborder membrane has also been cloned (EAAC1).[37] There are several types of glutamate transporters that have been cloned, but only EAAC1 is found in mammalian small intestine.[38,39]

Amino acid transport systems found in the basolateral membrane (see Table 8–1) are similar to those found in other nonintestinal cells. There have been very few studies on the ontogeny of basolateral transporters, and even less is known about their molecular characteristics compared to those of the brushborder amino acid transporters.[40] Two basolateral transport systems have been cloned. CAT-1 corresponds to y^+ and is also found in the basolateral membrane. ASCT1 and ASCT2 are two isoforms of a transporter family whose properties are similar to that found in transport system ASC.[34]

Peptide Transport

Transport of dipeptides and tripeptides constitutes an important pathway for absorbing products of protein digestion. The brushborder peptide transporters use the transmembrane electrochemical H gradient as the driving force. There seem to be at least two brushborder peptide transporters, PEPT1 and PEPT2, and both have been cloned.[41]

TABLE 8–1
Classification of Amino Acid Transport Systems in the Brushborder and Basolateral Membranes of Small Intestine

Transport System (name of cloned transporter)	Substrates	Dependence on Na^+ Gradient
Brushborder		
B	Dipolar α-amino acids	Yes
$B^{o,+}$	Dipolar α-amino acids	Yes
	Basic amino acids	
	Cystine	
$b^{o,+}$ (D2, rBAT, NBAT)	Dipolar α-amino acids	No
	Basic amino acids	
	Cystine	
y^+ (CAT1, CAT2A, CAT2B)	Basic amino acids	No
IMINO	Imino acids, aminoisobutyric acid	Yes
ß	ß-Amino acids, taurine	Yes
x^-_{AG} (EAAC1)	Acidic amino acids	Yes
Basolateral		
A	Dipolar α-amino acids	Yes
	Imino acids	
ASC (ASCT1, ASCT2)	Three- and four-carbon dipolar amino acids	Yes
asc	Three- and four-carbon dipolar amino acids	No
L	Bulky, hydrophobic, dipolar amino acids	No
y^+ (CAT1, CAT2A, CAT2B)	Basic amino acids	No

Adapted from Castagna et al.[34] and Ganapathy et al.[36]

PEPT1 is expressed in the kidney and the intestine, PEPT2 only in the kidney. There is a proximal-to-distal gradient in abundance of PEPT1 mRNA, which is most abundant in the duodenum. A peptide transporter that has facilitative transporter properties is thought to exist in the basolateral membrane of the small intestine.[42]

Bile Acid Transport

Intestinal transport of bile acids is an essential step in enterohepatic circulation of bile and is, therefore, important in fat absorption. Bile acids are absorbed from the intestinal lumen by a Na^+-dependent bile acid brushborder transporter located mainly in the ileum. This transporter has been cloned, and mRNA expression is greatest in the ileum and the kidney and is absent from the proximal small intestine.[43] This apical membrane Na^+-dependent bile acid transporter (ASBT) is homologous to, but distinct from, the basolateral Na^+-dependent bile acid transporter (BSBT) expressed mainly in hepatocytes.[44,45] Bile acid–binding proteins presumably transport bile acids in the cytosol, then an anion exchange protein carries bile acids across the basolateral membrane.[46]

In summary, there are brushborder and basolateral transport systems responsible for transcellular absorption of sugars, amino acids, peptides, and bile acids. Several of the associated transporters have been cloned, allowing for parallel studies on developmental changes in gene expression and in transporter abundance and activity.

METHODS OF MEASURING INTESTINAL TRANSPORT

Intestinal nutrient transport activity in the developing gut has been measured using a variety of methods, several of which are briefly described here.

In Vitro Techniques

The ability to transport against concentration gradients can be studied by determining whether isolated intestines can accumulate substrates at concentrations greater than those in the incubation medium or, in Ussing chamber preparations, whether these tissues can accumulate substrates in the serosal compartment at concentrations greater than those in the mucosal compartment. An Ussing chamber preparation can also be used to determine whether addition of substrate in the luminal or mucosal compartment can alter the transepithelial potential difference, which would be an indication of cotransport with ions. While these preparations can indicate the appearance of transport activity, they cannot provide accurate estimates of J_{max} (maximum transport rate) of transport activity. The maximum transport rate is usually determined by measuring initial uptake of a range of substrate concentrations into membrane vesicles or everted tissues. Changes in J_{max} are true indicators of changes in either transporter number or transporter turnover rate (amount of substrate absorbed by each transporter per unit time). A discussion of the everted tissue method may be found in Karasov and Diamond,[47] and that of the vesicle method in Hopfer.[35]

In Vivo Techniques

Measurements of transporter activity are sometimes made in vivo, although the breath hydrogen test is usually used to determine extent of malabsorption of ingested carbohydrates. Luminal and vascular perfusion in vivo of an intestinal segment is sometimes used to determine absorption rates.[48] The principle of these studies is to perfuse labeled substrate and saline into the lumen and then measure the substrate's appearance in the vascular bed, which is also perfused with saline. For studies on D-glucose transport, usually its nonmetabolizable but transportable analog, 3-O-methylglucose (3-OMG), is used to prevent the confounding effects of metabolism during in vivo experiments. Finally, absorption rates of 3-OMG have been measured in chronically-catheterized animals,[49] an approach that has the advantage of measuring transport without the added influence of anesthesia or surgery. The principle of these studies is to measure total (active plus passive) 3-OMG absorption, to calculate passive 3-OMG absorption estimated from the measured absorption of a nontransportable stereoisomer L-glucose, and then to calculate carrier-mediated uptake as the difference between total uptake and passive uptake.

REGULATORY MECHANISMS

Mechanisms underlying ontogenetic changes in intestinal nutrient transport vary, and are classified mainly as nonspecific or specific mechanisms. We refer the readers to Ferraris and Diamond[8] for a detailed discussion.

Nonspecific Mechanisms

Changes in Surface Area

Perhaps the most common mechanism influencing intestinal nutrient transport is a change in intestinal surface area or mucosal mass. In fact, the slope of double logarithmic plots of intestinal surface area (excluding area amplification by villi and microvilli) against body weight equals 0.7 to 1.0 in almost all species examined so far,[3,17] suggesting that intestinal surface area increases in direct or slightly less than direct proportion to increases in body weight. Thus, the single most important mechanism underlying dramatic increases in intestinal absorption is an increase in intestinal surface area. Conversely, declines in intestinal absorptive surface area, such as those observed during diarrhea or malnutrition, are accompanied by lower total absorptive capacities.

Changes in the Proportion of Transporting to Nontransporting Cells

This is, perhaps, the second most significant, though less heralded and less documented, nonspecific mechanism underlying changes in intestinal nutrient absorption. Intestinal cells typically differentiate from stem cells in the crypt and mature as they migrate up the villus column, and are eventually exfoliated from the villus tip. Newly born rats have very slow enterocyte migration rates (in the order of 22 days for weaning rats[50]). Hence, in young mammals, there is synthesis of new enterocytes, but little exfoliation of mature enterocytes, so that relatively more mature enterocytes occupy most of the villus column. As mammals grow older, the typical crypt-to-villus (CV) gradient in transport activity becomes more pronounced. In newborn pigs, cells all along the CV axis absorb nutrients; in contrast, only cells in the upper villus regions absorb nutrients in adults.[51] Another suite of changes in rates of enterocyte proliferation and migration up the villus during weaning is associated with shifts in the activities of brushborder membrane hydrolases and transporters. These processes probably underlie much of development-related, nonspecific decreases in nutrient absorption per mg tissue.

Changes in Plasma Membrane Lipid Composition

There are significant alterations in the lipid composition of brushborder and basolateral membranes during development.[52,53] Some of these occur with shifts in dietary inputs during gestation, lactation and weaning.[54] The changes in proportions of different fatty acids, types of phospholipid head groups, and in levels of cholesterol coincide with altered physical characteristics of the enterocyte membranes. The changes in membrane lipid composition and physical characteristics in turn can not only influence passive permeability of the membrane to various nutrients, but also affect the activity of transporters by altering turnover number or moles of substrate absorbed per mole of transporter per unit time.[55]

Other Nonspecific Adaptive Mechanisms

Changes in electrochemical gradient for Na^+ would alter the transport rate of any nutrient cotransported with Na^+. Glucagon enhances intestinal glucose transport by hyperpolarizing the membrane, thereby increasing the electrochemical gradient for the Na^+ and increasing glucose transport rate.[56] Changes in electrochemical gradient for Cl^- and other ions alter membrane potential, and affect the absorption of nutrients cotransported with ions. This is known for cystic fibrosis, which is associated with higher rates of intestinal glucose and alanine absorption, and presumably for other Na^+-coupled uptake processes as well. The increase in Na^+-coupled transport rates is speculated to be caused by the hyperpolarized resting membrane potential due to dysfunctional regulation of the Cl^- channel.[57]

Changes in paracellular permeability also affect transepithelial transport of nutrients. Transient changes in paracellular permeability, triggered by Na^+-dependent absorption of certain nutrients, result in solvent drag of other nutrients. This would nonspecifically and transiently alter the transport of nutrients crossing the epithelial layer by solvent drag.[22] The contribution of solvent drag to total absorption of nutrients is discussed in detail in other articles.[8,58]

Specific Mechanisms

Changes in Site Density of Intestinal Nutrient Transporters

This mechanism accounts for most adaptations involving a change in transport rate of a single nutrient or category of nutrients. Dietary carbohydrates increase the number of glucose-absorbing sites in mouse small intestine.[59,60] The decreasing, proximal-to-distal regional gradient in rates of glucose transport is correlated with a decreasing, proximal-to-distal gradient in site density of glucose transporters.[61,62]

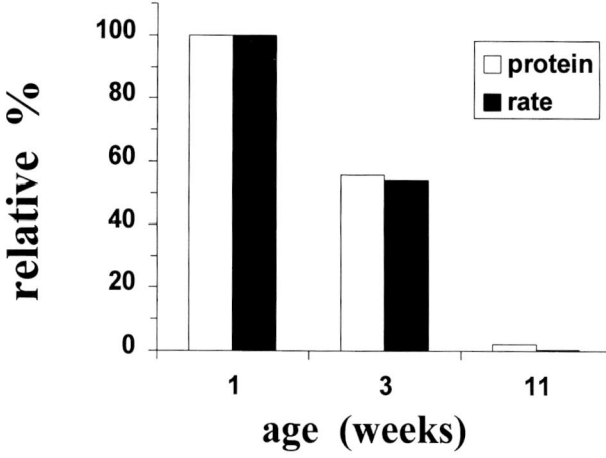

FIGURE 8–2. The developmentally related decline in glucose transport rate in sheep is tightly correlated with decreases in amounts of SGLT1 protein in the brushborder membrane. Rate of transport and amount of protein in 3- and 11-week-old lambs are expressed relative to those found in 1-week-old lambs. (Data from Shirazi-Beechey SP, Hirayama BA, Wang Y, et al. Ontogenic development of lamb intestinal sodium-glucose cotransporter is regulated by diet. J Physiol [Lond] 1991;437:699–708.)

During development, changes in amounts of transporter proteins are tightly correlated with changes in rates of intestinal transport of bile acids in rats[45] and of glucose in lambs (Figure 8–2[63]).

For some, but not all, transport systems, developmentally-related, specific changes in transporter activity are tightly correlated with changes in levels of mRNA coding for those transport systems. Changes in the steady-state levels of mRNA, in turn, are modulated by differences in transcription rates and mRNA stability.

Changes in Affinity Constants

These may occur during ontogenetic development, when one type of transporter is sequentially replaced by another type of transporter exhibiting different kinetic constants. For example, the ratio of galactose absorption to glucose absorption declines during early development in rats, rabbits, cats, and pigs, suggesting a sequential appearance of transporters, from one type having a lower affinity for galactose relative to glucose, to one having a greater affinity for galactose.[17,64,65]

Changes in Turnover Number

This mechanism has not been reported for brushborder transporters. Acute hyperglycemia, however, induces a 3.4× increase in J_{max} of basolateral glucose transport, but only a 1.5× increase in site density of transporters in rat enterocytes.[66,67] This suggests either that inactive transport sites were converted to active sites after short-term hyperglycemia, or that the turnover number of each site increased.

Expression of Transport Activity

Changes in intestinal nutrient transport in neonates arise mainly from changes in transport activity per cell (or per unit mucosal mass), and from changes in total number of cells or intestinal mass. It is important to distinguish the former mechanism, which is specific, from the latter mechanism, which is nonspecific and therefore affects the transport of all nutrients. When studying ontogeny of nutrient transport, it becomes apparent that the transport capacity of the small intestine can increase solely because intestinal mass increases. Ferraris and Diamond[8] provide a series of equations to distinguish the two mechanisms. Briefly, uptake (J) is often normalized to a measure of intestinal mass (wet weight, dry weight, amount of protein, amount of DNA), so that:

$$J \text{ per mg} = (\text{transporter copies per mg}) (v)$$

where v = the transporter turnover number as defined above, p. 127. Since v rarely changes, alterations in J per mg usually indicates changes in number of transporters per mg, and a significant increase in absorption rate per mg in the neonatal intestine indicates a developmentally related increase in number of transporters. Uptake should be determined at concentrations that yield J_{max}.[68]

Transport rate can also be normalized per unit length of intestine, so that:

$$J \text{ per cm} = (J \text{ per mg}) (\text{mg per cm})$$

Total uptake capacity (ΣJ) of the small intestine can be estimated either by multiplying J per mg by total intestinal weight, or J per cm by total intestinal length. Because of regional differences in absorption rates and mass per cm of intestine, it is more accurate to estimate ΣJ by determining uptake rates per cm in different regions, interpolating uptake rates between regions, and then summing over the length of the small intestine.

Although intestinal uptake capacity is highly informative, it is not particularly useful when uptake capacities of intestines from different species or from conspecific individuals differing in body weights are compared. Since neonatal animals grow rapidly in weight, it is often useful to normalize uptake capacity to body weight or, more accurately, to metabolic body weight (because metabolic rate increases with weight at approximately $BW^{0.75}$ among mammals).

GENERALIZED PATTERNS OF INTESTINAL NUTRIENT TRANSPORT DEVELOPMENT

Age-related changes in intestinal transport of nutrients can be separated into three main phases: prenatal, suckling, and then weaning and postweaning. The phases are separated by changes in dietary inputs, and during each phase the structural and functional characteristics of the intestine are matched to the demands associated with the specific types of dietary inputs. In this section we present a basic pattern of nutrient transporter development. We focus on recent findings (mainly since 1992), and supplement previous reviews of nutrient transporter development.[3,69,70]

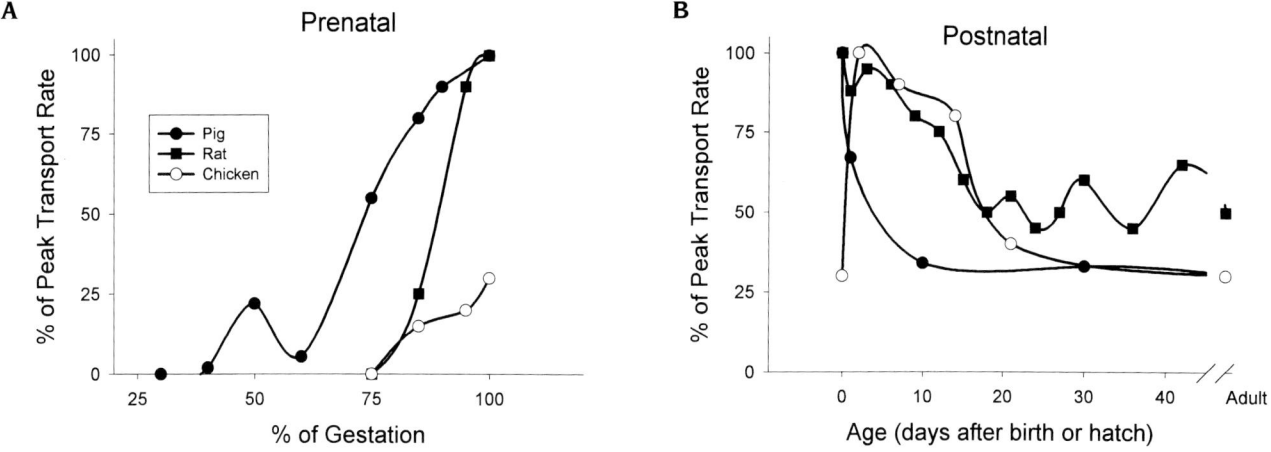

FIGURE 8–3. Ontogenetic changes in rates of brushborder glucose uptake by intact tissues during prenatal (A) and postnatal (B) development of pigs, rats, and chickens. Values are expressed as percentages of the highest reported rates of uptake during ontogenetic development. (Data from various sources.)

Much more is known about age-related changes in glucose uptake by the apical membrane than about those in any other nutrient or solute. Therefore, we first use glucose as a model solute to present ontogenetic development of brushborder membrane transport. Subsequent sections describe how this pattern varies between solutes, membrane domains, and species.

Prenatal Development

The first phase of intestinal apical glucose transporter development begins at the completion of intestinal organogenesis. The cells lining the primitive intestine differentiate into columnar enterocytes with microvilli and begin to express characteristic apical proteins,[71] including SGLT1.[70] Cytodifferentiation and expression of apical transporters are first seen in the proximal intestine, and proceed distally.

After their appearance, the number of transporters increases throughout the remainder of the gestation period (Figure 8–3). The underdeveloped intestines of premature infants and the associated problems of digestion and nutrition highlight the importance of the final stages of intestinal development. However, less is known about the changes in nutrient transport during the third trimester than for any other period of development. In vivo studies suggest absorptive capacities are lower in preterm infants relative to those delivered at term,[72] but definitive studies of transport functions are lacking. Difficulties associated with obtaining tissues from third trimester human fetuses have necessitated the use of animal models. The intestines of fetal pigs, the principal model, undergo rapid growth and dramatic increases in densities of SGLT1 between 74% of term and birth.[73]

Birth and Suckling

The next principal phase of intestinal development starts at birth and continues until the time of weaning. Newborns must consume and absorb relatively large volumes of milk to satisfy their high weight-specific requirements for energy and nutrients. Correspondingly, for all mammals studied, SGLT1 densities and rates of uptake are higher at birth than at any other age (see Figure 8–3B), whether normalized to tissue dimensions or apical membrane protein content. The high rates of transport at birth are partly explained by the presence of fully mature enterocytes along most of the CV axis of neonates. As a consequence, at birth the entire villus is capable of absorbing nutrients, not just, as is seen in older stages,[74] the upper third.

The conversion of the intestine from a relatively quiescent state during late gestation to being fully active after onset of suckling coincides with several dramatic changes in intestinal structure and functions. The most notable change is an increased mitotic activity in the crypts. The enterocytes that are produced after birth gradually replace those synthesized during gestation. This effectively dilutes the mature fetal enterocytes with immature adult-type enterocytes that have not yet fully expressed transport functions, and that also differ in several other characteristics.[75] The replacement of pig and rat fetal enterocytes requires up to 2 weeks, or longer, due to the long life span of the fetal enterocytes, compared to the 24 to 48 hour typical of adult enterocytes.[76] As the average age of the enterocytes declines, so do rates of glucose transport, and the characteristic distribution of carrier-mediated absorption along the CV axis is established.

Interpreting the postnatal shifts in SGLT1 abundance and activity[77] is made difficult by concurrent changes in mucosal mass.[78] Another complicating factor is postnatal changes in the chemical and physical characteristics of the apical membrane,[79,80] which may alter passive permeation of solutes and transporter functions.[81]

Weaning and Beyond

Another suite of changes in intestinal structure and functions begins at the end of suckling in preparation for the shift from milk to the adult diet. Rates of glucose transport decline after weaning, but the magnitude of decline varies widely and is closely related to adult feeding habits (see the next section, describing species differences). The changes after weaning are genetically programmed; they occur even if weaning is delayed. The declines in rates of uptake appear to be more of a nonspecific response to changes in cell kinetics and differentiation and villus maturation than to changes in the properties of absorption.[82]

In summary, studies of brushborder membrane glucose transport have revealed a basic pattern of developmental changes in densities and activities of the Na$^+$-dependent glucose transporter, changes that are matched to shifts in dietary inputs and in metabolic needs of the developing organism.

VARIATIONS ON A THEME: ALTERNATIVE PATTERNS OF TRANSPORTER DEVELOPMENT

This section is devoted to descriptions of the variations in the pattern of transporter development as they relate to different species, to different solutes and their associated transporters, and to different regions of the gastrointestinal tract.

Species Differences in Ontogenetic Development of Apical Glucose Transport

Animal models have provided valuable insights about the patterns and mechanisms of transporter development. The majority of animal models are mammals (rats, mice, guinea pigs, rabbits, pigs, sheep, cats, dogs, mink) because of their relevance to human development. There has also been an interest in defining patterns of transporter development in other vertebrate groups, including domesticated and wild birds, amphibians and fish, for comparative, biomedical and agricultural purposes. In this section, we highlight differences in ontogenetic development of glucose transport among species.

There are obvious genetic differences underlying the species-specific patterns of SGLT1 development. These can extend to variation within species, with genetic disorders providing dramatic examples.[83] Genetic selection for strains with higher growth rates has led to larger intestines that could have more transporters,[84] but has not yet influenced the types and energetics of transporters.[85]

Prenatal

Active glucose transport appears before birth in all species studied so far. However, the gestational age when brushborder glucose transport is first detected varies widely among mammals. A trend becomes evident when gestational age of appearance of transport activity in a species is expressed as a percentage of term and then plotted against gestational length for that species (Figure 8–4). Species with long gestations, such as humans and pigs, express transporters earlier than species with short gestations (e.g., rats and mice). Corresponding with the short incubation period of chickens (21 days), brushborder glucose and amino acid apical transport do not develop until just prior to hatch.

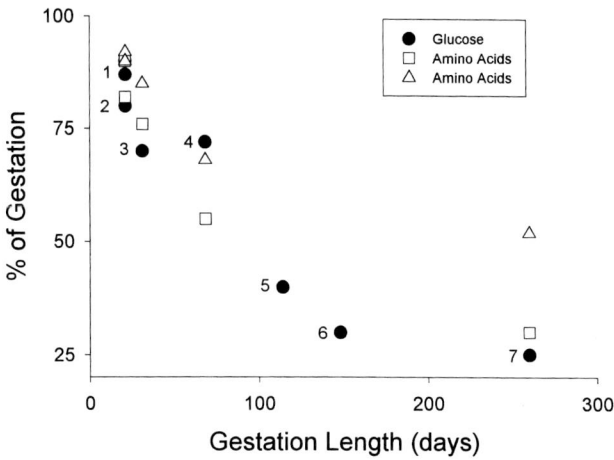

FIGURE 8–4. Initial appearance of brushborder glucose and amino acid transporters in the small intestine during fetal development of the rat and mouse (1), chicken (2), rabbit (3), guinea pig (4), pig (5), sheep (6), and human (7). Time of appearance is expressed as percentage of the normal gestation period. (Data from various sources.) Because of the number of amino acid transporters reported for rat, mouse, chicken, rabbit, guinea pig, and humans, we only show two amino acid transport systems. Within a species, a square represents the amino acid transport system appearing first; a triangle, the amino acid transport system appearing last. Note that brushborder amino acid transport, like glucose transport, appears before birth in all species.

Suckling

There are two basic responses of the mammalian intestine to the onset of suckling. For some species, there are rapid and dramatic changes in intestinal structure and functions. An excellent example is the hypertrophic (enlarged cells) and hyperplastic (more cells) responses of the neonatal dog and pig intestine that lead to nearly twofold increases in mucosal weight during the first 24 hours after birth.[17,70,86–88] Apparently, the production of transporters does not match the pace of anatomical (tissue) growth, resulting in postnatal declines in rates of transport per unit intestine. This suggests that the postnatal decline in glucose transport is not caused by a loss of the transporters present at birth, but instead by a "dilution" of mature, transporting enterocytes with immature enterocytes that have not yet acquired transport functions.

In other species, there are less dramatic postnatal increases in intestinal mass. The intestines of cats grow little during the first week after birth, and there is little if any postnatal decline in rates of glucose uptake.[65,89] The guinea pig, mouse, and rat intestine also grow slower during the suckling period than do those of dogs and pigs in the same period. Regardless of events during the time immediately after birth, by the end of suckling, rates of glucose uptake per unit intestine are lower than at birth.

In birds, rates of glucose transport decline after they begin to eat.[90,91] Unlike mammals, rates of glucose uptake in chickens do not reach a peak until 2 days after hatch, which coincides with the transition from yolk nutrition to complete dependence on exogenous food.[92]

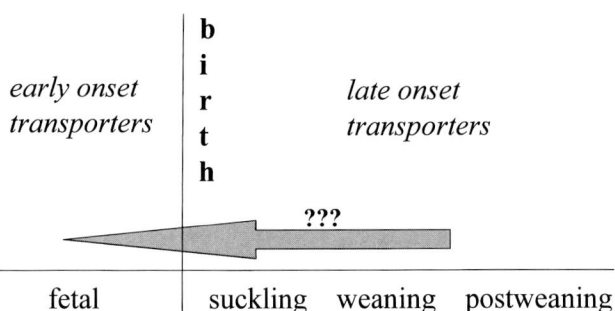

FIGURE 8–5. Intestinal nutrient transporters categorized according to the time of appearance of transporter activity during development. Glucose and amino acid transporters appear prenatally in all species studied so far. In contrast, fructose and bile acid transporters appear postnatally. It is not known whether these postnatal or late-onset transporters can be induced to appear earlier during development (*arrow*), much as dietary and hormonal manipulations can induce the precocious appearance of sucrase.

Weaning and Beyond

Changes in rates of glucose transport and densities of SGLT1 at the time of weaning reflect the evolutionary diet (species specialization towards a certain diet, e.g., herbivory) and digestive strategies of each species. The importance of genetic determinants is also apparent, in that the changes in transport functions occur even when the diet remains constant. This has been demonstrated for several nutrients in fish,[93] amphibians,[94] chickens,[77] and mammals.[95]

The postweaning changes in glucose transport are related to the evolutionary diet. Omnivores continue to eat a diet containing digestible carbohydrate and retain high densities of SGLT1 and rates of glucose transport, whereas in carnivores rates of glucose transport decline after weaning. Although ruminants eat large quantities of digestible carbohydrate, their intestines are not normally exposed to glucose and do not express appreciable levels of SGLT1.[63] Pinnipeds may provide an interesting, yet obscure, example of the relations between diet and expression of SGLT1. Unlike other mammals, the milk of pinnipeds does not contain lactose, and the carnivorous adult diet would contain only trace amounts of glucose. The a priori expectation is that expression and regulation of SGLT1 will be minimal throughout the life history of these species.

Different Solutes and Their Transporters

Intestinal nutrient transporters may be classified into two general categories (Figure 8–5): those that appear before birth (prenatal or early-onset transporters) and those that appear after birth (postnatal or late-onset transporters). In this section, we highlight how various transport systems differ in patterns of their ontogenetic development.

Sugars

Although SGLT1 is considered to be the principal apical membrane carrier for aldohexoses, one or more additional types of apical glucose transporters have been proposed to be present. Analyses of rates of glucose uptake in brushborder membrane vesicles (BBMVs) prepared from human fetuses have clearly revealed two transport systems. A high-affinity, low-capacity system, presumably SGLT1, is present throughout the small intestine, whereas a low-affinity, high-capacity system can be detected in the proximal intestine.[96,97] Similar findings have been reported for other mammals,[73,98–100] young ducks,[101] and fish.[102] The two transport systems are strategically distributed in various intestinal regions to allow rapid absorption of dietary sugars when present at high luminal concentrations in the proximal small intestine, and efficient "salvage" of sugars at low luminal concentrations in the distal regions.

The relative proportion of uptake via the two systems changes during development. In pigs, the percentage of glucose uptake via the low-affinity system declines shortly before birth.[73] In rats and mice, both systems can still be detected after birth, but the low-affinity system disappears at the time of weaning. Despite the abundant evidence derived from transport studies, it remains uncertain from biochemical studies whether there are multiple brush-border aldohexose transporters, each with different kinetic properties, or a single transporter (SGLT1) that exhibits different kinetic properties. A single type of transporter may exhibit different kinetics during the process of cell and/or protein maturation along the CV axis or in response to age-related shifts in apical membrane composition and fluidity.[99]

A second low-affinity and high-capacity apical sugar transporter, GLUT5, is specific for the ketohexose fructose.[103] A postnatal increase in GLUT5 expression would explain why older infants are better able to absorb, hence tolerate, dietary fructose than neonates.[104]

The increase in fructose transport at weaning in rodents corresponds with its appearance in the diet. However, the relationship with diet does not always match predictions. Suckling dogs and mink are not exposed to dietary fructose, yet both have the capacity to absorb fructose by a low-affinity carrier.[105,106] It is possible that GLUT5, or some other type of sugar transporter, is present before weaning, and may act as a low-affinity, low-specificity carrier for sugars. This would allow suckling dogs and mink to rapidly absorb the products of lactose hydrolysis. Corresponding with this speculation, the GLUT5 of rats apparently can function as a low-affinity glucose transporter.[107] However, this is not true for the GLUT5 of humans.[108]

Transcellular absorption of sugars requires a second set of transporters in the basolateral membrane. The onset of suckling triggers an increase in the basolateral transporter (GLUT2) densities, coinciding with a two- to threefold increase in glycolytic activities.[109] Postnatal changes in GLUT2 expression and activity have been directed more toward understanding the rapid and reversible regulation in response to dietary inputs, with little or nothing known about age-related changes in GLUT2 densities and/or regulation.

Amino Acids and Peptides

Although amino acids are considered to be important nutrients for intestinal cell metabolism,[110] less is known about age-related changes for the several classes of apical amino acid transporters. Further, because a suitable marker is not available to correct for passive diffusion of amino acids, reported rates of amino acid uptake by intact tissues include both carrier-mediated and carrier-independent pathways of absorption. Interpretations of age-related changes in amino acid uptake are further complicated by concurrent changes in intestinal dimensions and membrane protein content and permeability, which can change the relative importance of diffusion and carrier-mediated uptake. Despite these limitations, amino acid transport systems are known to vary among species and stages of development.[3] The increasing availability of molecular and genetic probes will enhance our understanding of amino acid uptake and age-related changes in the types, densities, and activities of the transporters. This section focuses on results obtained using BBMVs or intact tissues when measured over a wide range of concentrations, a protocol that allows investigators to calculate the saturable and carrier-independent pathways of absorption.

Apical amino acid transporters are first expressed prenatally (see Figure 8–4) at the same time as or shortly after the appearance of SGLT1.[3] Initial rates of leucine uptake per mg BBMV protein, hence densities of transporters, increase during the remainder of gestation in pigs, and the characteristic declining proximal-to-distal gradient of uptake is established before birth.[73] Unlike glucose transport, the main increase in leucine uptake occurs during the last 25 percent of gestation. Moreover, the magnitude of increase between first appearance and birth is much lower for leucine (1.9-fold) than it is for glucose (25-fold).

The highest rates of apical amino acid absorption are measured at birth, with subsequent declines during suckling and postweaning.[111] The postnatal decreases in transport rates tend to be steeper for essential amino acids. The most dramatic example is the apparent loss, shortly after birth, of the Na-dependent taurine transporter from the intestine of cats[112] and of other species (reviewed by O'Flaherty et al.[113]). Although intestinal taurine transport declines during postnatal development of mice and other species, the transporters are retained.[113,114]

Basolateral transporters play an important role in providing needed amino acids (e.g., glutamine) to the enterocytes from the blood between meals and in transporting dietary amino acids from the enterocytes to the portal circulation following a meal. Despite their obvious importance, age-related changes in the types, densities, and activities of the basolateral amino acid transporters have yet to be described.

Bile Acids

The transporters for bile acids have what appears to be a paradoxical pattern of development. They are absent during suckling, when fat intake is high and bile acid secretion and recycling should be maximal. Instead, the sodium-dependent bile acid transporters appear in the distal small intestine at the time of weaning,[45,115–117] when fat intake usually declines. Interestingly, feeding bile acids to sucklings may cause precocious expression of the bile acid transporters, though an induced diarrhea may be a causative factor.[118] Despite the lack of transporters during suckling, passive absorption of bile acids along the entire length of small intestine allows sucklings to recover and recycle the majority of secreted bile acids.[119] It is uncertain why expression of the transporters is delayed until weaning. It is possible the lack of transporters during suckling allows bile acids to enter the colon and thereby influence development of the enteric microbiota.

Regional Considerations

The transporters are generally not distributed evenly throughout the small intestine, and two gradients can be described. The first is the horizontal distribution from the pyloric sphincter and proceeding distally. The second pattern of distribution is the vertical arrangement of transporters along the CV axis. Both of these gradients change during development.

Development of Transport Systems in the Duodenum, Jejunum, and Ileum

Transporters are first detected in the apical membrane of the proximal intestine, and gradually appear distally as the wave of cytodifferentiation proceeds toward the ileum. During fetal development, transporters for sugars, amino acids, and other solutes are expressed in the colon of some species (dogs,[120] pigs,[69] sheep,[121] rats[122]). The most dramatic age-related redistribution of transporters along the proximal-to-distal gradient is the loss of the colonic nutrient transporters during the suckling period. In vivo studies have provided suggestive evidence that the neonatal colon also has a transient capacity to transport lactose.[72] Nutrient transporters can also be detected throughout the entire cecum of newly hatched chickens, but they become restricted to the proximal region, adjacent to the colon, within just a few days after onset of feeding.[123] Although apical transporters for sugars and amino acids disappear from the colon of mammals, those present in the basolateral membrane are retained.[121]

Compared to those in other regions, rates of transport are generally higher in the proximal intestine for sugars and peptides, and higher in the midintestine for amino acids. Other transporters, such as those for nucleosides, appear to be distributed evenly along the length of small intestine.[124] For most species, these regional patterns of transport develop before or shortly after birth and are retained throughout life. An interesting exception is the regional pattern of glucose accumulation by BBMV prepared from postnatal mink.[105] The proximal-to-distal, declining gradient in transporter activity so typical in other species is also present in adult mink; but during suckling and during weaning stages, rates of glucose accumulation per mg BBMV protein tend to be higher in the distal mink intestine.

Development of Transport Systems along the Crypt-Villus Axis

The CV distribution of transporters is sensitive to the proliferation and cytodifferentiation of enterocytes as these enterocytes emerge out of the crypts and migrate to the tip of the villus.[125] Therefore, age-related changes in rates of enterocyte proliferation and migration, such as those that occur after onset of suckling and again at weaning, will influence the abundance and relative proportions of different apical transporters.

Circadian Rhythm

Transporter expression is subject to a strong diurnal rhythm in adult rats.[126,127] Activities of intestinal disaccharidases[128] and the intestinal L-histidine transporter[129] are also subject to circadian rhythm in adult rats. Fructose transport rates and GLUT5 mRNA levels in weaning rats, however, do not follow any circadian rhythm.[130] This discrepancy between adult and weaning rats may be explained by the undeveloped physiological circadian rhythm at the age of weaning. Unlike adult rats that consume 90% of their food during the night,[19] rat pups feed virtually all the time. The typical rhythm of food intake of adults begins only when postweaning pups reach 29 days.[131]

Development of Transporters in Carnivores and Omnivores

The dietary shifts that occur during the evolution of a species influence three aspects of nutrient transport. In addition to determining when the various nutrient transporters are expressed and the basal levels of expression, the evolutionary diet determines the ability of species to adaptively modulate transport rates to match changes in diet composition. For example, the presence of varying amounts of carbohydrate in the diets of omnivores coincides with high densities of apical glucose transporters and with the ability to rapidly and reversibly modulate the densities of transporters. In contrast, carnivorous species have low basal densities of SGLT1. Moreover, members of families that are exclusively carnivores (e.g., cats and salmonids) have either lost or never acquired the ability to adaptively modulate densities of SGLT1.[93] Species that may be carnivores as adults but are members of families with omnivorous representatives (e.g., mink) may have low basal rates of glucose uptake, but these can be upregulated if glucose or other digestible carbohydrates are added to the diet. Ruminants are similar to mink in that basal SGLT1 expression is low, but it can be upregulated if glucose is infused into the intestine.[132]

Role of Early Onset Nutrient Transporters during Gestation

The appearance of nutrient transporters during gestation was initially considered to be a consequence of a pattern of development.[3] More recently, prenatal onset transporters (those that are expressed prior to birth or hatch) have been shown to be critical for normal fetal development (reviewed by Buddington[70]). After cytodifferentiation and expression of intestinal glucose and amino acid transporters, fetuses begin to swallow amniotic fluid. The low concentrations of sugars and amino acids in amniotic fluid have been calculated to provide between 10% and 14% of the fetus' requirements for energy and nutrients.[133] After 45 days of gestation, by which time pig fetuses have prenatal onset nutrient transporters and presumably have started to swallow amniotic fluid, there are changes in the concentrations of amino acids in the amniotic and allantoic fluids, and in the fetal and maternal plasma.[134] Some of the most dramatic changes and maternal-fetal differences are for concentrations of glutamine, which is known to be critical for fetal nitrogen metabolism, particularly by the developing intestine. Also to be considered are potentially biologically active molecules present in the amniotic fluid, which may modulate the genetic program of intestinal development.[135]

Effect of Dietary Shifts during Gestation

When the ability of fetuses to swallow amniotic fluid is prevented by esophageal ligation, growth and maturation of the intestine and fetus are slowed (reviewed by Trahair and Sangild[136]). Conversely, growth and maturation of the intestine can be accelerated by adding nutrients and/or growth factors to the amniotic fluid[137] and can induce higher rates of nutrient transport.[138] These latter findings have clinical implications for treatment of intrauterine growth retardation due to placental insufficiency. Further, the importance of luminal nutrition for intestinal development explains why the transition of premature infants to full enteral nutrition is accelerated when gradually increasing amounts of nutrients are fed. Therefore, the prenatal appearance of certain nutrient transporters may be a consequence of development, but is critical for normal development of the intestine and fetus. It is possible that fetal swallowing and processing of amniotic fluid is more important for species with long gestations.

Effects of Dietary Shifts during the Perinatal Period

The immediate and long-term influences of colostrum on postnatal intestinal growth, the brushborder membrane hydrolases, and macromolecular uptake are well known (reviewed by Kelly and Coutts[139]). Colostrum also induces expression of SGLT1,[88] and apparently within 6 hours after onset of feeding since comparable increases are not detected when pigs are fed milk replacer diets or an oral electrolyte solution or are food-deprived.[140] It has generally been considered that mature enterocytes, such as the fetal enterocytes present at birth, may have limited adaptive capacities. Instead, the influences of diet are manifested by altering rates of enterocyte production and migration, thereby nonspecifically changing transport rates, and by modulating the expression of various genes, thereby specifically changing transport rates.[141] Recent evidence indicates that at least SGLT1 densities in adult rats can be rapidly increased in response to in vivo exposure to the biologically active peptide GLP-2.[142]

Effect of Dietary Shifts during the Suckling Stage

After the short period of colostrum intake the diet of sucklings is mature milk, which is relatively constant in composition. Although there are differences in composition of milk of various species, there has probably been little change in milk composition during the recent evolution of each species. Therefore, it can be predicted that the ability of sucklings to adaptively modulate transport functions will be comparable to that of adults of species consuming diets that vary little in composition (e.g., carnivorous diets). This is the case for sucklings of pigs[143] and omnivorous mammals.[95] Only at a later stage of development, when diet can be expected to change and begin to vary in composition, as in the case of omnivorous diets, should the intestine change basal rates of transport and acquire the ability to adaptively modulate transport rates. The contrasting situation is evident for amphibians that have omnivorous tadpoles that metamorphose into carnivorous adults, at which time basal rates of glucose transport decline and the ability to adaptively modulate transport functions is lost.[94]

Despite the apparent lack of adaptive capacities to specifically modulate transport, changes in lipid composition of milk may nonspecifically alter transport rate. Feeding lactating rats lipids with different ratios of fatty acids alters milk composition and rates of sugar transport by their pups.[144] However, the same laboratory has found that feeding different proportions of saturated and unsaturated lipids does not influence sugar transport by sucklings, despite changing milk composition.[145]

The relationship between the densities of glucose transporters and intake of amino acid transporters and diet composition during development is not as distinct as that between glucose transporters and intake of carbohydrate. Because amino acids provide energy, and some are essential nutrients, all animals must consume and process adequate amounts of protein to satisfy requirements for growth and maintenance of tissues. Therefore, even though age-related shifts in ratios for rates of uptake for amino acids relative to glucose may coincide with changes in diet composition, these shifts are caused more by changes in rates of transport for glucose than for amino acids.

Effects of Shifts in Intestinal Luminal Bacterial Populations during Development

The relationship between age-related changes in diet and transport functions are generally attributed to nutrient composition. An often overlooked influence of diet involves how it affects the bacterial assemblages in the developing intestine, and how this could affect intestinal structure, and thereby nonspecifically alter transport functions.[146,147] At the time of weaning, changes in intestinal and villus dimensions and in rates of transport[17,69,82] are paralleled by shifts in bacterial populations.[148] In human infants, development of the ileal transporter system and associated enterohepatic recycling of bile acids may be dependent on acquisition of an enteric bacterial assemblage capable of transforming secreted bile acids.[149]

Intestinal Absorptive Capacities

The capacities of the entire length of small intestine to transport nutrients are of critical importance to developing animals, and highlight the relationship between the nutrient transporters and intestinal growth. When transport capacities (mmol per d) are exceeded by dietary loads, diarrhea may result. This is exemplified by the fructose intolerance of neonates.

After the initial appearance of transporters, the capacities of the fetal intestine to transport nutrients increase up to birth. This increased capacity is accomplished by a combination of increases in rates of transport per unit tissue and in intestinal growth. For example, intestinal mass and brushborder membrane protein, including the transporters, increase exponentially during gestation of pigs, with the greatest increase occurring between 60 percent of term and birth.[73] As a consequence, total transport capacities increase dramatically, far outpacing the increase in body weight.

Despite generalized declines in rates of nutrient transport per mg after onset of suckling, capacities of the intestine either increase or remain stable because of intestinal growth.[17] A similar pattern is known for lactase, which declines in specific activity during suckling and weaning, but total intestinal activity remains fairly stable.[150] Transport capacities continue to increase during the growth phase of animals, corresponding with ever-increasing dietary loads. However, as rates of body weight gain decline, there is a concurrent decrease in uptake capacities normalized to metabolic mass.[4] Once a stable, adult body weight is attained, transport capacities can decline, but remain responsive to changes in metabolic needs and dietary loads. By increasing metabolic expenditures and dietary inputs above normal during development, it is possible to accelerate the growth in intestinal mass and influence both the densities and characteristics of glucose transporters.[101]

MOLECULAR MECHANISMS UNDERLYING DEVELOPMENT OF TRANSPORT AND REGULATORY SYSTEMS

In this section, we compare the molecular mechanisms underlying the development of prenatal onset and postnatal onset transporters, and then of regulatory processes modulating their activity.

Prenatal Onset Transporters

Brushborder glucose and amino acid transporters are classical examples of prenatal onset transporters, as described above, pp. 130 to 134. For these transporters, transport mechanisms as well as regulatory mechanisms go through various stages of development.

Transport Mechanisms

Sugars. During neonatal stages, glucose and amino acid transport mechanisms have typically high specific activities, which subsequently and gradually decline to specific activities found in adults. In chicks, a decrease in site density of transporters underlies much of this developmentally-related decrease in brushborder glucose transport rates.[77] Changes in Na^+ permeability and membrane fluidity had no or modest effects, respectively, on glucose transport. In rats, this postweaning decline in transport activity is hardwired or genetically programmed, and is not dependent on removal of substrates from the lumen at the normal time of weaning. For example, rates of galactose transport in rats that are prevented from normal weaning by being fed dry milk are similar to those in rats that are allowed to wean normally onto a chow diet.[4] Unlike transport rate per mg tissue, which declines modestly with age, steady-state levels of SGLT1 mRNA do not change with developmental stage in rats, and are also genetically programmed,[151,152] as would be expected from the genetically programmed expression of transporter activity.

The hardwired development of SGLT1 activity and mRNA in rats contrasts with that of sheep. As lambs shift from maternal to ruminant nutrition, the amount of sugars in the gut decreases. From high rates found in lambs, transport rate per mg declines by about 200× during weaning, and this decrease is paralleled by an equally dramatic decrease in brushborder SGLT1 protein[63,153] (see Figure 8–2). In sharp contrast, mRNA levels decrease by only 4×. Prevention of weaning by providing lambs with milk-replacer diets maintains SGLT1 protein and activity at high levels, but there is no or little change in mRNA levels. This concordance between glucose transport rates and SGLT1 protein levels on one hand and disparity between transport rates and SGLT1 mRNA levels on the other is well documented, and occurs not only during normal ontogenetic development of Na$^+$-dependent glucose transport,[151,153] but also during maturation of Na$^+$-dependent glucose transport activity along the CV axis.[154,155] It also indicates that caution must be used when extrapolating mRNA abundance to transporter densities and functions.

GLUT2 protein and mRNA are already expressed at the blastocyst stage, well before organ differentiation.[156] Expression of GLUT2 at this embryonic stage may reflect an early homeostatic role for this transporter, which would allow embryos, and later the developing enterocytes, to obtain glucose from the circulation or maternally provided fluid.[156] There has been no study describing ontogenetic development of this transporter during suckling and weaning stage. In rats, levels of GLUT2 mRNA in the small intestine are either relatively constant from birth until postweaning[152] or increase gradually and modestly from birth until weaning.[151] In humans, levels of GLUT2 mRNA increase with development.[108]

In summary, ontogenetic development of SGLT1 at the molecular level differs between rats and sheep. In rats, glucose transport rates per mg decrease modestly, whereas SGLT1 mRNA levels do not change with development; both these events are hardwired. In sheep, the developmentally-related decrease in transport rates and protein levels is much more dramatic, but is reversible when glucose is infused luminally. In both species, marked and consistent differences in magnitude of changes in levels of mRNA and in rates of transport suggest that regulation is post-transcriptional. As with SGLT1, there are either no changes or only modest changes in levels of GLUT2 mRNA with development.

Amino acids. The pattern of basic amino acid transport per mg in rat intestine during development is similar to the expression of y$^+$ mRNA.[4,40] Levels of y$^+$ mRNA are high before birth in rats, coinciding with appearance of transporter activity in various species, as reviewed by Buddington and Diamond.[3] Levels of mRNA then decrease modestly during the suckling stage, and subsequently increase during weaning and postweaning stages. This pattern, however, differs from the typical neonatal-to-adult decline in transport rate observed for prenatal onset amino acid transporters (described above, pp. 128 to 134).[157] This underlines the difficulty in comparing total transport of an amino acid transportable by several systems to that of levels of protein or mRNA coding for a single transport system.

The molecular mechanisms underlying the developmental pattern of appearance of other amino acid transporters have not yet been studied. Concentrations of mRNA for the apical peptide transporter PEPT are known to peak 4 days after rats are born, with a subsequent decline to adult levels.[158]

Regulatory Mechanisms

The regulatory mechanisms modulating activity of these nutrient transporters are poorly developed shortly after birth. For example, brushborder glucose transporters may not be modulated by diet before completion of weaning in rats. Large changes in dietary glucose levels that typically induce twofold changes in brushborder glucose transport rates in adult rats and mice[95] do not alter rates of glucose transport and levels of SGLT1 mRNA in gavaged suckling and pellet-fed weaning rats.[4,152,159,160] Similarly, suckling pigs are unable to modulate rates and capacities of glucose and fructose transport to match changes in the levels of different carbohydrates in the diet.[143]

The ability to modulate transport functions is apparently acquired at the time of weaning. For example, brushborder glucose transport in sheep is responsive to luminal nutrients. Direct infusion of glucose into the intestinal lumen increases transporter number and transport rate in sheep.[161] The density of transporters is correlated with the amount of substrate needing to be absorbed by the intestine. In rats, the reasons for maintenance of high rates of activity of prenatal onset transporters throughout ontogeny and for absence of dietary regulation of these transporters during suckling are not clear. Perhaps consistency in composition of dietary intake in omnivorous rodents did not favor the evolution of mechanisms that would regulate intestinal transport during early development.

There has been no study of dietary regulation of basolateral glucose transport during development. Levels of GLUT2 mRNA, however, do not change with dietary carbohydrate levels in weaning rats.[152] On the other hand, in adult rats glucose transport rate and GLUT2 transporter sites in the basolateral membrane change with dietary carbohydrate levels.[162,163]

Brushborder glucose transport is also independent of certain hormones known to dramatically alter the development of intestinal brushborder hydrolases. Brushborder glucose absorption is similar among adrenalectomized weaning rats fed high-glucose and glucose-free diets and sham-operated litter mates also fed high-glucose and glucose-free diets.[5] Likewise, glucocorticoids are unlikely to play a major regulatory role in postnatal maturation of glucose transport in pigs.[164] Finally, intestinal glucose transport per mg of tissue was similar between hypothyroid and euthyroid pups (Monteiro and Ferraris, unpublished observations).

In summary, luminal nutrients specifically modulate SGLT1 transporter expression in postweaning sheep, but not in preweaning rats.

Postnatal Onset Transporters

Developmental changes and regulatory mechanisms vary for the different postnatal onset transporters.

Transport Mechanisms

GLUT5. In contrast to that of prenatal onset transporters, activity of postnatal onset transporters is much lower during suckling compared to during subsequent stages. In rats, expression of GLUT5 protein and mRNA increases parallel to rates of transporter activity: low levels during suckling and weaning, high levels after completion of weaning.[107,126,152]

ASBT. An abrupt increase in transporter number is the main mechanism underlying the abrupt increase in transport rate of bile acids by rat, dog, and human ileum during weaning.[165,166] Dramatic (100×) increases in steady-state levels of mRNA parallel the increase in transporter number that occurs, typically, between 17 and 19 days postparturition in rats. These ontogenetic differences in expression are regulated partly at the transcriptional level, as nuclear transcription rates increase 15× between 7 and 28 days.[166] The large increase in mRNA levels and the smaller increase in transcription rates suggest a potential role of mRNA stability in regulating transporter abundance.

Mechanisms underlying developmental regulation of GLUT5 and ASBT genes may be increases in transcription rates and mRNA stability. An important question in developmental biology is why bile acid and fructose transporter genes are expressed strongly only in later stages of development of many species.

Regulatory Mechanisms

Unlike those of prenatal onset transporters, regulatory mechanisms modulating the activity of postnatal onset transporters clearly respond to dietary signals. This observation then leads to a question not only of fundamental but also of clinical importance: whether these transporters can be expressed earlier during development not only by dietary but also by hormonal manipulations. Its clinical relevance arises from the need to overcome immature and limited absorptive functions exhibited by prematurely born infants.[16,167] To answer this question, GLUT5 and ASBT will be used as models representing postnatal onset transporters.

Mechanisms modulating ontogenetic expression of GLUT5. Intestinal fructose transport rates and GLUT5 mRNA levels, typically low throughout suckling and weaning stages and typically high after weaning, can be precociously enhanced by dietary or luminal signals.[152,160] The receptive age is sharply defined: while fructose transport rates can be enhanced during weaning (15 to 24 days), they cannot be enhanced during suckling (≤ 14 days).[161] Luminal signals are highly specific: only dietary fructose and sucrose can enhance fructose transport (Figure 8–6). Changes in

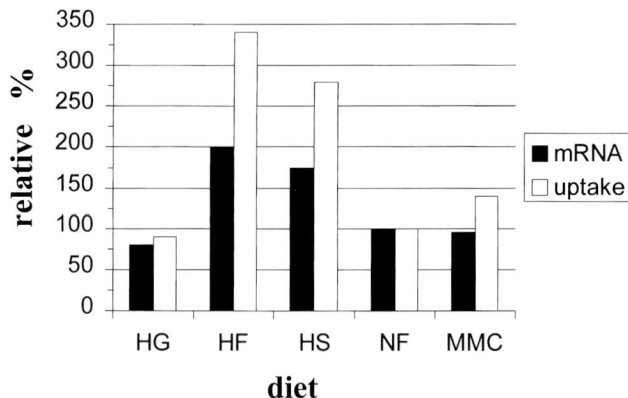

FIGURE 8–6. Enhancement of intestinal fructose transport rates and GLUT5 mRNA levels in 22-day-old weaning pups by precocious introduction of dietary fructose or sucrose. Transport rates and mRNA levels are each normally low until 28 to 30 days of age but can be increased dramatically by just 24 to 96 hours of feeding fructose-containing diets to 16- to 22-day-old pups. HG = high glucose; HF = high fructose; HS = high sucrose; NF = fructose free; MMC = littermates staying with the dam and subsisting on both milk and chow. Values are normalized to those observed in pups fed a fructose-free diet. (Data from Shu R, David ES, Ferraris RP. Precocious induction of intestinal fructose transport and GLUT5 expression in weaning rats. AM J Physiol 1997;272:G446–53.)

fructose absorption rates are tightly correlated with changes in levels of GLUT5 mRNA. The promoter region of GLUT5 contains a cAMP response element.[168]

The suckling-to-weaning transition (13 to 15 days) coincides with a large corticosterone surge;[169] increases in corticosterone levels may, therefore, play a major role in allowing substrate regulation of GLUT5 expression. Enhancement of fructose transport rates and GLUT5 mRNA levels by dietary fructose, however, is similar in adrenalectomized, weaning pups and in sham-operated litter mates,[5] suggesting that dietary induction in weaning rats is independent of corticosterone levels. Luminal fructose, and not endocrine or neurocrine signals, is apparently the only signal required to upregulate fructose transport and GLUT5 mRNA, since fructose feeding did not upregulate GLUT5 expression in bypassed loops of pups subjected to Thiry Vella surgery and subsequently fed high fructose diets (Figure 8–7).[39]

Glucocorticoids may play a role in permitting dietary regulation, though it is not required for regulation itself. When dexamethasone, a synthetic glucocorticoid, is given to suckling pups prior to gavage of fructose solutions, there are nonspecific increases in intestinal absorption of all nutrients. On top of this nonspecific increase, there is a pronounced, specific increase in fructose transport per mg in dexamethasone-treated suckling pups gavaged with high fructose, but not in litter mates gavaged with high glucose.[170] Hence, in suckling pups, precocious administration of exogenous glucocorticoids allows luminal fructose to regulate the GLUT5 gene; in weaning pups, GLUT5 is no longer responsive to glucocorticoids. Glucocorticoids

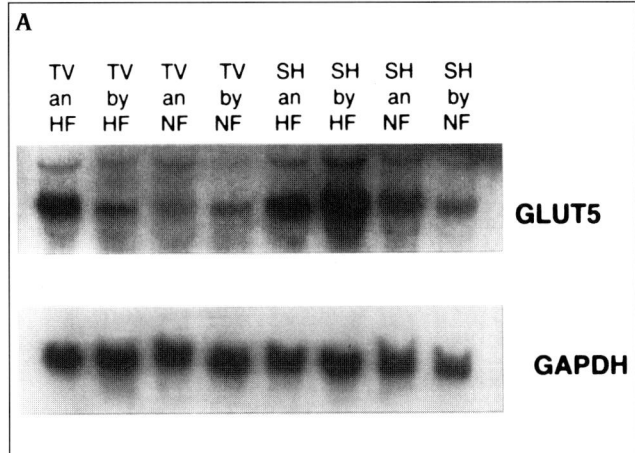
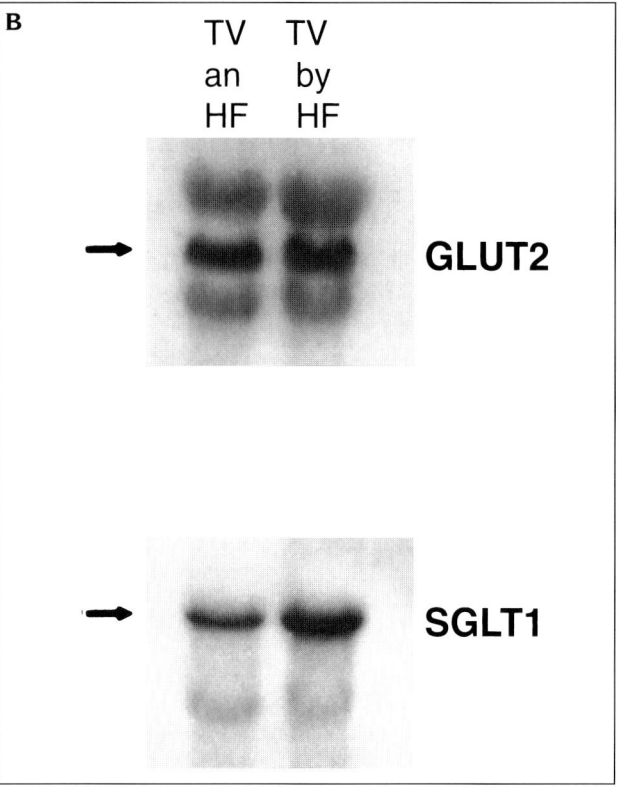

FIGURE 8–7A. Expression of GLUT5 mRNA (*top*) in the anastomosed (an) or bypassed (by) small intestine of rat pups subjected to Thiry Vella (TV) or sham (SH) surgery. Both ends of the bypassed loop in TV pups were exteriorized as stomas. The "bypassed region" in SH pups corresponded to the bypassed loop in TV pups, but instead of being exteriorized, it was reconnected to the remnant intestine (and thus was not actually bypassed). Pups were fed a high-fructose (HF) or fructose-free (NF) diet. GLUT5 mRNA levels and fructose transport rates (not shown) were higher in the anastomosed, compared to the bypassed, region of TV pups fed an HF diet. Levels of GLUT5 mRNA and rates of fructose transport (not shown) in the bypassed loop were similar to those in the anastomosed loop in TV pups fed NF. (From Shu R, David ES, Ferraris RP. Luminal fructose modulates fructose transport and GLUT5 expression in small intestine of weaning rats. Am J Physiol 1998;274:G232–9. Reprinted with permission from the American Physiological Society.)

FIGURE 8–7B. In contrast, levels of GLUT2 and SGLT1 mRNA were similar in anastomosed and bypassed intestinal regions of TV pups.

also promote a similar type of response in the sucrase-isomaltase gene: there is a permissive effect during suckling, and little or no effect during weaning.[171]

Dietary induction is independent of plasma thyroxine levels. Luminal fructose increases fructose transport rates and GLUT5 mRNA levels in euthyroid as well as in hypothyroid rat pups (Monteiro and Ferraris, unpublished observations).

Mechanisms modulating ontogenetic expression of ASBT. Like GLUT5, ASBT expression can be regulated by diet or hormones. Gavaging of taurocholate in 12-day-old rats induces precocious expression of ileal bile acid transport and hastens maturation of ileal villi.[118] Some of the increase is nonspecific (i.e., due to the stress of gavaging), but a significant portion is specific to taurocholate feeding. Pharmacologic doses of corticosteroids induce precocious development of bile acid transport when provided to pregnant rats or to suckling pups.[116,172]

In summary, prenatal or early-onset transporters are already significantly expressed before birth, but during suckling their expression may not be modulated by dietary or endocrine signals. In contrast, postnatal or late-onset transporters are expressed well after birth; and once present, their expression is specifically regulated not only by diet, but in some cases by endocrine signals as well.

CLINICAL CORRELATES OF NUTRIENT TRANSPORT DERANGEMENTS

Malabsorption of certain specific nutrients occurs in neonates mainly because active intestinal transport systems are either insufficient or absent. The inability of the intestinal mucosa to absorb a dietary nutrient is a result of conditions categorized as either congenital or acquired. A congenital condition of nutrient intolerance could be due to the deficiency (e.g., congenital glucose-galactose malabsorption) or diminished quantity (e.g., congenital short gut syndrome) of transporters. An acquired condition of nutrient malabsorption can be a consequence of different pathology (e.g., inflammatory bowel disease) that can lead to a temporary or even permanent loss of certain transporters. In both congenital and acquired defects, unabsorbed nutrients then pass through the entire length of the small intestinal tract, causing various biochemical and physiological effects in both the colon and distal small intestine.

Carbohydrate Malabsorption

The end-products of intestinal carbohydrate digestion are the monosaccharides glucose, galactose, and fructose. Normal intestinal absorption of the monosaccharides is important, because 24 to 50 percent of an infant's energy need is provided by dietary carbohydrates.[173]

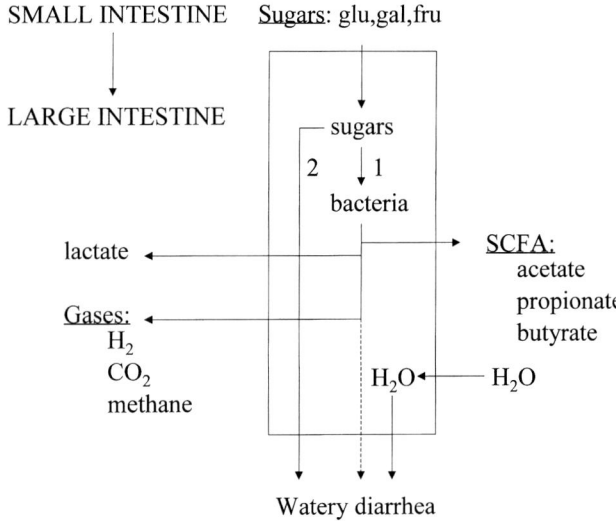

FIGURE 8–8. Consequences of malabsorbed carbohydrates. Pathway 1. Bacterial fermentation of unabsorbed sugars (glu = glucose; gal = galactose; fru = fructose) in the large intestine produces short chain fatty acids (SCFA), lactate, and various gases. Pathway 2. Unabsorbed sugars not fermented by colonic bacteria create a hyperosmolar colonic environment that draws water from the body and leads to a watery diarrhea.

Malabsorbed carbohydrates have two effects (Figure 8–8). First, colonic bacterial fermentation of sugars produces short-chain fatty acids (SCFAs: acetate, butyrate, propionate), lactate, and various gases, including hydrogen, carbon dioxide, and methane.[174,175] Short-chain fatty acids are important in maintaining the functional integrity of the colon.[176–179] Second, unfermented sugars increase the osmolality of luminal contents to values higher than those of plasma, thereby attracting water and eventually producing a watery diarrhea.[180,181] Ironically, as a consequence of this osmotic type of diarrhea, SCFAs may become malabsorbed because of rapid transit out of the colon. Fermentation might become disrupted because of a bacterial mass-dilution effect of the watery diarrhea, and a rapid transit time causing a bacterial flush out of the colon.[182]

In carbohydrate malabsorption, a watery diarrhea develops immediately or a few days after the ingestion of the unabsorbed substrate, and subsides when the offending sugar is removed from the diet.

Tests of Congenital Carbohydrate Malabsorption

The looseness of the stools and the frequency of stooling should be checked from the patient's clinical history. The presence of sugar in the stool can be determined by checking for significant levels of reducing substances. Metabolism of hydrolyzed sugars by colonic bacteria yields an acidic pH that can easily be tested with the use of Nitrazine paper (Squibb and Sons, Princeton, NJ). The techniques of breath H_2 and $^{13}CO_2$ tests detect and quantify H_2 and CO_2 gas produced by colonic bacterial fermentation.[183–186] A xylose tolerance test can also be used to test for malabsorption due to intestinal villous atrophy.[187] Intestinal biopsy is only indicated for confirmation of initial diagnosis.[188]

Congenital Carbohydrate Malabsorption

Glucose-galactose malabsorption (GGM), isolated fructose malabsorption, and fructose-glucose-galactose malabsorption have been reported.[189–192]

Glucose-galactose malabsorption. Glucose-galactose malabsorption (GGM) is the only genetically-established form of abnormal monosaccharide absorption in humans.[193,194] This autosomal recessive disorder of glucose and galactose absorption has been mapped to chromosome 22q13.1.[195] A missense mutation causing glucose and galactose malabsorption is the result of a G→A conversion at nucleotide position 92 that mutated Asp^{28}→Asn, rendering SGLT1 nonfunctional.[196] Martin et al.[197] have identified 31 new mutations of SGLT1 in 25 families with GGM. A total of 17 homozygous and 16 heterozygous mutations were observed, most of which were missense mutations and the remainder nonsense, frame shift, and splice-site mutations. Many missense mutations involve the insertion or deletion of charged and polar residues, and impair SGLT1 trafficking to the plasma membrane, the transport cycle, or both.

The main GGM symptom is severe watery diarrhea leading to dehydration, malnutrition, failure to thrive, and even death.[189] The stool is voluminous, has low pH because of fermentation of unabsorbed sugar, and has increased amounts of SCFA. Chemical analyses of stools in these patients will show the absence of lactose but will test positive for the monosaccharides glucose and galactose. Fructose, which is absorbed by GLUT5, is well tolerated. Symptoms are resolved after a diet free of lactose and sucrose is instituted. Prenatal screening for GGM is now available for suspected cases, and this will decrease postnatal morbidity associated with this condition.[198]

A much rarer form of total monosaccharide malabsorption, fructose-glucose-galactose malabsorption, whose rate of occurrence is unknown, has been reported, and its presentation is much more severe and life-threatening.[199] Profuse diarrhea develops immediately after sugar intake. Intestinal disaccharidase levels are usually normal, and all three monosaccharides are present in abundant quantities in the stool. Symptoms subside with complete elimination of sugars from the diet. The affected patient is managed with total parenteral nutrition (TPN) as a carbohydrate-free diet is introduced. This disorder may be due not to the absence of SGLT1 and GLUT5 at the brushborder membrane, but rather to a defect in the transport system that is shared by the three monosaccharides (i.e., GLUT2) at the basolateral membrane, where these monosaccharides are transported from the cytosol to the bloodstream. To date, documentation of this disorder is scanty.

Fructose malabsorption. Fructose, as a monosaccharide, is normally not a sugar component in a newborn's diet. But as a byproduct of the hydrolytic digestion of sucrose, there is an increased exposure to this sugar during infancy. Fructose malabsorption is a major cause of gastrointestinal distress in adults and a major culprit in functional or irritable bowel syndrome.[200–203] A possible explanation is the potential deficiency of the intestinal fructose transporter

GLUT5 in these patients. Because of the increasing rate of using fructose as a major sugar in fruit juices or as a sweetener in various dietary products, and because of the cultural trends of introducing these products at an earlier age, dietary fructose has been implicated as a significant cause of chronic nonspecific diarrhea of childhood, or "toddler's diarrhea." This phenomenon makes teleologic sense, since GLUT5, which is a late-onset transporter, is not fully elaborated until weaning. The infant's and toddler's intestines may be ill-prepared to handle dietary fructose. After fructose feeding, malabsorption of fructose occurs, followed by diarrhea.

Isolated fructose malabsorption is the result of genetic absence of the fructose transporter GLUT5. Diarrhea and abdominal colic are symptoms that disappear after a shift to a fructose-free diet. An autosomal recessive inheritance is postulated.[191] Breath H_2 test and, to a limited extent, $^{13}CO_2$ breath test have made clear these cases of deficient intestinal fructose absorption.[203]

Differential diagnoses. Defects in brushborder enzymes are, by far, the leading cause of carbohydrate intolerance across all age groups. The most prevalent carbohydrate malabsorption syndrome in man is the result of the developmental deficiency or absence of intestinal lactase activity.[204] The incidence of lactase deficiency ranges from 5 to 60%, depending on the race and population of patients.[205] Symptoms are usually alleviated by the provision of the enzyme lactase, which is involved in the disaccharide breakdown, or the elimination of the disaccharide lactose from the diet. Cystic fibrosis patients also exhibit gastrointestinal symptoms of abdominal distress and diarrhea that mimic carbohydrate malabsorption symptoms.[206,207] Gluten-induced enteropathy, although rare in neonates, is another condition that should be considered.[208,209]

Acquired Carbohydrate Malabsorption

Carbohydrate malabsorption may also arise from a variety of primary conditions:

1. An abnormally rapid intestinal transit time in diarrheal illnesses leads to nutrient malabsorption in general, and to carbohydrate malabsorption in particular.[210]
2. Following infectious viral or bacterial gastroenteritis, injury to the intestinal mucosa gives rise to a secondary brushborder disaccharidase deficiency, or to a temporary absence of sugar transporters due to exfoliated enterocytes. A denuded intestinal lining results from pathogens damaging the bowel wall, and leads to a diminished absorptive area and to compromised function of the remaining intestinal cells. In rotaviral enteritis, defective glucose transport is also the result of reduced disaccharidase and Na+-K+ ATPase activities. Glucose-stimulated Na+ transport is impaired in the small bowel epithelium after the virus invades the intestinal mucosa. Diarrhea and malabsorption follow.[211]
3. In neonates with necrotizing enterocolitis (NEC), there is intestinal mucosal destruction leading to a temporary deficiency of the mucosal brushborder enzymes involved in the hydrolysis of dietary sugars and of transporter proteins involved in absorption of monosaccharides. A decreased intestinal absorptive capacity heralds the onset of clinical symptoms of patients who later develop fulminant NEC.[212] Breath H_2 in NEC patients is also increased.[213]
4. Sugar intolerance should be considered in young children recovering from intestinal surgery. Diarrhea only develops when feeding is first initiated following a period of intravenous nutrition therapy or when a stronger feed is reintroduced. Reintroduction and rapid advancement of oral feedings after starvation or prolonged fasting also lead to malabsorption due to fasting-induced intestinal villous atrophy.[214,215]

Acquired short bowel syndrome is a result of radical surgery for conditions such as NEC (the leading cause of short bowel syndrome in infancy), intestinal atresias, midgut volvulus, extensive intestinal aganglionosis, and omphalocele-gastroschisis.[216,217] A substantial shortening of the small or large intestines may lead to malabsorption and, therefore, malnutrition.[218]

5. Inflammatory bowel diseases have associated villous atrophy, crypt hyperplasia, and increased intestinal permeability. When enteral nutrition is introduced, malabsorption occurs and diarrhea follows.[219]

In summary, carbohydrate malabsorption results from various congenital and acquired conditions that affect all ages and all stages of gut development. The significance of carbohydrate intolerance is that carbohydrates constitute a major proportion of the host's energy supply. Consequences of carbohydrate malabsorption include biochemical and physiological effects that can be life threatening.

Amino Acid Transport Abnormalities

Although the diet of newborns is only 8 to 10% protein, this intake is more than sufficient to maintain positive nitrogen balance. There are 10 to 15 inherited disorders of intestinal amino acid transport that have been identified.[220,221] Many more of these genetic abnormalities of amino acid transport involve the kidney and liver.[220] The well-described disorders of amino acid transport involving the small intestine, such as Hartnup disease and cystinuria, may not manifest overt symptoms of amino acid malabsorption because the affected amino acids are also absorbed in the form of peptides.[220] Additionally, more than one system may be involved in the transport of these amino acids.[36] Hence, the loss of the specific transport system may not significantly affect the overall transport of the particular amino acid into the cell because of the existence of these so-called "backup" systems (Figure 8–9). Amino acids transported as part of peptide chains are released intracellularly into free amino acids and get absorbed into the bloodstream. Within the cell, these amino acids may also link with other amino acids, and subsequently cross the basolateral membrane. Amino acid groups that share the same transporter, therefore, may not equally be affected by the deficiency of the shared transport system. Most inborn errors of intestinal amino acid transport may also be paralleled by concomitant deficiencies in the renal transport systems for the same group of amino acids affected, which may significantly influence their clinical presentation. Amino acid transport is affected in a process similar to that of sugar transport in diarrheal conditions due to brushborder damage or loss.[222] In rats with overwhelm-

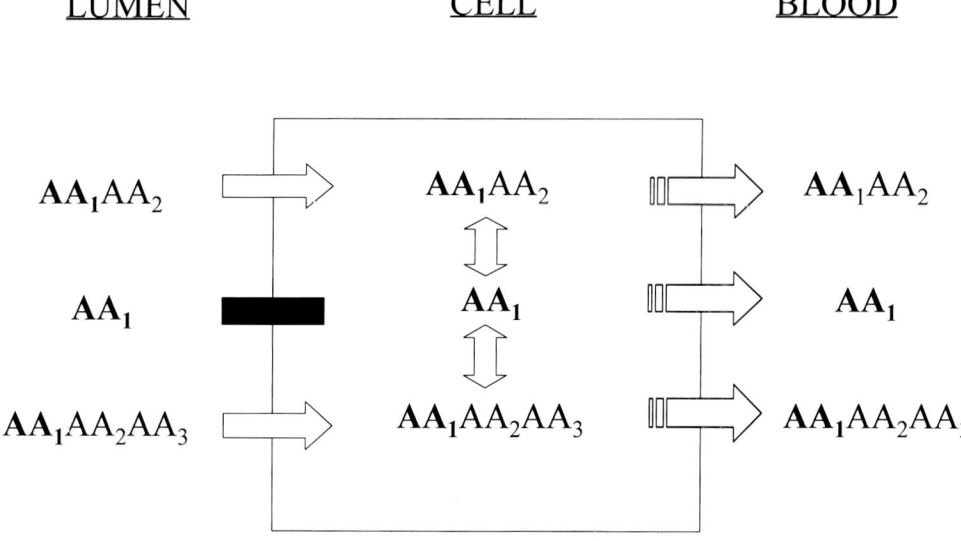

FIGURE 8–9. Schematic diagram of intestinal brushborder amino acid uptake by various transport systems. A defect (*solid rectangle*) in the brushborder transporter of a specific amino acid (AA_1) does not produce a deficiency because AA_1 can also be transported as part of a dipeptide (AA_1AA_2) or a tripeptide ($AA_1AA_2AA_3$) across the brushborder membrane (*open arrows*). The amino acid can then cross the basolateral membrane using transport systems (*dashed open arrows*) different from those in the brushborder membrane.

ing infection intestinal amino acid absorption is shown to be impaired.[223,224] To date, no genetic disorder of intestinal peptide transport has been reported.[36]

Bile Acid Transport Abnormalities

Bile acid malabsorption is often secondary to a diarrheal disease or to a partial or total resection of the terminal ileum. Bile acids are either passively absorbed along the length of the small intestine or actively assimilated by an active high-affinity transport system in the distal ileum.[225,226] Any disturbance of the former has insignificant consequences, while any disturbance of the latter may lead to malabsorption and, therefore, increased entry of bile acids into the colon, leading to diarrhea. Since the distal ileum plays a central role in the conservation of bile acids within the enterohepatic circulation, any disease involving the terminal ileum will result in abnormalities of bile acid absorption and metabolism. Enterohepatic circulation is, therefore, interrupted in such cases as ileal resection due to atresias or necrotizing enterocolitis and subsequent short bowel syndrome, intestinal bypass surgery, or in any inflammatory involvement of the terminal ileum. These conditions will lead to bile acid loss and subsequent bile acid diarrhea.[227,228] The rapid transit time in diarrheal illnesses also results in less time for bile acids to be absorbed.[225]

Congenital Short Bowel Syndrome

The diagnosis of congenital short bowel syndrome loosely includes various intestinal anomalies such as gastroschisis, atresias, malrotation, volvulus, and apple peel anomaly of the superior mesenteric artery.[229] The overall function of the gut is usually impaired. A dysmotile small intestine, a sequela of vascular insufficiency, presents as a functional bowel obstruction. The malabsorption picture arising from a dysmotile small intestine is a function of diminished surface area for absorption of nutrients. Once the dysmotile gut is challenged with luminal substrates, chronic severe diarrhea develops and failure to thrive ensues, unless optimal parenteral nutrition is provided. With gradual introduction and increase in the volume of feeds, intestinal adaptation, such as villous hyperplasia and increase in bowel length, eventually develops, leading to improved feeding tolerance.[230]

FUTURE DIRECTIONS

Little is known about development of intestinal nutrient transport; and much less is known about both molecular mechanisms underlying developmental patterns and regulatory mechanisms modulating intestinal nutrient transport during ontogeny. We conclude by providing research directions that are especially promising considering how little information there is about intestinal nutrient transport during development. Instead of giving an exhaustive list, we only suggest what we think are studies that should be conducted in the near future.

1. Cellular and molecular mechanisms underlying development of amino acid transport. We have described developmental patterns of intestinal amino acid transport, but, surprisingly, there is virtually no information about cellular and molecular mechanisms underlying development of this important class of transporters. Perhaps the reason for this neglect is that carrier-mediated transport of amino acids already occurs before birth. Nevertheless,

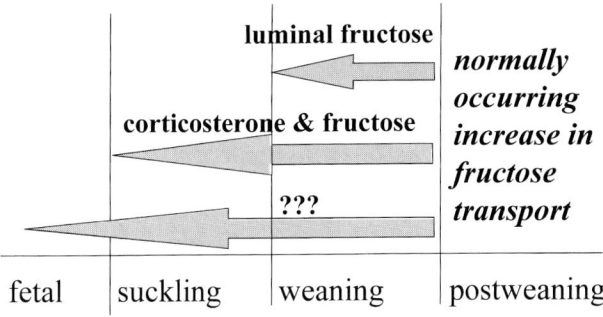

FIGURE 8–10. Dietary and hormonal manipulations can precociously enhance transport activity of GLUT5. Luminal fructose alone enhances activity of fructose transporters (and mRNA levels of GLUT5) during weaning (*top arrow*), but glucocorticoids are apparently needed before luminal fructose can enhance fructose transport in suckling pups (*middle arrow*). It is not known whether these manipulations can enhance fructose transport prenatally (*bottom arrow with question marks*).

greater understanding may lead to procedures that can enhance their activity in intestines of premature infants.

2. Developmental patterns of intestinal peptide transport. Not only are peptide transporters critical for providing the developing intestine with energy and essential nutrients; they are also important for absorption of b-lactam antibiotics[231] and possibly other peptide-like compounds.[232] Hence, age-related changes in peptide transporters could influence antibiotic efficacy.

3. Cellular and molecular mechanisms underlying development of brushborder glucose, fructose, and bile acid transport in the small intestine. Therapeutic peptides targeted to the bile acid transporter[233] may be effective only after infants have expressed ileal bile acid transporters. A key question for postnatal onset transporters such as GLUT5 and ASBT is whether they can be expressed earlier during development (Figure 8–10).

4. Developmental patterns of vitamin absorption. It is not known whether transport systems for certain vitamins or categories of vitamins develop prenatally or postnatally. This information is of clinical importance, since absorption of vitamins may prove limiting for infants who have higher daily requirements for these essential nutrients.

5. Developmental patterns of nutrient transport in the basolateral membrane. Almost nothing is known. Transporters in the basolateral membrane provide nutrients to enterocytes, and may prove important in the growth, maturation and differentiation of the intestinal mucosa.

6. There are three sources of the signals that trigger ontogenetic changes in transport functions. First, genetically-programmed timing mechanisms are present within the intestine. These are subject to modulation by another set of signals that originate from internal sites other than the intestine, such as glucocorticoids and thyroid hormones.[234] The role of these endocrine factors in regulating developmental appearance of transporters, especially during the suckling stage, remains largely unknown, in contrast to the very large literature on the effect of hormonal factors on brushborder hydrolases. The third source of signals is dietary, hence external, signals. Transport functions are known to be modulated by luminal nutrient levels.[235] Moreover, the biogenic amines that result from bacterial metabolism of dietary inputs can influence transport functions. Also to be considered are non-nutritive, biologically active substances present in dietary inputs, such as those in milk and amniotic fluid. There is a need to better understand the "windows of opportunity" during which the program of the developing intestine is responsive to the different signals that originate from the three sources.

7. The relationship between transporter functions and the chemical and physical characteristics of the membrane environment. It is uncertain how developmentally-related and diet-related shifts in membrane composition and physical features might influence transporter functions in the apical and basolateral membranes.

This work was supported by NIH grant AG11403, USDA grant 94-38500-0044, US Department of Commerce grant NA36-RG0505, and the UMDNJ Graduate School of Biomedical Sciences.

REFERENCES

1. Henning SJ, Rubin DC, Shulman RJ. Ontogeny of the intestinal mucosa. In: Johnson LR, editor. Physiology of the gastrointestinal tract. 3rd ed. New York: Raven Press; 1994. p. 571–610.
2. Henning SJ. Functional development of the gastrointestinal tract. In: Johnson LR, editor. Physiology of the gastrointestinal tract. 2nd ed. New York: Raven Press; 1987. p. 285–300.
3. Buddington RK, Diamond JM. Ontogenetic development of intestinal nutrient transporters. Annu Rev Physiol 1989; 51:601–19.
4. Toloza EM, Diamond J. Ontogenetic development of nutrient transporters in rat intestine. Am J Physiol 1992;263:G593–604.
5. Monteiro IM, Ferraris RP. Precocious enhancement of intestinal fructose uptake by diet in adrenalectomized rat pups. Pediatr Res 1997;41:1–7.
6. Crane RK. The physiology of the intestinal absorption of sugars. In: Jeanes A, Hodge J, editors. Physiological effects of food carbohydrates. Washington DC: American Chemical Society; 1975. p. 2–19.
7. Heird WC, Gomez MR. Total parenteral nutrition in necrotizing enterocolitis. Clin Perinatol 1994;21:389–409.
8. Ferraris RP, Diamond JM. Regulation of intestinal sugar transport. Physiol Rev 1997;77:257–302.
9. Unger A, Goetzman BW, Chan C, et al. Nutritional practices and outcome of extremely premature infants. Am J Dis Child 1986;140:1027–37.
10. Troche B, Harvey-Wilkes K, Engle WD, et al. Early minimal feedings promote growth in critically ill premature infants. Biol Neonate 1995;67:172–81.
11. Bhatia AM, Feddersen RM, Musemeche CA. The role of luminal nutrients in intestinal injury from mesenteric reperfusion and platelet-activating factor in the developing rat. J Surg Res 1996;63:152–6.
12. Romero R, Kleinman RE. Feeding the very low birth weight infant. Pediatr Rev 1993;14:123–32.

13. Shulman RJ, Feste A, Ou C. Absorption of lactose, glucose polymers or combination in premature infants. J Pediatr 1995;127:626–31.
14. Ehrhardt MA, Bell AW. Developmental increases in glucose transporter concentrations in the sheep placenta. Am J Physiol 1997;272:R1132–41.
15. Koldovsky O. Development of absorption of monosaccharides. In: Lebenthal E, editor. Human gastrointestinal development. New York: Raven Press; 1989. p. 437–49.
16. Carver JD, Barness LA. Trophic factors for the gastrointestinal tract. Clin Perinatol 1996;23:265–85.
17. Puchal AA, Buddington RK. Postnatal development of monosaccharide transport in pig intestine. Am J Physiol 1992;262:G895–902.
18. Madara JL, Trier JS. The functional morphology of the mucosa of the small intestine. In: Johnson L, editor. Physiology of the gastrointestinal tract. 2nd ed. New York: Raven Press, 1987. p. 1209–49.
19. Ferraris RP, Yasharpour S, Lloyd KCK, et al. Luminal glucose concentrations in the gut under normal conditions. Am J Physiol 1990;259:G822–37.
20. Toloza EM, Lam M, Diamond J. Nutrient extraction by cold-exposed mice: a test of digestive safety margins. Am J Physiol 1991;261:G608–20.
21. Diamond J. Evolutionary design of intestinal nutrient absorption: enough but not too much. News Physiol Sci 1991;6:92–6.
22. Pappenheimer JR. Physiological regulation of epithelial junctions in intestinal epithelia. Acta Physiol Scand 1988;133:43–51.
23. Pappenheimer JR. Paracellular intestinal absorption of glucose, creatinine, and mannitol in normal animals: relation to body size. Am J Physiol 1990;295:G290–9.
24. Pappenheimer JR. On the coupling of membrane digestion with intestinal absorption of sugars and amino acids. Am J Physiol 1993;265:G409–17.
25. Hediger MA, Coady MJ, Ikeda TS, Wright EM. Expression cloning and cDNA sequencing of the Na+/glucose cotransporter. Nature 1987;330:379–81.
26. Burant CF, Takeda J, Brot-Laroche E, et al. Fructose transport in human spermatozoa and small intestine is GLUT5. J Biol Chem 1992;267:14523–6.
27. Mueckler M. Facilitative glucose transporters. Eur J Biochem 1994;219:713–25.
28. Cheeseman CI. GLUT2 is the transporter for fructose across the rat intestinal basolateral membrane. Gastroenterology 1993;105:1050–6.
29. Pessin JE, Bell GI. Mammalian facilitative glucose transporter family: structure and molecular regulation. Annu Rev Physiol 1992;54:911–30.
30. Hediger MA, Rhoads RB. Molecular physiology of sodium-glucose cotransporters. Physiol Rev 1994;74:993–1026.
31. Thorens B. Glucose transporters in the regulation of intestinal, renal and liver glucose fluxes. Am J Physiol 1996;270:G541–53.
32. Wright EM, Hirsch JR, Loo DD, Zampighi GA. Regulation of sodium-glucose cotransporters. J Exp Biol 1997;200:207–83.
33. Munck BG. Transport of glycine and lysine on the chloride dependent beta alanine (BO+) carrier in rabbit small intestine. Biochim Biophys Acta 1955;1235:93–9.
34. Castagna M, Shayakul C, Trotti D, et al. Molecular characteristics of mammalian and insect amino acid transporters: implications for amino acid homeostasis. J Exp Biol 1997;200:269–86.
35. Hopfer U. Membrane transport mechanisms for hexoses and amino acids in the small intestine. In: Johnson LR, editor. Physiology of the gastrointestinal tract. Vol. 2. New York: Raven Press; 1987. p. 1499–526.
36. Ganapathy V, Brandsch M, Leibach FH. Intestinal transport of amino acids and peptides. In: Johnson LR, editor. Physiology of the gastrointestinal tract. New York: Raven Press; 1994. p. 1773–94.
37. Kanai Y, Hediger MA. Primary structure and functional characterization of a high-affinity glutamate transporter. Nature 1992;360:467–71.
38. Rothstein J, Martin L, Levey A, et al. Localization of neuronal and glial glutamate transporters. Neuron 1994;13:713–25.
39. Lehre K, Levy L, Ottersen O, et al. Differential expression of the two glial glutamate transporters in the rat brain: quantitative and immunocytochemical observation. J Neurosci 1995;15:1835–53.
40. Puppi M, Henning SJ. Cloning of the rat ecotropic retroviral receptor and studies of its expression in intestinal tissues. Proc Soc Exp Biol Med 1995;209:38–45.
41. Leibach FH, Ganapathy V. Peptide transporters in the intestine and the kidney. Annu Rev Nutr 1996;16:99–119.
42. Saito H, Inui KI. Dipeptide transporters in apical and basolateral membranes of the human intestinal cell line Caco-2. Am J Physiol 1993;265:G289–94.
43. Wong MH, Oelkers P, Craddock AL, Dawson PA. Expression cloning and characterization of the hamster ileal sodium-dependent bile acid transporter. J Biol Chem 1994;269:1340–7.
44. Hagenbuch B, Meier PJ. Molecular cloning, chromosomal localization, and functional characterization of a human liver sodium/bile acid cotransporter. J Clin Invest 1994;93:1326–31.
45. Christie DM, Dawson PA, Thevananther S, Shneider BL. Comparative analysis of the ontogeny of a sodium-dependent bile acid transporter in rat kidney and ileum. Am J Physiol 1996;271:G377–85.
46. Aldini R, Roda A, Montagnani M, Roda E. Bile acid structure and intestinal absorption in the animal model. Ital J Gastroenterol 1995;27:141–4.
47. Karasov WH, Diamond JM. A simple method for measuring intestinal glucose transport in vitro. Am J Physiol 1983;245:G445–62.
48. Hirsh AJ, Tsang R, Kammila S, Cheeseman CI. Effect of cholecystokinin and related peptides on jejunal transepithelial hexose transport in the Sprague Dawley rat. Am J Physiol 1996;271:G755–61.
49. Uhing MR, Kimura RE. Active transport of 3-O-methylglucose by the small intestine in chronically catheterized rats. J Clin Invest 1995;95:2799–805.
50. Altmann GG, Enesco M. Cell number as a measure of distribution and renewal of epithelial cells in the small intestine of growing and adult rats. Am J Anat 1967;121:319–36.
51. Smith MW. Autoradiographic analysis of alanine uptake by newborn pig intestine. Experientia 1981;37:868–70.
52. Schwarz SM, Hostetler B, Ling SC, Watkins JB. Intestinal membrane lipid composition and fluidity during development in the rat. Am J Physiol 1985;248:G200–10.
53. Schwarz SM, Bostwick HE, Danziger MD, et al. Ontogeny of basolateral membrane lipid composition and fluidity in small intestine. Am J Physiol 1989;257:G138–44.
54. Perin N, Keelan M, Jarocka-Cyrta E, et al. Ontogeny of intestinal adaptation in rats in response to isocaloric changes in dietary lipids. Am J Physiol 1997;273:G713–20.
55. Brasitus TA, Dudeja PK, Bolt MJ, et al. Dietary triacylglycerol modulates sodium-dependent D-glucose transport, fluidity and fatty acid composition of rat small intestinal brush-border membrane. Biochim Biophys Acta 1989;979:177–86.
56. Debnam ES, Sharp PA. Acute and chronic effects of pancreatic glucagon on sugar transport across the brushborder and basolateral membranes of rat jejunal enterocytes. Exp Physiol 1993;78:197–207.

57. Baxter PJ, Goldhill J, Hardcastle J, et al. Enhanced intestinal glucose and alanine transport in cystic fibrosis. Gut 1990; 31:817–20.
58. Pappenheimer JR, Volpp K. Transmucosal impedance of small intestine: correlation with transport of sugars and amino acids. Am J Physiol 1992;263:C480–93.
59. Ferraris RP, Villenas SA, Hirayama BA, Diamond J. Effect of dietary carbohydrate on intestinal glucose transporter site density along the crypt-villus axis. Am J Physiol 1992;262: G1060–8.
60. Ferraris RP, Diamond JM. Crypt/villus site of substrate-dependent regulation of mouse intestinal glucose transporters. Proc Natl Acad Sci U S A 1993;90:5868–72.
61. Ferraris RP, Diamond JM. Use of phlorizin binding to demonstrate induction of intestinal glucose transporters. J Membr Biol 1986;94:77–92.
62. Ferraris RP, Lee PP, Diamond JM. Origin of regional and species differences in intestinal glucose uptake. Am J Physiol 1989;257:G689–97.
63. Shirazi-Beechey SP, Hirayama BA, Wang Y, et al. Ontogenic development of lamb intestinal sodium-glucose cotransporter is regulated by diet. J Physiol (Lond) 1991;437:699–708.
64. Buddington RK, Diamond JM. Ontogenetic development of nutrient transporters in rabbit intestine. Am J Physiol 1990; 259:G544–55.
65. Buddington RK, Diamond JM. Ontogenetic development of nutrient transport in cat intestine. Am J Physiol 1992; 263:G605–16.
66. Cheeseman CI, Maenz DD. Rapid regulation of D-glucose transport in basolateral membrane of rat jejunum. Am J Physiol 1988;256:G878–83.
67. Maenz DD, Cheeseman CI. Effect of hyperglycemia on D-glucose transport across the brush border and basolateral membranes of rat small intestine. Biochim Biophys Acta 1986;860:277–85.
68. Diamond JM, Karasov WH. Effect of dietary carbohydrate on monosaccharide uptake by mouse small intestine in vitro. J Physiol (Lond) 1984;349:419–40.
69. Smith MW. Postnatal development of transport function in the pig intestine. Comp Biochem Physiol Comp Physiol 1988; 90A:577–82.
70. Buddington RK. Nutrition and ontogenetic development of the intestine. Can J Physiol Pharmacol 1994;72:251–9.
71. Rubin DC. Spatial analysis of transcriptional activation in fetal rat jejunal and ileal gut epithilium. Am J Physiol 1992; 263:G853–62.
72. Murray RD, Ailabouni AH, Powers PA, et al. Absorption of lactose from colon of newborn piglet. Am J Physiol 1991; 261:G1–8.
73. Buddington RK, Malo C. Intestinal brush-border membrane enzyme activities and transport functions during prenatal development of pigs. J Pediatr Gastroenterol Nutr 1996;23:51–64.
74. Smith MW. Autoradiographic analysis of alanine uptake by newborn pig intestine. Experientia 1981;37:868–70.
75. Smith MW, Peacock MA. Anomalous replacement of foetal enterocytes in the neonatal pig. Proc R Soc Lond B Biol Sci 1980;206:411–20.
76. Smith MW, Jarvis LG. Growth and cell replacement in the new-born pig intestine. Proc R Soc Lond B Biol Sci 1978; 203:69–89.
77. Vazquez CM, Rovira N, Ruiz-Gutierrez V, Planas JM. Developmental changes in glucose transport, lipid composition, and fluidity of jejunal BBM. Am J Physiol 1997;273: R1086–93.
78. Marti T, Gonzalez E, Vinardell MP. Elucidation of intestinal transport results as a function of age. Physiol Res 1996;45:31–7.
79. Omodeo-Sale F, Lindi C, Marciani P, et al. Postnatal maturation of rat intestinal membrane: lipid composition and fluidity. Comp Biochem Physiol A Comp Physiol 1991;100:301–7.
80. Schwarz SM, Ling S, Hostetler B, et al. Lipid composition and membrane fluidity in the small intestine of the developing rabbit. Gastroenterology 1984;86:1544–51.
81. Meddings JB, DeSouza D, Goel M, Thiesen S. Glucose transport and microvillus membrane physical properties along the crypt-villus axis of the rabbit. J Clin Invest 1990; 85:1099–107.
82. Miller BG, James PS, Smith MW, Bourne FJ. Effect of weaning on the capacity of pig intestinal villi to digest and absorb nutrients. J Agric Sci Camb 1986;107:579–89.
83. Reimer RA, Field CJ, McBurney MI. Ontogenetic changes in proglucagon mRNA in BB diabetes prone and normal rats weaned onto a chow diet. Diabetologia 1997;40:871–8.
84. Smith MW, Mitchell MA, Peacock MA. Effects of genetic selection on growth rate and intestinal structure in the domestic fowl (*Gallus domesticus*). Comp Biochem Physiol Comp Physiol 1990; 97A:57–63.
85. Fan YK, Croom WJ Jr, Eisen EJ, et al. Selection for growth does not affect apparent energetic efficiency of jejunal glucose uptake in mice. J Nutr 1996;126:2851–60.
86. Widdowson EM. Development of the digestive system: comparative animal studies. Am J Clin Nutr 1985;41:384–90.
87. Xu R-J, Mellor DJ, Tungthanathanich P, et al. Growth and morphological changes in the small and large intestine in piglets during the first three days after birth. J Dev Physiol 1992;18:161–72.
88. Zhang HC, Malo C, Buddington RK. Suckling induces rapid intestinal growth and changes in brush border digestive functions of newborn pigs. J Nutr 1997;127:418–26.
89. Buddington RK, Lepine AJ. Postnatal development of cat intestine: changes in dimensions and nutrient transport. FASEB J 1997;11:A34.
90. Obst BS, Diamond J. Ontogenesis of intestinal nutrient transport in domestic chickens (Gallus gallus) and its relation to growth. Auk 1992;109:451–64.
91. Jackson S, Diamond J. Ontogenetic development of gut function, growth, and metabolism in a wild bird, the red jungle fowl. Am J Physiol 1995;269:R1163–73.
92. Moreno M, Otero M, Tur JA, et al. Kinetic constants of alpha-methyl-D-glucoside transport in the chick small intestine during perinatal development. Mech Ageing Dev 1996;92:11–20.
93. Buddington RK, Chen JW, Diamond JM. Genetic and phenotypic adaptation of intestinal nutrient transport to diet in fish. J Physiol 1987;393:261–81.
94. Toloza EM, Diamond JM. Ontogenetic development of transporter regulation in bullfrog intestine. Am J Physiol 1990; 258:G770–3.
95. Ferraris RP, Diamond JM. Specific regulation of intestinal nutrient transporters by their dietary substrates. Annu Rev Physiol 1989;51:125–41.
96. Malo C. Kinetic evidence for heterogeneity in Na+-D-glucose cotransport systems in the normal human fetal small intestine. Biochim Biophys Acta 1988;938:181–8.
97. Malo C. Separation of two distinct Na+/D-glucose cotransport systems in the human fetal jejunum by means of their differential specificity for 3-O-methylglucose. Biochim Biophys Acta 1990;1022:8–16.
98. Harig JM, Barry JA, Rajendran VM, et al. D-glucose and L-leucine transport by human intestinal brush-border membrane vesicles. Am J Physiol 1989;256:G618–23.
99. Thomson ABR, Gardner MLG, Atkins GL. Alternate models for shared carriers or a single maturing carrier in hexose uptake into rabbit jejunum in vitro. Biochim Biophys Acta 1987;903:229–40.

100. Brot-Laroche E, Dao M, Alcalde A, et al. Independent modulation by food supply of two distinct sodium-activated D-glucose transport systems in the guinea pig jejunal brush-border membrane. Proc Natl Acad Sci U S A 1988;85:6370–3.
101. Thomas V, Pichon B, Crouzoulon G, Barre H. Effect of chronic cold exposure on Na-dependent D-glucose transport along small intestine in ducklings. Am J Physiol 1996;271: R1429–38.
102. Ahearn GA, Behnke RD, Zonno V, Storelli C. Kinetic heterogeneity of Na-D-glucose cotransport in the teleost gastrointestinal tract. Am J Physiol 1992;263:R1018–23.
103. Crouzoulon G, Korieh A. Fructose transport by rat intestinal brush border membrane vesicles. Effect of high fructose diet followed by return to standard diet. Comp Biochem Physiol Comp Physiol 1991;100A:175–82.
104. Hoekstra JH, van Kempen AAMW, Bijl SB, Kneepkens CMF. Fructose breath hydrogen tests. Arch Dis Child 1993; 68:136–8.
105. Elnif J, Malo C, Buddington RK. Intestinal absorption of amino acids and sugars during postnatal development of mink. FASEB J 1998;12:A369.
106. Buddington RK. Nutrient transport by canine intestine during postnatal development. FASEB J 1996;10:A122.
107. Rand EB, Depaoli AM, Davidson NO, et al. Sequence, tissue distribution, and functional characterization of the rat fructose transporter GLUT5. Am J Physiol 1993;264:G1169–76.
108. Davidson NO, Hausman AM, Ifkovits CA, et al. Human intestinal glucose transporter expression and localization of GLUT5. Am J Physiol 1992;262:C795–800.
109. Cherbuy C, Carcy-Vrillon B, Posho L, et al. GLUT2 and hexokinase control proximodistal gradient of intestinal glucose metabolism in the newborn pig. Am J Physiol 1997;272: G1530–9.
110. Reeds PJ, Burrin DG, Jahoor F, et al. Enteral glutamate is almost completely metabolized in first pass by the gastrointestinal tract of infant pigs. Am J Physiol 1996;270:E413–8.
111. Navab F, Winter CG. Effect of aging on intestinal absorption of aromatic amino acids in vitro in the rat. Am J Physiol 1988; 254:G630–6.
112. Wolffram S, Hagemann C, Scharrer E. Regression of high-affinity carrier-mediated intestinal transport of taurine in adult cats. Am J Physiol 1991;261:R1089–95.
113. O'Flaherty L, Stapleton PP, Redmond HP, Bouchier-Hayes DJ. Intestinal taurine transport: a review. Eur J Clin Invest 1997;27:873–80.
114. Barada K, Atallah JB, Nassar CF. Age influence on intestinal taurine transport in mice. Comp Biochem Physiol 1997; 118A:159–63.
115. De Belle RC, Vaupshas V, Vitullo B, et al. Intestinal absorption of bile salts: immature development in the neonate. Pediatrics 1979;94:472–6.
116. Little JM, Lester R. Ontogenesis of intestinal bile salt absorption in the neonatal rat. Am J Physiol 1980;239: G319–23.
117. Schwarz SM, Watkins JB, Ling SC. Taurocholate transport by brush-border membrane vesicles from the developing rabbit ileum: structure/function relationships. J Pediatr Gastroenterol Nutr 1990;10:482–9.
118. Shneider BL, Michaud GA, West AB, Suchy FJ. The effects of bile acid feeding on development of ileal bile acid transport. Pediatr Res 1993;33:221–4.
119. Stahl GE, Mascarenhas MR, Fayer JC, et al. Passive jejunal bile salt absorption alters the enterohepatic circulation in immature rats. Gastroenterology 1993;104:163–73.
120. Robinson JWL, Luisier A-L, Mirkovitch V. Transport of amino-acids and sugars by the dog colonic mucosa. Pflugers Arch 1973;345:317–26.
121. Scharrer E, Amann B. Evidence for carrier-mediated uptake of sugars at the serosal side of lamb colon mucosa. Pflugers Arch 1980;384:279–82.
122. Cato III A, Pollack GM, Brouwer KL. Age-dependent intestinal absorption of valproic acid in the rat. Pharm Res 1995; 12:284–90.
123. Planas JM, Villa MC, Ferrer R, Moret M. Hexose transport by chicken cecum during development. Pflugers Arch 1986; 407:216–20.
124. McCloud E, Mathis RK, Grant KE, Said HM. Intestinal uptake of uridine in suckling rats: mechanism and ontogeny. Proc Soc Exp Biol Med 1994;206:425–30.
125. Smith MW. Comparative aspects of enterocyte differentiation. In: Gilles R, Gilles-Baillien M, editors. Transport processes, iono- and osmoregulation. Berlin: Springer-Verlag;1985.
126. Castello AA, Guma L, Sevilla M, et al. Regulation of GLUT5 gene expression in rat intestinal mucosa: regional distribution, circadian rhythm, perinatal development and effect of diabetes. Biochem J 1995;309:271–7.
127. Corpe CP, Burant CF. Hexose transporter expression in rat small intestine: effect of diet on diurnal variations. Am J Physiol 1996;271:G211–6.
128. Stevenson NR, Sitren AS, Furuya A. Circadian rhythmicity in several small intestinal functions is independent of the use of the intestine. Am J Physiol 1980;238:G203–7.
129. Furuya S, Yugari Y. Daily rhythmic change in the transport of histidine by everted sacs of rat small intestine. Biochim Biophys Acta 1971;241:245–8.
130. Shu R, David ES, Ferraris RP. Luminal fructose modulates fructose transport and GLUT5 expression in small intestine of weaning rats. Am J Physiol 1998;274:G232–9.
131. Henning SJ, Chang SSP, Gisel EG. Ontogeny of feeding control in suckling and weanling rats. Am J Physiol 1979; 237:R187–91.
132. Dyer J, Barker PJ, Shirazi-Beechey SP. Nutrient regulation of the intestinal Na$^+$/glucose co-transporter (SGLT1) gene expression. Biochem Biophys Res Comm 1997;230:624–9.
133. Pitkin RM, Reynolds WA. Fetal ingestion and metabolism of amniotic fluid protein. Am J Obstet Gynecol 1975;123: 356–63.
134. Wu G, Bazer FW, Tou W. Developmental changes of free amino acid concentrations in fetal fluids of pigs. J Nutr 1996; 125:2859–68.
135. Gutierrez ED, Grapperhaus KJ, Rubin DC. Ontogenetic regulation of spatial differentiation in the crypt-villus axis of normal and isografted small intestine. Am J Physiol 1995; 269:G500–11.
136. Trahair JF, Sangild PT. Systematic and luminal influences on the perinatal development of the gut. Equine Vet J 1997; Suppl 24:40–50.
137. Trahair JF, Harding R, Bocking AD, et al. The role of ingestion in the development of the small intestine in fetal sheep. Q J Exp Physiol 1986;71:99–104.
138. Buchmiller TL, Fonkalsrud EW, Kim CS, et al. Upregulation of nutrient transport in fetal rabbit intestine by transamniotic substrate administration. J Surg Res 1992;52:443–7.
139. Kelly D, Coutts APG. Biologically active peptides in colostrum and milk. In: Laplace JP, Fevrier C, Barbeau A, editors. Digestive physiology of pigs. EAAP Pub # 88, 1997.
140. Zhang HC, Malo C, Buddington RK. Diet influences intestinal develpoment of pigs during the first 6 hours after birth. J Nutr 1998. [In press]
141. Smith MW. Diet effects on enterocyte development. Proc Nutr Soc 1992;51:173–8.
142. Cheeseman CI. Upregulation of sodium-dependent glucose transport across rat jejunal brush-border membrane vesicles induced by GLP-2 infusion *in vivo*. Am J Physiol 1998. [In press]

143. Vega YM, Puchal AA, Buddington RK. Intestinal amino acid and monosaccharide transport in suckling pigs fed replacers with different sources of carbohydrate. J Nutr 1992;122:2430–9.
144. Keelan M, Perin N, Clandinin MT, Thomson ABR. Intestinal transport in suckling rats is modified by feeding nursing mothers diets with lipids mimicking various artificial milks. Gastroenterology 1996;110:A810.
145. Perrin N, Keelan M, Jarocka-Cyrta E, et al. Ontogeny of intestinal adaptation in rats in response to isocaloric changes in dietary lipids. Am J Physiol 1997;273:G713–20.
146. Chu SH, Walker WA. Bacterial toxin interaction with the developing intestine. Gastroenterology 1993;104:916–25.
147. Alverdy J. The effect of nutrition on gastrointestinal barrier function. Semin Respir Infect 1994;9:248–56.
148. Swords WE, Wu C-C, Champlin FR, Buddington RK. Postnatal changes in selected bacterial groups of the pig colonic microflora. Biol Neonate 1993;63:191–200.
149. Boehm G, Braun W, Moro G, Minoli I. Bile acid concentrations in sureum and duodenal aspirates of healthy preterm infants. Biol Neonate 1997;71:207–14.
150. Buller HA, Koth MJC, Goldman DA, et al. Coordinate expression of lactase-phlorizin hydrolase mRNA and enzyme levels in rat intestine during development. J Biol Chem 1990;265:6978–83.
151. Miyamoto K, Hase K, Taketani Y, et al. Developmental changes in intestinal glucose transporter mRNA levels. Biochem Biophys Res Commun 1992;183:626–31.
152. Shu R, David ES, Ferraris RP. Precocious induction of intestinal fructose transport and GLUT5 expression in weaning rats. Am J Physiol 1997;272:G446–53.
153. Lescale-Matys L, Dyer J, Scott D, et al. Regulation of the ovine intestinal Na+/glucose co-transporter (SGLT1) is dissociated from mRNA abundance. Biochem J 1993;291:435–40.
154. Freeman TC, Wood IS, Sirinathsinghji DJS, et al. The expression of the Na+/glucose cotransporter (SGLT1) gene in lamb small intestine during postnatal development. Biochim Biophys Acta 1993;1146:203–12.
155. Smith MW, Turvey A, Freeman TC. Appearance of phloridzin-sensitive glucose transport is not controlled at mRNA level in rabbit jejunal enterocytes. Exp Physiol 1992;77:525–8.
156. Aghayan M, Rao LV, Smith RM, et al. Developmental expression and cellular localization of glucose transporter molecules during mouse preimplantation development. Development 1992;115:305–12.
157. Younoszai MK, Smith C, Finch MH. Comparison of in vitro jejunal uptake of L-valine and L-lysine in the rat during maturation. J Pediatr Gastroenterol Nutr 1985;4:992–7.
158. Miyamoto K, Shiraga T, Morita K, et al. Sequence, tissue distribution and development changes in rat intestinal oligopeptide transporter. Biochim Biophys Acta 1996;1305:34–8.
159. David ES, Cingari DS, Ferraris RP. Dietary induction of intestinal fructose absorption in weaning rats. Pediatr Res 1995;37:777–82.
160. David ES, Tran T, Ferraris RP. Can intestinal fructose transport be induced in suckling rats? FASEB J 1996;10:A704.
161. Shirazi-Beechey SP, Gribble SM, Wood IS, et al. Dietary regulation of the intestinal sodium-dependent glucose cotransporter (SGLT1). Biochem Soc Trans 1994;22:655–8.
162. Cheeseman CI, Harley B. Adaptation of glucose transport across rat enterocyte basolateral membrane in response to altered dietary carbohydrate intake. J Physiol 1991;437:563–75.
163. Burant CF, Saxena M. Rapid, reversible substrate regulation of fructose transporter (GLUT5) expression in rat small intestine and kidney. Am J Physiol 1994;267:G71–9.
164. Sangild PT, Sjostrom H, Noren O, et al. The prenatal development and glucocorticoid control of brush-border hydrolases in the pig small intestine. Pediatr Res 1995;37:207–12.
165. Barnard JA, Ghishan FK, Wilson FA. Ontogenesis of taurocholate transport by rat ileal brush border membrane vesicles. J Clin Invest 1985;75:869–73.
166. Shneider BL, Dawson PA, Christie D, et al. Cloning and molecular characterization of the ontogeny of a rat ileal sodium-dependent bile acid transporter. J Clin Invest 1995;95:745–54.
167. La Gamma EF, Brown LE. Feeding practices for infants weighing less than 1500 g at birth and the pathogenesis of necrotizing enterocolitis. Clin Perinatol 1994;21:271–306.
168. Mahraoui L, Takeda J, Mesonero J, et al. Regulation of impression of the human fructose transporter (GLUT5) by cyclic AMP. Biochem J 1994;340:169–75.
169. Henning SJ. Plasma concentrations of total and free corticosterone during development in the rat. Am J Physiol 1978;4:E451–6.
170. David ES, Bhagat D, Ferraris RP. Dexamethasone precociously induces intestinal sugar transport in suckling rats. Pediatr Res 1997;41:81A.
171. Nanthakumar NN, Henning SJ. Ontogeny of sucrase-isomaltase gene expression in rat intestine: responsiveness to glucocorticoids. Am J Physiol 1993;264:G306–11.
172. Barnard JA, Ghishan FK. Methylprednisolone accelerates the ontogeny of sodium-taurocholate cotransport in rat ileal brushborder membrane. Lab Clin Med 1986;108:545–55.
173. Lifschitz CH. Carbohydrate needs in preterm and term infants. In: Tsang R, Nichols B, editors. Nutrition during infancy. Philadelphia: Hanley and Belfus; 1988. p. 122–32.
174. Kien CL, Kepner J, Grotjohn K, et al. Stable isotope model for estimating colonic acetate production in premature infants. Gastroenterology 1992;102:1458–66.
175. Levitt MD. Production and excretion of hydrogen gas in man. N Engl J Med 1969;281:122-7.
176. Sakata T, von Engelhardt W. Stimulatory effect of short-chain fatty acids on epithelial cell proliferation in rat large intestine. Comp Biochem Physiol Comp Physiol 1983;74A:459–62.
177. Kripke SA, Fox AD, Berman JM, et al. Stimulation of intestinal mucosal growth with intracolonic infusion of short-chain fatty acids. J Parenteral Enteral Nutr 1989;13:109–16.
178. Koruda MJ, Rolandelli RH, Bliss DZ, et al. Parenteral nutrition supplemented with short-chain fatty acids: effect on the small bowel mucosa in normal rats. Am J Clin Nutr 1990;51:685–9.
179. Soergel KH. Colonic fermentation: metabolic and clinical implications. Clin Investigator 1994;72:742–8.
180. Holtug K, Clausen MR, Hove H, et al. The colon in carbohydrate malabsorption: short-chain fatty acids, pH, and osmotic diarrhea. Scand J Gastroenterol 1992;27:545–52.
181. Kien CL, Liechty EA, Myerberg DZ, Mullet MD. Dietary carbohydrate assimilation in the premature infant: evidence for a nutritionally significant bacterial ecosystem in the colon. Am J Clin Nutr 1987;46:456–60.
182. Kien CL. Digestion, absorption and fermentation of carbohydrates in the newborn. Clin Perinatol 1996;23:211–28.
183. Barr RG, Perman JA, Schoeller DA, Watkins JB. Breath tests in pediatric gastrointestinal disorders: new diagnostic opportunities. Pediatrics 1978;62:393–401.
184. King CE, Toskes PP. The use of breath tests in the study of malabsorption. Clin Gastroenterol 1983;12:591–610.
185. Solomons NW. Evaluation of carbohydrate absorption: the hydrogen breath test in clinical practice. Clin Nutr 1984;3:71–8.
186. Lifschitz CH, Boutton TW, Carrazza F, et al. A carbon-13 breath test to characterize glucose absorption and utilization in children. J Pediatr Gastroenterol Nutr 1988;7:842–7.
187. Christie DL. Use of the one-hour blood xylose test as an indicator of small bowel mucosal disease. J Pediatr 1978;92:725–8.

188. Vanderhoof JA, Hunt LI, Antonson DL. A rapid procedure for small intestinal biopsy in infants and children. Gastroenterology 1981;80:938–41.
189. Marks JF, Norton JB, Fordtran JS. Glucose-galactose malabsorption. J Pediatr 1966;69:225–8.
190. Schneider AJ, Kinter WB, Stirling CE. Glucose-galactose malabsorption. N Engl J Med 1966;274:305–12.
191. Wales JKH, Primhak RA, Rattenbury J, Taylor CJ. Isolated fructose malabsorption. Arch Dis Child 1990;65:227–9.
192. Iacono G, Carroccio A, Cavataio F, et al. Congenital fructose-glucose-galactose malabsorption. J Pediatr Gastroenterol Nutr 1995;21:95–9.
193. Desjeux JF, Turk E, Wright EM, et al. Congenital selective Na+ D-glucose cotransport defects leading to renal glycosuria and selective intestinal malabsorption of glucose and galactose. In: Metabolic basis of inherited disease. 7th ed. New York: McGraw-Hill; 1995. p. 2463–78.
194. Wright EM, Hirayama BA, Loo DDF, et al. Intestinal sugar transport. In: Johnson LR, editor. Physiology of the gastrointestinal tract. 3rd ed. New York: Raven Press; 1994. p. 1751–72.
195. Turk E, Klisak I, Bacallao R, et al. Assignment of the human Na+/glucose cotransporter gene SGLT1 to chromosome 22q13.1. Genomics 1993;17:752–4.
196. Turk E, Zabel B, Mundlos S, et al. Glucose/galactose malabsorption caused by a defect in the Na$^+$-glucose cotransporter. Nature 1991;28:354–6.
197. Martin MG, Turk E, Lostao MP, et al. Defects in Na$^+$-glucose cotransporter (SGLT1) trafficking and function cause glucose-galactose malabsorption. Nat Genet 1996;12:216–20.
198. Martin MG, Turk E, Kerner C, et al. Prenatal identification of a heterozygous status in two fetuses at risk for glucose-galactose malabsorption. Prenat Diagn 1996;16:458–62.
199. Riby JE, Fujisawa T, Kretchmer N. Fructose absorption. Am J Clin Nutr 1993;58 Suppl:748S–53S.
200. Fernandez-Banares F, Esteve-Pardo M, de Leon R, et al. Sugar malabsorption in functional bowel disease: clinical implications. Am J Gastroenterol 1993;88:2044–50.
201. Rumessen JJ, Gudmand-Hoyer E. Functional bowel disease: malabsorption and abdominal distress after ingestion of fructose, sorbitol and fructose-sorbitol mixture. Gastroenterology 1988;95:694–700.
202. Truswell AS, Seach JM, Thorburn AW. Incomplete absorption of pure fructose in healthy subjects and the facilitating effects of glucose. Am J Clin Nutr 1988;48:1424–30.
203. Hoekstra JH, van den Aker JHL, Kneepkens CMF, et al. Evaluation of $^{13}CO_2$ breath tests for the detection of fructose malabsorption. J Lab Clin Med 1996;127:303–9.
204. Lebenthal E, Ross TM, Nord KS, Branski D. Recurrent abdominal pain and lactose absorption in children. Pediatrics 1981;67:828–32.
205. Sahi T. Genetics and epidemiology of adult-type hypolactasia. Scand J Gastroenterol 1994;29 Suppl 202:7–20.
206. O'Brien S, Mulcahy H, Fenlon H, et al. Intestinal bile acid malabsorption and cystic fibrosis. Gut 1993;34:1137–41.
207. Hardcastle PT, Taylor CJ. Sodium/glucose cotransporter activity in cystic fibrosis. Arch Dis Child 1996;75:170.
208. Falchuk ZM. Update on gluten-sensitive enteropathy. Am J Med 1979;67:1085–96.
209. Mulder CJJ, van Bergeijk JD, Jansen TLTA, Uil JJ. Coeliac disease. Diagnostic and therapeutic pitfalls. Scand J Gastroenterol 1993;28Suppl200:42–7.
210. Sellin JH, Hart R. Glucose malabsorption associated with rapid intestinal transit. Am J Gastroenterol 1992;87:584–9.
211. Hamilton JR. Major symptoms and signs of digestive tract disorder. In: Behrman RE, Vaughan VC, Nelson WE, editors. Nelson textbook of pediatrics. 13th ed. Philadelphia: WB Saunders; 1987. p. 411–27.
212. Book LS, Herbst JJ, Jung AL. Carbohydrate malabsorption in necrotizing enterocolitis. Pediatr Diagnosis 1976;57:201–4.
213. Kirschner BS, Lahr C, Lahr D, et al. Detection of increased breath hydrogen in infants with necrotizing enterocolitis [abstract]. Gastroenterology 1977;72:1080.
214. Inoue Y, Grant JP, Snyder PJ. Effect of glutamine-supplemented total parenteral nutrition on recovery of the small intestine after starvation atrophy. J Parenteral Enteral Nutr 1993;17:165–70.
215. Ortega MA, Nunez MC, Suarez MD, et al. Age-related response of the small intestine to severe starvation and refeeding in rats. Ann Nutr Metab 1996;40:351–8.
216. Galea MH, Holliday H, Carachi R, Kapila L. Short-bowel syndrome: a collective review. J Pediatr Surg 1992;27:592–6.
217. Vanderhoof JA, Langnas AN, Pinch LW, et al. Short bowel syndrome. J Pediatr Gastroenterol Nutr 1992;14:359–70.
218. Bury KD. Carbohydrate digestion and absorption after massive resection of the small intestine. Surg Gynecol Obstet 1972;135:177–87.
219. Menzies IS, Turner MW. Intestinal permeability of molecules in health and disease. In: MacDonald TT, editor. Immunology of the gastrointestinal tract (Immunology and medicine series). Dordrech: Kluwer Academic Publishers; 1992.
220. Wellner D, Meister A. A survey of inborn errors of amino acid metabolism and transport in man. Annu Rev Biochem 1981;50:911–68.
221. Chung YC, Kim YS, Shadchehr A, et al. Protein digestion and absorption in human small intestine. Gastroenterology 1979;76:1415–21.
222. Khin MU. In vitro uptake of amino acids in the jejunal mucosa of patients with cholera. J Diarrhoeal Dis Res 1993;11:67–74.
223. Gardiner K, Barbul A. Intestinal amino acid absorption during sepsis. J Parenteral Enteral Nutr 1993;17:277–83.
224. Gardiner KR, Ahrendt GM, Gardiner RE, Barbul A. Failure of intestinal amino acid absorptive mechanisms in sepsis. J Am Coll Surg 1995;181:431–6.
225. Eusufzai S. Bile acid malabsorption in patients with chronic diarrhea. Scand J Gastroenterol 1993;28:865–8.
226. Hofmann AF. Intestinal absorption of bile acids and biliary constituents; the intestinal component of the enterohepatic circulation and the integrated system. In: Johnson LR, editor. Physiology of the gastrointestinal tract. 3rd ed. New York: Raven Press; 1994. p. 1845–67.
227. Eusufzai S. Bile acid malabsorption: mechanism and treatment. Dig Dis 1995;13:312–21.
228. Nyhlin H, Merrick MV, Eastwood MA. Bile acid malabsorption in Crohn's disease and indications for its assessment using SeHCAT. Gut 1994;35:90–3.
229. Hancock BJ, Wiseman NE. Lethal short-bowel syndrome. J Pediatr Surg 1990;25:1131–4.
230. Huysman WA, Tibboel D, Bergmeijer JH, Molenaar JC. Long-term survival of a patient with congenital short-bowel and malrotation. J Pediatr Surg 1991;26:103–5.
231. Yuasa H, Amidon GL, Fleisher D. Peptide carrier-mediated transport in intestinal brush border membrane vesicles of rats and rabbits cephradine uptake and inhibition. Pharm Res 1993;10:400–4.
232. Lipka E, Crison J, Amidon GL. Transmembrane transport of peptide-like compounds: prospects for oral delivery. J Contr Release 1996;39:121–9.
233. Kramer W, Wess G, Neckermann G, et al. Intestinal absorption of peptides by coupling to bile acids. J Biol Chem 1994;269:10621–7.
234. Collie NL. Hormonal regulation of intestinal nutrient absorption in vertebrates. Am Zool 1995;35:474–82.
235. Ferraris RP. Regulation of intestinal nutrient transport. In: Johnson LR, editor. Physiology of the gastrointestinal tract. 3rd ed. New York: Raven Press; 1994. p. 1821–44.

CHAPTER 9

Development of Innate Immunity in the Small Intestine

Andre J. Ouellette, PhD

Charles L. Bevins, MD, PhD

The intestinal epithelium is the largest surface where an organism interacts directly with the external environment. By its organization into villus projections, the surface area of the intestine is amplified anatomically to increase the luminal absorptive area. This sheet of epithelial cells is the sole barrier between the luminal contents and the circulation. Remarkably, the intestinal epithelium is renewed continually and rapidly throughout the lifetime of mammals.

The epithelial renewal process involves stem cell proliferation and cell migration. During their migration from crypts upward onto the villi, cells differentiate into enterocytes, enteroendocrine cells, or goblet cells. Subsequently, these cells undergo apoptosis in association with exfoliation into the lumen from the villus tips. Depending on the species, epithelial cells that leave the proliferative zone complete their life cycle in 2 to 5 days. Unlike these three epithelial lineages, a fourth lineage, the Paneth cells, undergo terminal differentiation during downward migration from the stem cell progenitors toward the base of the crypt.[1] In contrast to the short lifespan of the epithelial cells on villi, that of Paneth cells at the crypt base is 20 to 25 days.

The structural adaptations that have evolved to satisfy requirements for adequate nutrient absorption also increase the opportunity for colonization of the mucosal surface by microorganisms. The epithelium of the small bowel must execute its digestive and absorptive functions while inhibiting most microbes from establishing themselves as significant resident populations. For reasons that are not fully understood, the bacterial load in the small intestine is markedly lower than that of the colon and cecum, often containing 10^4 to 10^6 times fewer microbes per gram of tissue than are found distally. Many factors are thought to contribute to this physiologic situation, including the digestive and mucous secretions of the gastrointestinal tract, acquired immune responses, and gene-encoded antimicrobial peptides and proteins that serve as mediators of innate immunity.

Studies of acquired, or clonal, immune responses of the gut indicates that mammals commit extensive energy and resources to B cell–mediated humoral immunity through the transport of secretory IgA molecules across the epithelium to the gut lumen.[2,3] This component of enteric immunity is vital to mammalian intestinal host defense, as is evident by the protective effects of specific IgA introduced into mice. Furthermore, intraepithelial T cells reside on the villi interspersed among enterocytes and function in cell-mediated immunity.[4] Both of these arms of lymphocyte-mediated acquired immunity are initiated by specific antigens. Based on total numbers of lymphocytes, the gut may be considered the largest lymphoid organ of the body.

The kinetics of T-cell and B-cell responses, however, suggest that they may not be sufficiently rapid to control an acute bacterial infection. Accordingly, the sole reliance on adaptive immunity may permit microbes to overgrow the epithelium before an effective immune response can be mounted.[5] In this context, innate mucosal defenses would function as a first line of protection against deleterious microbial colonization (Figure 9–1).

Innate defenses encompass both physical and chemical barriers. Activities associated with the process of digestion and with the normal physiology of the gastrointestinal tract are likely to contribute to innate mucosal defenses that help control the small intestinal bacterial population. For example, gastric acidity, digestive enzymes, bile salts, peristalsis, mucus, the resident commensal flora, and the exfoliation of enterocytes during epithelial renewal may contribute effectively to the inhibition of microbial growth.

Studies performed in invertebrates, insects, amphibia, and teleosts show that species lacking clonal immune mechanisms respond to bacterial or fungal infection by releasing proteins and peptides that act immediately, directly, and effectively on invading microbes.[5–7] Preformed and rapidly inducible, these antimicrobial proteins and peptides protect against microbial colonization and invasion. Studies in many diverse species, including humans and other mammals, have shown that the production of antimicrobial proteins and peptides is a highly conserved host defense strategy in evolutionary terms.

With these considerations in mind and with the discovery that endogenous antimicrobial peptides are abundant constituents of granules in mammalian phagocytic cells,[8]

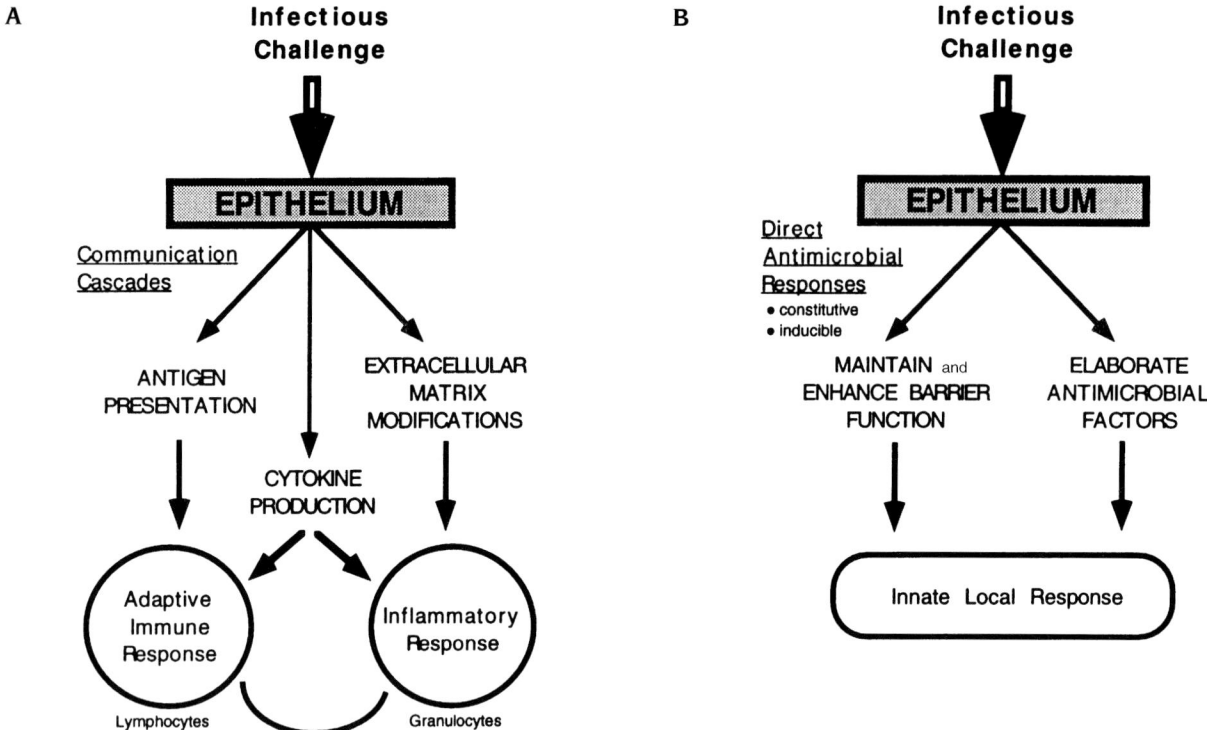

FIGURE 9–1. Roles of epithelial cells in mucosal host defense responses. A. Epithelial cells participate in the intercellular communication and coordination of the adaptive immune response. B, Epithelial cells actively participate in innate immune responses.

hypotheses that mammalian epithelia may employ preformed (or rapidly inducible) peptide antibiotics to provide a biochemical barrier to invading pathogens were developed.[9–12] A rich literature now supports that position.[6,13–20] This chapter will highlight relevant aspects of antimicrobial peptides within the theme of more general innate defenses of the mammalian intestinal mucosa.

INTESTINAL EPITHELIUM IN MUCOSAL IMMUNITY

Although the intestinal epithelium forms an important physical barrier for defense, what evidence supports the idea that these cells *actively* participate in host defense? Of the major epithelial cell lineages of the small bowel, three cell types—absorptive enterocytes, goblet cells, and Paneth cells—exhibit activities that implicate them in mucosal defense function (Figure 9–2). Intraepithelial lymphocytes, T cells, gut-associated lymphoid tissue, M cells, and the largely uncharacterized cell populations of the lamina propria will not be considered here, principally because they participate in acquired rather than innate immune responses, and each represents a topic beyond the scope of this chapter. We do not mean to imply, however, that the effectors and cells involved in acquired and innate immune function are compartmentalized or completely distinct from each other. These populations are likely to be highly interactive, exchanging molecular signals that influence challenges to the enteric immune system.

INTESTINAL EPITHELIAL CELL LINEAGES

The understanding of intestinal epithelial cell lineage determination has been advanced by four general investigational approaches: (1) analysis of normal intestinal ontogeny,[21–26] (2) epithelial differentiation in isografts of fetal mouse, rat, and human small intestine,[27–32] (3) reporter transgene expression controlled by promoters that are specifically active in particular epithelial cell lineages,[33–51] and (4) ablation or disruption of the epithelial cell phenotype by gene deletion or expression of cytotoxic transgenes that are controlled by lineage-specific gene promoters.[52–56] Each approach has yielded important information on cellular and molecular events pertinent to enteric innate immunity.

In rodents, the lineage determination begins in the third week of gestation, when the rodent gut endoderm remodels to form an epithelial monolayer that adheres to rudimentary villus projections. Endodermal cytodifferentiation first takes place in the duodenum then proceeds progressively in a wave-like fashion to the ileum. Crypt ontogeny in rodents occurs postnatally, as the intervillous epithelium matures during the first 2 weeks post partum.[57,58] At birth (day P1), the mouse epithelium is polyclonal and is derived from stem cells with multiple genotypes that are distributed throughout the epithelial sheet. By the end of the second week, crypts have become clonal through mechanisms that are not understood beyond the descriptive level. The adult epithelial sheet and its four lineages are continually regenerated from these monoclonal crypt stem cells although it is not known

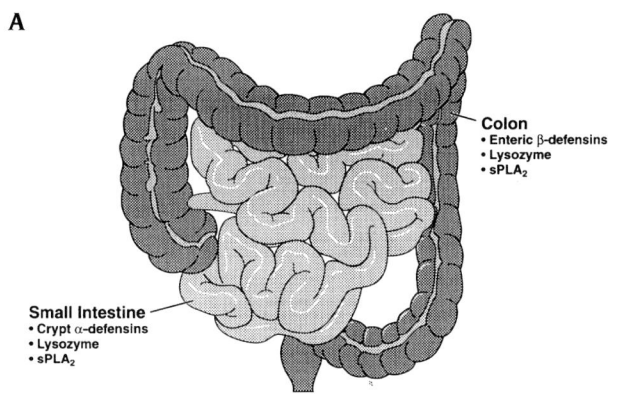

FIGURE 9-2. A, The primary peptide mediators of mucosal innate immunity are shown for the small intestine and colon. B, Microbial challenges in the alimentary tract and the epithelial cells that participate in the defense of the small intestinal mucosa. Schematic diagram of elongated alimentary tract highlighting large numbers of microbes (depicted as dots) that colonize the large intestine, fewer microbes that colonize the small intestine, and variable numbers of microbes that enter via the mouth. The top drawing depicts the mucosal surface of the small intestine in greater detail, to show amplification of the enteric surface area in the form of villi that project into the lumen. In the boxed region, the contributions of the major intestinal epithelial cell populations are summarized. Goblet cells, Paneth cells, M cells, and enterocytes contribute to host defense of this mucosal surface, as described in detail in the text.

whether crypts contain a single progenitor stem cell from which proliferative descendants arise or whether crypts are populated by several equivalent stem cells.

INTESTINAL GOBLET CELLS

Intestinal goblet cells are well-known for the production of a physical barrier between the epithelium and the contents of the lumen.[59–62] Goblet cell–secreted mucins are central in the establishment of this complex mucopolysaccharide barrier. Goblet cell numbers increase in inflammatory enteropathies, including ulcerative colitis, and goblet-cell hyperplasia is associated with episodes of inflammation that occur during parasitic infections.[63] Studies of rodents infected with *Trichinella spiralis* have implicated T-helper (Th) cells, particularly Th2 cell-derived mediators, as mediators of this goblet-cell hyperplasia.[64]

The goblet cell also secretes intestinal trefoil factor (mTFF3), a peptide containing three intramolecular disulfide bonds that form a trefoil-like motif.[65] Secreted mTFF3 is implicated in barrier function because mTFF3-deficient mice develop inflammatory bowel disease and megacolon and are severely immunocompromised when challenged with a chemical irritant to the epithelium, such as dextran sodium sulfate.[66] The mechanism(s) by which mTFF3 exerts these effects is unknown. The goblet-cell secretions probably function as a physical polymeric barrier that prevents microbial attachment and colonization rather than exerting direct killing effects on ingested microorganisms.[67]

ABSORPTIVE ENTEROCYTES

The apical secretion of secretory IgA by enterocytes is a classic example of epithelial participation in acquired immunity but a possible role for enterocytes in innate immunity has not gained much attention. However, exfoliating enterocytes may contribute to innate immunity by a novel mechanism. Extracts of human ileal mucosa were recently shown to contain an antimicrobial activity; after its purification from protein extracts and sequencing, the activity was found to be histone H1 and histone-derived peptide fragments.[68] That histones have antimicrobial activities in in vitro assays has been known since the 1950s, and histones H1 and H2b have been isolated as major peptide antibiotics of mouse macrophages.[69] At first glance, it is difficult to accept that key elements of nucleosome structure could participate in luminal innate immunity. However, immunochemistry has revealed that the histone antigen translocates from the nucleus to the cytoplasm in enterocytes during exfoliation-associated apoptosis. Histone also is released from villus epithelial cells undergoing apoptosis following dissociation from the lamina propria with ethylenediamine tetraacetic acid (EDTA) treatment.[68] The investigators of the study suggest that, since an estimated 10^{11} enterocytes exfoliate daily into the human small bowel, the contribution of their histones to mucosal immunity could be important, albeit secondary to their nuclear function (Figure 9–2B).

PANETH CELLS

Paneth cells are granulated secretory epithelial cells that reside at the base of the crypts of Lieberkühn in the small intestine of many species. In the 19th century, Schwalbe and Paneth first described granulated cells at the base of the "intestinal glands."[70,71] Paneth drew the large, apically-oriented granules as the hallmark of these cells, noting that they were specific to the crypts in the small intestine. Also, he suggested that their likely function was to secrete granules into the intestinal lumen.[71]

Early studies of Paneth cells focused on their striking morphology, and there was a considerable research effort to infer their function by histochemical approaches, including their avid staining by eosinophilic dyes, and by testing the differential solubility of their granules in organic and acidic solvents. Histochemical and biochemical analyses had shown that Paneth cell granules were rich in disulfide-containing proteins[72] and mucopolysaccharides. An apparent association between feeding and Paneth cell granule release was the focus of attention for years but studies by Trier and colleagues demonstrated that the synthesis and release of Paneth cell granules was independent of food injestion.[73,74] Consistent with this, recent experiments have shown that Paneth cells, which respond directly and dramatically to cholinergic agonists, do not respond to cholecystokinin.[75]

Insight into Paneth cell function was provided by studies of their protein secretions. The presence and release of Paneth cell lysozyme, an enzyme that hydrolyzes the peptidoglycan of bacterial cell walls, first implicated this epithelial cell lineage and its products in host defense.[76] Lysozyme, although found in macrophages and additional tissues, served as a useful marker for identifying agonists of Paneth cell secretion.[77–79]

The visualization of microorganisms within mouse Paneth cells by electron microscopy, led to the suggestion that Paneth cells might have a phagocytic role.[80,81] These images may represent bacteria that were phagocytosed, microbes that may have invaded Paneth cells, or organisms and soluble components of the crypt lumen that may have become internalized during the recycling of the apical membrane after granule release. The possible phagocytic function of Paneth cells remains controversial and is not widely accepted. Unlike neutrophils and macrophages, Paneth cells are nonmotile, specialized exocytic cells that resemble glands more than phagocytic white blood cells.

Paneth cells populate most crypts of the mouse small intestine.[82] Although they arise, as do all intestinal epithelial cell lineages, from mitotically active stem cells, Paneth cells mature below the proliferative zone, differentiating as they migrate downward.[83] Differentiation does not require luminal bacteria or dietary components because, histologically normal Paneth cells develop under germ-free conditions and also from murine or human fetal intestinal xenografts in nude mice.[30,84] Interestingly, Paneth cells in germ-free and normally reared mice and rats exhibit modest morphologic differences,[12,57] and oral administration of bacteria is reported to stimulate Paneth cell degranulation.[85] Paneth cell distribution is generally restricted to the small intestine, except in carcinoma or in severe inflammation such as occurs in Barrett's esophagus, Crohn's disease, gastritis, and ulcerative colitis.[86–91]

Antimicrobial Proteins and Peptides in Paneth Cells

Paneth cell granules are rich in a variety of antibiotic proteins and peptides, and the release of these granules onto the apical mucosal surface suggests that this secretion may contribute to active mucosal defense function.[92–94] For example, the granules of Paneth cells contain lysozyme, secretory phospholipase A_2 (sPLA$_2$), and α-defensins, which all have clear antimicrobial activities in vitro.[77,94,95] These markers of Paneth cells share a common feature—the same molecules or homologues from these gene families also are expressed in cells of myeloid lineage and packaged into granules. Given the role of neutrophils in host defense, it is likely that corresponding molecules released into the extracellular space by Paneth cells would also participate in innate immunity.

Exocytic Secretion by Paneth Cells

The molecular signals that mediate Paneth cell secretion are not completely understood. Cholinergic agonists have been reported to increase Paneth cell lysozyme secretion 20- to 40-fold,[77] and secretion is inhibited by atropine, a muscarinic antagonist.[96] Results of bethanechol or carbamylcholine administration also support the view that mouse intestinal Paneth cells have muscarinic receptors and suggest that secretion may be controlled by activation of G-proteins coupled to muscarinic receptors.[97,98] In perfusion studies, 10 mM NaF and 10 nM AlCl$_3$, which are nonspecific activators of many G-proteins, produced morphologic evidence of massive degranulation similar to that seen with 200 μM bethanechol. Although not conclusive, the findings are consistent with G-protein involvement.

In vitro, carbamylcholine exerts direct effects on isolated mouse intestinal crypts. Accumulation of cytosolic intracellular calcium (Ca^{++}) was induced in Paneth cells of isolated crypts but not in other cell populations of the crypt.[75] The pattern of Paneth cell cytosolic intracellular Ca^{++} flux was biphasic,[97] suggesting that the initial rise in cytosolic intracellular Ca^{++} depends on intracellular Ca^{++} stores and on the influx of calcium ion from the extracellular fluid. The investigators concluded that the second phase depended completely on Ca^{++} influx. Consistent with the notion that Paneth cell degranulation is not closely associated with feeding, administration of cholecystokinin had no effect on Paneth cell morphology or cytosolic intracellular Ca^{++} concentration.

Paneth Cell Differentiation and Ontogeny

Because many secretory products of Paneth cells are proteins with known roles in host defense, the mechanisms that regulate Paneth cell maturation are germane to understanding the development of innate immunity in the small bowel. To date, most insights are from studies of mice and rats, whose intestinal epithelium is immature at birth and undergoes extensive postnatal remodeling and crypt ontogeny during the first 3 postnatal weeks. This profile contrasts with human Paneth cells, which begin to develop during the first trimester of gestation, although levels of Paneth cell markers are several-fold lower in neonates than in adults.

The most highly differentiated Paneth cells are below the stem-cell zone at the base of the crypt.[57] A small percentage of crypt goblet cells, positioned above the stem-cell population in normal adult mice, contain small, electron-dense inclusions within the mucin granules. Also, crypt cells categorized as "intermediate," "granulomucous," or "transitional" also contain both mucins and electron-dense inclusions that are larger than those of granule goblet cells but smaller than the apical granules of the differentiating Paneth cells.[52] The next section will consider the responses of these intermediate cells to Paneth cell deficiency.

Paneth cell maturation has been investigated extensively during postnatal crypt ontogeny in normal and transgenic mice as well as in intestinal isografts. This lineage emerges coincident with cytodifferentiation of the fetal small intestinal endoderm, formation of crypts from an intervillous epithelium, and establishment of a stem cell hierarchy. Early in the differentiation process, Paneth cell markers accumulate in cells in the maturing epithelial monolayer.[52,57,99] During crypt expansion by fission in postnatal weeks 3 and 4, the number of Paneth cells per crypt increase markedly. Also during this phase of crypt ontogeny and multiplication, fucosylated and sialylated glycoconjugates become prominent components of Paneth cell granules and cytoplasm.[100] Phloxine-tartrazine, a histochemical stain that reacts strongly with adult Paneth cells and granulocytes containing cationic granules or inclusions, stains crypts of the proximal small bowel in 7-day-old mice; by 4 weeks of age, the staining pattern is the same as in adult mice.[52]

The α-defensins are expressed early in the morphogenesis and differentiation of mouse small intestine. Cells immunoreactive for cryptdin first appear interspersed in the epithelial sheet at embryonic day 15 (E15), coincident with conversion of the gut endoderm to a monolayer. Certain goblet cells also contain cryptdins later in gestation and in the newborn; approximately 10% of all goblet cells contain defensin at birth. These cells do not persist beyond the first postnatal week, after which cryptdin-positive cells resemble young Paneth cells in that they contain apical secretory granules.[57] Consistent with the proximal-to-distal progression of endodermal conversion, the number of immunopositive Paneth cells and the number of positive cells per crypt decrease progressively along the duodenal-ileal axis prior to the first 2 weeks. The expression patterns of other Paneth cell products occurs in parallel with cryptdin expression. For example, intestinal sPLA$_2$, a Paneth cell–specific marker in adult mice, is detected antigenically at 7 days of age.[57,101] Immunohistochemically, intestinal lysozyme is detected in Paneth cells at the base of developing crypts in 10-day-old mice, 3 days after sPLA$_2$ is first detected.[57] These findings suggest that Paneth cells that first produce lysozyme are already significantly well differentiated with respect to sPLA$_2$ and cryptdin expression. It is of interest, however, that sPLA$_2$ and lysozyme mRNA can be detected in the intestine of newborn mice, even though the peptides cannot be detected until days later.

Paneth cell differentiation occurs during crypt morphogenesis; however, whether the stimulus is programmed within the epithelium or induced by luminal or local paracrine or matrix factors derived from the mesenchyme is unknown. To address this issue, several research groups have used intestinal isografts to evaluate crypt ontogeny and lineage differentiation in a system where the gut is isolated from several of these potentially influential growth factors. In mouse, rat, and human implantation of intact fetal gut under the subcutaneous tissues of isogenic or athymic recipients results in morphogenesis that is positionally and morphologically correct.[27,30,32,84,102] Thus, the luminal presence of microflora, pancreatic or biliary secretions, or dietary constituents is not an essential effector of epithelial differentiation although these factors may indeed influence the developing epithelium in vivo. Although the appearance of Paneth cells is somewhat irregular with respect to the timing and sequential appearance of particular markers, relative to events in the intact small intestine of the newborn,[57] most implants appear normal within 2 to 3 weeks after placement in the subcutaneous space as does the proximal-distal gradient distribution of Paneth cells, the expression of known markers, and the anatomic positioning of Paneth cells. Because glucocorticoids and thyroid hormone induce the precocious appearance of markers for enterocytes,[103–106] perhaps the stress or the hormonal release associated with angiogenesis or surgery influences the timing of differentiation events in the implant system, as others have suggested. As is true for mouse tissue, colonic isografts lack Paneth cells throughout the implantation period.

With minor differences, Paneth cell appearance in germ-free and conventionally reared mice is essentially the same, with regard to their proteinaceous or glycoconjugate granule constituents. The exception is the expression of terminal α-fucose-containing glycoconjugates recognized by lectin *Anguilla anguilla* agglutinin (AAA).[100,107] In adult germ-free mice, Paneth cell granules and cytoplasm bind the lectin strongly but conventional mice show low levels of AAA staining, and when germ-free mice are repopulated with conventional flora, the normal pattern of AAA staining returns within 2 weeks. Thus, Paneth cell differentiation does not require the presence of the gut microflora although subtle changes in Paneth cell phenotype are detectable under germ-free conditions.

Disruption of Paneth Cell Biology in Mice

The creation of loss-of-function mutations to ablate particular cell types by introducing cytotoxic transgenes that are controlled by cell-specific gene promoters has led to valuable insights into interactions between cell populations. Such a transgenic approach has been used to induce Paneth cell deficiency.[52] The 5′-flanking region of the mouse cryptdin-2 gene (nucleotides −6500 to +34) was placed upstream of an attenuated diphtheria toxin A fragment coding sequence and upstream of the SV40 large T-antigen gene in a second set of mice. Transgenic mouse lines were established with the intention of directing expression of the toxic gene products specifically in the Paneth cell population and its precursors. Transgenic mice up to 6 to 8 weeks of age

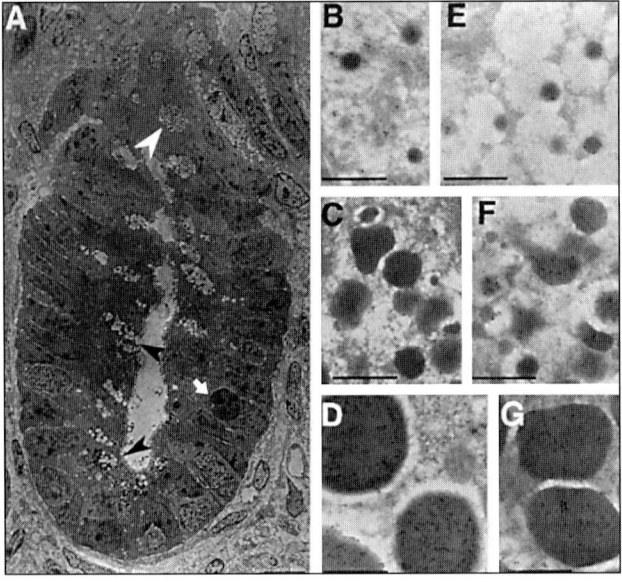

FIGURE 9–3. Mice expressing an SV-40 large T-antigen reporter transgene under control of the mouse cryptdin-2 gene promoter contain an amplified population of cryptdin- and secretory phospholipase A_2–producing intermediate and granule goblet cells. A, Transmission electron microscopy of a distal jejunal crypt showing ablation of mature Paneth cells. Numbers of intermediate cells (*solid arrowheads*) and granule goblet cells (*open arrowhead*) are increased on a per-crypt basis. The *open arrow* indicates an apoptotic cell. Bar = 4 μm. B to D, Electron microscopic immunohistochemical demonstration of $sPLA_2$ in the dense core granules in a granule goblet cell from the upper third of the crypt (B) and in intermediate cells located in the middle and lower thirds of the crypt (C and D, respectively). The sections were incubated with rabbit antiphospholipase A_2 antiserum and with gold-labeled goat antirabbit Ig. Bar = 1 μm. E to G, Electron microscopic immunohistochemical demonstration of cryptdin accumulation in core granules of a granule goblet cell positioned in the upper crypt (E) and in the secretory granules of intermediate cells located in the middle and lower thirds of the crypt (F and G, respectively). Sections were treated with rabbit anticryptdin and gold-labeled goat antirabbit Ig. Cryptdin and $sPLA_2$ are present only in cells containing electron dense cores, which become diminished in cells as they ascend the crypt-villus units. Villus goblet cells containing mucin globules that lack electron dense cores are not immunoreactive for $sPLA_2$ or cryptdin (data not shown). Bars = 1 μm. (With permission from Garabedian EM, Roberts LJJ, McNevin MS, Gordon JI. Examining the role of Paneth cells in the small intestine by lineage ablation in transgenic mice. J Biol Chem 1997;272:23729–40.)

contain Paneth cell–deficient crypts that are occupied by apparently undifferentiated crypt columnar cells (Figure 9–3). In these mice, there were no obvious effects on the proliferative capability or terminal differentiation programs of the other major epithelial lineages. Also, the crypts of mice maintained in a barrier facility had no evidence of colonization by commensal microflora of the gut as detected by silver staining.[52] Furthermore, in the transgenic mice expressing large T antigen, loss of recognizable Paneth cells coincided with an increased number of intermediate cells in the crypts that upregulated production of granules containing defensin. Thus, one outcome of these studies is the demonstration that Paneth cell deficiency induces the crypt intermediate cells to upregulate the production of gene products that are normally expressed only by the Paneth cell.

These observed phenotypes raise a number of issues. For example, in the absence of an exocytic pathway in the Paneth cells of disrupted crypts, it is possible that the epithelium continues to express Paneth cell genes. Similarly, the epithelium may produce antimicrobial peptides but release them constitutively rather than accumulating the peptides in granules for regulated secretion. Also, antimicrobial peptide genes that normally are not expressed by the small bowel epithelium may become activated subsequent to Paneth cell loss. It may be of interest to test the response of the gut epithelium of these transgenic mice to parasitic challenge such as infection with *T. spiralis* and treatments that induce changes in goblet cell and Paneth cell numbers.[64]

ANTIMICROBIAL PEPTIDES

Boman, author of the earliest studies of antimicrobial peptides in animals, traced the origins of the field of peptide antibiotics to Ehrlich, who sought to identify the "magic bullet" of chemotherapy.[13] That agent could be an immune substance, a natural product, or a chemical with the capability to kill a pathogenic microbe effectively without the host incurring unacceptable side effects. With Fleming's discovery of the lysozyme in 1922, a hydrolytic enzyme with substrate specificity for the peptidoglycan of bacterial cell walls, it became clear that vertebrate genomes could code for proteins that antagonized bacteria and could participate in host defense. Subsequently, the discovery of penicillin by Fleming and of gramicidin and tyrocidin from *Bacillus brevis* by Hotchkiss and Dubos stimulated the systematic screening of natural products and synthetic analogues for molecules with antibiotic properties. The impact of those efforts on world health has been enormous and tempered only by the emergence and dispersal of microbial species with resistance to most available antibiotics.

Within the past two decades, antimicrobial peptides have been identified from a broad range of sources. In general, antimicrobial peptides are distinguished from enzymatically assembled, amino acid–containing antibiotics by the fact that they are genetically encoded. Typically, genes that code for antimicrobial proteins and peptides are expressed by differentiated cell populations, including epithelia and phagocytes. In phagocytic cells, antimicrobial peptides are stored in granules and participate as primary mediators of nonoxidative microbial cell killing. In epithelial cells, peptides may be released constitutively, or they may accumulate in secretory granules for later release under the control of regulated exocytic pathways, as they do in Paneth cells.

The phylogenetic distribution is extensive for certain microbicidal peptide families. Examples include the fat body of many insect larvae, which induces antimicrobial peptide synthesis upon infection or exposure to lipopolysaccharide, the midgut of *Anopheles gambiae* and *Stomoxys calcitrans* which upregulate insect defensin gene expression after a blood meal, and winter flounder skin mucous cells which accumulate pleurocidin, a potent antibacterial peptide.[108,109] In frogs, the skin produces an endogenous antimicrobial peptide, magainin, one of the first antimicrobial peptides to be described.[11] Magainin also is found in specialized cells in the stomach and in glandular cells at the base of intestinal folds.[110–112] In humans, phagocytes, airway and reproductive epithelia, and Paneth cells produce a variety of gene-encoded antimicrobial peptides that function in host defense.

Antimicrobial Peptide Structure and Phylogeny

Antimicrobial peptides range from linear, α-helical molecules to dicyclic, β-sheet-containing peptides that contain up to three disulfide bonds and have no α-helical component.[17,113] Several authors have suggested grouping antimicrobial peptides on the basis of their biochemical composition or secondary structures into categories such as (1) linear, amphipathic α-helical molecules, (2) β-sheet-containing peptides with one or more disulfide bonds, (3) peptides lacking cysteine that contain high levels of one or more amino acids, and (4) those peptides that are less easily categorized.

Antimicrobial peptide families exist in species that span the evolutionary ladder. They are found in *Entamoeba* sp., insects, the horseshoe crab, plants, and in phagocytic leukocytes and epithelia of many vertebrates, including humans.[6,14,16,20,114–121] In mammals, the peptides generally function to kill ingested microbes intracellularly within the phagolysosomes or extracellularly via their release onto mucosal surfaces, where they may function as inhibitors of epithelial colonization.[122] That varied epithelia contribute to their own mucosal immunity is increasingly evident. This feature has broad phylogenetic distribution.

Cecropins and defensins, isolated from moth larvae and rabbit phagocytes, respectively, were the first gene-encoded, antimicrobial peptides whose primary structures were defined. A comparison of the insect cecropin peptide with mammalian neutrophilic defensins, now termed α-defensins, illustrates how the properties of antimicrobial peptides with reasonably similar activities can differ markedly. Cecropins are prototypes of the linear, amphipathic α-helical peptides, and they lack cysteine. In contrast, defensins consist of three strands of β-sheet structure that result from the formation of three intramolecular and invariant disulfide bonds between the six cysteine residues of the peptide. Thus, the primary, secondary, and tertiary structures of antimicrobial peptides may vary significantly. Despite this diversity of primary and secondary structures, antibiotic peptides are usually amphipathic, a feature that permits the peptides to disrupt the microbial cell membranes and kill microorganisms, perhaps by disabling or dissipating electrochemical gradients.[123,123–125]

DEFENSINS

Mammalian defensins consist of two closely related 3-4 kDa, cationic antimicrobial peptide families, the α- and β-defensins.[123] The α-defensins were among the first antimicrobial peptide families to be recognized and characterized and are major constituents of the primary granules of mammalian phagocytic leukocytes.[122,123,126–128] Certain α-defensins are stored in the azurophilic granules of neutrophils, where they may account for 5 to 18% of the total cellular protein.[129] It has been estimated that the fusion of a phagosome containing an ingested microorganism with the primary granule exposes the microorganism to defensin concentrations of at least 10 mg/mL.[129] Other α-defensins are abundantly expressed in Paneth cells, and their structure and biology will be discussed in some detail below.

The second family of defensins, the β-defensins, were discovered in cattle as antimicrobial peptides of neutrophil granules and of airway and lingual epithelial cells.[9,130,131] They have been identified in several mammalian and avian species and appear to be expressed by a greater variety of cell types than are the α-defensins. For example, in humans, β-defensin peptides or transcripts have been detected in the kidney, skin, pancreas, gingiva, salivary gland, cornea, and airway epithelium.[132–134] In cystic fibrosis, the ionic strength of airway surface fluid has been shown to inhibit human β-defensin (hBD)-1 antibacterial activity in vitro, and this inhibition has been implicated in the microbial pathogenesis associated with the disease.[135–137] There is, however, some controversy regarding the ionic strength of the airway fluid in both healthy individuals and those with cystic fibrosis and the relative contribution of hBD-1 to airway surface fluid defenses.[138] Accordingly, the role of hBD-1 in the pathophysiology of cystic fibrosis is uncertain. In the intestinal tract, significant expression of β-defensins have been reported in ruminants.[139–141] but not in other mammals. Recently, Diamond and Bevins reviewed the β-defensins.[142]

Defensin Structure

The α- and β-defensins both contain six cysteine residues which form three disulfide bonds. For α-defensins, specific and invariant disulfide bond pairings form between Cys1-Cys6, Cys2-Cys4, and Cys3-Cys5.[143] In the β-defensins, the pairing occurs between Cys1-Cys5, Cys2-Cys4, and Cys3-Cys6.[144] Although the Cys-Cys tridisulfide pairings of these two peptide families differ,[123,145] their folded conformations are remarkably similar.[145–147] Experimental refolding of α- and β-defensins synthesized in solid phase[18] suggests that these pairings are thermodynamically favorable. In addition to their topologic similarities, both peptide families have conserved glycine residues, and α-defensins have characteristic glycine, glutamic acid, and arginine residues at conserved positions.[148]

The folded conformation of the α-defensins consists of three β-strands and no α-helical content;[146,147] this highly constrained tertiary structure is required for antimicrobial activity.[123] The 1.9 Å crystal structure of the human neutrophil α-defensin HNP-3 is a noncovalent, amphipathic dimer in which arginine side chains lie equatorially above a hydrophobic surface consisting of apolar monomer side chains.[149] The amino and carboxyl termini of the monomers are clustered on the pole of the dimer opposite the hydrophobic face.[123,150] However, the solution structures of α-defensins from rabbit neutrophils show that those α-defensin peptides are monomeric. As described below, these structural differences are associated with major differ-

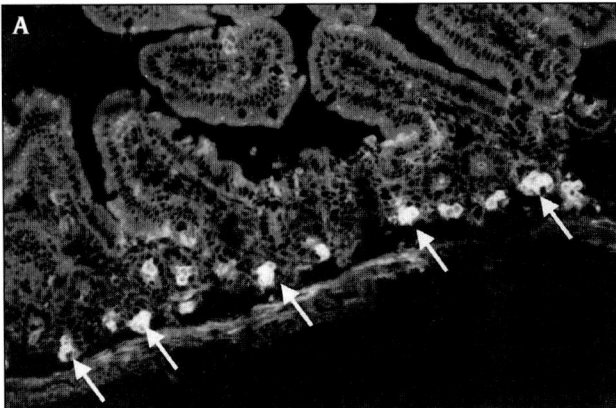 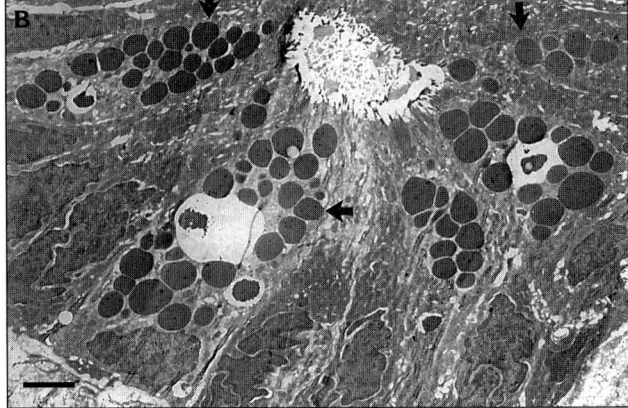

FIGURE 9–4. α-Defensins in mouse and human Paneth cell granules. A, Immunohistochemical detection of cryptdins in adult mouse small intestine as described.[99] Cryostat sections of periodate-lysine:paraformaldehyde-fixed mouse small intestines were cut at a thickness of 1 or 4 μm. Sections were incubated with PBS containing 1% BSA for 15 min prior to application of the primary rabbit polyclonal anticryptdin-1 antibody for 2 h at room temperature at a 1:100 dilution, washed, and treated with goat antirabbit IgG coupled to CY3 (Jackson Immunologicals,). As previously demonstrated,[82] cryptdins are present in Paneth cells at the base of the crypts of Lieberkühn in adult mouse small intestine (arrows). B, Transmission electron microscopic immunohistochemical analysis of HD-5 expression in the human ileal crypt. Granules rich in HD-5 immunogold staining are localized to Paneth cells (arrows). Bar = 2 μm. (Data from: Porter EM, Liu L, Oren A, et al. Localization of human intestinal defensin 5 in Paneth cell granules. Infect Immun 1997;65:2389–95.

ences in action and in the apparent mechanisms by which these peptides interact with reconstituted model membranes.

Defensin Mechanism of Microbial Cell Killing

Defensins are broadly effective against gram-positive and gram-negative bacteria, fungi, spirochetes, protozoa, and enveloped viruses.[151] The α-defensins from human and rabbit neutrophils both achieve cell killing by membrane disruption but by apparently different mechanisms. Human and rabbit human neutrophil α-defensins share extensive structural similarity with respect to conserved disulfide bonds, amphipathicity, and β-sheet backbones, yet as noted above, human HNP-2 peptide is a noncovalent dimer and rabbit α-defensin NP-1 is monomeric in solution.[146,147,152] The outer and inner membranes of Escherichia coli are permeabilized sequentially by the human neutrophil peptides, and these peptides induce the formation of ion channels in lipid bilayers.[153,154] Both these peptide-elicited effects are influenced by membrane energetics.[154] Dimeric HNP-2 forms large multimeric pores after insertion into model membranes. The diameter of the human neutrophilic defensin pore structure has been estimated to be 20 Å, on the basis of the defensin atomic structure and the deduced minimum pore diameter for sized dextran polymer release from preloaded membrane phospholipid vesicles.[149] A pore model in which six human neutrophil defensin dimers intercalate in the bilayer to form the pore annulus has been proposed and reviewed.[123] In sharp contrast, monomeric NP-1 causes graded leakage of dextran from phospholipid vesicles of the same composition. Thus, NP-1 does not induce stable multimeric pores but permeabilizes the membrane by generating large, short-lived defects in the phospholipid bilayer.[123,155] No similar detailed analysis of β-defensin activity is yet reported.

α-Defensins in Paneth Cells

In addition to neutrophils, α-defensins also are abundant constituents of Paneth cell granules.[156,157] In both humans and mice, in situ hybridization experiments have shown that enteric defensin transcripts are present in Paneth cells,[12,158,159] and antibodies to recombinant HD-5 and to synthetic cryptdin-1 react with Paneth cells in a highly specific fashion (Figure 9–4).

In mice, several α-defensin peptides are present in the small intestinal Paneth cells. Six mouse cryptdins have been purified to homogeneity from rinsed tissue by combined gel permeation chromatography and reverse-phase high-performance liquid chromatography (HPLC).[82,94,160] Peptide sequencing of these purified enteric defensins revealed several isoforms, and peptide recoveries from the intact small bowel showed that levels of intestinal isoforms differed, with approximately equivalent levels of cryptdins 1, 2, 5, and 6 and lower overall levels of cryptdins 3 and 4.[82] As a group, Paneth cell defensins have extended amino termini that are four to six residues longer than the average N-terminus of the leukocyte-derived defensins, but the role of the N-terminus has not been formally examined.

As expected, as constituents of Paneth cell secretory granules, the α-defensins are present in the lumen of the mouse small intestine. Peptides with charge-to-size ratios characteristic of defensins have been detected in the saline rinses of adult mouse jejunum and ileum by acid-urea polyacrylamide gel electrophoresis (PAGE).[82,94] Interestingly, direct electrophoretic comparison of putative luminal and tissue cryptdins has shown that many of the peptides do not comigrate, suggesting some modification of the luminal peptides. Cryptdins have been recovered from the washings of the jejunal and ileal lumen without administration of pharmacologic agents, demonstrating that the peptides are released and resist degradation in the intestinal lumen.[94]

Using the combined Bio-Gel P-60 and reverse-phase HPLC purification scheme used for the purification of cryptdin 1 to 6 tissue forms, luminal forms of cryptdins have been purified. Some luminal cryptdin peptides have primary sequences identical to the cellular cryptdins isolated from intestinal tissue, and their biochemical and antimicrobial properties are under investigation.[94]

Defensin precursors from Paneth cells and neutrophils are similar in their general features. All are synthesized as 85 to 100 amino acid pre-propeptides that contain canonical signal sequences, acidic propeptide segments of approximately 40 amino acids, and a mature peptide at the C-terminus of the pre-propeptide.[161] Human Paneth cell defensin precursors HD-5 and HD-6 show greater divergence than do the cryptdin precursors in the mouse.[158,159,162] In cells of myeloid origin, the α-defensin precursors appear to be cleaved within 4 to 24 hours after synthesis by sequential events that produce intermediates of 75 and 56 amino acids;[163-166] nearly all defensin exists in mature phagocytic cells as fully processed peptide. In mice, the pre-prosegments of cryptdin precursors are more highly conserved than the mature defensin peptide-coding regions, suggesting that the prosegment may be involved in defensin trafficking during granulogenesis. The details of Paneth cell α-defensin processing have not been reported.

Human Paneth cells express defensin genes at levels equivalent to those in the mouse[159] but in contrast to the numerous defensin isoforms in mouse Paneth cells, there are only two active cryptdin genes in the human Paneth cells.[162] Initial studies using immunologic detection of HD-5 peptides in postsurgical ileal neobladders and ileal tissue have revealed multiple forms processed at the N-terminus. In ileal neobladder urine, three forms were chemically characterized, representing amino acids 36 to 94, 56 to 94, and 63 to 94. The shortest form (63 to 94) is similar to a recombinant HD-5 peptide (64 to 94) which has broad-spectrum antimicrobial activity. In extracts from washed ileal tissue, two forms were characterized, amino acids 24 to 94 and 29 to 94. The activity of the isolated peptide isoforms remains to be tested. The detection of apparently propeptide forms suggests that human Paneth cells may store pro-HD-5 that is processed to mature peptide during or after exocytic secretion. Searching for HD-6 using characteristic chromatographic and electrophoretic properties of defensins, rather than the immunologic detection used for HD-5, revealed a mature peptide (amino acids 69 to 100) in both sources. Whether proforms predominate for this defensin in tissues will be important to determine when immunologic reagents become available.

Defensin Genes

Structure and Tissue Expression

The α-defensin genes characteristically have tissue-specific expression patterns. Although some genes are expressed in cells of myeloid lineage and others in Paneth cells, so far no single defensin gene has been found to be expressed in both types of cells.[122] A striking observation has emerged from analysis of the α-defensin gene structure in several species: all the α-defensin genes expressed in cells of hematopoietic origin have three exons but those genes expressed in Paneth cells have two. Highly similar exons in the hematopoietic and epithelial defensin genes of several mammalian species suggest that corresponding ancestral genes of each type existed prior to the evolutionary divergence of these species.

The two exons of the Paneth cell defensin genes are similar in organization and sequence to the second and third of the hematopoietic defensin genes. Isolation and characterization of complete genomic coding sequences for mouse cryptdins 1 to 6[167] (Darmoul et al., unpublished observations) and the human HD-5 and HD-6 genes[158,159] has shown that the 5′-untranslated region and the pre-prosegment of Paneth cell genes are encoded completely by exon 1. An additional intron interrupts the 5′-untranslated region of myeloid defensin genes analyzed from human,[168,169] guinea pig,[170] and rabbit.[171] In all cases, the most distal exon of the α-defensin genes codes for the functional peptide. Interestingly, for many of the mouse α-defensins, the N-terminal cryptdin residue is coded by the first complete codon of exon 2[167] but that is not the case with cryptdin-4 or with rabbit or human neutrophil α-defensins.[148,151] A model for a possible evolutionary history of the human defensin gene family has been proposed.[162]

The mechanisms that direct tissue-specific gene expression are unknown. In transgenic mice, a putative cryptdin-2 gene promoter is capable of directing the appropriate expression of reporter genes.[52,57] Lines of mice were produced that express transgenes consisting of 6.5 kb of DNA 5′- of the cryptdin-2 gene transcription start site, upstream of a human growth hormone (hGH) reporter gene. In several pedigrees of these transgenic mice, Paneth cells produce hGH appropriately and only in Paneth cells.[57] The phenotypes of mice expressing attenuated diphtheria toxin A fragment and SV40 large T antigen as reporter genes for this cryptdin-2 gene promoter[52] have been described in a previous section. Both RNA blot hybridization and reverse transcriptase polymerase chain reaction (RT-PCR) analyses showed that hGH mRNA expression in cryptdin-2/hGH transgenics was restricted to the small intestine and was consistent with the proximal-to-distal distribution of Paneth cells. Expression of the cryptdin-2/hGH transgene in newborn mice was detected in the proliferating and nonproliferating cells of the intervillous epithelium until approximately 5 days of age and became restricted to Paneth cells later in crypt ontogeny. In adults, expression was restricted to Paneth cells. Thus, the 6.5 kb of DNA, upstream of the cryptdin-2 gene transcription start site, is sufficient to direct cryptdin gene expression in Paneth cells.[57] In normal mouse embryos, an anticryptdin antibody stains cells in the undifferentiated intervillous epithelium coincident with remodeling of the endoderm to form a monolayer in the third week of gestation. Although levels are low, PCR-based assays detect cryptdin mRNAs in 1-day-old mice (Figure 9–5A), and DNA sequence analysis has confirmed the presence of several cryptdin-coding sequences in the small bowel of the newborn, of which cryptdin-6 represents 60% of the clones analyzed.[99] It seems unlikely that cryptdin-expressing cells in the neonatal epithelial monolayer are progenitors of adult intestinal Paneth cells because transgenics that are Paneth cell deficient throughout crypt ontogeny develop normally.[52]

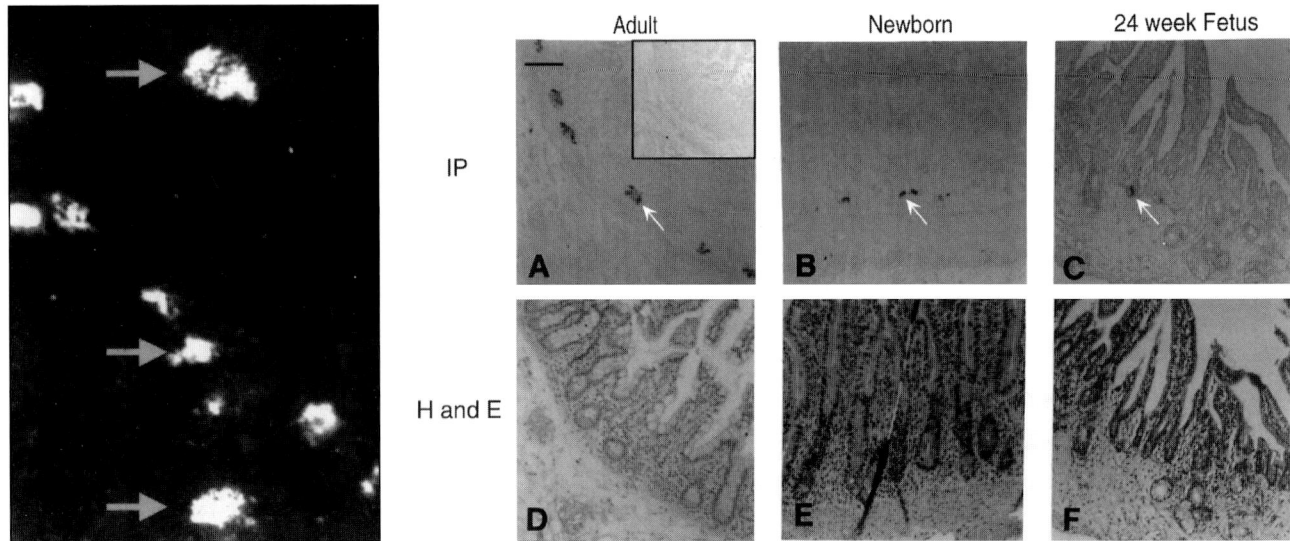

FIGURE 9–5. A. α-Defensin gene expression in developing murine and human small intestine. *Left panel*, Immunohistochemical detection of cryptdins in the small intestine of a newborn mouse. In contrast to their localization in Paneth cell granules in adult mice (Figure 9–4), cryptdin-positive cells in the intestine of 1-day-old mice are scattered throughout the developing epithelium[99] (*arrows*). No immunoreactivity was detected using preimmune serum. *Right panel*, HD-5 peptide expression in human small intestinal development. Terminal ileum tissue was stained with polyclonal rabbit HD-5 antiserum in (A) adult, (B) term newborn, and (C) 24-week fetus, using a counterstain of light green. Arrows denote positive staining of Paneth cells by polyclonal HD-5 antibody. Control slide of adult tissue was stained with preimmune serum and counterstained with light green (A, *inset*). Parallel tissue sections were stained with hematoxylin and eosin (D,E,F). Bar = 100 microns. (With permission from Salzman NH, Polin RA, Harris MC, et al. Enteric defensin expression in necrotizing enterocolitis. Pediatr Res 1998;40:22–6.)

Interestingly, transgenic nursing mouse pups carrying an HD-5 gene construct express the peptide in Paneth cells at low levels, with a rapid increase during the weaning period[172] a developmental sequence very similar to that of endogenous mouse cryptdin gene expression.[12,99,173,174]

In mice, at least one Paneth cell α-defensin gene is expressed differentially along the longitudinal axis of the murine small intestine. Cryptdin-4 mRNA is not detectable in the proximal small bowel, increasing to maximal levels in the distal ileum. In contrast, cryptdin-1 and cryptdin-5 mRNA content is equivalent in the duodenum, jejunum, and ileum.[175] The distribution of cryptdin-4 mRNA correlates with the greater number of bacteria found in the distal intestine, revealing a level of heterogeneity that is not morphologically apparent. It seems unlikely that microbial antigens or metabolic products stimulate selective accumulation of cryptdin-4 mRNA since the positional specificity of cryptdin-4 gene expression is the same in gnotobiotic mice as in mice with normal flora (Ouellette et al., unpublished observations). Cryptdin-4 is the most active mouse Paneth cell α-defensin isoform in assays conducted in vitro[94] although it is difficult to assess the relative activities of peptides isolated from different sources and characterized by different research groups. Given its pattern of differential expression, cryptdin-4 may contribute to innate immunity specifically in the distal small bowel, particularly where the bacteria are greatest in number.

The α-defensin transcripts and peptides described originally in human and mouse Paneth cells also are expressed in reproductive epithelium of those species. In mice, mRNA was detected by RT-PCR amplification and the peptides have been localized to the Sertoli's and Leydig's cells of the testis by immunoperoxidase staining with an anticryptdin-1 antibody.[176] In 15P-1 cells, a mouse Sertoli's cell line, α-defensin expression was inducible both by coculture with germ cells and by administration of the nerve growth factor,[176] a mediator of spermatid and Sertoli's cell interactions. In humans, mRNA corresponding to Paneth cell α-defensins were detected by RT-PCR in the endocervix, endometrium, and chorion as well as in an endometrial cell line; DNA analysis of the amplified sequences showed that some were HD-5 variants with 1 to 3 nucleotide substitutions,[177] which may be allelic variants in the human population. Also, immunohistochemical experiments have detected the HD-5 peptide in the endocervical epithelium,[178] demonstrating that it is produced in the human female genitourinary tract epithelium. In addition, two rabbit α-defensins with primary structures very different from the known rabbit myeloid α-defensins have been isolated from the kidney,[179,180] suggesting that there are α-defensins specific to the renal epithelium as well.

Expression during Development

Defensin-encoding mRNAs accumulate during intestinal development, and their appearance coincides with Paneth cell differentiation during intestinal crypt ontogeny.[12,57] The α-defensins are expressed early in the morphogenesis and differentiation of the murine small intestine. Cryptdin immunoreactivity is initially detected as the gut endoderm converts to a monolayer of epithelium at gestational day 15. During postnatal week 1, cryptdin immunoreactivity is observed in cells that resemble young Paneth cells. In situ hybridization experiments have shown that approximately

10% of crypts in 10-day-old mice are positive for cryptdin mRNA but by day 15, all crypts are positive and Paneth cell numbers in the proximal and distal small intestine are comparable. In adult mice, every crypt, regardless of its position along the length of the small bowel, is positive for α-defensin as assessed immunohistochemically or by RT-PCR.[82,94] In 42-day-old adult mice, there are an average of three cryptdin-positive cells per duodenal crypt, and ileal crypts each contain an average of five Paneth cells.[57] By day 42, the cryptdin-positive goblet cells occasionally seen in younger animals are absent from the duodenum, jejunum, and ileum.

In mice, a subset of cryptdin genes are differentially expressed during postnatal crypt ontogeny (see Figure 9–5A). As studies of mice expressing the cryptdin-2 promoter-hGH reporter transgene construct predicted,[57] cryptdin mRNAs are readily detected in the intestinal RNA in the newborn by RT-PCR[99] although they cannot be detected by conventional northern blot analysis.[12,99,174] Cryptdin-6 is the most frequent Paneth cell α-defensin cDNA cloned from intestinal RNA from newborn mice. The mRNAs that code for the Paneth cell markers lysozyme, matrilysin, and CRS1C also are detectable at birth.[99,181]

In humans, the genes encoding HD-5 and HD-6 are expressed in the developing fetus as early as 13.5 weeks of gestation, as detected by RT-PCR. This expression coincides with the appearance of Paneth cells in early ontogeny.[172] Whereas HD-5 mRNA was detected in both small intestine and colon, HD-6 was found only in the small intestine.[172] By 17 weeks' gestation, both HD-5 and HD-6 mRNA were detected by RT-PCR only in the small intestine (Figure 9–5B). At 24 weeks, HD-5 and HD-6 mRNA were detectable by northern blot hybridization but at levels approximately 200-fold lower than in the adult mice.[172] There is immunohistochemical evidence of intracellular HD-5 peptide in Paneth cells at 24 weeks gestation.[182] The intracellular peptide level generally correlates with mRNA levels during development. The physiologic significance of low-level defensin expression in human fetal intestine is not yet clear. However, the expression of defensins in utero, in the absence of stimulation by any inflammatory or infectious source, suggests constitutive expression of human Paneth cell defensin genes, similar to that in mice. This idea is consistent with the notion that enteric α-defensins, similar to the hematopoietic α-defensins, have constitutive levels of expression and are part of a developmental program of the highly differentiated cells in which they are expressed.

Expression in Necrotizing Enterocolitis

Necrotizing enterocolitis (NEC) affects newborn infants, particularly those born prematurely, but the precise cause is unknown.[183,184] Although controversial, a leading hypothesis suggests a link between infection and NEC.[185] The disease usually involves the terminal ileum and results in necrosis with hemorrhage, mucosal edema, and limited inflammation.[186] The higher incidence of NEC in premature newborns[187,188] may be related to the immaturity of local innate defenses.[185]

In cases of NEC, the level of enteric defensin mRNA expression is significantly elevated over that observed in controls.[182] This suggests that defensin expression can be induced by an exogenous stimulus provided by the process of NEC. In these experiments, the number of Paneth cells is increased approximately two-fold in NEC compared with controls, suggesting that the disease process may promote the differentiation of the crypt stem cells to produce greater numbers of Paneth cells.[182] Interestingly, the intracellular level of HD-5 peptide as detected by immunohistochemistry appeared unchanged despite an increase in HD-5 mRNA in the NEC samples. The implications of this paradoxical observation are not clear. Immunohistochemical detection of secretory proteins is an observation of a steady-state process and does not directly reflect levels of peptide production unless there is no degradation or secretion of the peptide. One interpretation is that the defensin peptides are being actively secreted in response to the ongoing disease process. Alternatively, defensin mRNA translation may be reduced in NEC compared with controls. Future studies of the regulation and secretion of Paneth cell defensins should shed light on these various possibilities. Nevertheless, these experiments support an association between enteric defensin expression and NEC, suggesting that enteric defensins may be involved in the pathophysiology of NEC. The low level of HD-5 and HD-6 expression during fetal life as compared with term newborns and adults may reflect one aspect of immature intestinal innate defenses and possibly be one factor that predisposes humans to NEC.

Chromosomal Map Location and Evolution

Paneth cell defensin genes are closely linked at chromosomal loci that include the myeloid defensin genes. The two human Paneth cell defensin genes map to 8p21-8pter,[162] the cytogenetic location of the myeloid defensin genes at 8p23;[189] in mice, the α-defensin genes are syntenic with those in humans, mapping to the proximal region of chromosome 8.[190,191] The proximity of cryptdin genes in mice is evident from several instances in which two complete genes have been isolated on several different 20 kb bacteriophage genomic clones (Huttner KM, Ouellette AJ, unpublished observations). For example, complete cryptdin-3 and cryptdin-5 genes, cryptdin-4 and cryptdin-5 genes, and cry-i and CRS1C[174] genes have been found paired on several different phage isolates (Ouellette AJ, Huttner KM, unpublished observations). Because coisolated family members have divergent second exons, the mouse linkage data demonstrate that evolutionarily distant cryptdin genes may be only a few kilobases apart on the physical map.

To delineate the possible evolutionary relationships of the defensin genes, the nucleotide sequence of the introns were compared using a dot-matrix Pustell analysis of nucleotide similarity.[162] Intron sequences were used for this analysis because they are likely to be relatively free of the evolutionary pressure of selection. In the case of the introns of human enteric defensins, a modest but relatively uniform sequence identity (54%) is seen along a diagonal through the entire intron region. This pattern is consistent with the possibility of duplication of a common ancestral gene and subsequent accumulation of nucleotide changes over evolutionary time. The introns of mouse enteric defensin genes 3, 5, and 6 are all highly similar (85%), suggesting that they arose from a more recent gene duplication event.[167] Comparison of the murine and human enteric genes shows a low degree of similarity (~38%), distributed evenly throughout the intron sequence.

An unexpected pattern of nucleotide similarity emerged when the human enteric and hematopoietic α-defensin genes were similarly compared.[162] In the comparison with HD-5, the region of highest similarity lies at the 5' portion of the intron and the adjoining exon but in the comparison with HD-6, the region of high similarity lies at the 3' portion of the intron and the adjoining downstream exon. Analogous patterns of similarity were apparent from the comparison of HD-5 and HD-6 with rabbit hematopoietic defensins. In contrast, when the hematopoietic genes were compared with one another, high nucleotide similarity was uniformly distributed throughout the intron (human versus human [76%] and human versus rabbit [59%]). Together, these findings suggest that the human and rabbit hematopoietic genes were recently derived from a common ancestral gene, and that the two human epithelial genes are more distantly related. The findings also suggest a complex relationship between the hematopoietic and the epithelial genes.

A model was proposed to account for the various patterns of sequence similarity revealed in these alignments. The model suggests that (1) an early duplication of a primordial defensin gene yielded the ancestral genes of present day HD-5 and HD-6 in a head-to-tail array. Each of these genes then accumulated nucleotide changes with a relatively uniform distribution over evolutionary time; (2) more recently, a subsequent homologous, but unequal, meiotic cross-over event generated a derivative chromosome containing the two original genes and a new gene composed of a hybrid of sequences from the two parental genes. This hybrid gene then served as the ancestor to the present-day hematopoietic genes and acquired the characteristic upstream exon and promoter of the hematopoietic defensin genes through a translocation event. Over time, this ancestral hematopoietic gene accumulated further sequence changes but retained the interesting pattern of sequence similarity, where the high nucleotide similarity of HD-5 is seen with the 5' portion of the hematopoietic genes, and the high similarity of HD-6 is seen with the 3' portion of these genes and; (3) given the previous two features, much more recent duplication events could then have yielded the hematopoietic defensin genes.

This model, although speculative, offers a plausible mechanism for the various nucleotide similarities observed, including the high similarity between the hematopoietic defensin genes (within and between species), the less pronounced nucleotide similarity of the enteric defensin genes, and the unusual pattern of similarity between the enteric and hematopoietic defensin genes. Finally, these sequence comparisons, independent of the proposed model, suggest that epithelial defensin genes predate the hematopoietic genes in evolution.

Antimicrobial Activity of Paneth Cell Defensins

Paneth cell α-defensins are microbicidal against *E. coli*. Although an early report showed that cryptdin-1 was active only against an attenuated *Salmonella typhimurium* mutant but not against the parental strain,[82] cryptdins 2 and 6 were shown to kill *Listeria monocytogenes*, *E. coli*, and *S. typhimurium*.[160] Under optimized pH and ionic conditions, all cryptdins were found to possess activity against *E. coli* ML35, *Staphylococcus aureus*, and *S. typhimurium*.[94] Among the murine Paneth cell α-defensins, cryptdins 4 and 5 have greater activity than the other four cryptdin isoforms in agar diffusion assays.[94] Relative to the activity of rabbit neutrophil defensin NP-1, cryptdin-5 was approximately five times more active at concentrations in the 100 µg/mL range, and cryptdin-4 had 50-fold greater activity than NP-1 at 100-300 µg/mL.[94]

Recombinant human Paneth cell HD-5 is active against several bacterial species and also against the fungus *Candida albicans*. The recombinant HD-5 peptide retains activity even after partial proteolysis, evidence that this peptide could function within the hostile environment of the intestinal lumen.[192] The recombinant HD-5 peptide tested was deduced from the cDNA sequence but its relation to the actual peptide in human small intestine is unclear since the N-terminus of the natural peptide remains to be clarified.

Selective Activity of Murine α-Defensins

The murine cryptdin isoforms are a group of closely related α-defensins that should be useful for analyzing structure-activity relationships in this peptide family. For example, cryptdins 1, 2, 3, and 6 differ from each other in sequence only by 1 to 4 amino acids, yet these primary structural features result in peptides with dramatically different activities in vitro. For example, cryptdin-2, which differs from cryptdin-3 only by a T10K replacement, was nonbactericidal for *E. coli*.[94] In contrast, cryptdin-3 was a potent microbicide against *E. coli*. A different pattern of target-specific activity was observed with respect to the sensitivity of *Giardia lamblia* trophozoites to cryptdin exposure.[193] In those experiments, cryptdins 2 and 3 were highly active against this intestinal protozoan in vitro but cryptdins 1 and 6 had little or no effect on trophozoite survival. Cryptdin-2 and 3 also share the ability to elicit chloride ion secretion when applied apically to monolayers of T84 cells.[194] When administered apically to the cells, cryptdins 2 or 3, but not cryptdin-1 or cryptdins 4 to 6, elicited a reversible, dose-dependent Cl⁻ secretory effect that ceased rapidly upon dilution. The only consistent difference between the active and inactive peptides is Arg 15 in the active peptides and Gly 15 in the inactive ones.

Cryptdin-4 is the most cationic of the cryptdins, and it is the first defensin peptide with a chain-length variation between the fourth and fifth cysteine residues.[82] In vitro, cryptdin-4 has the greatest combined bacteriostatic and bactericidal activity of the murine enteric defensins.[94] In studies of cryptdins isolated from rinses of the murine small intestinal lumen, a cryptdin-4 variant lacking the N-terminal Gly residue was recovered.[195] Interestingly, the des-Gly cryptdin-4 peptide lacked antibacterial activity against *E. coli* and an attenuated strain of *S. typhimurium*. Thus, it appears that the length of the N-terminus may be a factor in the ability of this peptide class to kill certain microbial targets. A systematic analysis of the effects of amino acid substitutions in cryptdin isoforms on antimicrobial activity against a variety of microorganisms is likely to reveal potential structure-function relationships in these peptides and perhaps in defensins in general.

The structural basis for the functional differences of the cryptdin-1-like isoforms appears to reside among a small number of surface-accessible residues. This conclusion is based on an analysis of structural models of the four cryptdins generated using the crystallographic backbone of the homologous human defensin HNP-3.[150,156] Amino acid side chains specific to individual isoforms were predicted to be surface exposed by homology and positioned near turns in the backbone. Possibly, the predicted topologic differences influence the ability of specific side chains of certain isoforms to interact with particular substituents of target cell membranes. Because the constituent membrane phospholipids strongly affect peptide-membrane interactions,[196] such modeling may help to explain the differential activities of individual peptides against particular microorganisms, for example, the inability of a bactericidal peptide to kill a eukaryotic target cell.

FUTURE PERSPECTIVES

Significant contributions to this area are likely to come from studies of mice and other species making the transition from germ-free to colonized states. For example, the kinetics of mucosal barrier establishment in the small bowel of the newborn is not understood in cellular or molecular terms, and mechanisms that influence or determine Paneth cell differentiation are unknown. The impact of microbes in the intestinal lumen on this epithelial maturation may be profound. Analysis of Paneth cell–deficient mice also should help clarify the role of Paneth cells in innate immunity and compensatory responses to their absence.[52] The phenotypes of mice deficient in Paneth cell–specific gene products should also reveal important insight into gut physiology. As they have in the past, defensins and their genes may serve as useful markers in determining mechanisms of epithelial cell differentiation and lineage determination, particularly in humans. An understanding of the details of defensin biosynthesis and regulation will help define the role of these peptides and that of Paneth cells in the establishment of enteric mucosal defense.

REFERENCES

1. Bjerknes M, Cheng H. The stem-cell zone of the small intestinal epithelium. IV. Effects of resecting 30% of the small intestine. Am J Anat 1981;160:93–103.
2. Neutra MR, Pringault E, Kraehenbuhl JP. Antigen sampling across epithelial barriers and induction of mucosal immune responses. Annu Rev Immunol 1996;14:275–300.
3. Trahair JF, Neutra MR, Gordon JI. Use of transgenic mice to study the routing of secretory proteins in intestinal epithelial cells: analysis of human growth hormone compartmentalization as a function of cell type and differentiation. J Cell Biol 1989;109:3231–42.
4. Lundqvist C, Baranov V, Hammarström S, et al. Intra-epithelial lymphocytes. Evidence for regional specialization and extrathymic T cell maturation in the human gut epithelium. Int Immunol 1995;7:1473–87.
5. Boman HG. Antibacterial peptides: key components needed in immunity. Cell 1991;65:205–7.
6. Ganz T, Lehrer RI. Antimicrobial peptides of vertebrates. Curr Opin Immunol 1998;10:41–4.
7. Zasloff M. Antibiotic peptides as mediators of innate immunity. Curr Opin Immunol 1992;4:3–7.
8. Lehrer RI, Ganz T. Defensins: endogenous antibiotic peptides from human leukocytes. Ciba Foundation Symposium 1992;171:276–93.
9. Diamond G, Zasloff M, Eck H, et al. Tracheal antimicrobial peptide, a cysteine-rich peptide from mammalian tracheal mucosa: peptide isolation and cloning of a cDNA. Proc Natl Acad Sci U S A 1991;88:3952–6.
10. Stolzenberg ED, Anderson GM, Ackermann MR, et al. Epithelial antibiotic induced in states of disease. Proc Natl Acad Sci U S A 1997;94:8686–90.
11. Zasloff M. Magainins, a class of antimicrobial peptides from Xenopus skin: isolation, characterization of two active forms, and partial cDNA sequence of a precursor. Proc Natl Acad Sci U S A 1987;84:5449–53.
12. Ouellette AJ, Greco RM, James M, et al. Developmental regulation of cryptdin, a corticostatin/defensin precursor mRNA in mouse small intestinal crypt epithelium. J Cell Biol 1989;108:1687–95.
13. Boman HG. Opening remarks. In: Marsh J, Goode JA, editors. Antimicrobial peptides. Chichester: John Wiley & Sons Ltd; 1994. p. 1–4.
14. Broekaert WF, Cammue BPA, De Bolle MFC, et al. Antimicrobial peptides from plants. Crit Rev Plant Sci 1997;16:297–323.
15. Lehrer RI, Ganz T. Endogenous vertebrate antibiotics—defensins, protegrins, and other cysteine-rich antimicrobial peptides. Ann N Y Acad Sci 1996;797:228–39.
16. Meister M, Lemaitre B, Hoffmann JA. Antimicrobial peptide defense in *Drosophila*. Bioessays 1997;19:1019–26.
17. Nissen-Meyer J, Nes IF. Ribosomally synthesized antimicrobial peptides: their function, structure, biogenesis, and mechanism of action. Arch Microbiol 1997;167:67–77.
18. Selsted ME. Investigational approaches for studying the structures and biological functions of myeloid antimicrobial peptides. In: Setlow, JK, editor. Genetic engineering. Principles and methods. New York, NY: Plenum Press; 1993. p. 131–47.
19. Tomita M, Takase M, Wakabayashi H, Bellamy W. Antimicrobial peptides of lactoferrin. Adv Exp Med Biol 1994; 357:209–18.
20. Zanetti M, Gennaro R, Romeo D. Cathelicidins: a novel protein family with a common proregion and a variable C-terminal antimicrobial domain. FEBS Lett 1995;374:1–5.
21. Louvard D, Kedinger M, Hauri HP. The differentiating intestinal epithelial cell: establishment and maintenance of functions through interactions between cellular structures. Annu Rev Cell Biol 1992;8:157–95.
22. Plateroti M, Freund JN, Leberquier C, Kedinger M. Mesenchyme-mediated effects of retinoic acid during rat intestinal development. J Cell Sci 1997;110:1227–38.
23. Simon-Assmann P, Kedinger M. Heterotypic cellular cooperation in gut morphogenesis and differentiation. Semin Cell Biol 1993;4:221–30.
24. Mahida YR, Galvin AM, Gray T, et al. Migration of human intestinal lamina propria lymphocytes, macrophages and eosinophils following the loss of surface epithelial cells. Clin Exp Immunol 1997;109:377–86.
25. Fritsch C, Simon-Assmann P, Kedinger M, Evans GS. Cytokines modulate fibroblast phenotype and epithelial-stroma interactions in rat intestine. Gastroenterology 1997;112:826–38.

26. Orian-Rousseau V, Aberdam D, Fontao L, et al. Developmental expression of laminin-5 and HD1 in the intestine: epithelial to mesenchymal shift for the laminin gamma2 chain subunit deposition. Dev Dyn 1996;206:12–23.
27. Gutierrez ED, Grapperhaus KJ, Rubin DC. Ontogenic regulation of spatial differentiation in the crypt-villus axis of normal and isografted small intestine. Am J Physiol Gastrointest Liver Physiol 1995;269:G500–11.
28. Molmenti EP, Perlmutter DH, Rubin DC. Cell-specific expression of α_1-antitrypsin in human intestinal epithelium. J Clin Invest 1993;92:2022–34.
29. Rubin DC. Spatial analysis of transcriptional activation in fetal rat jejunal and ileal gut epithelium. Am J Physiol 1992;263:G853–63.
30. Rubin DC, Roth KA, Birkenmeier EH, Gordon JI. Epithelial cell differentiation in normal and transgenic mouse intestinal isografts. J Cell Biol 1991;113:1183–92.
31. Rubin DC, Swietlicki E, Gordon JI. Use of isografts to study proliferation and differentiation programs of mouse stomach epithelia. Am J Physiol 1994;267:G27–39.
32. Rubin DC, Swietlicki E, Roth KA, Gordon JI. Use of fetal intestinal isografts from normal and transgenic mice to study the programming of positional information along the duodenal-to-colonic axis. J Biol Chem 1992;267:15122–33.
33. Cheng L, Qian SJ, Rothschild C, et al. Alteration of the binding specificity of cellular retinol-binding protein II by site-directed mutagenesis. J Biol Chem 1991;266:24404–12.
34. Cohn SM, Roth KA, Birkenmeier EH, Gordon JI. Temporal and spatial patterns of transgene expression in aging adult mice provide insights about the origins, organization, and differentiation of the intestinal epithelium. Proc Natl Acad Sci U S A 1991;88:1034–8.
35. Cohn SM, Simon TC, Roth KA, et al. Use of transgenic mice to map cis-acting elements in the intestinal fatty acid binding protein gene (Fabpi) that control its cell lineage-specific and regional patterns of expression along the duodenal-colonic and crypt-villus axes of the gut epithelium. J Cell Biol 1992;119:27–44.
36. Crossman MW, Hauft SM, Gordon JI. The mouse ileal lipid-binding protein gene: a model for studying axial patterning during gut morphogenesis. J Cell Biol 1994;126:1547–64.
37. Gordon JI. Intestinal epithelial differentiation: new insights from chimeric and transgenic mice. J Cell Biol 1989;108:1187–94.
38. Gordon JI, Schmidt GH, Roth KA. Studies of intestinal stem cells using normal, chimeric, and transgenic mice. FASEB J 1992;6:3039–50.
39. Hansbrough JR, Fine SM, Gordon JI. A transgenic mouse model for studying the lineage relationships and differentiation program of type II pneumocytes at various stages of lung development. J Biol Chem 1993;268:9762–70.
40. Hansbrough JR, Fine SM, Roth KA, Gordon JI. A transgenic mouse model for studying differentiation programs and lineage relationships in the developing mouse pulmonary epithelium. Chest 1992;101:6S–7S.
41. Hermiston ML, Gordon JI. Organization of the crypt-villus axis and evolution of its stem cell hierarchy during intestinal development. Am J Physiol Gastrointest Liver Physiol 31 1995;268:G813–22.
42. Hermiston ML, Green RP, Gordon JI. Chimeric-transgenic mice represent a powerful tool for studying how the proliferation and differentiation programs of intestinal epithelial cell lineages are regulated. Proc Natl Acad Sci U S A 1993; 90(19):8866–70.
43. Kim SH, Roth KA, Moser AR, Gordon JI. Transgenic mouse models that explore the multistep hypothesis of intestinal neoplasia. J Cell Biol 1993;123:877–93.
44. Lorenz RG, Gordon JI. Use of transgenic mice to study regulation of gene expression in the parietal cell lineage of gastric units. J Biol Chem 1993;268:26559–70.
45. Roth KA, Gordon JI. Spatial differentiation of the intestinal epithelium: analysis of enteroendocrine cells containing immunoreactive serotonin, secretin, and substance P in normal and transgenic mice. Proc Natl Acad Sci U S A 1990; 87:6408–12.
46. Roth KA, Hermiston ML, Gordon JI. Use of transgenic mice to infer the biological properties of small intestinal stem cells and to examine the lineage relationships of their descendants. Proc Natl Acad Sci U S A 1991;88:9407–11.
47. Simon TC, Gordon JI. Intestinal epithelial cell differentiation: new insights from mice, flies and nematodes. Curr Opin Genet Dev 1995;5:577–86.
48. Simon TC, Roth KA, Gordon JI. Use of transgenic mice to map cis-acting elements in the liver fatty acid-binding protein gene (*Fabpl*) that regulate its cell lineage-specific, differentiation-dependent, and spatial patterns of expression in the gut epithelium and in the liver acinus. J Biol Chem 1993;268: 18345–58.
49. Lambert M, Colnot S, Suh E, et al. cis-acting elements and transcription factors involved in the intestinal specific expression of the rat calbindin-D9k gene-binding of the intestine-specific transcription factor Cdx-2 to the TATA box. Eur J Biochem 1996;236:778–88.
50. Traber PG. Epithelial cell growth and differentiation .5. Transcriptional regulation, development, and neoplasia of the intestinal epithelium. Am J Physiol Gastrointest Liver Physiol 1997;273:G979–81.
51. Tung J, Markowitz AJ, Silberg DG, Traber PG. Developmental expression of SI is regulated in transgenic mice by an evolutionarily conserved promoter. Am J Physiol Gastrointest Liver Physiol 1997;273:G83–92.
52. Garabedian EM, Roberts LJJ, McNevin MS, Gordon JI. Examining the role of Paneth cells in the small intestine by lineage ablation in transgenic mice. J Biol Chem 1997; 272:23729–40.
53. Hermiston ML, Gordon JI. Inflammatory bowel disease and adenomas in mice expressing a dominant negative N-cadherin. Science 1995;270:1203–7.
54. Hermiston ML, Wong MH, Gordon JI. Forced expression of E-cadherin in the mouse intestinal epithelium slows cell migration and provides evidence for nonautonomous regulation of cell fate in a self-renewing system. Genes Dev 1996;10:985–96.
55. Li Q, Karam SM, Gordon JI. Simian virus 40 T antigen-induced amplification of pre-parietal cells in transgenic mice. Effects on other gastric epithelial cell lineages and evidence for a p53-independent apoptotic mechanism that operates in a committed progenitor. J Biol Chem 1995;270:15777–88.
56. Wong MH, Hermiston ML, Syder AJ, Gordon JI. Forced expression of the tumor suppressor adenomatosis polyposis coli protein induces disordered cell migration in the intestinal epithelium. Proc Natl Acad Sci U S A 1996;93:9588–93.
57. Bry L, Falk P, Huttner K, et al. Paneth cell differentiation in the developing intestine of normal and transgenic mice. Proc Natl Acad Sci U S A 1994;91:10335–9.
58. Gordon JI, Hooper LV, McNevin MS, et al. Epithelial cell growth and differentiation .3. Promoting diversity in the intestine: conversations between the microflora, epithelium, and diffuse GALT. Am J Physiol Gastrointest Liver Physiol 1997;273:G565–70.
59. Bansil R, Stanley E, Lamont JT. Mucin biophysics. Annu Rev Physiol 1995;57:635–57.
60. Ishikawa N, Horii Y, Oinuma T, et al. Goblet cell mucins as the selective barrier for the intestinal helminths: T-cell-inde-

pendent alteration of goblet cell mucins by immunologically 'damaged' *Nippostrongylus brasiliensis* worms and its significance on the challenge infection with homologous and heterologous parasites. Immunology 1994;81:480–6.
61. Manjili MH, France MP, Sangster NC, Rothwell TL. Quantitative and qualitative changes in intestinal goblet cells during primary infection of *Trichostrongylus colubriformis* high and low responder guinea pigs. Int J Parasitol 1998;28:761–5.
62. Tuccari G, Barresi G. Simultaneous demonstration of mucins and lysozyme in duodeno-jejunal biopsies of coeliac infants. Basic Appl Histochem 1984;28:177–82.
63. Fujino T, Ichikawa H, Fukuda K, Fried B. The expulsion of *Echinostoma trivolvis* caused by goblet cell hyperplasia in severe combined immunodeficient SCID mice. Parasite 1998;5:219–22.
64. Ishikawa N, Wakelin D, Mahida YR. Role of T helper 2 cells in intestinal goblet cell hyperplasia in mice infected with *Trichinella spiralis*. Gastroenterology 1997;113:542–9.
65. Thim L. A new family of growth factor-like peptides. 'Trefoil' disulphide loop structures as a common feature in breast cancer associated peptide (pS2), pancreatic spasmolytic polypeptide (PSP), and frog skin peptides (spasmolysins). FEBS Lett 1989;250:85–90.
66. Mashimo H, Wu DC, Podolsky DK, Fishman MC. Impaired defense of intestinal mucosa in mice lacking intestinal trefoil factor. Science 1996;274:262–5.
67. Kindon H, Pothoulakis C, Thim L, et al. Trefoil peptide protection of intestinal epithelial barrier function: cooperative interaction with mucin glycoprotein. Gastroenterology 1995;109:516–23.
68. Rose FR, Bailey K, Keyte JW, et al. Potential role of epithelial cell-derived histone H1 proteins in innate antimicrobial defense in the human gastrointestinal tract. Infect Immun 1998;66:3255–63.
69. Hiemstra PS, Eisenhauer PB, Harwig SSL, et al. Antimicrobial proteins of murine macrophages. Infect Immun 1993;61:3038–46.
70. Schwalbe G. Bietrage zur Kenntniss der Drusen in den Darmwandungen, in's Besondere der Brunner'schen Druden. Arch f Mikr Anat 1872;8:92–114.
71. Paneth J. Uweber die secernirenden Zellen des Dunndarm-Epithels. Arch f Mikr Anat 1888;31:113–91.
72. Selzman HM, Liebelt RA. Localization of sulfhydryl and disulfide groups of protein in Paneth cell secretion of the mouse intestine. J Histochem 1962;10:106.
73. Staley MW, Trier JS. Morphologic heterogeneity of mouse Paneth cell granules before and after secretory stimulation. Am J Anat 1965;117:365–83.
74. Trier JS, Lorenzsonn V, Groehler K. Pattern of secretion by Paneth cells of the small intestine of mice. Gastroenterology 1967;53:(2)240–9.
75. Satoh Y, Habara Y, Ono K, Kanno T. Carbamylcholine- and catecholamine-induced intracellular calcium dynamics of epithelial cells in mouse ileal crypts. Gastroenterology 1995;108:1345–56.
76. Ghoos Y, Vantrappen G. The cytochemical localization of lysozyme in Paneth cell granules. Histochem J 1971;3:175–8.
77. Peeters TL, Vantrappen GR. The Paneth cell: a source of intestinal lysozyme. Gut 1975;16:553–8.
78. Peeters TL, Vantrappen GR. Purification and partial characterization of lysozyme from mouse small intestine. Experientia 1976;32:1125–6.
79. Vantrappen GR, Peeters TL. Proceedings: the production of lysozyme by the Paneth cell. Gut 1974;15:826–7.
80. Erlandsen SL, Chase DG. Paneth cell function: phagocytosis and intracellular digestion of intestinal microorganisms. II. Spiral microorganism. J Ultrastructural Res 1972;41:319–33.

81. Erlandsen SL, Chase DG. Paneth cell function: phagocytosis and intracellular digestion of intestinal microorganisms. I. *Hexamita muris*. J Ultrastructure Res 1972;41:296–318.
82. Selsted ME, Miller SI, Henschen AH, Ouellette AJ. Enteric defensins: antibiotic peptide components of intestinal host defense. J Cell Biol 1992;118:929–36.
83. Cheng H, Merzel J, Leblond CP. Renewal of Paneth cells in the small intestine of the mouse. Am J Anat 1969;126:507–25.
84. Winter HS, Hendren RB, Fox CH, et al. Human intestine matures as nude mouse xenograft. Gastroenterology 1991;100:89–98.
85. Satoh Y. Effect of live and heat-killed bacteria on the secretory activity of Paneth cells in germ-free mice. Cell Tissue Res 1988;251:87–93.
86. Albedi FM, Lorenzetti E, Contini M, Nardi F. Immature Paneth cells in intestinal metaplasia of gastric mucosa. Appl Pathol 1984;2:43–8.
87. Frydman CP, Bleiweiss IJ, Unger PD, et al. Paneth cell-like metaplasia of the prostate gland. Arch Pathol Lab Med 1992;116:274–6.
88. Matsubara F. Morphological study of the Paneth cell. Paneth cells in intestinal metaplasia of the stomach and duodenum of man. Acta Pathol Jpn 1977;27:677–95.
89. Rubio CA, Kanter L, Björk J, et al. Paneth cell-rich flat adenoma of the rectum: report of a case. Jpn J Cancer Res 1996;87:109–12.
90. Rubio CA, Porwit-McDonald A, Rodensjö M, Duvander A. A method of quantitating Paneth cell metaplasia of the stomach by image analysis. Anal Quant Cytol Histol 1989;11:115–8.
91. Symonds DA. Paneth cell metaplasia in diseases of the colon and rectum. Arch Pathol 1974;97:343–7.
92. Satoh Y, Ishikawa K, Tanaka H, et al. Immunohistochemical observations of lysozyme in the Paneth cells of specific-pathogen-free and germ-free mice. Acta Histochem 1988;83:185–8.
93. Lacasse J, Martin LH. Detection of CD1 mRNA in Paneth cells of the mouse intestine by in situ hybridization. J Histochem Cytochem 1992;40:1527–34.
94. Ouellette AJ, Hsieh MM, Nosek MT, et al. Mouse Paneth cell defensins: primary structures and antibacterial activities of numerous cryptdin isoforms. Infect Immun 1994;62:5040–7.
95. Harwig SSL, Tan L, Qu X-D, et al. Bactericidal properties of murine intestinal phospholipase A_2. J Clin Invest 1995;95:603–10.
96. Satoh Y. Atropine inhibits the degranulation of Paneth cells in ex-germ-free mice. Cell Tissue Res 1988;253:397–402.
97. Gesase AP, Satoh Y, Ono K. G-protein activation enhances Ca^{+2}-dependent lipid secretion of the rat harderian gland. Anat Embryol (Berl) 1995;192:319–28.
98. Satoh Y, Ishikawa K, Oomori Y, et al. Bethanechol and a G-protein activator, NaF/AlCl3, induce secretory response in Paneth cells of mouse intestine. Cell Tiss Res 1992;269:213–20.
99. Darmoul D, Brown D, Selsted ME, Ouellette AJ. Cryptdin gene expression in developing mouse small intestine. Am J Physiol Gastrointest Liver Physiol 1997;272:G197–206.
100. Bry L, Falk PG, Midtvedt T, Gordon JI. A model of host-microbial interactions in an open mammalian ecosystem. Science 1996;273:1380–3.
101. Desai SJ, Mulherkar R, Wagle AS, Deo MG. Ontogeny of enhancing factor in mouse intestines and skin. Histochemistry 1991;96:371–4.
102. Rubin DC, Ong DE, Gordon JI. Cellular differentiation in the emerging fetal rat small intestinal epithelium: mosaic patterns of gene expression. Proc Natl Acad Sci U S A 1989;86:1278–82.
103. Henning SJ. Biochemistry of intestinal development. Environ Health Perspect 1979;33:9–16.

104. Henning SJ. Development of the gastrointestinal tract. Proc Nutr Soc 1986;45:39–44.
105. Martin GR, Henning SJ. Relative importance of corticosterone and thyroxine in the postnatal development of sucrase and maltase in rat small intestine. Endocrinol 1982;111:912–8.
106. McDonald MC, Henning SJ. Synergistic effects of thyroxine and dexamethasone on enzyme ontogeny in rat small intestine. Pediatr Res 1992;32:306–11.
107. Gordon JI, Hooper LV, Bry L, et al. Interactions between epithelial cells and bacteria, normal and pathogenic response. Science 1997;276:965.
108. Lehane MJ, Wu D, Lehane SM. Midgut-specific immune molecules are produced by the blood-sucking insect *Stomoxys calcitrans*. Proc Natl Acad Sci U S A 1997;94:11502–7.
109. Dimopoulos G, Richman A, Muller HM, Kafatos FC. Molecular immune responses of the mosquito *Anopheles gambiae* to bacteria and malaria parasites. Proc Natl Acad Sci U S A 1997;94:11508–13.
110. Moore KS, Bevins CL, Brasseur MM, et al. Antimicrobial peptides in the stomach of *Xenopus laevis*. J Biol Chem 1991;266:19851–7.
111. Moore KS, Bevins CL, Tomassini N, et al. A novel peptide-producing cell in *Xenopus*: multinucleated gastric mucosal cell strikingly similar to the granular gland of the skin. J Histochem Cytochem 1992;40:367–78.
112. Reilly DS, Tomassini N, Bevins CL, Zasloff M. A Paneth cell analogue in *Xenopus* small intestine expresses antimicrobial peptide genes: conservation of an intestinal host-defense system. J Histochem Cytochem 1994;42:697–704.
113. Boman HG. Peptide antibiotics and their role in innate immunity. Annu Rev Immunol 1995;13:61–92.
114. Bevins CL. Antimicrobial peptides as agents of mucosal immunity. In: Marsh J, Goode JA, editors. Antimicrobial peptides. Chichester: John Wiley & Sons; 1994. p. 250–69.
115. Boman HG. Peptide antibiotics: holy or heretic grails of innate immunity? Scand J Immunol 1996;43:475–82.
116. Bower CK, Daeschel MA, McGuire J. Protein antimicrobial barriers to bacterial adhesion. J Dairy Sci 1998;81:2771–8.
117. Gallo RL, Huttner KM. Antimicrobial peptides: an emerging concept in cutaneous biology. J Invest Dermatol 1998;111:739–43.
118. Ganz T, Lehrer RI. Antimicrobial peptides of leukocytes. Curr Opin Hematol 1997;4:53–8.
119. Ganz T, Weiss J. Antimicrobial peptides of phagocytes and epithelia. Semin Hematol 1997;34:343–54.
120. Moore AJ, Beazley WD, Bibby MC, Devine DA. Antimicrobial activity of cecropins. J Antimicrob Chemother 1996;37:1077–89.
121. Schroeder JM. Epithelial peptide antibiotics. Biochem Pharmacol 1999;57:121–34.
122. Selsted ME, Ouellette AJ. Defensins in granules of phagocytic and non-phagocytic cells. Trends Cell Biol 1995;5:114–9.
123. White SH, Wimley WC, Selsted ME. Structure, function, and membrane integration of defensins. Curr Opin Struct Biol 1995;5:521–7.
124. Lee DG, Shin SY, Maeng CY, Hahm KS. Cecropin A melittin hybrid peptide exerts its antifungal effects by damaging on the plasma membranes of *Trichosporon beigelii*. Biotechnol Lett 1998;20:211–4.
125. Wenk MR, Seelig J. Magainin 2 amide interaction with lipid membranes: calorimetric detection of peptide binding and pore formation. Biochemistry 1998;37:3909–16.
126. Lehrer RI, Selsted ME, Szklarek D, Fleischmann J. Antibacterial activity of microbicidal cationic proteins 1 and 2, natural peptide antibiotics of rabbit lung macrophages. Infect Immun 1983;42:10–4.
127. Selsted ME, Brown DM, DeLange RJ, Lehrer RI. Primary structures of MCP-1 and MCP-2, natural peptide antibiotics of rabbit lung macrophages. J Biol Chem 1983;258:14485–9.
128. Lehrer RI, Ganz T, Selsted ME. Defensins: endogenous antibiotic peptides of animal cells. Cell 1991;64:229–30.
129. Ganz T, Selsted ME, Szklarek D, et al. Defensins. Natural peptide antibiotics of human neutrophils. J Clin Invest 1985;76:1427–35.
130. Schonwetter BS, Stolzenberg ED, Zasloff MA. Epithelial antibiotics induced at sites of inflammation. Science 1995;267:1645–8.
131. Selsted ME, Tang YQ, Morris WL, et al. Purification, primary structures, and antibacterial activities of beta-defensins, a new family of antimicrobial peptides from bovine neutrophils. J Biol Chem 1993;268:6641–8.
132. McCray PB Jr, Bentley L. Human airway epithelia express a β-defensin. Am J Respir Cell Mol Biol 1997;16:343–9.
133. Zhao CQ, Wang I, Lehrer RI. Widespread expression of beta-defensin hBD-1 in human secretory glands and epithelial cells. FEBS Lett 1996;396:319–22.
134. Bensch KW, Raida M, Mägert H-J, et al. hBD-1: A novel β-defensin from human plasma. FEBS Lett 1995;368:331–5.
135. Goldman MJ, Anderson GM, Stolzenberg ED, et al. Human β-defensin-1 is a salt-sensitive antibiotic in lung that is inactivated in cystic fibrosis. Cell 1997;88:553–60.
136. Bals R, Goldman MJ, Wilson JM. Mouse β-defensin 1 is a salt-sensitive antimicrobial peptide present in epithelia of the lung and urogenital tract. Infect Immun 1998;66:1225–32.
137. Bals R, Wang X, Wu Z, et al. Human beta-defensin 2 is a salt-sensitive peptide antibiotic expressed in human lung. J Clin Invest 1998;102:874–80.
138. Knowles MR, Robinson JM, Wood RE, et al. Ion composition of airway surface liquid of patients with cystic fibrosis as compared with normal and disease-control subjects. J Clin Invest 1997;100:2588–95.
139. Tarver AP, Clark DP, Diamond G, et al. Enteric beta-defensin: molecular cloning and characterization of a gene with inducible intestinal epithelial cell expression associated with *Cryptosporidium parvum* infection. Infect Immun 1998;66:1045–56.
140. Huttner KM, Brezinski-Caliguri DJ, Mahoney MM, Diamond G. Antimicrobial peptide expression is developmentally regulated in the ovine gastrointestinal tract. J Nutr 1998;128:297S.
141. Huttner KM, Lambeth MR, Burkin HR, et al. Localization and genomic organization of sheep antimicrobial peptide genes. Gene 1998;206:85–91.
142. Diamond G, Bevins CL. Beta-defensins: endogenous antibiotics of the innate host defense response. Clin Immunol Immunopathol 1998;88:221–5.
143. Selsted ME, Harwig SS. Determination of the disulfide array in the human defensin HNP-2. A covalently cyclized peptide. J Biol Chem 1989;264:4003–7.
144. Tang YQ, Selsted ME. Characterization of the disulfide motif in BNBD-12, an antimicrobial beta-defensin peptide from bovine neutrophils. J Biol Chem 1993;268:6649–53.
145. Zimmermann GR, Legault P, Selsted ME, Pardi A. Solution structure of bovine neutrophil β-defensin-12: the peptide fold of the β-defensins is identical to that of the classic defensins. Biochemistry 1995;34:13663–71.
146. Skalicky JJ, Selsted ME, Pardi A. Structure and dynamics of the neutrophil defensins NP-2, NP-5, and HNP-1: NMR studies of amide hydrogen exchange kinetics. Proteins 1994;20:52–67.
147. Pardi A, Zhang XL, Selsted ME, et al. NMR studies of defensin antimicrobial peptides. 2. Three-dimensional struc-

tures of rabbit NP-2 and human HNP-1. Biochemistry 1992; 31:11357–64.
148. Kagan BL, Ganz T, Lehrer RI. Defensins: a family of antimicrobial and cytotoxic peptides. Toxicology 1994;87:131–49.
149. Wimley WC, Selsted ME, White SH. Interactions between human defensins and lipid bilayers: evidence for formation of multimeric pores. Protein Science 1994;3:1362–73.
150. Hill CP, Yee J, Selsted ME, Eisenberg D. Crystal structure of defensin HNP-3, an amphiphilic dimer: mechanisms of membrane permeabilization. Science 1991;251:1481–5.
151. Martin E, Ganz T, Lehrer RI. Defensins and other endogenous peptide antibiotics of vertebrates. J Leukoc Biol 1995;58:128–36.
152. Zhang XL, Selsted ME, Pardi A. NMR studies of defensin antimicrobial peptides. 1. Resonance assignment and secondary structure determination of rabbit NP-2 and human HNP-1. Biochemistry 1992;31:11348–56.
153. Lehrer RI, Barton A, Ganz T. Concurrent assessment of inner and outer membrane permeabilization and bacteriolysis in *E. coli* by multiple-wavelength spectrophotometry. J Immunol Methods 1988;108:153–8.
154. Lehrer RI, Barton A, Daher KA, et al. Interaction of human defensins with *Escherichia coli*. Mechanism of bactericidal activity. J Clin Invest 1989;84:553–61.
155. Hristova K, Selsted ME, White SH. Interactions of monomeric rabbit neutrophil defensins with bilayers: comparison with dimeric human defensin HNP-2. Biochemistry 1996;35:11888–94.
156. Ouellette AJ, Selsted ME. Paneth cell defensins: endogenous peptide components of intestinal host defense. FASEB J 1996;10(11):1280–9.
157. Porter EM, Liu L, Oren A, et al. Localization of human intestinal defensin 5 in Paneth cell granules. Infect Immun 1997;65:2389–95.
158. Jones DE, Bevins CL. Defensin-6 mRNA in human Paneth cells: implications for antimicrobial peptides in host defense of the human bowel. FEBS Lett 1993;315:187–92.
159. Jones DE, Bevins CL. Paneth cells of the human small intestine express an antimicrobial peptide gene. J Biol Chem 1992;267:23216–25.
160. Eisenhauer PB, Harwig SS, Lehrer RI. Cryptdins: antimicrobial defensins of the murine small intestine. Infect Immun 1992;60:3556–65.
161. Ganz T, Lehrer RI. Defensins. Curr Opin Immunol 1994;6:584–9.
162. Bevins CL, Jones DE, Dutra A, et al. Human enteric defensin genes: chromosomal map position and a model for possible evolutionary relationships. Genomics 1996;31:95–106.
163. Liu L, Ganz T. The proregion of human neutrophil defensin contains a motif that is essential for normal subcellular sorting. Blood 1995;85:1095–103.
164. Valore EV, Martin E, Harwig SS, Ganz T. Intramolecular inhibition of human defensin HNP-1 by its propiece. J Clin Invest 1996;97:1624–9.
165. Michaelson D, Rayner J, Couto M, Ganz T. Cationic defensins arise from charge-neutralized propeptides: a mechanism for avoiding leukocyte autocytotoxicity? J Leukoc Biol 1992;51:634–9.
166. Valore EV, Ganz T. Posttranslational processing of defensins in immature human myeloid cells. Blood 1992;79:1538–44.
167. Huttner KM, Selsted ME, Ouellette AJ. Structure and diversity of the murine cryptdin gene family. Genomics 1994;19:448–53.
168. Linzmeier R, Michaelson D, Liu L, Ganz T. The structure of neutrophil defensin genes. FEBS Lett 1993;326:299–300.
169. Sadro LC, Tremblay A, Solomon S, Palfree RG. Differential expression of corticostatins/defensins: higher levels of CS-4 (NP-2) transcripts compared with CS-6 (NP-5) in rabbit lung. Biochem Biophys Res Commun 1993;190:1009–16.
170. Nagaoka I, Someya A, Iwabuchi K, Yamashita T. Structure of the guinea pig neutrophil cationic peptide gene. FEBS Lett 1992;303:31–5.
171. Ganz T, Rayner JR, Valore EV, et al. The structure of the rabbit macrophage defensin genes and their organ-specific expression. J Immunol 1989;143:1358–65.
172. Mallow EB, Harris A, Salzman N, et al. Human enteric defensins—gene structure and developmental expression. J Biol Chem 1996;271:4038–45.
173. Ouellette AJ, Cordell B. Accumulation of abundant messenger ribonucleic acids during postnatal development of mouse small intestine. Gastroenterology 1988;94:114–21.
174. Ouellette AJ, Lualdi JC. A novel mouse gene family coding for cationic, cysteine-rich peptides. Regulation in small intestine and cells of myeloid origin [published erratum appears in J Biol Chem 1994;269:18702]. J Biol Chem 1990;265:9831–7.
175. Darmoul D, Ouellette AJ. Positional specificity of defensin gene expression reveals Paneth cell heterogeneity in mouse small intestine. Am J Physiol Gastrointest Liver Physiol 34 1996;271:G68–74.
176. Grandjean V, Vincent S, Martin L, et al. Antimicrobial protection of the mouse testis: synthesis of defensins of the cryptdin family. Biol Reprod 1997;57:1115–22.
177. Svinarich DM, Wolf NA, Gomez R, et al. Detection of human defensin 5 in reproductive tissues. Am J Obstet Gynecol 1997;176:470–5.
178. Quayle AJ, Porter EM, Nussbaum AA, et al. Gene expression, immunolocalization, and secretion of human defensin-5 in human female reproductive tract. Am J Pathol 1998;152:1247–58.
179. Bateman A, MacLeod RJ, Lembessis P, et al. The isolation and characterization of a novel corticostatin/defensin-like peptide from the kidney. J Biol Chem 1996;271:10654–9.
180. Wu ER, Daniel R, Bateman A. RK-2: a novel rabbit kidney defensin and its implications for renal host defense. Peptides 1998;19:793–9.
181. Wilson CL, Heppner KJ, Rudolph LA, Matrisian LM. The metalloproteinase matrilysin is preferentially expressed by epithelial cells in a tissue-restricted pattern in the mouse. Mol Biol Cell 1995;6:851–69.
182. Salzman NH, Polin RA, Harris MC, et al. Enteric defensin expression in necrotizing enterocolitis. Pediatr Res 1998;44:20–6.
183. Brown EG, Sweet AY. Neonatal necrotizing enterocolitis. Pediatr Clin North Am 1982;29:1149–70.
184. Kliegman RM. Models of the pathogenesis of necrotizing enterocolitis. J Pediatr 1990;117:S2–5.
185. Polin RA, Pollack PF, Barlow B, et al. Necrotizing enterocolitis in term infants. J Pediatr 1976;89:460–2.
186. Ballance WA, Dahms BB, Shenker N, Kliegman RM. Pathology of neonatal necrotizing enterocolitis: a ten-year experience. J Pediatr 1990;117:S6–13.
187. Kliegman RM. Neonatal necrotizing enterocolitis: bridging the basic science with the clinical disease. J Pediatr 1990;117:833–5.
188. Kliegman RM, Walker WA, Yolken RH. Necrotizing enterocolitis: research agenda for a disease of unknown etiology and pathogenesis. Pediatr Res 1993;34:701–8.
189. Sparkes RS, Kronenberg M, Heinzmann C, et al. Assignment of defensin gene(s) to human chromosome 8p23. Genomics 1989;5:240–4.
190. Ouellette AJ, Pravtcheva D, Ruddle FH, James M. Localization of the cryptdin locus on mouse chromosome 8 [published erratum appears in Genomics 1992;12:626]. Genomics 1989;5:233–9.

191. Lin MY, Munshi IA, Ouellette AJ. The defensin-related murine CRS1C gene: expression in Paneth cells and linkage to *Defcr*, the cryptdin locus. Genomics 1992;14:363–8.
192. Porter EM, van Dam E, Valore EV, Ganz T. Broad-spectrum antimicrobial activity of human intestinal defensin 5. Infect Immun 1997;65:2396–401.
193. Aley SB, Zimmerman M, Hetsko M, et al. Killing of *Giardia lamblia* by cryptdins and cationic neutrophil peptides. Infect Immun 1994;62:5397–403.
194. Lencer WI, Cheung G, Strohmeier GR, et al. Induction of epithelial chloride secretion by channel-forming cryptdins 2 and 3. Proc Natl Acad Sci U S A 1997;94:8585–9.
195. Ouellette AJ, Hsieh MM, Selsted ME. Structure and function of cryptdins isolated from mouse small intestinal lumen [abstract]. Gastroenterology (Suppl) 1996;110:(4)A985.
196. Hristova K, Selsted ME, White SH. Critical role of lipid composition in membrane permeabilization by rabbit neutrophil defensins. J Biol Chem 1997;272:24224–33.

CHAPTER 10

Ontogeny of T Lymphocytes within the Human Intestine

Duncan Howie, PhD

Thomas T. MacDonald, PhD, FRCPath

The newborn mammal is immediately exposed to a plethora of pathogenic and nonpathogenic microorganisms, in addition to numerous food antigens. In order to deal with these, the immune system of the gut must be developed enough to respond appropriately; yet it must be specifically unresponsive to foods. There is now a great deal of evidence that both of these processes are controlled by T cells. The immune system of the gut (GALT) develops during gestation such that at birth it is capable of responding, albeit temporarily less effectively than in the adult. The three arms of the GALT—lamina propria lymphocytes (LPL), intraepithelial lymphocytes (IEL) and Peyer's patches—develop at different stages of fetal ontogeny, as described below. In this chapter, the development of the gut immune system will be described, first, by site, with lamina propria, Peyer's patches, and IEL development analyzed. The molecular development and acquisition of T-cell receptor $\alpha\beta$ and $\gamma\delta$ complexity in the gut is then outlined, and the gut expression of HLA molecules, crucial in presentation of antigens to T cells, is described. Finally, the development of functional immunocompetence of T cells in the intestine during gestation and following birth will be addressed.

Much of the current information on T-cell development and function has been obtained via the study of T-cell subset and activation markers. The T-cell surface molecules described in this chapter are outlined in Table 10–1 along with their major functions. The cytokines mentioned in the text that are important for T-cell development and function are also shown in Table 10–1.

DEVELOPMENT OF HUMAN GUT-ASSOCIATED LYMPHOID TISSUE

Development of Lamina Propria Lymphocytes

In order to put the development of gut T cells in context, it is first necessary to briefly describe the composition of T cells in postnatal gut. In normal, healthy adults, T cells are present in the lamina propria and epithelium of the intestine. Adult lamina propria T cells are predominantly CD4+, $\alpha\beta$ TCR+.[1,2] Since they are probably derived from Peyer's patch blasts, they are all $\alpha 4\beta 7$+, although approximately 30% also express $\alpha E\beta 7$.[3] $\gamma\delta$ T cells are very uncommon.[4] They have an activated phenotype, being L-selectin[lo], CD69+, CD45RO+, CD25+, and FAS+.[5–9] A subpopulation are also FASL+. FAS crosslinking on lamina propria T cells rapidly leads to apoptosis.[9] Lamina propria CD8+ T cells are also CD45RO+ and express high levels of $\alpha E\beta 7$.[3] It is currently unclear if lamina propria CD8+ T cells are resident or are in transit to the epithelium. Since it has been established for many years that T blasts from the mesenteric lymph nodes preferentially lodge in the lamina propria and do not leave, for the lamina propria not to fill up with T cells there must be extensive cell death. Activated T cells are programmed to die unless rescued by antigen or a common γ chain cytokine, such as IL-2, IL-7, or IL-15,[10] and the expression of FAS and FASL on lamina propria T cells suggests that most lamina propria T cells die in situ. IL-7 is made by intestinal epithelial cells, and lamina propria T cells have functional IL-7 receptors.[11] However, the interactions between survival factors, such as IL-7, and death factors, such as FAS, has not been well explored in lamina propria T cells.

T cells in the human fetal intestine have some remarkable phenotypic similarities to the "memory activated" phenotype of adult gut lymphocytes, despite the absence of luminal antigen. Large numbers of fetal gut T cells have markers of activation and memory, and there are also immature T-cell subsets rarely seen in postnatal gut. In the absence of luminal antigen, however, it is likely that the phenotypic similarities between fetal and adult LPLs can be attributed to entirely different stimuli. While stimulation by luminal antigen is clearly responsible for the "memory activated" phenotype of adult LPLs, recent data provide evidence that in the human fetus, local differentiation of T-cell progenitors in the intestine causes them to express markers normally associated with activation, just as in the thymus.[12]

B and T cells are present, although scarce, in fetal lamina propria from 12 to 14 weeks gestation,[13] and their number increases with gestational age (Figure 10–1). Eosinophils and granulocytes appear from 19 weeks, later than their appearance in blood, where they are first seen at 13 weeks.[14,15] Large numbers of T cells in the fetal lamina propria express activation antigens, HLA-DR (20 to 30%), αEβ7 (HML-1, CD103, 30 to 40%) and have a low or undetectable expression of L-selectin. Surprisingly, no T cells in the fetal intestine express α4β7, which is known to be important in T-cell binding to MAdCAM (mucosal addressin cell adhesion molecule), which is expressed on gut endothelial cells, allowing extravasation into the gut. In addition, up to 70% of fetal LPLs express the CD45RO isoform of the common leukocyte antigen, commonly associated with memory T cells that have previously undergone antigenic stimulation.[12] Between 10 and 30% of T lymphocytes in the fetal lamina propria are actively dividing, and T blasts are abundant (Figure 10–2). T cells of both CD4 and CD8 subsets are in cell cycle. This is not the case in postnatal gut, where adult IELs and LPLs are predominantly in Go phase of the cell cycle, and proliferating T cells are only seen in the Peyer's patches, where they are presumably responding to gut antigens.[16] The presence of activated, dividing T cells in the fetal intestine in the absence of luminal microorganisms or food antigens is paradoxical. It is

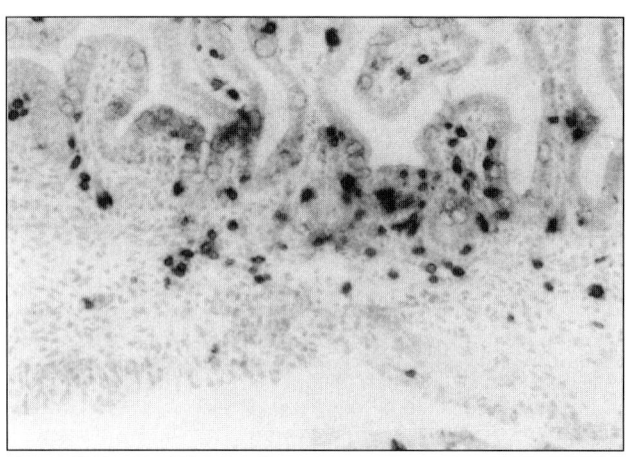

FIGURE 10–1. Cryostat section of 18-week fetal human small intestine stained with monoclonal anti-CD3. CD3+ T cells can be seen scattered throughout the lamina propria and in the epithelium. (Immunoperoxidase, original magnification × 200.)

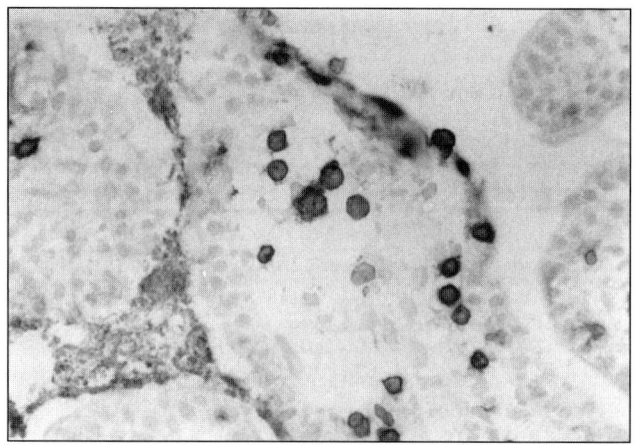

FIGURE 10–2. Cryostat section of 18-week fetal human small intestine stained with monoclonal anti-CD3. Large T cells with a blast-like morphology in addition to smaller quiescent T cells are clearly visible. (Immunoperoxidase, original magnification × 400.)

TABLE 10–1
T-cell Surface Markers and Their Functional Significance and the Cytokines Important in the Development and Function of Intestinal T Cells

Cell Surface Markers	Major Functions
CD4	T-cell ligand for MHC class II and marker of T-helper cells.
CD8	T-cell ligand for MHC class I and marker of cytotoxic/suppressor cells.
TCRαβ γδ	T-cell receptors for antigen.
α4β7	T-cell ligand for homing to the gut mediated by MAdCAM expressed on gut endothelial cells.
αEβ7 (CD103,HML-1)	T-cell ligand for E-cadherin expressed on gut epithelium. Expressed by majority of intestinal IELs.
L-selectin	T-cell ligand for carbohydrate moieties of glycoproteins expressed on high endothelial venules. Downregulation of L-selectin is indicative of T-cell activation.
CD69	T-cell activation marker.
CD45RO	Marker of memory T cells, binds CD22 on B cells; function of this interaction unknown.
CD25	IL-2 receptor, marker of activated T cells.
FAS (CD95, Apo-1)	Present on many cell types, initiates apoptosis on expressing cells after engagement with FAS ligand.
FAS-L (CD95L)	FAS ligand, expressed by cytotoxic T cells. Induces apoptosis in target cells after engagement of FAS on surface of target cell.
HLA DR, DP, DQ	MHC class II molecules; expression on T cells associated with activation.
CD7	T-lineage marker, expressed on all T cells and developing thymocytes.
CD8αα	Dimer of CD8 alpha chain, expressed by a large proportion of extrathymically-derived gut IELs in mice.
Cytokines	Major Functions
IL-2	T-cell growth factor produced by activated T cells.
IL-7	T-cell and early thymocyte growth factor, essential for maturation of immature thymocytes, produced by thymic stromal cells and gut epithelial cells.
IL-15	T- and B-cell growth factor, similar effects to IL-2.
IFN-γ	Cytokine produced by activated T cells; multiple effects including up-regulation of MHC class II on antigen-presenting cells and gut epithelial cells.
TNF-α	Product of activated monocytes/macrophages, multiple downstream effects in inflammatory responses.

possible that T cells in the gut prior to birth are subject to continuous stimulation by self-antigens and are undergoing selection in a manner similar to the extrathymic differentiation that has been observed in mice. In support of this hypothesis, T cells undergoing apoptosis (programmed cell death) are detectable in the fetal lamina propria by immunocytochemistry.[12] In addition, molecular evidence that T-cell receptor (TCR) recombination is occurring in situ in the intestine prior to birth is now emerging, and is discussed later in this chapter.

The fetal gut lamina propria also contains numerous T-cell subsets not seen in adults. There is a significant population of CD3+4-8- double-negative T cells (up to 20% of fetal LPLs), which is not seen postnatally. The function of these double-negative T cells in the fetus and the adult is unknown; however, a similar population of T cells has been observed in the peripheral immune system of mice and humans.[17,18] The peripheral blood double-negative T cells predominantly express an invariant TCR Vα rearrangement Vα24JαQ coupled to Vβ11 in humans and Vα14Jα28 coupled to either Vβ8, 7, or 2 in mice. Some of these cells coexpress the NK cell marker NKR-P1(NK1.1), and have thus been described as "natural T cells."[19] These cells are unique in responding with a very strong Th-2 (IL-4) cytokine profile in mice and a Th-0 (IL-4 & IFN-γ) cytokine profile in humans without the need for previous antigenic priming.[19,20] This ability to produce a rapid IL-4 response has been proposed to be important for induction of Th-2 responses.

An additional difference between the fetal and adult gut T cell populations is the abundance of CD3-7+ cells in the fetal gut lamina propria but not in the adult. CD7 is a lineage marker expressed on T cells from the earliest T-cell precursors, the expression of which diminishes slightly with maturation.[21] As such, it is a good marker for early T-lineage cells prior to the expression of more mature T-cell markers such as CD3, CD4, or CD8. CD3-7+ cells are abundant in fetal lamina propria, where they constitute almost 20% of all CD7+ cells.

CD8+ T cells in the fetal lamina propria are unique in expressing the CD8αα homodimer.[22] These CD8αα T cells are predominantly TCRα-β+, and make up almost 50% of the CD8+ lamina propria lymphocytes, and are numerous in the epithelium. In mice it is well established that CD8αα T cells are thymus-independent, arising from the bone marrow, and undergoing local expansion in the gut. It is likely that the CD8αα T cells in the fetal gut undergo similar pathways of maturation.

B cells in the adult lamina propria are mostly IgA-secreting plasma cells.[23] Stimulation by exogenous antigen is not thought to occur in the fetus, and consequently there are no lamina propria plasma cells. This situation changes after birth with exposure to dietary and microbial antigen, and by 12 days of age there are IgA and IgM+ B cells in the lamina propria, with IgA cells predominating after 3 months.[24]

Development of Intraepithelial Lymphocytes

In normal adults IELs are predominantly CD3+CD8+ TCRαβ+ with a memory phenotype (CD45RO+). These cells are mostly αEβ7+, binding to E-cadherin expressed by gut epithelial cells. Upon activation with IL-2 and alloantigen in vitro, these IELs develop cytotoxic function.[25] However, the phenotype of adult IELs in vivo is more consistent with resting cytolytic T cells. Adult small- and large-intestinal IELs do not express markers associated with cytolytic activity, such as granzyme B, perforin, FASL, and TNFα.[26] After isolation and activation, however, they upregulate these cytolytic effector molecules.[26] The epithelium of the intestine first contains lymphocytes at around 11 weeks gestation.[27–29] The number of CD3+ IELs increases in a linear fashion during gestation, so that at 27 weeks of gestation the numbers of IELs are approximately 70% of that seen in infants. Half of fetal IELs are subset-negative (CD3+4-8-) in comparison to adult IEL, where this subset comprises only around 6%.[30] CD3+TCRαβ+ IELs also express CD8αα homodimers.[22] Between 5 and 10% of fetal CD3+ IELs are in cell cycle.[12] T cells expressing the αβ TCR predominate in the blood and gut epithelium, comprising around 90% of CD3+ T cells in each compartment.[4,31,32] The other 10% express the γδTCR. In the adult, γδ T cells using Vδ2 predominate in the blood, and Vδ1 is predominant in the gut; Vδ2 is absent in the thymus.[33] The γδ population in the IEL, as in the blood, is included in the CD4-8- population; since this IEL population in the fetus is greater than in the adult, one would expect a higher proportion of γδ+ T cells in fetal IEL, but this is not the case. In the fetus the γδ population is exclusively Vδ2+, and comprises around 25% of the CD3+ population. It appears, therefore, that there is a population of CD4-8- IELs in the fetus that do not express the γδ heterodimer. Because Vδ2 is absent from the thymus, it has been suggested that this CD4-8- Vδ2-expressing IEL subset is extrathymically derived, undergoing local differentiation and expansion in situ from bone marrow progenitors without the need for the thymus microenvironment.[33,34] The CD3-7+ T cell population, abundant in the lamina propria, is almost absent from the epithelium. The reason for this dichotomy of CD3-7+ expression between the lamina propria and epithelium is unknown. It is possible that CD3-7+ cells in the lamina propria represent precursors of CD3+ cells that go on to populate the epithelium.

Table 10–2 summarizes the similarities and differences between lamina propria and epithelial T cells in the fetal and postnatal gut.

Development of Peyer's Patches

The first organized Peyer's patches appear at around 18 to 19 weeks gestation, and in the fetus as in the adult, predominate in the ileum. The number of Peyer's patches increases to around 100 throughout the gut at birth, to around 250 in the mid-teens, and decreases steadily to about 100 at 90 years of age.[35,36] Immunocytochemistry has enabled the development of Peyer's patches in the fetus to be tracked. The first signs of development of the Peyer's patch anlagen appears at 11 weeks gestation when subepithelial accumulations of CD4+, CD3-, HLA-DR+, and DP+, but not DQ+ accessory cells, are present.[13] No markers of other lymphoid lineages are detectable on these cells at this time. By 14 weeks gestation T cells can be seen in loose aggregates without defined structure; most of these T cells are CD4+. By 16 weeks gestation,

TABLE 10-2
Comparison of the Phenotype of Fetal and Adult IELs and LPLs Highlighting Differences and Similarities between the Two Populations

IEL	Fetus	Adult
Similarities		
CD4+	10%	10%
CD8+	40%	90%
TCR αβ	90%	90%
CD45RO+	70%	100%
CD7+3-	<2%	<2%
TCR γδ (% of CD3+)	10%	10%
TCR δ2	present	present
Differences		
TCR δ1	absent	present
CD3+4-8- (% of CD3+)	50%	6%
CD3+/Ki67+	5–10%	0%
CD8 αα+	detectable	absent

LPL	Fetus	Adult
Similarities		
CD4+	50%	50%
CD8+	30%	30%
αEβ7+	30%	50%
CD45RO+	60–70%	100%
CD3+/HLA-DR+	25%	26%
L-selectin	low	low
Differences		
CD3+/Ki67+	20–30%	absent
α4β7+	absent	100%
CD3+4-8- (% of CD3+)	up to 20%	absent
CD3-7+ (% of CD7+)	up to 20%	absent
CD8αα (% of CD8+)	50%	rare

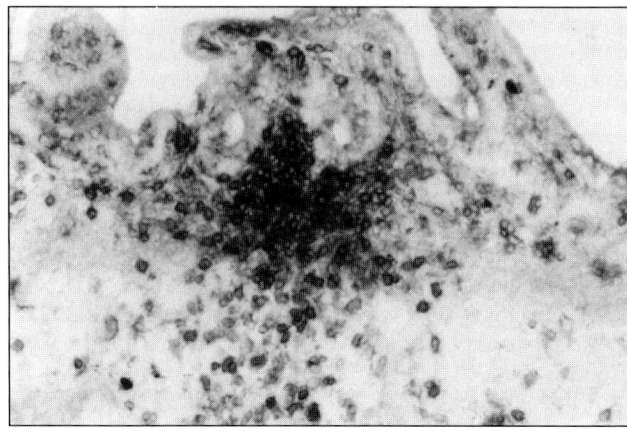

FIGURE 10–3. Cryostat section of 16-week fetal human small intestine stained with monoclonal anti-CD3. Large subepithelial accumulations of CD3+ cells probably represent the initial stages of Peyer's patch development. (Immunoperoxidase, original magnification × 200.)

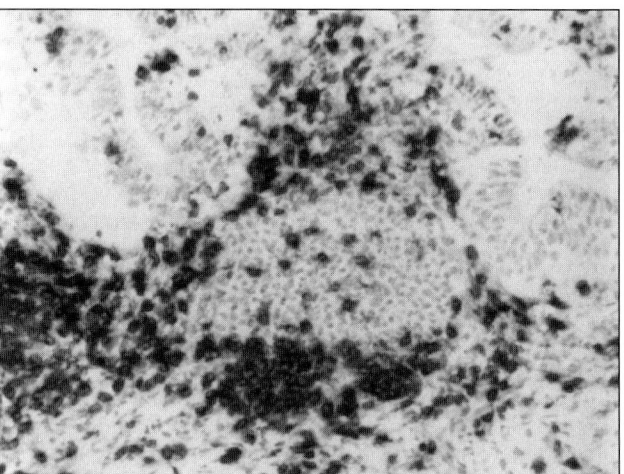

T-cells

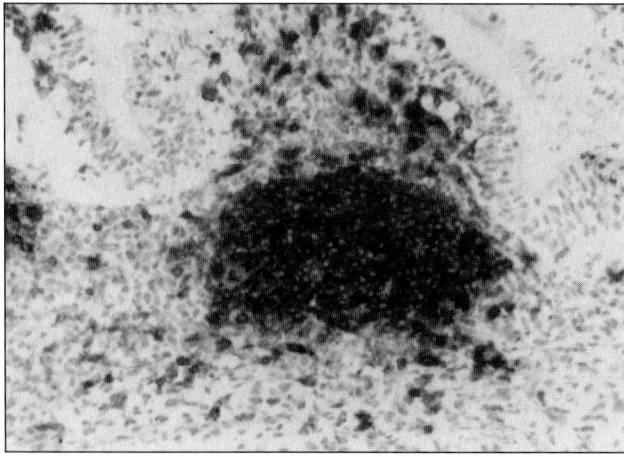

B-cells

FIGURE 10–4. Serial cryostat sections of 18-week fetal human small intestine stained with monoclonal anti-CD3 (T cells) and monoclonal anti-CD22 (pan-B cell) showing a Peyer's patch with a clearly defined T-cell zone and B-cell follicle. No germinal centers are seen in Peyer's patches prior to birth. (Immunoperoxidase, original magnification × 200.)

larger accumulations of T cells can be seen (Figure 10–3). In serial sections, some B cells are present in the same area. B cells expressing IgM and IgD along with mature B cell markers CD19, CD20, and CD22 are present at 16 weeks, but there is no zonation into B- and T-cell areas. The B cells seen in the Peyer's patches at this time are a relatively mature population in comparison to the pre-B cells detectable in the fetal spleen and lymph nodes from 7 to 8 weeks, and the B cells seen in the bone marrow and fetal liver from 7.5 weeks, which express cytoplasmic IgM but no surface immunoglobulin or other B-cell markers.[37]

At around 19 weeks, structures that more closely resemble adult Peyer's patches, with zonation into T- and B-cell areas, emerge (Figure 10–4). The B cells in the follicles surround follicular dendritic cells. This is not the case in postnatal Peyer's patches, where follicular dendritic cells are not seen in primary follicles. At 19 weeks gestation, as at 16 weeks, the T cells surrounding the B-cell follicle are mostly CD3+CD4+, with scattered CD8+ T cells. The T cells at 19 weeks gestation express HLA-D antigens, which in adult T cells is associated with activation; however, since there are very few CD3+ cells expressing KI67, a marker of proliferating cells and little IL-2 receptor expression on these cells, it is unlikely that this represents functional activation.

Macrophages are present in the follicles at 19 weeks gestation.[38] In the T-cell zone of the follicle and in the surrounding microenvironment, macrophages with dendritic cell morphology predominate. These cells do not express lysozyme or RFD7, both markers of scavenger macrophages, and are not present in the dome area, where the follicle-associated epithelium allows passage of antigens from the lumen into the Peyer's patch.[27] These cells may be differentiating into follicular dendritic cells that later will present antigen to follicular T cells. Macrophages in the dome area and follicle express the p150-95 component of CD11 that is expressed on all mature macrophages. This discrimination between dome dendritic cells and macrophages in the surrounding microenvironments is apparent at 19 weeks gestation. At around 17 weeks gestation the epithelium overlying the developing Peyer's patch changes from a columnar orientation, normally seen covering the villi outwith the Peyer's patches, to cuboidal.[36,39] At this time M cells can be seen in the follicle-associated epithelium, with their characteristic de-differentiated microvilli or microfolds. These embryonic M cells start to be invaded by T and B cells at 19 weeks gestation, to form the characteristic pockets of M cells surrounded by lymphocytes that are seen in postnatal gut.[37] In the absence of luminal microflora or food antigens, however, no germinal centers are seen in fetal Peyer's patches; but these form rapidly after birth following microbial colonization of the gut.[39,40]

It has recently been demonstrated that formation of Peyer's patch M cells from columnar epithelial cells is mediated in part by Peyer's patch B cells.[41] In this study it was shown that de-differentiation, reorganization of the brush-border, and transport of microparticles and *Vibrio cholerae* bacteria across a differentiated colonic epithelial cell line could be induced by coculture with Peyer's patch B cells. It is possible that the differentiation of M cells in the developing Peyer's patch is also induced by B cells.

ONTOGENY OF T CELL–RECEPTOR REPERTOIRE DEVELOPMENT IN FETAL INTESTINAL T CELLS

T cells recognize antigen bound to MHC class I and II molecules expressed by antigen-presenting cells. They have the capacity to recognize an enormous range of potential antigens, both foreign and self, via the TCR. The TCR is a heterodimer consisting of either an α and β or a γ and δ chain. Variability of the TCR arises from recombination of multiple germline-encoded DNA segments. These segments are termed variable (V), diversity (D), and joining (J) genes. Random recombination of these gene-segments, combined with the action of enzymes that add and delete nucleotides from the joining ends of these segments, results in an almost limitless number of potential different TCR sequences that can be expressed. The human TCRα and β loci contain 32 Vα subfamilies, almost 60 Jα segments, 26 Vβ subfamilies, 2 Dβ segments, and 13 Jβ segments. The area of greatest variability in the TCR is in the region where the V, D, and J coding ends join; this region is termed the CDR3 (complementarity determining region 3). Analysis of the variability of this region of the TCR can provide useful information about the potential antigen recognition of the TCR, and also of the activity of the enzymes that add and delete nucleotides from the germline encoded V, D, and J regions during recombination. Due to the central role of T cells in both peripheral and intestinal immunity, it is crucially important that the T cells of the gut have functional and varied TCR expression by birth.

Adult intestinal mucosa contains T cells of the $\alpha\beta$ and $\gamma\delta$ lineages.[42] T cells bearing $\gamma\delta$ TCRs develop in the thymus as a separate lineage from those bearing $\alpha\beta$ TCRs, as described earlier in the chapter[43–45] and in the gut are located preferentially in the paracellular space between the columnar epithelial cells covering the villi,[46] whereas TCR$\alpha\beta$ cells are located both in the lamina propria and epithelium. The ligands that both $\alpha\beta$ and $\gamma\delta$ T cells recognize in the gut are only partly understood. As described later, MHC class II molecules are expressed on fetal intestine epithelial cells in the second trimester. It is not known whether fetal-gut T cells expressing $\alpha\beta$ TCRs can recognize and respond to peptides associated with these class II molecules; however, $\gamma\delta$ T cells in the gut have recently been shown to recognize and respond cytolytically to the stress-induced MHC class I-like molecules MICA and MICB expressed by human intestinal epithelial cell lines.[47] As described below, however, TCR $\alpha\beta$+ and $\gamma\delta$+ cells are present from the second trimester onwards, and their diversity changes fundamentally from fetal to postnatal life.

Development of the Gut $\alpha\beta$ TCR Repertoire

Fetal intestinal LPL and IEL contain detectable mRNA for rearranged TCR β loci as early as 13 weeks gestation, but the number of TCR Vβ family members that are present is limited.[48] The number increases with gestation, so that at birth all 26 Vβ families are detectable as rearranged mRNA transcripts. Analysis of the CDR3 regions of these Vβ transcripts by CDR3 spectratyping and DNA sequencing reveals that they are diverse, with numerous nontemplated N region additions. IEL Vβ CDR3s are more restricted in repertoire up to around 19 weeks of gestation, when they become more diverse.

There is a marked disparity between expression of TCRβ chains and TCRα in the fetal intestine. Rearranged TCRα chains are undetectable until around 16 weeks of gestation, and even then the repertoire of expressed TCRVα chains is very limited. Expression of TCRβ in the absence of TCRα is strong evidence that TCR locus recombination may be occurring in situ in the intestine before birth. Random-anchored PCR and RACE (rapid amplification of cDNA ends) analysis of TCRα transcripts in the human fetal intestine reveals that a large majority of rearranged TCRα transcripts before 16 weeks gestation are recombined to an immature precursor segment that replaces Vα. This segment is termed T early alpha (TEA). The TEA locus is located 3' of Cδ and 5' of the most upstream Jα.[49] TEA has been postulated to have a role in opening of the TCR locus for subsequent rearrangement,[50–52] and has been reported to be expressed on thymocytes prior to the onset of TCRVα recombination with rearranged TCRJ-C segments.[50] In addition, many of the rearranged TCRα transcripts detectable around 16 weeks of gestation have joining segments correctly spliced to constant regions, but not recombined with TCR Vα. These transcripts initiate upstream of the Jα loci, and may be the result of initiation of transcription of the partially rearranged TCRα genes prior to full recombination of J-C joins with the Vα

loci.[53–55] TEA becomes less predominant with increasing gestational age, when more fully rearranged TCRα transcripts can be detected. Functionally rearranged TCRα transcripts are detectable earlier in LPLs than IELs; by 23 weeks gestation, however, TCRα transcripts with productively rearranged TCR V-J-C segments are detectable in both compartments. TEA is also detected in adult LPL and IELs.

In addition to TEA as the sole TCRα transcript in IELs and as the predominant TCRα transcript in the gut up to 16 weeks gestation, a new "T early β" transcript (TEB) has been identified as a major TCRβ transcript in the fetal intestine from 14 weeks gestation onwards.[48] Expression of this immature transcript in the gut is evidence that for many αβ T cells, TCRβ recombination has not yet occurred, and like the TCRα locus, may be doing so in the intestine. TEB, like TEA, is also expressed in fetal blood, and in adult IELs and LPLs in addition to the thymus.

The repertoire of adult intestinal αβ TCRs is remarkably different to that seen in the fetus. Adult IELs express an oligoclonal repertoire of αβ TCRs,[56–59] dominant clones being seen along the length of the gut.[59] These are thought to be derived from an expansion of a limited number of T-cell clones in the Peyer's patches prior to dissemination throughout the intestine. The ligands that drive this oligoclonal expansion have yet to be elucidated, but it has been shown that CD8+ IELs can recognize and respond with a cytotoxic response to antigen presented on the MHC I-like nonpolymorphic CD1 molecules CD1a, CD1b, CD1c, and CD1d.[56] CD1d is constitutively expressed on gut epithelial cells, and CD1a-c can be expressed during gut inflammation, infection, or neoplastic transformation.[60] It is very likely that the oligoclonal expansion of IELs bearing αβ TCRs is antigen-driven, as the fetal intestinal lumen is effectively sterile until birth, and both fetal LPL and IEL populations use a diverse and polyclonal array of αβ TCRs.[12,48]

Development of the Gut γδ TCR Repertoire

γδ T cells arise in the fetal liver and thymus at 6 to 8 weeks gestation,[61–63] and are detectable in the gut at 14 weeks gestation,[4] where they are located predominantly in the epithelium and comprise 10 to 30% of the IELs of the fetus.[4] By adulthood the proportion of γδ IELs remains around 2% in the small intestine[42,64] and up to 15 to 20% in the colon.[4,64,65] However, important changes in the complexity and clonality of the TCRδ repertoire occur in this period. Complexity and specificity of the TCRγδ heterodimer is largely contributed by the CDR3 region of the delta chain, which is produced by random joining of the V, D, and J segments in addition to random N-region nontemplated nucleotide insertion and insertion at the coding joints of nucleotides palindromic to the coding ends of the V, D, and J segments (P additions[66]). The CDR3 region of the TCRδ chain is generally longer and more variable in length than the α or β chains, and it has been suggested that the ligands for the γδ TCR are soluble non-MHC bound antigens, with the γδ TCR recognizing these in a fashion similar to immunoglobulin antigen binding.[67]

The TCRδ repertoire of fetal intestinal T cells in the second trimester of gestation is polyclonal, with numerous different CDR3 lengths being observed; however, sequence analysis reveals that the junctional regions of the CDR3 region at this time are limited by a lack of N-region additions at the joining ends of the V, D, and J segments.[68] In addition, numerous template-encoded P additions are seen at the junctions between the V, D, and J regions. Also, numerous identical TCRDV2 transcripts resembling the canonical sequences described in mice can be observed in different fetuses.[68] In the early period after birth (1 day to 4 weeks) the repertoire of expressed TCRδ transcripts remains polyclonal, but the junctional regions become more complicated, with numerous N-region nucleotide insertions in addition to P additions. After birth, the TCRδ repertoire becomes increasingly restricted, such that at midadolescence the limited diversity of TCRδ usage is comparable to that of adults in their sixtieth year of life. It is possible that the increasing restriction of the TCRδ repertoire in the gut with increasing age is caused by a change in the diversity of the ligands, but these have not been identified.

The traditional view of TCRδ usage in the adult intestine and peripheral immune compartments has been that Vδ1 is the predominantly used TCR Vδ chain in the gut and that Vδ2 is predominant in the periphery, where the TCR Vδ repertoire has been described as highly diverse.[69–71] Recent studies describing adult gut and peripheral blood TCR Vδ clonality and diversity have revealed that both the colon and peripheral blood Vδ repertoires are oligoclonal irrespective of whether Vδ1, 2, or 3 is used.[72–74] Moreover, in contrast to previous reports, it is now known that Vδ1, 2, and 3 are used by γδ T cells in the colon, and that despite the potential of TCR Vδ loci for great junctional diversity, TCR Vδ diversity in the blood and colon is highly restricted. This oligoclonal restriction of TCRδ is unique to each individual, and the clones in blood and intestine are separate. The dominant clones are also stable over time in each individual, being detected consistently over a 16-month period. This phenotype of stable clones scattered over long distances of the colon has been suggested to occur due to positive selection of a limited number of TCRδ-expressing T cells on gut-specific ligands prior to dissemination throughout the body and homing back to the gut via the α4β7-MAdCAM interaction, and not due to continuous in situ V(D)J recombination, which would be expected to produce a more polyclonal distribution of TCRδ usage.[74]

Table 10–3 summarizes the molecular features of the αβ and γδ TCR repertoire in the intestine from fetal to adult development.

MHC CLASS II EXPRESSION IN THE HUMAN FETAL INTESTINE

In order for T cells to be able to recognize and respond to antigens, the antigens have to be presented as peptides associated with class I or class II MHC. CD4+ T helper cells are restricted to recognition of antigen in the context of MHC II. Thus, for effective T cell-mediated immunity in the neonatal intestine, intestinal MHC class II+ accessory cells are required.

HLA-D+ accessory cells are intimately associated with the gut from the earliest stages of development. From the stage at which villi form early in gestation, HLA-D+ cells are seen in the lamina propria. HLA-DR and DP+ lamina propria cells

TABLE 10–3
Changes in Intestinal αβ and γδ TCR Diversity during Development

Age of Development	T Cell Receptor Expression	
	αβ	γδ
5–16 weeks	Rearranged TCRβ mRNA detectable at 13 weeks	10–30% IELs express γδ TCR at 14 weeks
	Polyclonal TCRβ usage	Polyclonal γδ expression
	Extensive N-region addition	Simple V(D)J junctions without N region additions
	No TCRα rearrangement	
	IEL Vβ expression more restricted than LPL	
	TEA & TEB expression abundant	
	Incomplete TCRα J-C rearrangements transcribed	
16 weeks to term		
	TEA less common	Polyclonal δ repertoire expressed
	TEB less common	No N-region additions
	Rearranged V-J-Cα transcripts detectable	Template encoded P additions at V(D)J joins
	TCRα transcripts restricted in diversity before 23 weeks	Canonical Vδ2 transcripts detectable
Birth to teens		
	TEA and TEB less abundant though still detectable	(1 day–4 weeks) N region additions detectable at V(D)J junctions
	All TCR Vβ and Vα segments used	Polyclonal TCR Vδ usage at birth becoming oligoclonal with time
	Polyclonal TCR Vαβ usage at birth, IELs becoming oligoclonal with age	TCRδ expression oligoclonal by mid-teens
Adulthood		
	TEA and TEB rare but detectable	γδ T cells 5-10% IELs
	αβ TCR IELs oligoclonal with identical dominant clones throughout the gut	Highly restricted TCRδ expression
	LPLs polyclonal	Identical dominant clones throughout the gut
		Clonality stable over time (>1 year)

with a macrophage-like morphology are present in the gut from 11 weeks gestation,[38] but HLA-DQ+ cells are not observed until 14 weeks of gestation. HLA-DR+ cells in the fetal lamina propria consist of macrophages and CD3+ T cells. The HLA-DR+ macrophage population in the fetal intestine is heterogeneous with respect to surface marker expression.[38] All cells within lymphoid aggregates of fetal ileum, from 16 weeks gestation onwards, are also HLA-DR+.

In the adult gut HLA-D antigens are expressed on small intestinal villus epithelial cells, but not generally on crypt epithelial cells.[75] They are not expressed on colonic epithelial cells,[76] but their expression can be induced by the products of activated T cells.[77] HLA-D antigens can be found on crypt epithelial cells adjacent to lymphoid follicles and on crypt epithelium in inflammatory bowel disease.[77,78] MHC class II molecules can be upregulated on columnar epithelial cells in the gut following immune stimuli.

In the fetal intestine HLA-D antigens are absent from the epithelium until 17 to 18 weeks of gestation, when they are present at the tips of the villi. With increasing age, expression of HLA-D is seen from the base to the tip of the villi. It is interesting that HLA-DR expression on fetal gut epithelium is most commonly seen at the tips of the villi. These epithelial cells are the oldest on the villus, and have presumably had the longest time to respond to any factors responsible for HLA induction. It is known that expression of HLA-D antigens on epithelial cells and epithelial cell turnover in the fetal gut are increased dramatically following stimulation of lamina propria T-cells with polyclonal T-cell activators such as pokeweed mitogen.[79] Interferon gamma is at least partly responsible for the observed MHC-II upregulation on fetal gut epithelial cells, as the supernatants from fetal gut explants treated with polyclonal T-cell activators induce MHC-II upregulation on colonic HT-29 cell lines, which is reversible on addition of anti-IFN-γ antibodies.[79] Also in adults, intestinal epithelium associated with Peyer's patches overlying the lymphoid follicle and immediately adjacent crypt cells is HLA-DR+. This is in contrast to the epithelium at the other side of the crypt from the Peyer's patch, derived from the same enteroblastic progenitor cells, which is HLA-DR–.[76] There have been conflicting reports on the expression of HLA-D region antigens on fetal gut epithelium, with some groups failing to detect any HLA-D molecules on these cells.[80] This is most likely due to differences in methodology with the use of different monoclonal antibodies.

FUNCTIONAL CHARACTERISTICS OF FETAL INTESTINAL T CELLS

With the ability to maintain premature infants at increasingly shorter gestational ages, it is important to have a full understanding of the immunocompetence of both the mucosal and systemic immune system of the fetus. Due to the obvious constraints of performing in vivo experiments with developing human intestine, the two main sources of information available on the functional capabilities of intestinal T cells prior to birth are limited studies of premature neonates, and experiments where intestinal T cells of fetal gut are stimulated in explant culture with mitogens, bacterial superantigens, or anti-CD3 monoclonal antibodies.[78,81] In these experiments it has been shown that the T cells in the fetal gut are capable of responding vigorously to lectins, superantigen, or anti-CD3 treatment, producing a largely Th-1 response, with IL-2 and IFN-γ being secreted into the organ culture supernatants.[81] In older specimens of intestine, with more T cells, more cytokines are produced. Activation of fetal lamina propria T cells with the superantigen *Staphylococcus aureus* enterotoxin B (SEB) or pokeweed mitogen (PWM) results in tissue injury, with epithelial shedding and loss of villi in intestine greater than 16 weeks gestation, and more moderate changes in younger specimens.[78,81] Activation of fetal intestinal T cells with SEB has been shown to occur largely through cells expressing the T-cell receptor beta chain Vβ3.[81] Upon activation, fetal intestinal T cells express CD25 and HLA-DR antigens. The mucosal damage and Th-1 cytokine production caused by treatment of explants with SEB or PWM is cyclosporin-A sensitive, showing that it is a T cell-mediated response.[78]

Analysis of the cellular and humoral immune competence of premature neonates indicates that they have the ability to respond to novel antigens with both delayed type hypersensitivity reactions and immunoglobulin production. Premature infants at 30 weeks of gestation challenged with DNCB give a delayed-type hypersensitivity (DTH) response. However, the response is more variable in preterm neonates than in infants of 2 to 12 months, in that some preterm neonates do not respond, but all infants respond positively to DNCB challenge.[82] Newborn infants are also able to reject skin allografts, indicating the functional competence of their cellular immune response.[83]

The mucosal immune system develops in parallel with the systemic immune system, and it is likely that the development of functional capability of cells in the periphery also occurs in the gut mucosa.

DEVELOPMENT OF INTESTINAL T CELLS AFTER BIRTH

Studies addressing the maturity of the immune system of the gut in neonates have relied mainly on the study of salivary IgA production as a measure of the secretory IgA response. Data are limited on T-cell development and function in the gut immediately after birth. At birth, concurrent with population of the lumen with bacteria, Peyer's patches develop germinal centers with plasmablasts.[39] The development of both the cellular and humoral immune response starts at birth and takes some months to mature. Interferon-γ and interleukin-4 (IL-4) production by neonatal peripheral T cells in response to PHA or concanavalin A (Con A) is markedly reduced in comparison to adult T cells.[84,85] This innate T-cell deficiency of the neonate is at a pretranslational level, as protein and mRNA transcripts for IFN-γ are comparably low.[85] It is not known, however, if this temporary functional deficiency of the peripheral T-cell pool is reflected in functional inactivity of gut T cells at this time. Certainly studies on direct activation of lamina propria T cells in explants of fetal intestine suggest that they are capable of a vigorous response. Numerous studies have addressed the development of IELs during late gestation and in the early postnatal period. As mentioned, expansion of IEL numbers occurs during late gestation, so that at 27 weeks gestation IEL numbers are roughly 70% of those in infants. It has been shown that orally-enterally fed infants have higher IEL numbers in the ileum than those given TPN, suggesting a role for luminal antigens in postnatal IEL expansion.[86] Also, full term neonates have significantly higher numbers of IELs than premature neonates. After birth there is a rapid expansion in IEL numbers, and infants in their second year have approximately three times as many IELs as neonates. It is likely that the stimulus for this rapid expansion is luminal antigen.[87]

CONCLUSION

The gut mucosal immune system develops during fetal life from the eleventh week of gestation onwards. During the second trimester there are less lymphocytes in the gut than are seen postnatally, but by 19 weeks Peyer's patches with T- and B-cell areas are present, and from the twelfth week onwards the gut epithelium and lamina propria is populated with T lymphocytes. The mRNA transcripts of the T-cell receptors αβ and γδ can be detected in the intestine from the fourteenth week of gestation onwards; these are largely productively rearranged, and their repertoire is polyclonal, increasing in N region diversity with gestation. There is some evidence that T-cell receptor αβ rearrangement may be occurring in situ, judging by the lag in detectable TCRα transcripts in the fetal gut and the presence of immature TCR transcripts "T early alpha" and "T early beta." Functionally, B cells in the intestine in premature neonates are capable of forming plasmablasts in response to infection,[40] and T cells in the fetal intestine are mature and able to secrete Th-1 cytokines upon activation.

Duncan Howie was the recipient of a PhD scholarship from the Special Trustees of St. Bartholomew's Hospital.

REFERENCES

1. Janossy G, Tidman N, Selby WS, et al. Human T lymphocytes of inducer and suppressor type occupy different microenvironments. Nature 1980;288:81–4.
2. Brandtzaeg P, Bosnes V, Halstensen TS, et al. T lymphocytes in the human gut epithelium preferentially express the alpha/beta antigen receptor and are often CD45/UCHL-1-positive. Scand J Immunol 1989;30:123–8.
3. Farstad IN, Halstensen TS, Lien B, et al. Distribution of β7 integrins in human intestinal mucosa and organised gut-associated lymphoid tissue. Immunology 1996;89:227–37.
4. Spencer J, Diss TC, Isaacson PG, MacDonald TT. Expression of disulphide and non-disulphide linked forms of the gamma/delta T cell receptor in human small intestinal epithelium. Eur J Immunol 1989;19:1335–8.
5. Berg M, Murakawa Y, Camerini D, James SP. Lamina propria lymphocytes are derived from circulating cells that lack the leu-8 lymph node homing receptor. J Immunol 1991;101:90–9.
6. Halstensen TS, Farstad IN, Scott H, et al. Intraepithelial TcRαβ+ lymphocytes express CD45RO more often than the TcRγδ counterparts in coeliac disease. Immunology 1990;71:460–6.
7. Schieferdecker HL, Ullrich R, Hirseland H, Zeitz M. T cell differentiation antigens on lymphocytes in the human intestinal lamina propria. J Immunol 1992;149:2816–22.
8. Boirivant M, Pica R, DeMaria R, et al. Stimulated human lamina propria T cells manifest enhanced Fas-mediated apoptosis. J Clin Invest 1996;98:2616–22.
9. De Maria R, Boirivant M, Cifone MG, et al. Functional expression of Fas and Fas ligand on human gut lamina propria T lymphocytes: a potential role for acidic sphingomyelinase pathway in normal immunoregulation. J Clin Invest 1996;97:316–22.
10. Akbar AN, Borthwick NJ, Wickremasinghe RG, et al. Interleukin-2 receptor common gamma chain signaling cytokines regulate activated T cell apoptosis in response to growth factor withdrawal: selective induction of anti-apoptotic (bcl-2, bcl-xL) but not pro-apoptotic (bax, bcl-xS) gene expression. Eur J Immunol 1996;26:294–9.

11. Watanabe M, Ueno Y, Yajima T, et al. Interleukin 7 is produced by human epithelial cells and regulates the proliferation of intestinal mucosal lymphocytes. J Clin Invest 1995;95: 2945–53.
12. Howie D, Spencer J, DeLord D, et al. Extrathymic T cell differentiation in the human intestine early in life. J Immunol 1998. [In press]
13. Spencer J, MacDonald TT, Finn T, Isaacson PG. Development of Peyer's patches in human fetal terminal ileum. Clin Exp Immunol 1986;64:536–43.
14. Spencer J, MacDonald TT, Isaacson PG. Development of human gut-associated lymphoid tissue. In: McGhee JR, Mestecky J, Ocra PL, Bienenstock J, editors. Recent advances in mucosal immunology. Advances in experimental medicine and biology, 216. New York, London: Plenum Press; 1987. p. 1421.
15. Playfair JHL, Wolfendale MR, Kay HEM. The leukocytes of peripheral blood in the human fetus. Br J Haematol 1963; 9:336–44.
16. Fell JM, Walker-Smith JA, Spencer J, MacDonald TT. The distribution of dividing T cells throughout the intestinal wall in inflammatory bowel disease. Clin Exp Immunol 1996;104: 280–5.
17. Lantz O, Bendelac A. An invariant T cell receptor α chain is used by a unique subset of major histocompatibility complex class-I specific CD4+ and CD4-8- T cells in mice and humans. J Exp Med 1994; 80:1097–106.
18. Porcelli S, Yockey CE, Brenner MB, Balk SP. Analysis of T cell antigen receptor (TCR) expression by human peripheral blood CD4-8- alpha/beta T cells demonstrates preferential use of several V beta genes and an invariant TCR alpha chain. J Exp Med 1993;178:1–16.
19. Prussin C, Foster B. TCR Vα24 and Vβ11 coexpression defines a human NK1 T cell analogue containing a unique Th0 subpopulation. J Immunol 1997;159:5862–70.
20. Yoshimoto T, Bendelac A, Watson C, et al. Role of NK1.1+ T cells in a Th2 response and in immunoglobulin E production. Science 1995;270:1845–7.
21. Haynes BF, Denning SM, Le PT, Singer KH. Human intrathymic T cell differentiation. Semin Immunol 1990;2:66–77.
22. Latthe M, Terry L, MacDonald TT. High frequency of CD8α/α homodimer bearing T cells in human fetal intestine. Eur J Immunol 1994;24:1703–5.
23. Brandtzaeg P. Research in gastrointestinal immunology. State of the art. Scand J Gastroenterol 1985;20:137–56.
24. Perkkio M, Savilahti E. Time of appearance of immunoglobulin-containing cells in the mucosa of the neonatal intestine. Pediatr Res 1980;14:953–55.
25. Ebert EC. Do the CD45RO+CD8+ intestinal intraepithelial T lymphocytes have the characteristics of memory cells? Cell Immunol 1993;147:331–40.
26. Chott A, Gerdes D, Spooner A, et al. Intraepithelial lymphocytes in normal human intestine do not express proteins associated with cytolytic function. Am J Pathol 1997;151: 435–42.
27. Orlic D, Lev R. An electron microscopic study of intraepithelial lymphocytes in human fetal small intestine. Lab Invest 1977;37:554–61.
28. Spencer J, MacDonald TT. Ontogeny of human mucosal immunity. In: MacDonald TT, editor. Ontogeny of the immune system of the gut. Boca Raton: CRC Press; 1990. p. 23.
29. Spencer J, Dillon SB, Isaacson PG, MacDonald TT. T cell subclasses in fetal human ileum. Clin Exp Immunol 1986;65:553–8.
30. Spencer J, MacDonald TT, Diss TC, et al. Changes in intraepithelial lymphocyte subpopulations in coeliac disease and enteropathy associated T cell lymphoma (malignant histiocytosis of the intestine). Gut 1989;30:339–46.
31. Brenner MB, McLean J, Dialynas DP, et al. Identification of a putative second T cell receptor. Nature 1986;322:145–9.
32. Faure F, Jitsukawa S, Triebel F, Hercend T. Characterisation of human peripheral lymphocytes expressing the gamma/delta complex with monoclonal antibodies. J Immunol 1988; 141:3356–60.
33. Bottino C, Tambussi G, Ferrini S, et al. Two subsets of human T lymphocytes expressing gamma/delta antigen receptor are identifiable by monoclonal antibodies directed to two distinct molecular forms of the receptor. J Exp Med 1988;168: 491–505.
34. Spencer J, Finn T, Isaacson PG. Gut-associated lymphoid tissue: a morphological and immunocytochemical study of the human appendix. Gut 1985;26:672–9.
35. Cornes JJ. Number, size and distribution of Peyer's patches in the human small intestine. Gut 1965;6:225–9.
36. Owen RL, Jones AL. Epithelial cell specialization within human Peyer's patches. An ultrastructural study of intestinal lymphoid follicles. Gastroenterology 1974;66:189–203.
37. Moxey PC, Trier JS. Specialized cell types in the human fetal small intestine. Anat Rec 1978;191:269–85.
38. Spencer J, MacDonald TT, Isaacson PG. Heterogeneity of non lymphoid cells expressing HLA-D region antigens in human fetal gut. Clin Exp Immunol 1987;67:415–24.
39. Bridges RA, Condie RM, Zak SJ, Good RA. The morphologic basis of antibody formation development during the neonatal period. J Lab Clin Med 1959;53:331–57.
40. Silverstein AM, Lukes RJ. Fetal response to antigenic stimulus. 1. Plasmacellular and lymphoid reactions in the human fetus to intrauterine infections. Lab Invest 1962;11:918–32.
41. Kerneis S, Bogdanova A, Kraehenbuhl JP, Pringault E. Conversion by Peyer's patch lymphocytes of human enterocytes into M cells that transport bacteria. Science 1997;277:949–52.
42. Trejdosiewicz LK, Smart CJ, Oakes DJ, et al. Expression of T-cell receptors TcR1 (γ/δ) and TcR2 (α/β) in the human intestinal mucosa. Immunology 1989;68:7–12.
43. Haas W, Tonegawa S. Development and selection of γ/δ T cells. Curr Opin Immunol 1992;4:147–55.
44. Haas W, Pereira P, Tonegawa S. γ/δ cells. Annu Rev Immunol 1993;11:637–85.
45. Itohara S, Mombaerts P, Lafaille J, et al. T cell receptor δ gene mutant mice: independent generation of $\alpha\beta$ T cells and programmed rearrangements of γ/δ TCR genes. Cell 1993;72: 337–48.
46. Ullrich R, Schieferdecker HL, Ziegler K, et al. γ/δ T cells in the human intestine express surface markers of activation and are preferentially located in the epithelium. Cell Immunol 1990;128:619–27.
47. Groh V, Steinle A, Bauer S, Spies T. Recognition of stress-induced MHC molecules by intestinal epithelial γ/δ T cells. Science 1998;279:1737–40.
48. Koningsberger JC, Chott A, Logtenberg T, et al. TCR expression in human fetal intestine and identification of an early T cell receptor β-chain transcript. J Immunol 1997;159:1775–82.
49. Wilson A, de Villartay J, Robson MacDonald H. T cell receptor δ gene rearrangement and T early α (TEA) expression in immature $\alpha\beta$ lineage thymocytes: implications for $\alpha\beta$/$\gamma\delta$ lineage commitment. Immunity 1996;4:37–45.
50. de Villartay J, Lewis D, Hockett RD, et al. Deletional rearrangement in the human T cell receptor α chain locus. Proc Natl Acad Sci U S A 1987;84:8608–12.
51. de Villartay J, Cohen DI. Gene regulation within the TCR α/δ locus by specific deletion of the TCRδ cluster. Res Immunol 1990;141:618–23.
52. Shimizu T, Takeshita S, Muto M, et al. Mouse germline transcript of TCRα joining region and temporal expression in ontogeny. Int Immunology 1993;5:155–60.

53. Yoshikai Y, Kimura N, Toyonaga B, Mak TW. Sequences and repertoire of human T cell receptor alpha chain variable region genes in mature T lymphocytes. J Exp Med 1986;164:90–103.
54. Roman-Roman S, Ferradini L, Azocar J, et al. Studies on the human T cell receptor alpha/beta variable region genes. I. Identification of 7 additional V alpha subfamilies and 14 J alpha gene segments. Eur J Immunol 1991;21:927–33.
55. Ricken G, Pluschke G, Krawinkel U. T cell receptor alpha chain germ line transcripts from activated lymphocytes. Immunol Lett 1992;32:97–8.
56. Balk SP, Ebert EC, Blumenthal RL, et al. Oligoclonal expansion and CD1 recognition by human intestinal intraepithelial lymphocytes. Science 1991;253:1411–5.
57. Van Kerckhove C, Russell GJ, Deusch K, et al. Oligoclonality of human intestinal intraepithelial cells. J Exp Med 1992;175:57–63.
58. Blumberg RS, Yockey CE, Gross GG, et al. Human intestinal intraepithelial lymphocytes are derived from a limited number of T cell clones that utilize multiple V beta T cell receptor genes. J Immunol 1993;150:5144–53.
59. Gross GG, Schwartz VL, Stevens C, et al. Distribution of dominant T cell receptor beta chains in human intestinal mucosa. J Exp Med 1994;180:1337–44.
60. Janeway C, Jones B, Hayday A. Specificity and function of T cells bearing gamma delta receptors. Immunol Today 1988;9:73–6.
61. Krangel MS, Yssel H, Brocklehurst C, Spits H. A distinct wave of human T cell receptor γ/δ lymphocytes in the early fetal thymus: evidence for controlled gene rearrangement and cytokine production. J Exp Med 1990;172:847–59.
62. Poggi A, Sargiacomo M, Biassoni R, et al. Extrathymic differentiation of T lymphocytes and natural killer cells from human embryonic liver precursors. Proc Natl Acad Sci U S A 1993;90:4465–9.
63. McVay LD, Carding SR. Extrathymic origin of human γ/δ T cells during fetal development. J Immunol 1996;157:2873–82.
64. Jarry A, Cerf-Bensussan N, Brousse N, et al. Subsets of CD3+ (T cell receptor α/β or γ/δ) and CD3- lymphocytes isolated from normal human gut epithelium display phenotypical features different from their counterparts in peripheral blood. Eur J Immunol 1996;20:1097–103.
65. Deusch K, Luling F, Reich K, et al. A major fraction of human intraepithelial lymphocytes simultaneously express the γ/δ T cell receptor, the CD8 accessory molecule and preferentially uses the Vδ1 gene segment. Eur J Immunol 1991;21:1053–9.
66. Lafaille JJ, Decloux A, Bonneville M, et al. Junctional sequences of T cell receptor γ/δ genes: implications for γ/δ T cell lineages and for a novel intermediate of V(D)J joining. Cell 1989; 59:859–70.
67. Rock EP, Sibbald PR, Davis MM, Chien YH. CDR3 length in Ag specific immune receptors. J Exp Med 1994;179:323–8.
68. Holtmeier W, Witthöft T, Hennemann A, et al. The TCR-δ repertoire in human intestine undergoes characteristic changes during fetal to adult development. J Immunol 1997;158:5632–41.
69. Ohmen JD, Barnes PF, Uyemura K, et al. The T cell receptor of human gamma/delta T cells reactive to *Mycobacterium tuberculosis* are encoded by specific V genes but diverse V-J junctions. J Immunol 1991;147:3353–9.
70. Uyemura K, Deans RJ, Band H, et al. Evidence for clonal selection of gamma/delta T cells in response to a human pathogen. J Exp Med 1991;174:683–92.
71. Tamura N, Holroyd KJ, Banks T, et al. Diversity in junctional sequences associated with the common Vγ9 and Vδ2 gene segments in normal blood and lung compared with the limited diversity in a granulomatous disease. J Exp Med 1990;172:169–81.
72. Loh EY, Elliott JF, Cwirla S, et al. Polymerase chain reaction with single sided specificity: analysis of the T cell receptor delta chain. Science 1989;243:217–20.
73. Chowers Y, Holtmeier W, Harwood J, et al. The Vδ1 T cell receptor repertoire in human small intestine and colon. J Exp Med 1994;180:183–90.
74. Holtmeier W, Yehuda C, Lumeny A, et al. The δ T cell receptor repertoire in human colon and peripheral blood is oligoclonal irrespective of V region usage. J Clin Invest 1995;96:1108–17.
75. Scott H, Solheim BG, Brandtzeag P, Thorsby E. HLA-DR like antigens in the epithelium of the human small intestine. Scand J Immunol 1980;12:77–82.
76. Spencer J, Finn T, Isaacson PG. Expression of HLA-DR antigens on epithelium associated with lymphoid tissue in the human gastrointestinal tract. Gut 1986;27:153–7.
77. Selby WS, Janossy G, Mason DY, Jewell DP. Expression of HLA-DR antigens by colonic epithelium in inflammatory bowel disease. Clin Exp Immunol 1983;53:614–8.
78. MacDonald TT, Spencer J. Evidence that activated mucosal T cells play a role in the pathogenesis of enteropathy in human small intestine. J Exp Med 1988;167:1341–9.
79. MacDonald TT, Weinel A, Spencer J. HLA-DR expression on human fetal intestinal epithelium. Gut 1988;29:1342–8.
80. Russell GJ, Bhan AK, Winter HS. The distribution of T and B lymphocyte populations and MHC class II expression in human fetal and postnatal intestine. Pediatr Res 1990;27:239–44.
81. Lionetti P, Spencer J, Breese E, et al. Activation of Vβ3+ T cells and tissue damage in human small intestine induced by the bacterial superantigen *Staphylococcus aureus* enterotoxin B. Eur J Immunol 1993;23:664–8.
82. Uhr JW, Dancis J, Grantz Neumann CG. Delayed type hypersensitivity in premature neonatal humans. Nature 1960;187:1130–1.
83. Fowler R, Schubert WK, West CD. Acquired partial tolerance to homologous skin grafts in the human infant at birth. Ann N Y Acad Sci 1960;87:403–28.
84. Lewis DB, Larsen A, Wilson CB. Reduced interferon-gamma mRNA levels in human neonates. J Exp Med 1986;163:1018–23.
85. Wilson CB, Westall J, Johnston L, et al. Decreased production of interferon gamma by human neonatal cells: intrinsic and regulatory deficiencies. J Clin Invest 1986;77:860–7.
86. Machado CSM, Rodrigues MAM, Maffei AVC. Assessment of gut intraepithelial lymphocytes during late gestation and the neonatal period. Biol Neonate 1994;66:324–9.
87. Machado CSM, Rodrigues MAM, Maffei AVC. Gut intraepithelial lymphocyte counts in neonates, infants and children. Acta Paediatr 1994;83:1264–7.

CHAPTER 11

Development of B Lymphocytes within the Mucosal Immune System

Alistair J. Ramsay, PhD

Kenneth W. Beagley, PhD

The concept of a mucosal immune system, with functions at least partly independent of the systemic immune system, was initially proposed by Besredka in 1919.[1] He demonstrated that rabbits were protected from fatal dysentery if given oral inocula of killed *Shigella* bacillus, regardless of specific serum antibody titers. However, not until 1963 was this local immune system characterized in a molecular sense, when Tomasi showed that mucosal fluids contained high levels of a new immunoglobulin isotype, termed immunoglobulin (Ig) A.[2] In contrast, this isotype was found only at low levels in the serum. Furthermore, mucosal IgA was found to contain a secretory component[2] and a J chain that linked two Ig monomers together.[3] These components appear to distinguish IgA in external secretions, now known as secretory (s)IgA, from serum IgA. The development of antisera for IgA and secretory component facilitated detailed studies of the GI tract and other mucosal tissues, which revealed that great numbers of IgA B lymphocytes localized in the lamina propria near the mucosal surface, whereas secretory component was found to occur adjacent to epithelial cells. Thus, it appeared that sIgA was produced locally and bound to secretory component prior to its appearance in secretions.[4] These findings set the scene for development of a new field in immunology, and one of seemingly critical importance, given that our initial encounter with over 90% of the pathogens to which we are exposed occurs at mucosal surfaces. Indeed, the mucosal immune system has recently been the subject of considerable interest in light of the human immunodeficiency virus (HIV) pandemic, although much remains to be clarified, particularly of the events underlying mucosal immunoregulation.

THE MUCOSAL IMMUNE SYSTEM

Epithelial tissues comprising an area of up to 400 m² overlie the mucosae in adult humans. The mucosa-associated lymphoid tissues (MALT) are the major inductive sites for IgA responses in mammals. They appear to have three major functions: (1) to protect mucosae against invasion and colonization; (2) to block uptake of undegraded dietary and microbial antigens; and (3) to prevent the development of harmful immune responses should such antigens penetrate the mucosal barrier.[5] As mucosae are continually exposed to foreign matter, MALT must regulate appropriate effector mechanisms to optimize responses and avoid local tissue damage. MALT consist of: discrete lymphoid compartments, such as the Peyer's patches of the small intestine; other isolated lymphoid follicles and the appendix (all comprising GALT); the components of nasopharyngeal lymphoid tissues, including Waldeyer's ring of tonsillar tissue, collectively referred to here as NALT; bronchus-associated lymphoid tissues (BALT); and tissues in the genito-urinary tract. It is in these sites that local immune responses are initiated and are mediated by the great numbers of lymphoid cells migrating to the mucosal parenchyma. The putative link between these tissues is often termed the "common mucosal immune system," whereby immunocytes sensitized at one site, particularly GALT, may transfer immunity after homing to other mucosal and glandular sites.[6,7] This concept is discussed in more detail below. The migration of B and T lymphocytes from MALT to mucosal effector tissues, particularly the GI, respiratory, and reproductive tracts, forms the basis of the adaptive mucosal immune response. Collectively, MALT comprise up to 75% of the organized lymphoid tissues in humans, other primates, mice, rats, and rabbits. That mammals are highly dependent on the mucosal immune system for protection is indicated by the fact that most microorganisms either invade via mucosae or populate these surfaces as normal flora. Protection at mucosal surfaces is due in part to the local production of IgA antibodies by IgA-producing cells in lamina propria and glandular acinar regions. The greatest collection of immunocompetent T lymphocytes occurs in the GI tract, where GALT provides the precursor B and T lymphocytes destined for lamina propria, tissues that contain more than 10^{10} IgA-producing B lymphocytes per meter of human intestine.[8] Local T lymphocytes of the CD4-positive (CD4+) and CD8+ phenotype also populate these tissues, and mediate helper and cytotoxic effector functions, respectively. Early studies in athymic or thymectomized animals demonstrated a requirement for T lymphocytes in the regulation of IgA responses.[9,10] Their regulatory functions are due largely to the secretion of soluble hormone-like molecules, termed cytokines, which bind to high-affinity receptors on other immunocytes and regulate their development, activation, and differentiation. Together, T lymphocytes and the variety of cytokines they secrete regulate IgA synthesis in mucosal tissues, and as a result of these interactions, up to 3 to 4 g of IgA is secreted daily into the human GI tract.[7]

Gut-associated lymphoid tissues are the best characterized of the organized mucosal lymphoid tissues, and comprise the small intestinal Peyer's patches and large numbers of single lymphoid follicles scattered throughout the gut wall. It is useful to distinguish GALT as inductive immune tissues, where mature B and T lymphocytes and antigen-presenting cells first encounter foreign antigens, from the effector regions, such as the lamina propria, where B and T lymphocytes that leave GALT reside and mediate mucosal immune responses.[11] Intraepithelial lymphocytes, which populate the epithelial cell layer, represent another major component of the GI immune system. This population, some cells of which provide helper factors for local B lymphocyte antibody production,[12] is made up largely of T lymphocyte phenotypes, and accordingly is considered in detail elsewhere in this volume.

INDUCTIVE TISSUES OF THE GASTROINTESTINAL TRACT

The Peyer's patches of the small intestine and the lymphoid follicles associated with the large bowel constitute the major inductive sites in the GI tract. As illustrated in Figure 11–1, Peyer's patches consist of anatomically and functionally distinct regions: a specialized dome epithelium, a follicular B-cell zone, and a parafollicular T-cell-enriched area.[11] The dome epithelium consists of specialized antigen-sampling cells, termed microfold (M) cells, or follicle-associated epithelial (FAE) cells, which take up lumenal antigen and transport it into the underlying patches.[13–16] Microfold cells possess small microvilli and thin processes extending around lymphocytes, and do not appear to degrade antigen, but rather pass it on to the underlying cells closely associated with the M-cell basolateral surface.[14] It may be that discrimination between food antigens and potential pathogens occurs at the level of the M cells, where the former remain unprocessed while the latter are recognized and processed as foreign. Antigens taken up by M cells include soluble proteins, viruses, and enterobacteria. Lymphoid follicles containing germinal centers occur beneath the dome and are thought to be sites of high-level antibody isotype switching and affinity maturation, giving rise to large numbers of lymphocytes bearing surface IgA.[17,18] This process is facilitated by the retention and presentation of antigen on follicular dendritic cells. The follicles do not appear directly to give

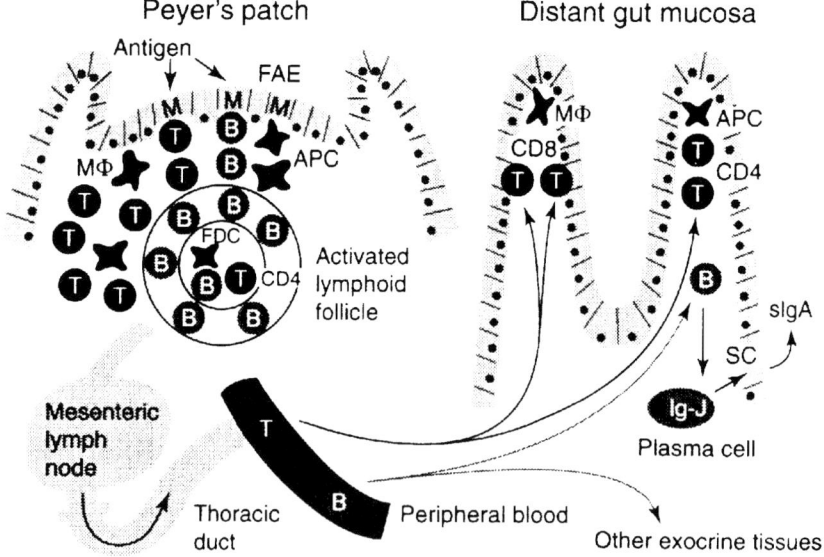

FIGURE 11–1. Induction of intestinal immune responses in Peyer's patches and resultant cell traffic in the mucosal immune system. Peyer's patches consist of a specialized follicle-associated epithelium (FAE) through which lumenal antigen is sampled and taken up by macrophages (MΦ) and other specialized antigen-presenting cells (APC) and presented to adjacent T and B lymphocytes. Lymphoid follicles are activated by this process, and specific memory B lymphocytes are generated following their exposure to antigen on follicular dendritic cells (FDC) in the presence of CD4+ T helper lymphocytes. Primed B and T lymphocytes mature further in the draining mesenteric lymph nodes and migrate, via the thoracic duct, into the peripheral circulation, from where they extravasate in mucosal tissues, predominantly the intestinal lamina propria, following their recognition of molecules on local endothelial cells. After further differentiation under the influence of APC, T lymphocytes and their secreted products in these tissues, mucosal B lymphocytes secrete specific Ig, predominantly polymeric IgA, which is transported into the lumen as secretory (s)IgA after binding secretory component (SC) synthesized in epithelial cells. (With permission from Brandtzaeg P. Basic mechanisms of mucosal immunity—a major adaptive defense system. Immunologist 1995;3:89–96. Hogrefe & Huber Publishers, Seattle, Toronto, Bern, Gottingen)

rise to high numbers of antibody-producing cells, unlike systemic lymphoid tissues. The adjacent zones contain a full complement of T lymphocyte subtypes, and over half are CD4+ helper T lymphocytes, whereas CD8+ T lymphocytes are also present in abundance.[8] With the aid of local macrophages and dendritic cells, antigen-specific B lymphocytes are generated, leave the Peyer's patches, migrate through the systemic circulation via the efferent lymphatics and thoracic duct, and eventually home back to mucosal effector tissues, particularly, but not exclusively, to the lamina propria of the GI tract (see Figure 11–1).

Effector Tissues of the Gastrointestinal Tract and Secretory Immunoglobulin A

The lamina propria of the GI tract is the only tissue where large numbers of antibody-secreting B lymphocytes (plasma cells) are found under normal physiologic conditions.[19] Up to 90% of these cells produce antibodies of the IgA isotype, and due to a lifespan limited to 5 to 9 days,[20] at least in mice, they are continuously replaced by precursors from the Peyer's patches. It is generally assumed that migrating B lymphocytes bearing IgA molecules on their surface rapidly differentiate into IgA plasma cells in the lamina propria on encountering local T-helper lymphocytes and the cytokines they produce. The antigen-dependent regulation of mucosal B lymphocyte responses is discussed in more detail in a subsequent section of this chapter. More work is needed to fully characterize the lymphoid cells present in GI lamina propria. For example, the roles of major histocompatibility complex (MHC) class II-positive B lymphocytes and macrophages in activating local CD4+ T lymphocytes should receive more emphasis. The proportion of T lymphocytes among immune cells in GI lamina propria has been estimated at between 40% and 90%, the variability most likely being due to the different techniques used for identification.

Two subclasses of IgA have been identified in humans and differ in several respects. Immunoglobulin A1 possesses a 13-amino acid proline-rich sequence in its hinge region and represents the site of cleavage by IgA proteases.[21] This region is lacking in the IgA2 molecule, which is thereby resistant to the activity of these enzymes, produced by a range of bacteria.[22] It would appear, therefore, that an abundance of IgA2 in secretions should be advantageous, particularly in light of evidence that cleavage products of IgA1 may coat potentially pathogenic bacteria and protect them from attack by other antibody molecules.[23] Interestingly, in this respect, there appears to be a marked disparity in the distribution of IgA1 and A2 subclasses between different mucosal tissues, with the former predominating in the respiratory and upper digestive tracts, and the latter more abundant in the distal gut.[24] Most serum IgA is monomeric and is produced in the bone marrow, although small amounts of polymeric IgA are found in serum, most likely following spillover from mucosal sites. Secretory IgA is a dimer of about 390,000 molecular weight; and the associated J chain, which is not homologous to the Ig or secretory component, although apparently not a member of the immunoglobulin superfamily, does have a domain structure with similarities to the classic Ig domain.[25] The J chain is probably required for polymer formation in B lymphocytes, and its complexing with monomeric IgA to form dimers occurs immediately prior to secretion. The J chain provides a conformation to IgA (and IgM) that is necessary for noncovalent binding to secretory component.[26]

The primary role of secretory antibodies, and sIgA in particular, is to act in concert with the many innate immune mechanisms that function at mucosae to prevent microorganisms from invading the body and to neutralize toxins. This process of immune exclusion generally occurs in the absence of inflammation, as local inflammatory responses could be disastrous given the volume of antigenic material to which mucosae are exposed. For this reason, it is important that sIgA antibodies do not bind complement via the classic pathway. Thus, these molecules provide an early line of defense for the body, and are produced by the multitude of activated B lymphocytes that migrate to secretory mucosae and exocrine glands and localize beneath the epithelial basement membrane. Here, IgA is produced largely in dimeric form,[3] and reaches the lumen by active transport through secretory epithelial cells.[24] Secretory antibodies must function in a highly proteolytic environment, and the intrinsic resistance of these molecules is enhanced by their binding of the secretory component. As a result of these processes, sIgA antibody is present at the point of initial contact with pathogens, particularly viruses and bacteria, and their multivalency makes them very effective at neutralization. However, the mechanisms by which sIgA molecules neutralize microorganisms are not entirely clear. Simple binding of these molecules, so that their penetration is prevented, is clearly an oversimplification. Recent studies have shown that IgA may form immune complexes in the mucosal lamina propria,[24] and is also able to bind viruses within infected epithelial cells.[27] In addition, influenza viruses bound by sIgA may, nevertheless, enter receptive cells via the plasma membrane and reach the nucleus; however, viral mRNA is not transcribed from such virions.[28] Secretory IgA molecules may also prevent a variety of bacteria from infecting mucosal epithelia via carbohydrate-specific interactions that occur independently of specific antibody activity. For example, mannose-containing oligosaccharide side chains on the IgA heavy chain are recognized by specific lectins on bacterial fimbriae,[29] whereas IgA molecules also mediate local antibacterial cytotoxic activity, particularly against invasive bacterial species, by binding Fc receptors on monocytes and CD4+ T lymphocytes.[30]

ONTOGENY OF B LYMPHOCYTES

Stem Cells

The cells of the immune system responsible for antibody production are termed B lymphocytes to denote their origins in the avian bursa of Fabricius and mammalian adult bone marrow.[31] Seminal studies in chickens led to the concept that B lymphocyte development occurred in the specific tissue microenvironment of the bursa and could be separated from the development of other lymphocytes.[32] Thus, removal of the bursa early in life severely impairs B lymphocyte development and the capacity to mount a humoral response, whereas the ability to reject skin grafts and to mount a delayed-type hypersensitivity response remains intact.[33] In mammals, the development of B lymphocytes is not absolutely dependent on a single tissue such as the bursa. In mice, B lymphocytes are produced in both the fetal liver, the spleen, and possibly in the blood islands of the yolk sac.[34] In adult life, cells with the characteristics of pre-B lymphocytes (producing heavy, but not light, immunoglobulin chains) are easily identified in the bone marrow but not in the spleen.[35] Thus, specific tissues absolutely required for B lymphocyte development do not appear to exist in mammals, unlike birds. However, at certain times during development, B lymphocyte-specific microenvironments may be found in several different tissues.

The central paradigm underpinning the study of hematopoiesis is that all myeloid and lymphoid cells (including B lymphocytes) develop from multipotential stem cells. These cells must have both the capacity to "self renew" (i.e., to continually give rise to new stem cells throughout life), and the ability to differentiate along multiple lineage pathways following their receipt of appropriate signals, such as lineage-specific cytokines and/or signaling from specialized stromal cells within the bone marrow microenvironment. The existence of multipotential stem cells was first demonstrated in adoptive transfer systems. Donor bone marrow cells carrying radiation-induced karyotypic changes or retroviral markers[36,37] were transferred in limiting numbers to recipients whose lymphoid systems had been destroyed by whole-body irradiation. When the full complement of blood cells had developed in the recipients, their lymphoid tissues were examined for cells that had arisen from the marked stem cells. Some individual animals had myeloid (nonlymphoid) cells that shared the same marker, others had B and T lymphocytes that were clonally related, and in further groups of the mice, all of the blood cells shared the same marker and appeared, therefore, to be the progeny of a single transferred cell. Although the "lymphoid stem cell" has not been formally identified, its existence is supported by a number of observations.[38] In the transfer studies outlined above, the finding that only B and T lymphocytes were clonally related in some recipients of marked bone marrow cells implies a shared precursor. Both cell types rearrange antigen receptor genes and are absent in certain immunodeficiencies, such as in mice with severe combined immunodeficiency (SCID). The development of both lineages is also impaired in interleukin (IL)-7 gene knockout mice,[39] further supporting a common precursor. In vitro studies in a number of laboratories have also identified cells with the potential to give rise to B lymphocytes as well as cells of other lineages: for example, macrophages. This suggests that the lymphoid stem cell may represent the first differentiation step along the lymphoid differentiation pathway.

A major advance that enabled investigators to study the process of lymphopoiesis was the development of in vitro tissue culture systems, such as that developed by Whitlock and Witte in 1984.[40] These systems allowed researchers to dissect the microenvironment of the bone marrow in order to understand the complex regulatory signals involved in controlling B lymphocyte development. These early in vitro studies clearly demonstrated that signals delivered by soluble factors and cell-cell interactions between the developing lymphoid cells and stromal support cells were both essential for the successful development of B lymphocytes.[41,42] Indeed, IL-7, stem cell factor (SCF), c-kit ligand, steel factor, and IL-11, in various combinations, have all been shown to support different stages of B lymphocyte development in vitro (reviewed[43]). It should be noted, however, that bone marrow stromal cell clones may produce at least 12 cytokines in culture, and thus the above-mentioned list is likely to be incomplete.

In most studies, the stromal support cultures contained a mixture of cell types, including adventitial reticular cells, epithelial cells, fibroblasts, and immature macrophages.[44] Stromal cell cultures have been cloned, and homogeneous cell lines developed.[45–47] Many of these cloned cells are preadipocytes that retain the ability to turn reversibly into fat cells.[48] No single cell type or clone, however, has the ability to replace all of the support functions provided by the heterogeneous stromal support cultures used in earlier studies. This requirement for multiple cell types to support B lymphocyte lymphopoiesis in vitro is consistent with in vivo observations: that the most immature B lymphocyte precursors are found in the subendosteal region, whereas more mature progeny migrate toward the central sinuses; and that distinct stromal cells may exist in each of these regions.[49] Lymphocyte precursors adhere tightly to stromal cells in long-term bone marrow cultures, whereas monoclonal antibodies to two cell adhesion molecules, vascular lymphocyte-associated antigen (VLA)-4, and vascular cell adhesion molecule (VCAM)-1, were shown to block this binding and to inhibit lymphopoiesis, presumably by disrupting communication between pre-B lymphocytes and stromal cells.[50,51] Both of these molecules are constitutively expressed in murine bone marrow, and have also been shown to be important for the development of human B lymphocytes. Antibodies against the CD44 surface marker have also been shown to disrupt lymphoid cell development if added early to long-term bone marrow cultures,[51] indicating that this molecule is also important in cell-cell signaling during B lymphopoiesis.

Recent findings that several growth factors (eg., granulocyte colony stimulating factor, macrophage colony stimulating factor, IL-7, SCF), once secreted, are quickly immobilized onto components of the extracellular matrix (ECM), such as heparin sulphate,[52] suggest another form of interaction that may be essential for controlling lymphopoiesis. Receptors on developing lymphoid cells may be activated by ECM-associated cytokines in addition to the soluble cytokines mentioned above. From this overview, it is apparent that B lymphocyte development occurs in a complex microenvironment in bone marrow, as shown in Figure 11–2. This process is under the control of: (1) cell-cell interactions between stromal elements and developing lymphoid cells; (2) soluble cytokines secreted either by cells within the bone marrow itself or by other immune cells, such as activated T lymphocytes; and (3) ECM-associated cytokines that may also be produced within bone marrow or in the periphery. It appears that all three control mechanisms are required for successful B lymphocyte development.

Generation of Antibody Diversity

Perhaps the most remarkable feature of B lymphocytes is their inherent ability to express an extremely large ($>10^8$) repertoire of antibodies, each with different antigen-

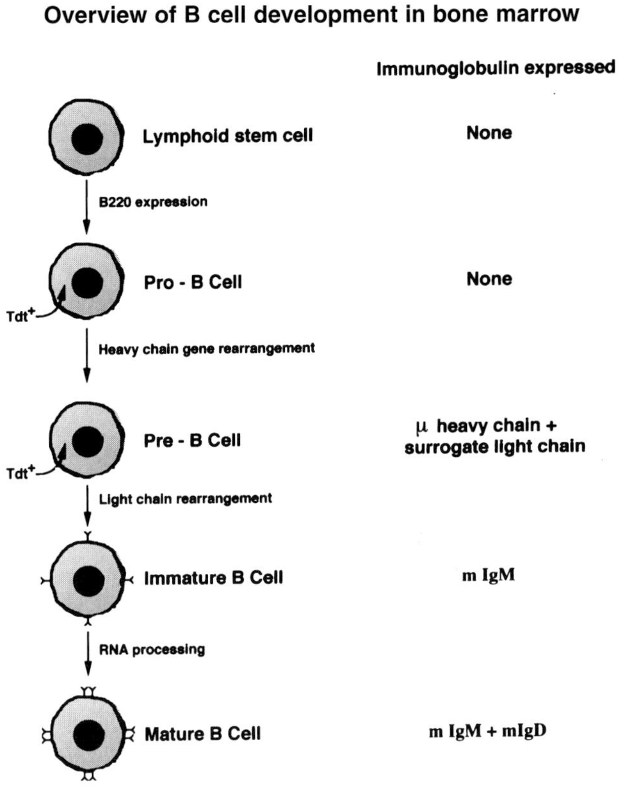

Overview of B cell development in bone marrow

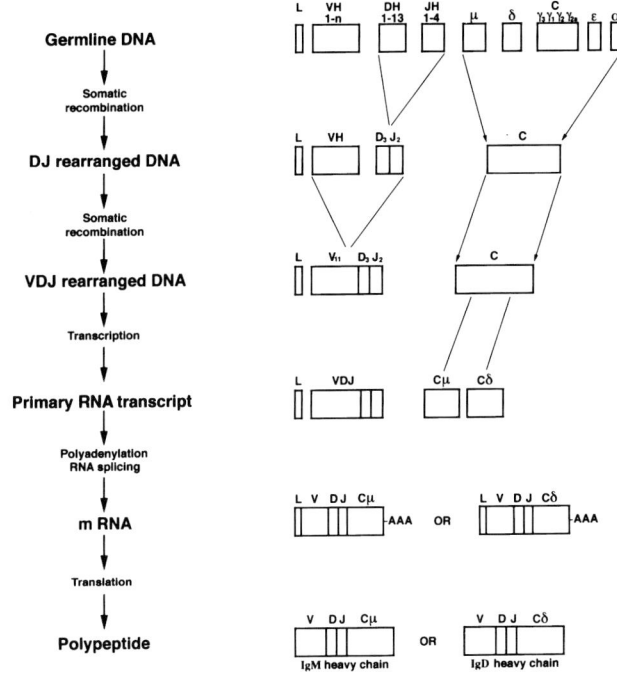

FIGURE 11-2. Overview of B-cell development in the bone marrow. Lymphoid stem cells undergo antigen-independent gene rearrangement within their heavy- and light-chain gene loci. This process results in virgin B cells expressing both membrane-bound IgD and IgM, which enter the circulating B-cell pool.

FIGURE 11-3. Heavy-chain Ig gene rearrangement in the mouse. Two DNA joinings are required to generate a functional heavy-chain gene. First, D_H to J_H joining occurs (in this case D_3 to J_2), and is followed by V_H to $D_H J_H$ joining (in this case V_{11} to $D_3 J_2$). Following this process, the constant region (C) gene sequences (encoded by several exons), together with a leader sequence (L), are spliced to the rearranged variable region gene during processing of the primary RNA transcript. Translation of these mRNAs results in B cells expressing membrane-bound IgD and IgM.

combining sites. This involves the random shuffling of multiple germline gene segments that encode both the heavy and light Ig chains during B lymphocyte development in the bone marrow.[53] This process occurs in a carefully regulated progression, so that an immunocompetent B lymphocyte will contain a single functional variable-region DNA sequence encoding an Ig heavy chain and a single functional variable-region DNA sequence encoding an Ig light chain. Combination of these two gene sequences results in a B lymphocyte committed to recognition of a single specific antigen. Thus B (and T) lymphocytes are unique among vertebrate cells, in that they contain chromosomal DNA that is no longer identical to germline DNA.

As sequence data on immunoglobulins accumulated, it became obvious that, in addition to explaining the great diversity of Ig molecules, models of antibody production had also to explain the association of a variable amino terminal region together with a constant carboxy-terminal end in both heavy and light chains, and also the existence of different isotypes with the same antigenic specificity resulting from association of a given variable region with different heavy chains. In a classic paper published in 1965, Dryer and Bennett[54] proposed that each heavy and light chain is encoded by two separate genes: one encoding the variable region, and one encoding the constant region. Although at odds with the then-current dogma of one gene-one protein, studies in the succeeding 30 years have proved this theory essentially correct, although somewhat simplified. A brief overview of the mechanisms underlying the generation of antibody diversity is given below. For more detailed descriptions, readers are referred to several recent reviews.[55–59]

The κ and λ light chains and the heavy chains of Ig molecules are encoded by separate gene loci located on different chromosomes. Both light-chain DNAs comprise three gene families: V (variable), J (joining), and C (constant). Heavy (H)-chain gene DNA is made up of V, J, and C gene families, together with a fourth, D (diversity) loci. In germline DNA, each of these loci is made up of multiple coding segments separated by noncoding regions. Production of Ig requires that these gene segments are rearranged to produce functional heavy- and light-chain Ig genes. The process begins with H-chain gene rearrangement, as shown in Figure 11–3. A D_H gene segment moves next to, and joins, a J_H gene segment. This $D_H J_H$ segment then joins with one member of the V_H gene family to form a $V_H D_H J_H$ gene segment, together with a short 5' L (leader) exon that codes for the entire variable region of the immunoglobulin heavy chain. This is separated from a number of C region genes by an intron. A promoter sequence is located upstream of the heavy-chain leader sequence. Similar rearrangement occurs between V and J gene segments in both the κ and λ light-chain gene loci. Flanking each of the germline V, D, and J gene segments are unique recombination signal sequences (RSS) made up of conserved palindromic heptamer and AT-rich nonamer sequences separated by either 12 or 23 base pairs. In germline heavy-chain DNA, one RSS is found at 3' of each V gene segment, 5' of each J gene segment, and both sides of each D gene segment. These RSS serve as signals for the recombination process, and their separation distance (equivalent to either one or two turns of the DNA helix) ensures that VJ and VDJ joining occurs rather than joining of segments from the same gene family. The V-(D)-J recombination is catalyzed by a group of enzymes collectively known as V-(D)-J recombinases, which are unique to cells of the B and T lymphocyte lineage. Further diversity within variable regions is achieved by the random addition of up to 15 nucleotides at junctions between V, D, and J segments. Addition of these N-nucleotides is catalyzed by the enzyme, terminal deoxynucleotidal transferase (Tdt), also unique to lymphoid cells. If heavy-chain gene rearrangement is successful, RNA polymerase can bind to the promoter sequence and transcribe the entire heavy-chain gene. Both the Cμ and Cδ gene segments are transcribed in developing B lymphocytes in bone marrow. Differential polyadenylation and RNA splicing removes introns and processes the primary transcript to generate mRNA encoding either Cμ or Cδ. If successful, recombination is achieved within both the heavy- and light-chain loci. The combination of these products results in a B lymphocyte expressing both IgM and IgD with identical antigenic specificity on its surface. Surface expression of complete Ig signals the cessation of VDJ recombination, and these B lymphocytes are then ready to leave the bone marrow and enter the periphery, where their future development depends on encounter with antigen, as discussed below.

B Lymphocytes

The developmental pathways for B lymphocytes outlined in the preceding section describe the origin of the majority of these cells in mice. A second population of B lymphocytes, also found in mice, differ significantly from the majority in: their tissues of origin; their use of particular V gene families and N region addition during development of their antigenic repertoire; their capacity for self-renewal; and their patterns of tissue distribution and expression of phenotypic markers. In the following discussion, conventional B lymphocytes that develop in the bone marrow are defined as B2 lymphocytes, while the minority subset are defined as B1 lymphocytes. The B1 lymphocytes have been further subdivided into B1a and B1b cell subsets. These appear to be functionally and phenotypically indistinguishable, except for their expression of CD5 surface markers: B1a cells being CD5+, while B1b lymphocytes are CD5–. The B1 lymphocytes are likely to be important cells within the mucosal immune system, as they have been shown to selectively populate the intestinal lamina propria in allotype chimeric mice, and also when adoptively transferred to SCID mice, in both cases giving rise to IgA-secreting cells. While there is no dispute over the existence of two subsets of B lymphocytes fulfilling the criteria listed above, there is, nevertheless, considerable controversy as to

TABLE 11-1
Surface Antigen Expression by Murine B1 and B2 B Lymphocytes

Surface Antigen	B1 Lymphocytes	B2 Lymphocytes
IgM	+++	+
IgD	+/– to +	+++
CD5	+(On B1a), –(on B1b)	–, (May be induced by "T-independent" antigens)
CD11b (MAC 1)	+(In peritoneum)	–
CD23 (FcεR)	–	++
B220 (RA3-6B2)	+	+++
IL-5 receptor	+	Inducible

whether these subsets constitute separate lineages, or occur as a result of stimulation by different types of antigen. A brief description of the data supporting each of these arguments is presented below; however, for more detail readers are referred to a recent review of these issues.[60]

Expression of the CD5 molecule (Ly-1, Leu-1), a marker formerly thought to be restricted to helper T lymphocytes, on a number of mouse and human B lymphocyte tumors was first reported in the early 1980s.[61,62] Since then, other phenotypic differences between B1 lymphocytes and conventional B2 lymphocytes have been noted, as outlined in Table 11-1. The B1 lymphocytes in the peritoneal cavity were shown to be IgM^{Hi}-IgD^{Lo}, CD11b (Mac 1)+, $B220^{Lo}$, to spontaneously express the IL-5R and to be negative for CD23 (FcεR). These cells were also shown to be most abundant in peritoneal and pleural cavities, but constituted a minor fraction of splenic B lymphocytes, and were rarely detected in other lymphoid tissues such as lymph nodes and Peyer's patches. In addition, B1 lymphocytes are found in small numbers in the thymus,[63] salivary glands, and female reproductive tract. In humans these cells show less tissue specificity, making up 10 to 25% of the B lymphocyte pool found in adult peripheral blood and lymphoid organs.[62] Conventional B2 lymphocytes are IgM^{Lo}-IgD^{Hi}, CD5–, CD11b–, $B220^{Hi}$, CD23+ and usually only express IL-5R following activation. In terms of development, fetal omentum is able to reconstitute B1 but not B2 lymphocytes,[64,65] whereas in most studies, adult bone marrow is able to reconstitute B2 but not B1 lymphocytes,[66] although this has recently been disputed.[67]

The B1 lymphocytes are, in fact, self-replenishing throughout adult life, as demonstrated in adoptive transfer studies, where FACS-sorted B1 lymphocytes completely and permanently reconstituted the B1 population.[68] The B1 lymphocytes produce a large component of the serum IgM pool,[69] but also make significant contributions to serum IgG3 and IgA levels.[70-72] In addition, these cells may home to the intestinal lamina propria and make a significant contribution to mucosal IgA responses.[72,73] A small number of peritoneal cavity B1 lymphocytes (<5% in BALB/c mice) appear to have actually undergone isotype switching to IgA.[72] During Ig gene rearrangement, B1 lymphocytes use only a restricted number of available V region genes:[74,75] e.g., the two-to-three member V_H11 gene family is represented in 5 to 20% of Ig rearrangements found in peritoneal cavity B1 lymphocytes. Furthermore, V-(D)-J rearrangement in B1 lymphocytes, particularly in late fetal and early postnatal life, is characterized by absence or reduced levels of N region addition, consistent with findings that Tdt is not expressed by fetal progenitors of B1 lymphocytes.[76,77] Modification of antibody responses by somatic mutation, following antigen activation, is also reduced in B1 lymphocytes compared to B2 lymphocytes,[62,78] although this may not apply in the case of the IgA+ B1 lymphocytes found in mucosal sites. The B1 cell antigenic repertoire appears skewed toward T-independent antigens associated with microorganisms and some autoantigens. For example, B1 lymphocytes contribute most of the antibody response to antigens such as phosphorylcholine (PC), α1-3 dextran, *Salmonella*, and phosphatidylcholine found on bromelain-treated mouse erythrocytes.[62,79] Many of the antibodies produced by B1 lymphocytes appear to be low-affinity and polyspecific (natural antibodies), differentiating them from the high-affinity, fine-specificity antibodies produced by B2 lymphocytes.[62,79] It should be noted, however, that B1 lymphocytes are capable of making T-dependent responses to certain antigens such as PC-KLH.[80] Based on these data, Herzenberg and colleagues have suggested that B1 lymphocytes represent a separate lineage of B lymphocytes. In their model, evolution has resulted in the emergence of a series of hemopoietic stem cells that give rise to functionally distinct layers of the immune system,[81] in which B1 lymphocytes represent the most primitive B lymphocyte lineage. These cells arise from stem cells in fetal omentum and early fetal liver, and are maintained throughout life by self-renewal (stem cells committed to this lineage are not retained in adult bone marrow). They produce broadly reactive, low-affinity antibodies using mainly germline V gene sequences. These antibodies are constitutively expressed in serum (and possibly mucosal secretions), and are directed toward antigens found on microbial pathogens. B1 lymphocytes are home to mucosal surfaces where these microbes are likely to be encountered. Implicit in this hypothesis is that all of the features that distinguish B1 lymphocytes are programmed in the progenitor cells prior to Ig gene rearrangement. These are the characteristics that would be predicted for a primitive form of humoral immunity, and conventional B2 lymphocytes are predicted to have arisen later in evolution and their responses superimposed on those of B1 lymphocytes.

The alternative hypothesis of B1 cell origin holds that both lineages develop from a common lymphoid precursor, and that the form of antigen involved in triggering the newly arisen B lymphocyte determines the developmental pathway of that particular cell.[82] This hypothesis also holds that commitment to either the B1 or B2 lymphocyte pathway can occur only after Ig gene rearrangement. The experimental basis was provided by Wortis and colleagues, who reported that normal splenic B lymphocytes that were CD5−, IgM^{Lo}-IgD^{Hi}, and CD23+ assumed the phenotype of B1 lymphocytes (CD5+, IgM^{Hi}-IgD^{Lo}, CD23−) following culture with anti-IgM antibodies and IL-6.[83] Based on these observations, it was proposed that cross-linking of surface Ig by TI-2 antigens in the absence of T lymphocyte helps lead to a B1 developmental pathway, whereas cognate interaction with a T-helper cell, without crosslinking of Ig, leads to the B2 pathway. This hypothesis is supported by findings that: (1) TI-2 antigens induce largely IgM responses that are rarely mutated (i.e., typical of B1 Ig); (2) mice with the Xid defect are unable to mount TI-2 responses and are deficient in B1 lymphocytes;[84,85] and (3) mice treated from birth with anti-IL-10 antibodies are deficient in B1 lymphocytes and fail to respond to PC and α1-3 dextran.[69] This hypothesis is at odds, however, with findings in BALB/c mice stimulated with the TI-2 antigen TNP-Ficoll, which indicate that greater than 90% of responding B lymphocytes are CD5−.[86] In addition, there is some evidence that crosslinking of surface Ig in the absence of cognate T lymphocyte help results in negative selection either by deletion or anergy.[87,88] We also have recently found that B1 cell numbers are increased in IL-6 gene knockout mice, an observation difficult to reconcile with the need for IL-6 in the induction of CD5 expression on B2 lymphocytes as described by Wortis and colleagues.

Clarification of the exact origins of B1 lymphocytes will obviously require detailed analyses of differences in gene expression between fetal and adult B lymphocyte progenitors. However, B1 lymphocytes in both mouse and man clearly have the ability to switch to IgA antibody production and to migrate to mucosal tissues such as the intestinal lamina propria. A greater understanding of the biology of these cells will aid our understanding of mucosal immunity.

ANTIGEN-DEPENDENT MUCOSAL B LYMPHOCYTE DEVELOPMENT

The induction of mucosal IgA antibodies, at least by conventional B lymphocytes, is highly dependent on help provided by CD4+ T lymphocytes generated in MALT and the costimulatory molecules and cytokines they express (reviewed[89]). Antigen-specific activation of B lymphocytes in MALT apparently leads to Ig heavy-chain switching, resulting in the expression of surface IgA by IgM-bearing B lymphocytes. Interactions of CD28 and CD40 ligand molecules on the surface of local T lymphocytes with the B7 molecules on antigen-presenting cells and CD40 on B lymphocytes, respectively, provide the critical co-stimulatory signals for this process.[90] Cytokines regulate the early stages of lymphocyte development, and following encounter with antigen mediate the process of isotype switching, whereby genes encoding the μ heavy chain are replaced with a downstream heavy-chain gene (γ1, γ2, γ3, γ4, ε, or α). Finally, following isotype switching, these factors direct the differentiation of B lymphocytes to antibody-secreting cells.

The description of two subsets of CD4+ T helper (Th) cells, defined by their pattern of cytokine secretion and biologic activity, has been important for understanding the regulation of both mucosal and systemic immune responses.[91] The so-called Th1 cells secrete IL-2, interferon-γ, and tumor necrosis factor, and typically provide help for the development of cell-mediated immunity against viruses and intracellular bacteria. In contrast, Th2 cells secrete IL-4, IL-5, IL-6, IL-10, and IL-13 and provide help for antibody synthesis, particularly the IgG1, IgE, and IgA isotypes. While this classification has largely stood the test of time, with some modifications,[92] a further population with a composite cytokine secretion profile, termed Th0 cells, has now been identified.[93,94] The cytokine milieu in which T lymphocytes are activated and subsequently differentiate are crucial factors in determining their phenotype (reviewed[95]). Indeed,

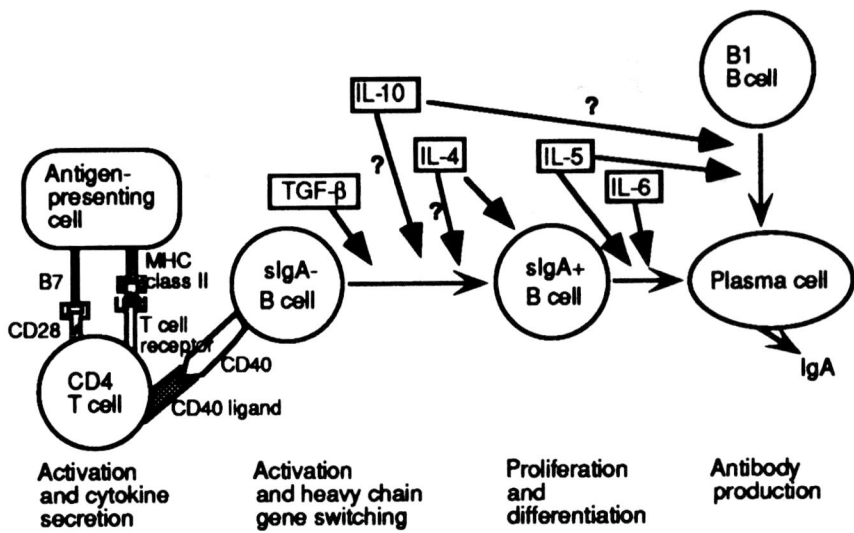

FIGURE 11–4. Putative cellular and cytokine interactions in the development of mucosal IgA antibody production in mice. Antigen is processed in MALT by antigen-presenting cells (APC) and presented to naive CD4+ T-helper cells in the context of MHC class II molecules. The T lymphocyte activation is dependent on costimulatory interaction between the B7 and CD28 molecules. Activated T lymphocytes and other local cell populations secrete a variety of cytokines important for antibody production. Further costimulatory interactions between the CD40 molecule and its ligand, together with TGFβ production, are crucial for Ig heavy chain switching, while other cytokines drive subsequent steps in the differentiation of IgA B lymphocytes. Interleukin-4 and IL-10 are thought to play a role in this process, however, the evidence is unclear. Interleukin-5, and possibly IL-10, drive the development of B1 B lymphocytes, which may give rise to IgA-producing cells, although their repertoire is thought to be skewed toward T-independent antigens. (Adapted from Brandtzaeg P. Basic mechanisms of mucosal immunity—a major adaptive defense system. Immunologist 1995;3:89–96.)

the cytokines IL-12 and IL-4 may direct naive T lymphocytes down the Th1 or Th2 pathways, respectively, while later in their development interferon (IFN)-γ and IL-10 may direct the expansion of Th1 and Th2 cells, respectively. The Th1 and Th2 cells are found in approximately equal numbers in MALT,[96] but in effector tissues, T lymphocyte cytokine production is strongly biased toward Th2 responses.[96–98] The important roles thought to be played by Th cells and other immune cell populations and their secreted products in directing the development of mucosal antibody responses are shown diagrammatically in Figure 11–4 and discussed in detail below.

Cellular Regulation of Immunoglobulin A Responses in Mucosa-Associated Lymphoid Tissues

The studies of Strober and colleagues originally demonstrated a role for Peyer's patch T lymphocytes in the process of antibody isotype switching to IgA production.[99,100] These workers showed that cloned T lymphocytes derived from Peyer's patches increased the frequency of surface IgA-bearing cells in cultures of lipopolysaccharide-stimulated splenic B lymphocytes, unlike splenic T-lymphocyte clones. Cognate interactions between these "switch" T lymphocytes and the stimulated B lymphocytes were required for switching to occur, but this process did not induce the actual secretion of IgA antibodies. The demonstration of a role for a second type of T-helper lymphocyte in directing antigen-specific IgA responses in murine Peyer's patch soon followed, and it became clear that the activity of these cells could be mediated by their soluble secreted factors.[101–103] These helper cells directed IgA production only by surface IgA-bearing B lymphocytes, indicating their provision of help only to switched, mature B lymphocytes. Dendritic cells resident in Peyer's patches may also regulate B lymphocyte switching to IgA. Clusters of activated Peyer's patch T lymphocytes and dendritic cells in culture with B lymphocytes from either spleen or Peyer's patch were shown to direct the production of up to a hundredfold more IgA than splenic clusters of these cells.[104] The T lymphocytes and dendritic cells from MALT could also mediate these effects in pre-B lymphocyte cultures, suggesting that the source of the dendritic cells may be a crucial factor in switching and the secretion of mucosal IgA antibodies.[105]

Antibody Isotype Switching in Mucosa-Associated Lymphoid Tissues

After their activation by antigen, B lymphocytes bearing surface IgM and IgD markers may switch to the expression of a different heavy-chain constant region (C_H), resulting in changes in the class of antibody synthesized and in the effector function of the antibody produced.[106] The specificity of antigen binding is unaltered, as the expressed V(D)J region and light chain remain unchanged. The change in antibody class involves recombination between DNA segments (switch or S regions) that are located just upstream of C_H genes, and it occurs, for most isotypes, when upstream and downstream S regions join in such a way that a DNA loop is formed that contains the intervening C_H genes to be deleted. Switch recombination occurs in mature B lymphocytes following their exposure to antigen; indeed, the resultant heavy-chain class is strongly influenced by the nature of the antigen.[106] Both T lymphocyte-dependent and independent antigens appear to induce switching in conjunction with both cytokines and cognate signals (from T lymphocytes and Ig crosslinking in the former and crosslinking in the latter). In vivo, antibody class switching usually begins in the periarteriolar lymphoid sheaths and in germinal centers about 6 days after B lymphocyte activation by T lymphocyte-dependent antigens, and occurs simultaneously with somatic mutation.[107] For a more detailed description of the molecular mechanisms underlying isotype switching in general, the reader is referred to a recent comprehensive review.[108]

In addition to isotype switching induced by cognate interaction with T lymphocytes, effectively through CD40-CD40 ligand binding,[109] this process is also mediated via the activity of cytokines, particularly IFN-γ, IL-4, and transforming growth factor (TGF)-β, in combination with "noncognate" activational signals. Cytokine-induced switching is preceded by the induction of germline transcripts corresponding to the Ig isotype to which the B lymphocyte will switch. Thus, IL-4 induces IgG1 and IgE germline transcripts in human B lymphocytes prior to the expression of these isotypes,[110] whereas mice deficient for IL-4 production (IL-4$^{-/-}$) cannot express IgE, but have only reduced expression of the IgG1 isotype.[111,112] The IFN-γ induces isotype switching to IgG2a in mouse B lymphocytes,[113] although this effect is less dramatic than IL-4-mediated switching to IgG1 and IgE, but may inhibit the latter or, indeed, germline IgA transcripts and switching to IgA.[114] Mice that lack receptors for IFN-γ display reduced antimicrobial IgG2a production.[115]

In vitro evidence in favor of IL-4 as an important IgA switch factor[116,117] has not been borne out in IL-4$^{-/-}$ mice, in which neither IgA antibody levels nor numbers of IgA-secreting cells in the lungs or small intestinal lamina propria differed from wild-type mice that had not been deliberately immunized.[118] Thus, the ability of mucosal B lymphocytes to undergo switching to IgA production does not depend on the presence of IL-4; however, the IL-4$^{-/-}$ mice did have significantly smaller and fewer small intestinal Peyer's patches than wild-type mice, and very poor germinal center development.[119] The IL-4$^{-/-}$ mice were also unable to mount intestinal IgA responses following oral immunization with soluble proteins in the face of a strong response to cholera toxin given as a component of the inoculum. This defect was apparently due to their failure to fully develop the antigen-specific Th2 cells and B lymphocytes required to induce germinal center activity in the gut, rather than defective IgA isotype switching in the absence of IL-4.[119]

Transforming growth factor-β has recently emerged as a key cytokine for IgA isotype switching. Germline IgA transcripts and subsequent switching to IgA are induced by this factor in both murine and human B lymphocytes following treatment with lipopolysaccharide or CD40 ligand.[114,120] Transforming growth factor-β acts on surface IgM$^+$, sIgA$^-$ lymphocytes: thus, its role probably does not extend to post-switch differentiation. It induces human germline transcripts for both IgA1 and IgA2 B lymphocytes stimulated with *Branhamella catarrhalis*, a bacterium associated with the upper respiratory tract,[121] and switching to IgA by CD4 T lymphocyte- and mitogen-activated human B lymphocytes.[122] It appears, however, that the switching effects mediated by this factor may not be restricted to IgA. Transforming growth factor-β selectively promoted increases in murine germline $C_{H\gamma}2b$ RNA levels and IgG2b isotype secretion by IgM$^+$, IgG2b$^-$ B lymphocytes, while neutralization of this factor reduced secretion of all IgG subclasses by murine B lymphocytes.[123] Thus, it appears that following activation with appropriate B lymphocyte stimuli, TGF-β induces isotype switching to both IgA and IgG2b, but may also enhance the secretion of all IgG subclasses in a manner independent of class switching. Transforming growth factor-β-induced IgA-switching is consistent with the observation that the TGF-β response element is located proximally to the Iα gene segment in B lymphocytes; however, this gene sequence is not exclusively associated with the α heavy-chain gene, but is also found upstream of other C_H genes.[123] Indeed, the possibility arises that the primary stimulus may also influence isotype switching, while TGF-β appears to be crucial for IgA isotype switching in vitro, this does not occur in experimental situations with all B-lymphocyte mitogens.[90,124]

The tissue-specific nature of IgA switching is a further issue bearing on the role of TGF-β as an IgA switch factor. Immunoglobulin A B lymphocyte development occurs only in Peyer's patch germinal centers and in similar structures elsewhere in MALT, whereas TGF-β is produced by both lymphoid and nonlymphoid cells in many tissues. In addition, up to 70% of Peyer's patch germinal center B lymphocytes are surface IgA$^+$, however in vitro studies indicate that the frequency of IgA switching is only about 3%.[125–127] It has recently been shown that TGF-β, IL-4, and IL-5 together induced surface IgA$^+$ B lymphocyte populations of up to 20%,[120] and it may be that synergy between these, and possibly other factors, is important in vivo. It is clear that IL-4 and IL-5 may increase switch recombination other than by regulating germline transcripts; however, the mechanisms underlying these effects are, as yet, poorly understood.[114,120]

B Lymphocyte Homing in the Mucosal Immune System

Following their activation, proliferation, and partial differentiation in MALT, both B and T cells migrate to regional lymph nodes, and after further differentiation travel through efferent lymphatics and the thoracic duct into the peripheral circulation, from where they home to the lamina propria of various mucosal tissues. The maturation of IgA B cells from GALT and BALT into blasts with this migratory capacity occurs, respectively, in draining mesenteric and mediastinal lymph nodes, whereas cells from NALT and other components of MALT may also mature in local draining nodes.[128,129] It is clear, however, that migratory cells from GALT and BALT are capable of migration either to the gut or the respiratory tract,[6,130] although mesenteric node blasts appear to preferentially migrate to gut rather than lung, and the reverse is true for cells from mediastinal nodes.[131] Nev-

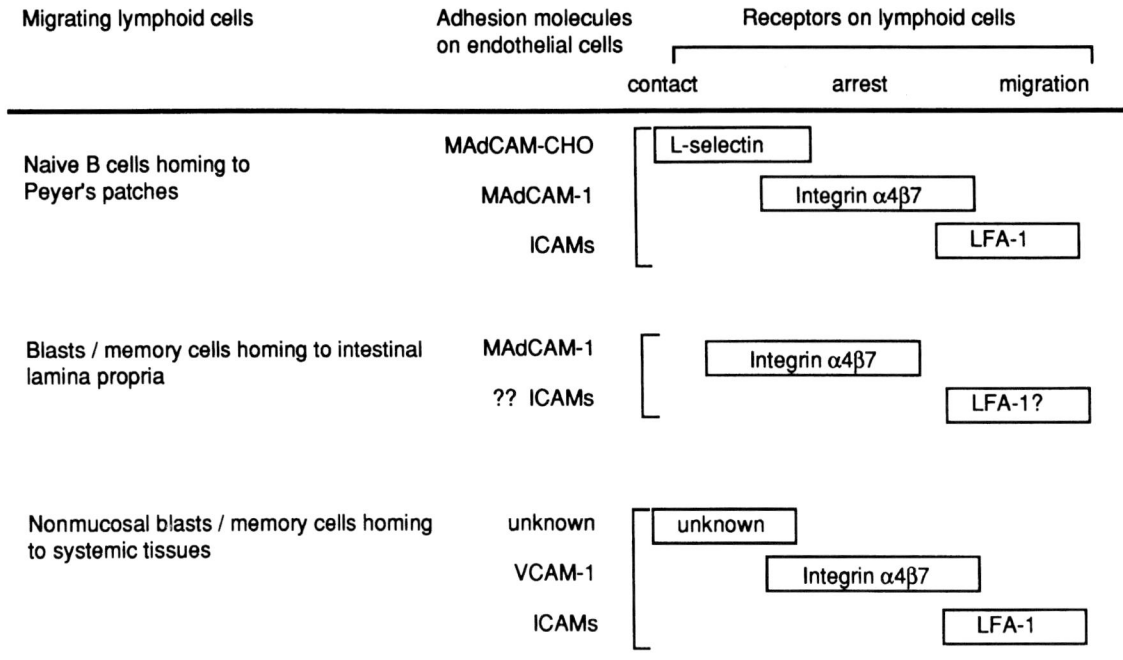

FIGURE 11–5. Cell surface adhesion interactions underlying the homing of mucosal lymphocytes. Receptors expressed on the surface of naive mucosal lymphocytes and mucosal blast cells adhere to specialized ligands on endothelial cells in MALT and intestinal lamina propria prior to their extravasation. Different homing ligands are recognized by nonmucosal lymphocytes. Quantitative as well as qualitative regulation of lymphocyte receptor expression is important in differential cell migration as described in the text. (Adapted from Butcher EC, Picker LJ. Lymphocyte homing and homeostasis. Science 1996;272:60–6.)

ertheless, antigen-specific blasts from either source may localize in the intestine,[131,132] bronchi,[131] salivary glands,[133] mammary glands,[131,134] and uterus.[131] These observations led to the proposition of a "common mucosal immune system," whereby cells sensitized at one site in MALT could settle in many different mucosal tissues through shared surface markers and/or other recognition signals for localization. Such widespread dissemination from a single source would appear to represent a highly attractive basis for mucosal vaccination strategies, as discussed below; although several lines of evidence indicate restrictions on the extent of cellular traffic between mucosal organs. Certainly, local preferences appear to exist for B cells from GALT and BALT,[131] while intestinal blasts tend to localize in the immunized region of the jejunum or colon after migration in the peripheral circulation.[135] Initial localization may occur independently of the presence of specific antigen,[132,136] although both antigen and local specific T-cell populations may be important for localization and/or retention of mucosal B cells.[132,136,137]

The molecular basis for the localization patterns of mucosal immunocytes, indeed for lymphocyte homing in general, involves the expression of different cell surface adhesion molecules that engage, in multistep sequences, corresponding determinants (often referred to as addressins) expressed by vascular endothelial cells, as shown in Figure 11–5. Soluble factors, including cytokines and growth factors such as IL-2, IL-10, TGF-β, vasoactive intestinal peptide, and hepatocyte growth factor, have also been implicated in the regulation of lymphocyte homing,[138] while it is becoming clear that chemokines, particularly due to their capacity for binding glycosaminoglycans, may play a major role in attracting circulating cells to endothelia.[139–141] This discussion focuses largely on mechanisms underlying the homing behavior of mucosal immunocytes; however, readers may also be interested in a recent comprehensive review of the molecular processes of lymphocyte homing in general.[138]

Mature lymphocytes generally recirculate continuously from blood to tissue and back into the bloodstream once or twice per day,[142] although in this respect significant differences exist between naive and antigen-stimulated memory cell populations. Naive lymphocytes exhibit reasonably homogeneous patterns of recirculation through secondary lymphoid tissues such as Peyer's patches, tonsils, lymph nodes, and spleen, where antigen is encountered.[143] In contrast, the migratory behavior of memory lymphocytes is highly heterogeneous, and occurs not only through lymphoid tissues but also through "effector" tissues such as mucosal lamina propria, skin, and joints.[143]

Localization of these cells may be tissue-selective and highly restricted, so that they target sites where they will re-encounter antigen or are adapted to perform their functions. The homing of IgA B lymphocytes to mucosal lamina propria is an excellent example of this process, which mediates, at one level, the specialization of regional immune responses. The extravasation of mucosal B lymphocytes has been shown to involve, in particular, recognition of the mucosal addressin cell adhesion molecule (MAdCAM)-1 on local endothelial cells by the integrin α4β7 on the migrating cell,[144] although certain cells, predominantly mucosal T lymphocytes that express αEβ7 integrin, appear to migrate deeper into intestinal tissues and may be retained by the binding of this molecule to E-cadherin expressed on local epithelial cells.[145]

The process of lymphocyte recruitment may be conveniently separated into four successive steps.[138] The first is primary adhesion and rolling on the vascular endothelial cell surface, in which constitutive lymphocyte receptors interact with vascular ligands. This step is highly transient and reversible, and may be followed by a rapid lymphocyte activation phase (lasting seconds) in which lymphocyte surface receptors, perhaps including chemokine receptors,[146] trigger integrin adhesion to vascular ligands. Thirdly, an activation-dependent arrest phase may occur, which is reversible over several minutes and involves integrin binding; and, finally, in the presence of appropriate cellular signals, diapedesis and extravasation may follow.

In situ studies in murine intestinal tissues have recently served to clarify processes whereby naive lymphocytes home to Peyer's patches while antigen-stimulated mucosal memory cells target the intestinal lamina propria.[146,147] Peyer's patch high endothelial venules (HEV) display a unique suite of homing markers (L-selectin ligand^{Low}, MAdCAM-1^{Hi}, intracellular adhesion molecule [ICAM]-1$^+$, and ICAM-2$^+$) that necessitate the sequential engagement of L-selectin to initiate contact, α4β7 integrin to slow rolling, and leukocyte function antigen (LFA)-1 and α4β7 for arrest. Members of the α4 integrin family do not appear to be involved in the homing of naive lymphocytes to nonmucosal peripheral lymph nodes, as their HEV do not express MAdCAM-1. Levels of α4β7 integrin expression on naive lymphocytes are insufficient for their direct binding to the MAdCAM-1$^+$, L-selectin ligand$^-$ HEV in intestinal lamina propria, ensuring their access to MALT but not to mucosal lamina propria effector sites. However, α4β7 integrin^{Hi} mucosal memory blasts may interact with lamina propria venules using this integrin alone.[147] It appears that mucosal homing determinants are shared among Peyer's patches, mesenteric lymph nodes, and the intestinal lamina propria,[143,144] and further sets of these molecules may be shared by NALT, BALT, and their associated mucosal effector tissues. Further studies of these molecular relationships will be important to facilitate the development of more effective mucosal vaccination strategies, particularly for immunity at sites such as the respiratory and reproductive tracts.

Role of Cytokines in Mucosal B Lymphocyte Terminal Differentiation

Following their migration from MALT into mucosal effector tissues, primed IgA B lymphocytes undergo further differentiation into plasma cells. Local T lymphocyte-derived IL-5, IL-6, and IL-10 are thought to be important mediators in this process and are abundantly produced in these tissues. Early in vitro studies showed that soluble factors produced by murine T lymphocytes were able to enhance the production of IgA in cultures of B lymphocytes from either Peyer's patch or spleen. One of the factors responsible for this activity was subsequently shown to be IL-5,[148] a cytokine originally identified for its growth and differentiation influence on B lymphocytes and eosinophils. The removal of surface IgA$^+$ B lymphocytes from the cultures abrogated these effects, indicating that IL-5 was acting on IgA-committed B lymphocytes.[149,150] Thus, murine IL-5 apparently has no activity on surface IgA$^-$ B lymphocytes, but has been shown to increase IgA reactivity of activated mucosal sIgA$^+$ B lymphocytes, either alone[149] or in synergy with IL-4,[151] IL-6,[152] or TGF-β.[126]

On this basis, IL-5, while not apparently promoting a switch to IgA, has been regarded as an IgA B lymphocyte terminal differentiation factor, inducing surface IgA$^+$ B lymphocytes in cell cycle to differentiate into IgA-producing cells. In support of this contention, IL-5-secreting Th2 lymphocytes are present at high frequency in IgA effector sites of murine mucosal tissues,[96–98] whereas vector-expressed IL-5 selectively enhances antigen-specific IgA reactivity at murine mucosae following local immunization.[153] In contrast, human IL-5 appears to have relatively little effect on IgA B lymphocyte differentiation, although human B lymphocytes that are activated by exposure to the bacterium *Branhamella catarrhalis* can be induced to secrete IgA in the presence of IL-5.[154] However, this effect could not be demonstrated using a variety of more conventional B-lymphocyte mitogens: emphasizing, once again, the important role of the primary activation signal for B-lymphocyte differentiation. Despite this in vitro evidence supporting a role for IL-5 in mucosal IgA B lymphocyte development, particularly in mice, our recent studies in IL-5-deficient animals have indicated no real deficiency in their ability to mount mucosal IgA responses to conventional antigens.[155] Indeed, numbers of IgA-staining B lymphocytes in intestinal lamina propria were similar in IL-5$^{-/-}$ and wild-type mice that had not been deliberately immunized, and no significant defects were found in small intestinal IgA responses in IL-5 mutants given local inocula of a variety of antigens, including the dietary protein ovalbumin, influenza virus, or vaccinia virus. Evidence that IL-5 influences the development of the B1 cell subset,[156] and that peritoneal B1 cells give rise to a significant proportion of IgA B lymphocytes in intestinal lamina propria,[157] prompted us to analyze this population in IL-5$^{-/-}$ mice. A 50% reduction in B1 cell numbers was found in both the peritoneal cavity and gut of these animals, and this was reflected functionally in reduced antiphosphorylcholine antibody levels in intestinal fluids following challenge with attenuated *Salmonella typhimurium*.[73] Thus IL-5, which is produced in abundance in mucosal effector tissues such as intestinal lamina propria, may direct the development of switched surface IgA-bearing mucosal B lymphocytes, as evidenced by in vitro studies, but is not obligatory for this process in vivo, except, perhaps, in the case of B1 lymphocytes.

Interleukin-6 is a multifunctional factor, secreted by many cell types, that was originally identified by its ability to induce the terminal differentiation of B lymphocytes.[158] Interleukin-6 enhances antibody secretion by activated B lymphocytes in vitro, but does not appear to enhance their differentiation, a proposition confirmed in transgenic (IL-6-overexpressing) mice, which display a massive tissue plasmacytosis, with IgG1 levels elevated by up to 400-fold and much smaller increases in other IgG isotypes.[159] Interleukin-6 was originally implicated in mucosal immunoregulation through its marked and selective enhancement of IgA production in vitro by IgA-switched B lymphocytes but not by surface IgA$^-$ B lymphocytes,[160] and appears, in this respect, to be a significantly more potent factor than IL-5 in mice. The presence in mucosal tissues of T lymphocytes, macrophages, and other cells with the potential for IL-6 production in vitro,[161,162] and the widespread distribution of cells containing IL-6 mRNA in intestinal lamina propria,[98] are also consistent with an important role for this factor in regulating the effector stage of IgA responses. In addition, B lymphocytes from human appendix are stimulated by IL-6 to secrete both IgA1 and IgA2 antibodies in the absence of any other in vitro stimulation.[161] Thus, IL-6 appears to play an important role in directing the terminal differentiation of IgA$^+$ B cells in both mice and humans.

Mice lacking IL-6 function had normal levels of B lymphocytes but a reduction in total T lymphocyte numbers, and whereas total serum immunoglobulin levels were similar in IL-6$^{-/-}$ mutants and their wild-type littermates, the mutants had impaired serum IgG antibody responses following virus infection.[163] Their secretion of cytokines other than IL-6 appeared not to be affected. In the absence of deliberate immunization, however, IL-6$^{-/-}$ mice had up to 50% fewer IgA$^+$ intestinal B lymphocytes than wild-type mice, indicative of a role for this factor in IgA B lymphocyte development in vivo.[164] Many of the residual IgA-positive cells in the mutant mice stained diffusely and appeared to represent B1 cells, distinct from conventional Peyer's patch B lymphocytes, and originating in the peritoneal cavity.[165] Recently, we have found that these cells respond to microbial antigens, such as bacterial lipopolysaccharide and phosphorylcholine, develop normally, and are fully functional in the absence of IL-6. More important, however, are the consequences of IL-6 deficiency for the development of mucosal IgA antibody responses to conventional B lymphocyte antigens by B lymphocytes from MALT. When immunized locally, IL-6$^{-/-}$ mice mounted deficient mucosal IgA responses to ovalbumin in the small intestine, and both IgA and IgG responses to vaccinia virus in the respiratory tract.[164] However, as shown in Figure 11–6, the ability of IL-6$^{-/-}$ mice to mount sustained mucosal antibody responses was fully restored following local administration of recombinant vaccinia viruses engineered to express IL-6.[164] While vector-encoded IL-6 promoted the development of lung IgA precursor cells, which are of mucosal origin, it clearly also provided proliferative signals for plasma cell precursors entering the lung from systemic immune sites, as shown by the restoration of IgG responses in IL-6$^{-/-}$ mice. In addition, while enzyme-linked immunosorbent assay (ELISA) titers of specific IgA and IgG antibodies were negligible in bronchial lavage fluids from IL-6$^{-/-}$ mice given vaccinia virus, strong responses, similar to those found in wild-type mice, were detected in IL-6$^{-/-}$ mice given the IL-6-expressing recombinant virus. These findings provide strong evidence that IL-6 plays a major role in the development of mucosal antibody responses to virus infection. Deficient mucosal IgA responses were also found in IL-6$^{-/-}$ mice challenged mucosally with *Candida albicans*,[166] although not in those given *Helicobacter felis* or soluble protein together with the mucosal adjuvant cholera toxin.[167] Thus, IL-6 may play an important role in the development of IgA B lymphocytes, depending on the nature of the stimulating antigen, but less so for B1 cells, which apparently respond to a different set of antigens than conventional B lymphocytes.

MODULATION OF MUCOSAL B LYMPHOCYTE RESPONSES

Mucosal Vaccination

The development of effective mucosal vaccination strategies has attained a high priority with the advent of the HIV pandemic. Nearly all pathogens, including HIV, enter the body via mucosal surfaces, and are thereby exposed initially to the mucosal immune system. This section summarizes the status of mucosal vaccination, with emphasis on antibody responses. Readers are referred to recent review articles and monographs for a more detailed description of mucosal vaccination.[168–172]

The potential importance of vaccine-induced mucosal antibody responses has been amply illustrated by recent indications that over 80% of HIV transmission occurs through heterosexual intercourse. Indeed, current thinking holds that the route of virus dissemination after mucosal infection involves a stepwise spread from mucosal draining lymph nodes to distant systemic lymphoid tissues, and therefore that systemic immune responses alone may not be sufficient to prevent genital transmission of the virus (reviewed[173]). While the development of both systemic and mucosal cytotoxic T cells will almost certainly be crucial targets for effective vaccination against HIV, stimulation of secretory IgA antibodies in tissues most at risk for virus transmission (i.e., genito-urinary mucosae) may also be important for the prevention of infection. Specific antiviral mucosal IgA antibodies have been shown to protect against mucosal infection with several different viruses,[174] and may neutralize viruses either in extracellular fluids or intracellularly.[175] A recent study involving 16 couples, in which one member had remained seronegative despite many years of exposure to an HIV-infected partner, also points to the potential importance of specific mucosal IgA antibody lev-

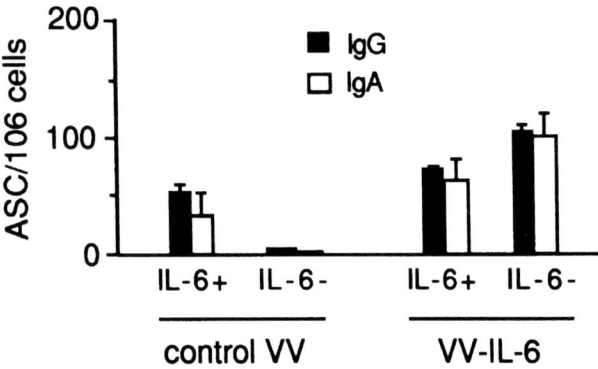

FIGURE 11–6. The influence of IL-6 on antiviral IgA and IgG responses in vivo. Wild-type (IL-6$^+$) or IL-6-deficient (IL-6$^-$) mice were given intranasal inocula of 10^7 plaque-forming units of recombinant vaccinia virus (VV) 10 days prior to analyses of numbers of virus-specific IgA and IgG antibody-secreting cells (ASC) by ELISPOT. The markedly deficient responses seen in the IL-6$^-$ mice were dramatically restored when these mice were given vaccinia virus constructs engineered to express this factor.

els as a correlate of protection against virus transmission.[176] Indeed, 82% of the seronegative partners had HIV-specific IgA, but not IgG, antibodies in vaginal fluids.

A great number of approaches have been used in attempts to elicit effective mucosal immune responses by vaccination but with varying degrees of success. Parenteral administration of antigens is rarely effective for the induction of good mucosal immunity, and it is now widely thought that direct stimulation of MALT is required. Both living and nonliving vaccine preparations have been applied to mucosal surfaces with mixed results. A major problem in this respect has been the effective targeting of antigens to MALT and/or their persistence in an immunogenic form in the harsh, proteolytic mucosal environment. This has often resulted in low-level or poorly persistent mucosal immune responses, particularly to nonreplicating antigens, even following the administration of large (milligram to gram) and multiple doses. Protective vehicles, including liposomes, biodegradable microspheres (usually polymers of DL-lactide-co-glycolide), and immunostimulatory complexes, have been developed to address the problems of antigen degradation and targeting;[169] however, the methods required for their preparation can lead to denaturation. However, mucosal lectins having immunostimulatory properties, such as cholera toxin, an extremely potent mucosal adjuvant,[177] and the heat-labile enterotoxin of *Escherichia coli*, have been shown to promote both mucosal and systemic antibody responses when conjugated to, or even simply co-delivered with, a variety of antigens.

Perhaps more promisingly, a wide range of recombinant vectors, either live, attenuated viral and bacterial contructs or nonreplicating DNA vaccines, have recently been used to deliver vaccine antigens to mucosal surfaces.[5,169–171,178–180] Viruses with known mucosal tropism, including adenoviruses, polioviruses, and poxviruses, and which permit the insertion of genes encoding relatively large antigens (or combinations of antigens), are held to have great promise as mucosal immunogens. However, the balance between attenuation of the vector and adequate expression and immunogenicity of encoded antigen is not always easy to achieve with such constructs. Similar constraints apply to a range of bacterial vectors, based on *Salmonella, Shigella, Escherichia coli, Lactobacillus, Vibrio cholerae,* or *Mycobacteria,* that have been developed for mucosal immunization. In these cases, additional problems to be overcome relate to the inappropriate form in which the encoded antigen is often expressed by such constructs. Deoxyribonucleic acid vaccines have also recently been shown, by ourselves and others, to prime for mucosal immune responses following either mucosal or systemic administration.[178,179,181,182] While the development of improved targeting techniques will be an obvious priority for mucosal DNA vaccination, the recent use of bacterial carriers to deliver these constructs into mucosal antigen-presenting cells in GALT represents a promising advance.[183] There is also ample evidence that coexpression of genes encoding cytokines along with heterologous vaccine antigens in a variety of recombinant vectors may boost vaccine-induced mucosal immune responses. Our recent studies have shown that the delivery of cytokines in this manner in DNA vaccines and/or different poxvirus vectors, particularly factors of importance at mucosae, such as IL-6, both enhances and sustains mucosal antibody responses.[89,153,164,178,179]

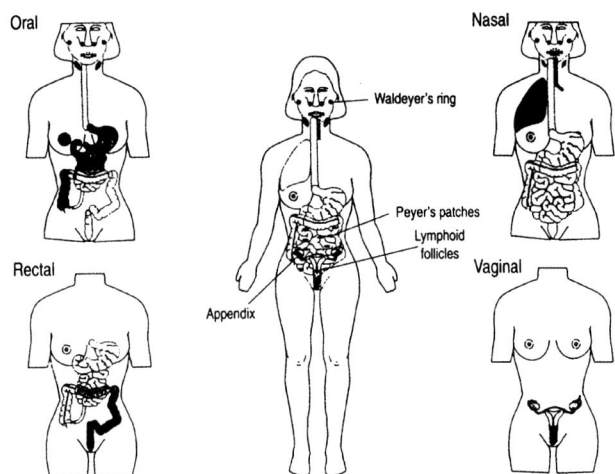

FIGURE 11–7. The common mucosal immune system and regionalized restrictions on cell migration in response to immunization. Specific IgA B lymphocytes disseminate preferentially to certain mucosal tissues, dependent on the site of initial encounter with antigen, where they mature into plasma cells and produce sIgA. While mucosal lymphocytes appear to exhibit largely regional preferences following immunization with nonreplicating immunogens, further migration pathways have come to light, particularly with the use of different vaccination regimens, e.g., specific IgA responses in the reproductive tract following intranasal delivery of antigen conjugated to cholera toxin or encoded in consecutively-delivered DNA and poxvirus vectors, as described in the text. (With permission from Czerkinsky C, Holmgren J. The mucosal immune system and prospects for anti-infectious and anti-inflammatory vaccines. Immunologist 1995;3:97–103. Hogrefe & Huber Publishers, Seattle, Toronto, Bern, Gottingen)

The existence of a common mucosal immune system is another factor with important implications for the development of mucosal vaccine strategies. Early studies seemed to indicate that the antigenic experience of a particular inductive site in MALT may be widely transferred to other mucosae through the migration and localization of primed immunocytes.[168] More recent work, however, has indicated that a degree of subcompartmentalization may exist within this system.[5] As shown in Figure 11–7, it appears, at least in the case of nonreplicating antigens, that oral vaccination induces strong IgA antibody responses in the small intestine, the ascending colon, and in certain distant exocrine glands, including the mammary and salivary glands.[5] However, relatively poor IgA responses appear to be induced in the distal large intestine, tonsillar tissues, or female genito-urinary tract. Similarly, immunization of MALT in the upper respiratory tract elicited antibodies in the airways, saliva, and nasal secretions, but no obvious responses were found in the gut.[184] Rectal and cervicovaginal antibody responses were clearly induced by local immunization of these tissues or their draining lymph nodes,[5,185] although little if any responses were found elsewhere. However, a promising recent development apparently exploits a novel pathway of cellular migration within the common mucosal immune system. This has come from the demonstration that antigens conjugated to the β-subunit of cholera toxin are able to induce specific IgA antibody

TABLE 11–2
Mechanisms Underlying the Induction of Oral Tolerance

Antigen Dose	Mechanism of Oral Tolerance

Multiple low dose, e.g., 5 × 1 mg (mouse)	1. Suppression
	    Transferable with CD4 T lymphocytes (mouse), CD8 T lymphocytes (rat)
	    Mediated by suppressive cytokines, e.g., TGF-β, IL-4, IL-10

Large bolus, e.g., 1 × 20 mg (mouse)	2. Anergy
	    Decreased IL-2 production upon re-exposure to antigen
	    Reversible by exogenous IL-2

5 × 5-500 mg (mouse)	3. Deletion Apoptosis

responses both locally and in the reproductive tract following their intranasal administration.[186,187] We have recently developed a mucosal prime-boost strategy, involving the delivery of DNA vaccines and poxvirus vectors, which also induces strong and persistent IgA antibody responses, not only in the respiratory tract, but also at distant mucosae, including the gut and reproductive tract (Ramsay, unpublished data). At a mucosal level, the capacity of a vaccine strategy such as this to produce effective immune responses in the reproductive and upper respiratory tracts and in the gut following intranasal delivery is highly attractive. It may be of particular relevance for immunization against sexually-transmitted diseases, and in underdeveloped countries, where the intestinal barrier caused by large loads of commensal and pathogenic microorganisms carried by many individuals, particularly children, appears to have diminished the immunogenicity of several common oral vaccines. Clearly, these findings signal a need for more research into the extent of cellular migration within the common mucosal immune system in order to best exploit its potential for site-specific vaccination.

Oral Tolerance

In contrast to vaccine-induced mucosal responsiveness, oral tolerance is defined as a state of immunologic unresponsiveness to an antigen induced by the feeding of that antigen.[188] Recent studies have shown that such a state of tolerance can also be induced by application of antigen to other mucosal surfaces, such as the nasal and respiratory tract mucosa.[189,190] However, most of what we currently know of mucosal tolerance comes from studies of fed antigen.[191] The need for this form of immune response is apparent when one considers that, on a daily basis, huge amounts of foreign antigenic material, in the form of food, transverse the gut, and are potentially exposed to GALT. This antigen load greatly exceeds the 3 to 4 g of IgA that is secreted daily into the adult intestine,[19] and if an active immune response was mounted against these antigens, it would have the potential to impair the nutrient absorptive function of the intestinal mucosa, as occurs in conditions such as celiac disease. As elsewhere in the immune system, the context or form in which an antigen is encountered is a major determinant of the resulting immune response. Thus, in the intestine, foreign antigens such as infectious microorganisms are recognized and elicit strong immune responses aimed at their elimination. Food antigens are also recognized, but elicit a response aimed at minimizing potential immune damage to the mucosal surface. Recent data show that this downregulation of responsiveness is an active process, and not simply the absence of an immune response.

Oral tolerance is specific for the antigen that is fed, and as a result both cell-mediated and humoral immunity are suppressed.[192] There appears to be a gradient of sensitivity to oral tolerance induction, with delayed type hypersensitivity responses mediated by Th1 cells being the most susceptible to tolerization.[193,194] This makes sense in terms of protecting the mucosal epithelium, in that this form of immune response has the greatest potential to damage epithelial tissues. This is exemplified in the TNBS (trinitrobenzene sulfonic acid) colitis model, where prior feeding of the hapten trinitrophenol (TNP) reduces the severity of colitis following TNBS enema.[195] The types of antigens known to induce oral tolerance include several eukaryotic proteins, contact allergens such as TNP, heterologous erythrocytes, and some killed viruses.[196] Interestingly, all of these are T-dependent antigens. The T-independent antigens do not appear to induce oral tolerance,[197] further indicating that this tolerance induction represents an immune response involving T-lymphocyte activation. Oral tolerance does not result in complete suppression of immunity.[198] Studies in mice indicate that humoral responses are reduced by approximately tenfold in animals fed antigen prior to systemic immunization compared to animals that were not fed. This state of induced nonresponsiveness is not permanent, lasting several months in mice before waning.

Several different mechanisms are thought to underlie the induction of oral tolerance, as shown in Table 11–2. The major determinant of which mechanism is induced appears to be antigen dose.[199] Oral tolerance has been shown to be mediated by clonal deletion, by clonal anergy, and by the induction of regulatory T lymphocytes secreting inhibitory cytokines. Each of these mechanisms targets helper T lymphocytes (Th1 more than Th2): thus, the resultant reduction in levels of humoral immunity is due to a reduction in T lymphocyte help rather than direct tolerization of B lymphocytes.

Studies in mice have shown that feeding of multiple low doses of antigen (5 × 1 mg), may induce regulatory T lymphocytes secreting the cytokines TGF-β, IL-10, and IL-4 in various combinations.[191] These cells appear to be CD4+ in the mouse, but may be CD8+ in the rat, and have been isolated from Peyer's patches and mesenteric lymph nodes, with the former being the more likely tissue of origin. The mechanisms by which these cells are induced are unknown; however, the critical regulatory events must occur in the Peyer's patch microenvironment, where the choice of active immunity or oral tolerance is made. Indeed, antigen targeting to Peyer's patches is essential for the induction of both types of response. It may be that different forms of antigen target distinct populations of antigen-presenting cells, leading to immunity or tolerance. Indeed, while soluble ovalbumin induces tolerance, ovalbumin given in liposomes induces both humoral and cellular immune responses (Beagley, unpublished data).

Feeding of a single large dose of antigen (20 mg in mice) induces oral tolerance via the induction of anergy in responsive cells. This mechanism of oral tolerance may involve uptake of antigen via epithelial cells rather than by Peyer's patches. Gut epithelial cells express both class I and class II MHC antigens, but may lack expression of the costimulatory B7 molecules (CD80-CD86).[200] Stimulation of T lymphocytes via the T cell receptor:MHC-antigen interaction (signal 1), in the absence of a B7:CD28 interaction (signal 2), is known to induce anergy in naive T lymphocytes. Antigen presentation by intestinal epithelial cells in vitro has also been shown to preferentially induce suppressor cells.[201,202] Nevertheless, there is, as yet, no direct in vivo evidence to implicate epithelial cells in the induction of oral tolerance.

Although oral tolerance is clearly controlled at the level of the T lymphocyte, a greater understanding of mechanisms underlying the induction of either tolerance or immunity is obviously essential for the development of effective oral vaccines aimed at inducing protective IgA responses. It should also be noted that oral feeding of antigen in animal models of autoimmunity has been shown to delay the onset, and/or reduce the severity, of disease (reviewed[203]). Once again, a greater understanding of the mechanisms underlying the induction of oral tolerance will be required before this treatment can be used successfully in humans.

DISEASES OF THE GASTROINTESTINAL TRACT INVOLVING ALTERED B LYMPHOCYTE FUNCTION

The greatest numbers of immune cells are found at mucosal surfaces, particularly the GI tract, as these sites represent the interface between external and internal environments. Cells of the GALT are continuously in contact with massive antigenic stimuli: mainly food-derived antigens in the small bowel and bacterial products in the large bowel. As such, many local immune cells have phenotypic characteristics of activated immunocytes. The sum total of the mucosal immune response must be an appropriate balance between active immunity, essential for protection, and low or no responses to certain antigens, a state essential for the maintenance of nutrient uptake. Not surprisingly, changes in immune function in the gut are often associated with various disease states that affect this organ. Some of these conditions are characterized by altered humoral immunity, and will be described briefly in this section.

Immunoglobulin A Deficiency

Immunoglobulin A deficiency (IgAD) occurs in approximately one in 600 individuals of European descent and sufferers are defined as having a serum IgA concentration of less than 50 µg per ml.[204,205] Affected individuals are usually also deficient in secretory IgA antibodies. In addition, 20 to 30% of IgAD patients also have defects in IgG subclasses, particularly IgG2 and IgG4.[206,207] Problems associated with IgAD range from asymptomatic individuals, at one end of the spectrum, through to patients with frequent sinopulmonary infections, GI disorders, allergies, and autoimmune diseases. Gastrointestinal infections in IgAD individuals include acute diarrheal illnesses, caused by both bacteria and viruses, and chronic diarrhea, caused by *Giardia lamblia*.[204,208] Other infections associated with IgAD include recurrent upper and lower respiratory tract infections, ear infections, sinusitis, bronchitis, and chronic infections of skin and mucosal surfaces caused by *Candida albicans*. The most severe infections usually occur in individuals who also have associated IgG deficiency.

Immunoglobulin A-deficient individuals have a higher incidence of autoimmune conditions, such as systemic lupus erythematosus, rheumatoid arthritis, Sjögren's syndrome, celiac disease, and insulin-dependent diabetes mellitus.[209] Not surprisingly, they produce antibodies against a variety of tissue autoantigens. These patients also make increased titers of antibodies against a variety of food antigens, and have increased incidences of allergic conditions, such as asthma, eczema, and allergic rhinitis.[210,211] Interestingly, many IgAD individuals make anti-IgA antibodies of the IgE or IgG isotypes,[212] which may predispose them to anaphylactic shock should they receive blood for some unrelated condition.

Immunoglobulin A-deficiency is due to the failure of IgM$^+$ cells to differentiate into IgA-secreting plasma cells; however, the precise underlying mechanisms are unknown. Most IgAD individuals have normal levels of IgM$^+$-IgD$^+$ B lymphocytes and normal levels of other isotypes in their serum. The reduced numbers of circulating IgA$^+$ cells in these patients suggest a defect at the level of isotype switching.[213] This hypothesis is supported by the reduced serum levels of TGF-β also found in some, but not all, IgAD individuals,[214] and remains attractive due to the demonstrated role of TGF-β in isotype-switching to IgA.[106,215] Alternatively, there may be defects in post-switch terminal differentiation to IgA-secreting plasma cells. The pathogenesis of IgAD remains unclear, despite increased recent research efforts in normal and genetically manipulated animals.

Celiac Disease

Celiac disease (gluten-sensitive enteropathy, celiac sprue) is characterized by damage to the small intestinal mucosa and malabsorption caused by hypersensitivity to gluten (gliadin) found in wheat, barley, and rye. The disease is most common in Caucasians, and the lesion is restricted to the small intestine and consists of villous atrophy marked by blunted and shortened, or even totally absent, villi.[216] The epithelium consists of disorganized, morphologically abnormal epithelial cells and elongated crypts in which immature epithelial cells are generated at a greatly increased rate. Symptoms commonly appear during the first 3 years of life after the introduction of cereals into the diet. A second peak incidence occurs during the third decade. Active celiac disease is characterized by a B and T lymphocyte infiltrate. The B lymphocytes in the lesion secrete IgA, IgG, and IgM, but the increase in IgG and IgM-secreting cells is disproportionately greater than the increase in IgA-secreting cells.[216–218] Up to 10% of these cells secrete antibodies specific for gliadin and mostly of the IgG isotype. In addition, complement deposits are often found in the subepithelial layer, suggesting that IgG-activated, complement-mediated epithelial damage may be an important cause of disease. Antibodies to gliadin are also present in sera from most patients with active disease. The IgA levels tend to fall when these individuals are placed on a gluten-free diet; however, serum IgG antigliadin antibodies may persist at low levels for up to 20 years. Interestingly, selective IgA deficiency is 10 times as frequent in celiac disease patients as in normal individuals. Treatment for most patients currently consists of a lifelong elimination from the diet of all gluten-containing foods.

Inflammatory Bowel Disease

Inflammatory bowel disease (IBD) consists of two separate conditions: ulcerative colitis (UC) and Crohn's disease (CD), which are both chronic inflammatory disorders of the intestine of unknown origin. Both conditions are characterized by intense active infiltration of macrophages and lymphocytes, including plasma cells, characteristic of chronic inflammation,[219] and also exhibit acute inflammatory components, such as continued influx of neutrophils from the circulation into the inflamed mucosa and thence into the intestinal lumen. Ulcerative colitis is characterized by diffuse mucosal ulcers restricted mainly to the mucosa, while CD often results in formulation of transmural granulomas. While acute intestinal inflammation, which is self-limiting, is a normal component of host defence, an unresolved question in IBD concerns the chronicity of this process and why it fails to resolve. A number of abnormalities in B lymphocyte numbers and function are known to occur in IBD. Numbers of spontaneous IgG-secreting B lymphocytes are increased more than those secreting other isotypes in IBD lesions.[220,221] While IgA is the predominant isotype in normal intestinal mucosae, IgA-secreting B lymphocyte numbers are decreased in IBD lesions. Immunoglobulin A antibodies normally prevent entry of lumenal antigen in the mucosa by a process of aggregation and immune exclusion, rather than by induction of an inflammatory response, which as a result of complement activation might cause localized tissue damage. Increased spontaneous secretion of IgM, IgG, and IgA by peripheral blood B lymphocytes has also been demonstrated in new-onset IBD patients.[221] Not only is IgG (and IgM) secretion greatly increased in IBD lesions, but changes in IgA subclass secretion have also been noted.[222–224] Immunoglobulin A2 is the predominant IgA subclass produced in normal intestinal mucosa; however, in IBD patients, secretion of IgA1 is increased and makes up from 70 to 75% of total IgA antibody levels. Decreased J-chain expression by both IgA1- and IgA2-secreting B lymphocytes has also been demonstrated in colonic mucosa from both UC and CD patients.[225] In addition, the presence of a variety of antibodies against self tissues and/or intestinal bacteria have been reported in IBD

(reviewed[219]), while antibodies against colon tissues were found in both UC and CD and were shown to crossreact with *Escherichia coli* 0-14 antigens.[226,227] This finding has led to the hypothesis that antibodies induced by *E. coli* may contribute to epithelial cell damage through crossreactivity. However, many of these antibodies could not activate complement, nor could they kill epithelial cells in vitro,[228] raising questions as to whether they played a causal role in IBD. It has also been shown that anticolon antibodies are not specific for IBD, suggesting that their production may be secondary to ongoing epithelial damage. Lymphocytotoxic antibodies[229] have also been described in those with IBD, while antineutrophil cytoplasmic antibodies appear to be present in the majority of UC patients.

REFERENCES

1. Besredka A. De la vaccination contre les etats typhoides par voie buccale. Ann Inst Pasteur 1919;33:882–903.
2. Chodirker WB, Tomasi TB Jr. Gamma globulins: quantitative relationships in human serum and nonvascular fluids. Science 1963;142:1080–1.
3. Halpern MS, Koshland ME. Novel subunit in secretory IgA. Nature 1970;223:1276–9.
4. Tomasi TB Jr, Tan EM, Solomon A, Prendergast RA. Characteristics of an immune system common to certain external secretions. J Exp Med 1965;121:101–24.
5. Czerkinsky C, Holmgren J. The mucosal immune system and prospects for anti-infectious and anti-inflammatory vaccines. Immunologist 1995;3:97–103.
6. Rudzik R, Clancy RL, Perey DY, et al. Repopulation with IgA-containing cells of bronchial and intestinal lamina propria after transfer of homologous Peyer's patch and bronchial lymphocytes. J Immunol 1975;114:1599–604.
7. Mestecky J. The common mucosal immune system and current strategies for induction of immune responses in external secretions. J Clin Immunol 1987;7:265–76.
8. Brandtzaeg P. Overview of the mucosal immune system. Curr Top Microbiol Immunol 1989;146:13–25.
9. Crewther P, Warner NL. Serum immunoglobulins and antibodies in congenitally athymic (nude) mice. Aust J Exp Biol Med Sci 1972;50:625–35.
10. Clough JD, Mims LH, Strober W. Deficient IgA antibody responses to arsanilic acid bovine serum albumin (BSA) in neonatally thymectomized rabbits. J Immunol 1971;106:1624–9.
11. McGhee JR, Mestecky J, Elson CO, Kiyono H. Regulation of IgA synthesis and immune response by T cells and interleukins. J Clin Immunol 1989;9:175–99.
12. Fujihashi K, Taguchi T, Aicher WK, et al. Immunoregulatory functions for murine intraepithelial lymphocytes: gamma/delta T cell receptor-positive (TCR+) T cells abrogate oral tolerance, while alpha/beta TCR+ T cells provide B cell help. J Exp Med 1992;175:695–707.
13. Bockman DE, Cooper MD. Pinocytosis by epithelium associated with lymphoid follicles in the bursa of Fabricius, appendix, and Peyer's patches. An electron microscopic study. Am J Anat 1973;136:455–77.
14. Owen RL, Jones AL. Epithelial cell specialization within human Peyer's patches: an ultrastructural study of intestinal lymphoid follicles. Gastroenterology 1974;66:189–203.
15. Neutra MR, Phillips TL, Mayer EL, Fishkind DJ. Transport of membrane-bound macromolecules by M cells in follicle-associated epithelium of rabbit Peyer's patch. Cell Tissue Res 1987;247:537–46.

16. Amerongen HM, Weltzin R, Farnet CM, et al. Transepithelial transport of HIV-1 by intestinal M cells: a mechanism for transmission of AIDS. J AIDS 1991;4:760–5.
17. Lebman DA, Griffin PM, Cebra JJ. Relationship between expression of IgA by Peyer's patch cells and functional IgA memory cells. J Exp Med 1987;166:1405–18.
18. Craig SW, Cebra JJ. Peyer's patches: an enriched source of precursors for IgA-producing immunocytes in the rabbit. J Exp Med 1971;134:188–200.
19. Mestecky J, MeGhee JR. Molecular and cellular interactions involved in IgA biosynthesis and immune response. Adv Immunol 1987;40:153–245.
20. Mattioli CA, Tomasi TB Jr. The life span of IgA plasma cells from the mouse intestine. J Exp Med 1973;138:452–60.
21. Tomasi TB. An overview of the mucosal system. In: Ogra PL, Lamm ME, McGhee JR, et al., editors. Handbook of mucosal immunology. San Diego: Academic Press; 1994. p. 3–8.
22. Plaut AG. The IgA1 proteases of pathogenic bacteria. Annu Rev Microbiol 1983;37:603–22.
23. Kilian M, Reinholdt J, Mortensen SB, Sorenson CH. Perturbation of mucosal immune defence mechanisms by bacterial IgA proteases. Bull Eur Physiopathol Respir 1983;19:99–104.
24. Brandtzaeg P. Basic mechanisms of mucosal immunity—a major adaptive defense system. Immunologist 1995;3:89–96.
25. Pumphrey RSH. Computer models of the human immunoglobulins. Immunol Today 1986;7:206–11.
26. Hauptman SP, Tomasi TB Jr. Mechanism of immunoglobulin A polymerization. J Biol Chem 1975;250:3891–6.
27. Mazanec MB, Nedrud JG, Kaetzel CS, Lamn ME. A three-tiered view of the role of IgA in mucosal defense. Immunol Today 1993;14:430–5.
28. Dimmock NJ, Taylor JP, Carver AS. Interaction of neutralised influenzae virus with avian and mammalian cells. In: Compas RW, Bishop DWL, editors. Segmented negative strand viruses. New York: Raven Press; 1993. p. 355–65.
29. Wold AE, Mestecky J, Tomana M. Secretory immunoglobulin A carries oligosaccharide receptors for *Escherichia coli* type 1 fimbrial lectin. Infect Immun 1990;58:3073–7.
30. Kilian M, Mestecky J, Russell MW. Defense mechanisms involving Fc-dependent functions of immunoglobulin A and their subversion by immunoglobulin A proteases. Microbiol Rev 1988;52:296–303.
31. Roitt IM, Greaves MF, Torrigiani G, Brostoff J, Playfair JH. The cellular basis of immunological responses. A synthesis of some current views. Lancet 1969;2:367–71.
32. Glick B, Chang TS, Jaap RG. The bursa of Fabricius and antibody production. Poult Sci 1956;35:224–6.
33. Cooper MD, Raymond DA, Peterson RD, et al. The functions of the thymus system and the bursa system in the chicken. J Exp Med 1966;123:75–102.
34. Owen JJ, Cooper MD, Raff MC. In vitro generation of B lymphocytes in mouse foetal liver, a mammalian 'bursa equivalent.' Nature 1974;249:361–3.
35. Gathings WE, Lawton AR, Cooper MD. Immunofluorescent studies of the development of pre-B cells, B lymphocytes and immunoglobulin isotype diversity in humans. Eur J Immunol 1977;7:804–10.
36. Abramson S, Miller RG, Phillips RA. The identification in adult bone marrow of pluripotent and restricted stem cells of the myeloid and lymphoid systems. J Exp Med 1977;145:1567–79.
37. Lemischka IR, Raulet DH, Mulligan RC. Developmental potential and dynamic behavior of hematopoietic stem cells. Cell 1986;45:917–27.
38. Kincade PW, Phillips RA. B lymphocyte development. Fed Proc 1985;44:2874–81.
39. von Freeden-Jeffry U, Vieira P, Lucian LA, et al. Lymphopenia in interleukin (IL)-7 gene-deleted mice identifies IL-7 as a nonredundant cytokine. J Exp Med 1995;181:1519–26.
40. Whitlock CA, Robertson D, Witte ON. Murine B cell lymphopoiesis in long term culture. J Immunol Methods 1984;67:353–69.
41. Kincade PW, Lee G, Pietrangeli CE, et al. Cells and molecules that regulate B lymphopoiesis in bone marrow. Annu Rev Immunol 1989;7:111–43.
42. Kincade PW, Witte PL, Landreth KS. Stromal cell and factor-dependent B lymphopoiesis in culture. Curr Top Microbiol Immunol 1987;135:1–21.
43. Cumano A, Kee BL, Ramsden DA, et al. Development of B lymphocytes from lymphoid committed and uncommitted progenitors. Immunol Rev 1994;137:5–33.
44. Kincade PW, Lee G, Paige CJ, Scheid MP. Cellular interactions affecting the maturation of murine B lymphocyte precursors in vitro. J Immunol 1981;127:255–60.
45. Collins LS, Dorshkind K. A stromal cell line from myeloid long-term bone marrow cultures can support myelopoiesis and B lymphopoiesis. J Immunol 1987;138:1082–7.
46. Whitlock CA, Witte ON. Long-term culture of murine bone marrow precursors of B lymphocytes. Methods Enzymol 1987;150:275–86.
47. Pietrangeli CE, Hayashi S, Kincade PW. Stromal cell lines which support lymphocyte growth: characterization, sensitivity to radiation and responsiveness to growth factors. Eur J Immunol 1988;18:863–72.
48. Gimble JM. The function of adipocytes in the bone marrow stroma. New Biologist 1990;2:304–12.
49. Rolink A, Melchers F. Molecular and cellular origins of B lymphocyte diversity. Cell 1991;66:1081–94.
50. Ryan DH, Nuccie BL, Abboud CN, Winslow JM. Vascular cell adhesion molecule-1 and the integrin VLA-4 mediate adhesion of human B cell precursors to cultured bone marrow adherent cells. J Clin Invest 1991;88:995–1004.
51. Miyake K, Medina KL, Hayashi S, et al. Monoclonal antibodies to Pgp-1/CD44 block lympho-hemopoiesis in long-term bone marrow cultures. J Exp Med 1990;171:477–88.
52. Lobb RR, Harper JW, Fett JW. Purification of heparin-binding growth factors. Anal Biochem 1986;154:1–14.
53. Hozumi N, Tonegawa S. Evidence for somatic rearrangement of immunoglobulin genes coding for variable and constant regions. Proc Natl Acad Sci U S A 1976;73:3628–32.
54. Dryer WJ, Bennett JC. The molecular basis of antibody formation. Proc Natl Acad Sci U S A 1965;54:864.
55. Staudt LM, Lenardo MJ. Immunoglobulin gene transcription. Annu Rev Immunol 1991;9:373–98.
56. Schatz DG, Oettinger MA, Schlissel MS. V(D)J recombination: molecular biology and regulation. Annu Rev Immunol 1992;10:359–83.
57. Lewis SM. The mechanism of V(D)J joining: lessons from molecular, immunological, and comparative analyses. Adv Immunol 1994;56:27–150.
58. Alt FW, Oltz EM, Young F, et al. VDJ recombination. Immunol Today 1992;13:306–14.
59. Chen J, Alt FW. Gene rearrangement and B-cell development. Curr Opin Immunol 1993;5:194–200.
60. Herzenberg LA, Kantor AB. B-cell lineages exist in the mouse. Immunol Today 1993;14:79–83.
61. Wang CY, Good RA, Ammirati P, et al. Identification of a p69,71 complex expressed on human T cells sharing determinants with B-type chronic lymphatic leukemic cells. J Exp Med 1980;151:1539–44.
62. Kipps TJ. The CD5 B cell. Adv Immunol 1989;47:117–85.

63. Miyama-Inaba M, Kuma S, Inaba K, et al. Unusual phenotype of B cells in the thymus of normal mice. J Exp Med 1988;168:811–6.
64. Solvason N, Lehuen A, Kearney JF. An embryonic source of Ly1 but not conventional B cells. Int Immunol 1991;3:543–50.
65. Solvason N, Kearney JF. The human fetal omentum: a site of B cell generation. J Exp Med 1992;175:397–404.
66. Kantor AB, Stall AM, Adams S, et al. Adoptive transfer of murine B-cell lineages. Ann N Y Acad Sci 1992;651:168–9.
67. Huang CA, Henry C, Iacomini J, et al. Adult bone marrow contains precursors for CD5+ B cells. Eur J Immunol 1996;26:2537–40.
68. Hayakawa K, Hardy RR, Stall AM, et al. Immunoglobulin-bearing B cells reconstitute and maintain the murine Ly-1 B cell lineage. Eur J Immunol 1986;16:1313–6.
69. Ishida H, Hastings R, Kearney J, Howard M. Continuous anti-interleukin 10 antibody administration depletes mice of Ly-1 B cells but not conventional B cells. J Exp Med 1992;175:1213–20.
70. Kroese FG, Butcher EC, Stall AM, et al. Many of the IgA producing plasma cells in murine gut are derived from self-replenishing precursors in the peritoneal cavity. Int Immunol 1989;1:75–84.
71. Sidman CL, Shultz LD, Hardy RR, et al. Production of immunoglobulin isotypes by Ly-1+ B cells in viable motheaten and normal mice. Science 1986;232:1423–5.
72. Beagley KW, Murray AM, McGhee JR, Eldridge JH. Peritoneal cavity CD5 (B1a) B cells: cytokine induced IgA secretion and homing to intestinal lamina propria in SCID mice. Immunol Cell Biol 1995;73:425–32.
73. Bao S, Beagley KW, Murray AM, et al. Intestinal IgA plasma cells of the B1 lineage are IL-5 dependent. Immunology 1998;94:181–8.
74. Andrade L, Huetz F, Poncet P, et al. Biased VH gene expression in murine CD5 B cells results from age-dependent cellular selection. Eur J Immunol 1991;21:2017–23.
75. Mageed RA, MacKenzie LE, Stevenson FK, et al. Selective expression of a VHIV subfamily of immunoglobulin genes in human CD5+ B lymphocytes from cord blood. J Exp Med 1991;174:109–13.
76. Gu H, Forster I, Rajewsky K. Sequence homologies, N sequence insertion and JH gene utilization in VHDJH joining: implications for the joining mechanism and the ontogenetic timing of Ly1 B cell and B-CLL progenitor generation. EMBO J 1990;9:2133–40.
77. Gu H, Forster I, Rajewsky K. Study of murine B-cell development through analysis of immunoglobulin variable region genes. Ann N Y Acad Sci 1992;651:304–10.
78. Lalor PA, Morahan G. The peritoneal Ly-1 (CD5) B cell repertoire is unique among murine B cell repertoires. Eur J Immunol 1990;20:485–92.
79. Kantor AB, Herzenberg LA. Origin of murine B cell lineages. Annu Rev Immunol 1993;11:501–38.
80. Taki S, Schmitt M, Tarlinton D, et al. T cell-dependent antibody production by Ly-1 B cells. Ann N Y Acad Sci 1992;651:328–35.
81. Herzenberg LA, Kantor AB, Herzenberg LA. Layered evolution in the immune system. A model for the ontogeny and development of multiple lymphocyte lineages. Ann N Y Acad Sci 1992;651:1–9.
82. Haughton G, Arnold LW, Whitmore AC, Clarke SH. B-1 cells are made, not born. Immunol Today 1993;14:84–7.
83. Cong YZ, Rabin E, Wortis HH. Treatment of murine CD5− B cells with anti-Ig, but not LPS, induces surface CD5: two B-cell activation pathways. Int Immunol 1991;3:467–76.
84. Hardy RR, Hayakawa K, Parks DR, Herzenberg LA. Demonstration of B-cell maturation in X-linked immunodeficient mice by simultaneous three-colour immunofluorescence. Nature 1983;306:270–2.
85. Mond JJ, Lees A, Snapper CM. T cell-independent antigens type 2. Annu Rev Immunol 1995;13:655–92.
86. Hayakawa K, Hardy RR, Honda M, et al. Ly-1 B cells: functionally distinct lymphocytes that secrete IgM autoantibodies. Proc Natl Acad Sci U S A 1984;81:2494–8.
87. Goodnow CC, Brink R, Adams E. Breakdown of self-tolerance in anergic B lymphocytes. Nature 1991;352:532–6.
88. Hartley SB, Crosbie J, Brink R, et al. Elimination from peripheral lymphoid tissues of self-reactive B lymphocytes recognizing membrane-bound antigens. Nature 1991;353:765–9.
89. Ramsay AJ. Genetic approaches to the study of cytokine regulation of mucosal immunity. Immunol Cell Biol 1995;73:484–8.
90. Defrance T, Vanbervliet B, Briere F, et al. Interleukin 10 and transforming growth factor beta cooperate to induce anti-CD40-activated naive human B cells to secrete immunoglobulin A. J Exp Med 1992;175:671–82.
91. Mosmann TR, Coffman RL. Two types of mouse helper T cell clones—implications for immune regulation. Immunol Today 1987;8:223–7.
92. Mosmann TR, Schumacher JH, Street NF, et al. Diversity of cytokine synthesis and function of mouse CD4+ T cells. Immunol Rev 1991;123:209–29.
93. Firestein S, Roeder WD, Laxer JA, et al. A new murine CD4+ T cell subset with an unrestricted cytokine profile. J Immunol 1989;143:518–25.
94. Street NE, Schumacher JH, Fong TA, et al. Heterogeneity of mouse helper T cells: evidence from bulk cultures and limit dilution cloning for precursors of TH1 and TH2 cells. J Immunol 1990;144:1629–39.
95. Seder RA, Paul WE. Acquistion of lymphokine-producing phenotype by CD4+ T cells. Annu Rev Immunol 1994;12:635–73.
96. Taguchi T, McGhee JR, Coffman RL, et al. Analysis of Th1 and Th2 cells in murine gut-associated tissues. Frequencies of CD4+ and CD8+ T cells that secrete IFN-gamma and IL-5. J Immunol 1990;145:68–77.
97. Xu-Amano J, Kiyono H, Jackson RJ, et al. Helper T cell subsets for immunoglobulin A responses: oral immunization with tetanus toxoid and cholera toxin as adjuvant selectively induces Th2 cells in mucosa associated tissues. J Exp Med 1993;178:1309–20.
98. Bao S, Goldstone S, Husband AJ. Localization of IFN-gamma and IL-6 mRNA in murine intestine by in situ hybridization. Immunology 1993;80:666–70.
99. Kawanishi H, Saltzman LE, Strober W. Characteristics and regulatory function of murine Con A-induced, cloned T cells obtained from Peyer's patches and spleen: mechanisms regulating isotype-specific immunoglobulin production by Peyer's patch B cells. J Immunol 1982;129:475–83.
100. Kawanishi H, Saltzman L, Strober W. Mechanisms regulating IgA class-specific immunoglobulin production in murine gut-associated lymphoid tissues. II. terminal differentiation of post switch sIgA-bearing Peyer's patch B cells. J Exp Med 1983;158:649–69.
101. Kiyono H, McGhee JR, Monsteller LM, et al. Isotype-specificity of helper T cell clones. Peyer's patch Th cells preferentially collaborate with mature IgA B cells for IgA responses. J Exp Med 1984;159:798–811.
102. Kiyono H, Monsteller-Barnum LM, Pitts AM, et al. Isotype-specific immunoregulation: IgA binding factors produced by Fcα receptor-positive T cell hybridomas regulate IgA responses. J Exp Med 1985;161:731–747.

103. Kiyono H, McGhee JR, Mosteller LM, et al. Murine Peyer's patch T cell clones. Characterization of antigen-specific helper T cells for immunoglobulin A responses. J Exp Med 1982;156:1115–30.
104. Spalding D, Williamson SI, Koopman WJ, McGhee JR. Preferential induction of polyclonal IgA secretion by murine Peyer's patch dendritic cell-T cell mixtures. J Exp Med 1984;160:941–6.
105. Spalding DM, Griffin JA. Different pathways of differentiation of pre-B cell lines are induced by dendritic cells and T cells from different lymphoid tissues. Cell 1986;44:507–15.
106. Stavnezer J. Immunoglobulin class switching. Curr Opin Immunol 1996;8:199–205.
107. Jacob J, Kassir R, Kelsoe G. In situ studies of the primary immune response to (4-hydroxy-3-nitrophenyl)acetyl. I. The architecture and dynamics of the responding cell populations. J Exp Med 1991;173:1165–75.
108. Stavnezer J. Antibody class switching. Adv Immunol 1996;61:79–146.
109. Cooke MP, Health AW, Shokat KM, et al. Immunological signal transduction guides the specificity of B cell-T cell interactions and is blocked in tolerant self-reactive B cells. J Exp Med 1994;179:425–34.
110. Isakson PC, Pure E, Vitetta ES, Krammer PH. T cell-derived B cell differentiation factor(s). Effect on the isotype switch of murine B cells. J Exp Med 1982;155:734–48.
111. Kuhn R, Rajewsky K, Muller W. Generation and analysis of interleukin-4 deficient mice. Science 1991;254:707–10.
112. Kopf M, LeGros G, Bachmann M, et al. Disruption of the murine IL-4 gene blocks Th2 cytokine responses. Nature 1993;362:245–48.
113. Snapper CM, Paul WE. Interferon-gamma and B cell stimulatory factor-1 reciprocally regulate Ig isotype production. Science 1987;236:944–7.
114. Shockett P, Stavnezer J. Effect of cytokines on switching to IgA and α germline transcripts in the B lymphoma I.29μ: transforming growth factor-β activates transcription of the unrearranged Cα gene. J Immunol 1991;147:4374–83.
115. Huang S, Hendriks W, Althage A, et al. Immune response in mice that lack the interferon-γ receptor. Science 1993;259:1742–5.
116. Lin Y, Shockett P, Stavnezer J. Regulation of the antibody class switch to IgA. Immunol Res 1991;10:376–80.
117. Wakatasuki Y, Strober W. Effect of downregulation of germline transcripts on immunoglobulin A isotype differentiation. J Exp Med 1993;178:129–38.
118. Ramsay AJ, Bao S, Beagley KW, et al. Cytokine gene knockout mice—lessons for mucosal B-cell development. In: Kagnoff MF, Kiyono H, editors. Essentials of mucosal immunology. San Diego: Academic Press; 1996. p. 247–61.
119. Vajdy M, Kosco-Vilbois MH, Kopf M, et al. Impaired mucosal immune responses in interleukin 4-targeted mice. J Exp Med 1994;181:41–53.
120. McIntyre TM, Kehry MR, Snapper CM. Novel in vitro model for high-rate IgA class switching. J Immunol 1995;154:156–61.
121. Islam KB, Nilsson L, Sideras P, et al. TGF-beta 1 induces germ-line transcripts of both IgA subclasses in human B lymphocytes. Int Immunol 1991;3:1099–106.
122. van Vlasselaer P, Punnonen J, de Vries JE. Transforming growth factor-beta directs IgA switching in human B cells. J Immunol 1992;148:2062–7.
123. McIntyre TM, Klinman DR, Rothman P, et al. Transforming growth factor beta 1 selectivity stimulates immunoglobulin G2b secretion by lipopolysaccharide-activated murine B cells. J Exp Med 1993;177:1031–7.
124. van den Wall Bake AW, Black KP, Kulhavy R, et al. Transforming growth factor-beta inhibits the production of IgG, IgM, and IgA in human lymphocyte cultures. Cell Immunol 1992;144:417–28.
125. Butcher EC, Rouse RV, Coffman RL, et al. Surface phenotype of Peyer's patch germinal center cells: implications for the role of germinal centers in B cell differentiation. J Immunol 1982;129:2698–707.
126. Coffman RL, Lebman DA, Shrader B. Transforming growth factor beta specifically enhances IgA production by lipopolysaccharide-stimulated murine B lymphocytes. J Exp Med 1989;170:1039–44.
127. Lebman DA, Lee FD, Coffman RL. Mechanism for transforming growth factor beta and IL-2 enhancement of IgA expression in lipopolysaccharide-stimulated B cell cultures. J Immunol 1990;144:952–9.
128. Nair PN, Schroeder HE. Duct-associated lymphoid tissue (DALT) of minor salivary glands and mucosal immunity. Immunology 1986;57:171–180.
129. Phillips-Quagliata JM, Lamm ME. Lymphocyte homing to mucosal effector sites. In: Ogra PL, Lamm ME, McGhee JR, et al., editors. Handbook of mucosal immunology. San Diego: Academic Press; 1994. p. 225–39.
130. Rudzik O, Perey DYE, Bienenstock J. Differential IgA repopulation after transfer of autologous and allogeneic rabbit Peyer's patch cells. J Immunol 1975;114:40–4.
131. McDermott MR, Bienenstock J. Evidence for a common mucosal immune system. I. Migration of B immunoblasts into intestinal, respiratory and genital tissues. J Immunol 1979;122:1892–98.
132. Guy-Grand D, Griscelli C, Vassalli P. The gut associated lymphoid system: nature and properties of the large dividing cells. Eur J Immunol 1974;4:435–43.
133. Montgomery PC, Ayyildiz A, Lemaitre-Coelho IM, et al. Induction and expression of antibodies in secretions: the ocular immune system. Ann N Y Acad Sci 1983;409:428–40.
134. Roux ME, McWilliams M, Phillips-Quagliata JM, Lamm ME. Origin of IgA-secreting cells in the mammary gland. J Exp Med 1977;146:1311–22.
135. Pierce NF, Cray WC Jr. Determinants of localization and duration of a specific mucosal IgA plasma response in enterically immunized animals. J Immunol 1982;128:1311–15.
136. Husband AJ. Kinetics of extravasation and redistribution of IgA-specific antibody containing cells in the intestine. J Immunol 1982;128:1355–9.
137. Dunkley ML, Husband AJ. The role of non-B cells in localizing an IgA plasma cell response in the intestine. Reg Immunol 1991;3:336–40.
138. Butcher EC, Picker LJ. Lymphocyte homing and homeostasis. Science 1996;272:60–6.
139. Tanaka Y, Adams DH, Shaw S. Proteoglycans on endothelial cells present adhesion-inducing cytokines to leukocytes. Immunol Today 1993;14:111–5.
140. Granowitz EV, Clark BD, Mancilla J, Dinarello CA. Interleukin-1 receptor antagonist competitively inhibits the binding of interleukin-1 to the type II interleukin-1 receptor. J Biol Chem 1991;266:14147–50.
141. Gilat D, Hershkoviz R, Mekori YA, Vlodavsky Lider O. Regulation of adhesion of CD4+ T lymphocytes to intact or heparinase-treated subendothelial extracellular matrix by diffusible or anchored RANTES and MIP-1 beta. J Immunol 1994;153:4899–906.
142. Ford WL, Gowans JL. Traffic of lymphocytes. Semin Hematol 1969;6:67–83.
143. Butcher EC. The regulation of lymphocyte traffic. Curr Top Microbiol Immunol 1986;128:85–122.

144. Picker LJ. Control of lymphocyte homing. Curr Opin Immunol 1994;6:390–406.
145. Cepek KL, Shaw SK, Parker CM, et al. Adhesion between epithelial cells and T lymphocytes mediated by E-cadherin and the αEβ7 integrin. Nature 1994;372:190–3.
146. Bargatze RF, Jutila MA, Butcher EC. Distinct roles of L-selectin and integrins alpha 4 beta 7 and LFA-1 in lymphocyte homing to Peyer's patch-HEV in situ: the multistep model confirmed and refined. Immunity 1995;3:99–108.
147. Berlin C, Bargatze RF, Campbell JJ, et al. Alpha 4 integrins mediate lymphocyte attachment and rolling under physiologic flow. Cell 1995;80:413–22.
148. Coffman RL, Shrader B, Carty J, et al. A mouse T cell product that preferentially enhances IgA production. I. Biologic characterization. J Immunol 1987;139:3685–90.
149. Beagley KW, Eldridge JH, Kiyono H, et al. Recombinant murine IL-5 induces high rate IgA synthesis in cycling IgA-positive Peyer's patch B cells. J Immunol 1988;141:2035–42.
150. Lebman DA, Coffman RL. The effects of IL-4 and IL-5 on the IgA response by murine Peyer's patch B cell subpopulations. J Immunol 1988;141:2050–6.
151. Murray PD, McKenzie DT, Swain SL, Kagnoff MF. Interleukin 5 and interleukin 4 produced by Peyer's patch T cells selectively enhance immunoglobulin A expression. J Immunol 1987;139:2669–74.
152. Kunimoto DY, Nordan RP, Strober W. IL-6 is a potent cofactor of IL-1 in IgM synthesis and of IL-5 in IgA synthesis. J Immunol 1989;143:2230–5.
153. Ramsay AJ, Kohonen CM. Interleukin-5 expressed by a recombinant virus vector enhances specific mucosal IgA responses in vivo. Eur J Immunol 1993;23:3141–5.
154. Beagley KW, Kiyono H, Alley CD, et al. Isolation of Peyer's patch T cell subsets involved in isotype specific immunoregulation. Adv Exp Med Biol 1987;216A:177–83.
155. Kopf M, Brombacher F, Hodgkin PD, et al. IL-5-deficient mice have a developmental defect in CD5+ B-1 cells and lack eosinophilia but have normal antibody and cytotoxic T cell responses. Immunity 1996;4:15–24.
156. Vaux DL, Lalor PA, Cory S, Johnson GR. In vivo expression of interleukin 5 induces an eosinophilia and expanded Ly-1B lineage populations. Int Immunol 1990;2:965–71.
157. Pecquet SS, Ehrat C, Ernst PB. Enhancement of mucosal antibody responses to *Salmonella typhimurium* and the microbial hapten phosphorylcholine in mice with X-linked immunodeficiency by B-cell precursors from the peritoneal cavity. Infect Immun 1992;60:503–9.
158. Okada M, Sakaguchi N, Yoshimura N, et al. B cell growth factors and B cell differentiation factor from human T hybridomas. Two distinct kinds of B cell growth factor and their synergism in B cell proliferation. J Exp Med 1983;157:583–90.
159. Suematsu S, Matsuda T, Aozasa K, et al. IgG1 plasmacytosis in interleukin 6 transgenic mice. Proc Natl Acad Sci U S A 1989;86:7547–51.
160. Beagley KW, Eldridge JH, Lee F, et al. Interleukins and IgA synthesis. Human and murine interleukin 6 induce high rate IgA secretion in IgA-committed B cells. J Exp Med 1989;169:2133–48.
161. Fujihashi K, McGhee JR, Lue C, et al. Human appendix B cells naturally express receptors for and respond to interleukin 6 with selective IgA1 and IgA2 synthesis. J Clin Invest 1991;88:248–52.
162. Mega J, McGhee JR, Kiyono H. Cytokine- and Ig-producing T cells in mucosal effector tissues: analysis of IL-5- and IFN-gamma-producing T cells, T cell receptor expression, and IgA plasma cells from mouse salivary gland-associated tissues. J Immunol 1992;148:2030–9.
163. Kopf M, Baumann H, Freer G, et al. Impaired immune and acute phase responses in IL-6-deficient mice. Nature 1994;368:339–42.
164. Ramsay AJ, Husband AJ, Ramshaw IA, et al. The role of interleukin-6 in mucosal IgA antibody responses in vivo. Science 1994;264:561–3.
165. Beagley KW, Bao S, Ramsay AJ, et al. IgA production by peritoneal cavity B cells is IL-6 independent: implications for intestinal IgA responses. Eur J Immunol 1995;25:2123–6.
166. Romani L, Mencacci A, Cenci E, et al. Impaired neutrophil response and CD4+ T helper cell 1 development in interleukin 6-deficient mice infected with *Candida albicans*. J Exp Med 1996;183:1345–55.
167. Bromander AK, Ekman L, Kopf M, et al. IL-6-deficient mice exhibit normal mucosal IgA responses to local immunizations and *Helicobacter felis* infection. J Immunol 1996;156:4290–7.
168. Mestecky J, Moldoveanu Z, Novak M, Compans RW. Mucosal immunity and strategies for novel microbial vaccines. Acta Paediatr Jpn 1994;36:537–44.
169. Michalek SM, Eldridge JH, Curtiss R, Rosenthal KL. Antigen delivery system: new approaches to mucosal immunization. In: Ogra PL, Lamm ME, McGhee JR, editors. Handbook of mucosal immunology. San Diego: Academic Press; 1994. p. 373–90.
170. Levine MM, Dougan G. Optimism over vaccines administered via mucosal surfaces. Lancet 1998;351:1375–6.
171. Service RF. Research news. Triggering the first line of defence. Science 1994;265:1522–4.
172. Ada GL, Ramsay AJ. Vaccines, vaccination and the immune response. Philadelphia: Lippincott-Raven; 1997.
173. Miller CJ, McGhee JR. Progress towards a vaccine to prevent sexual transmission of HIV (commentary). Nat Med 1996;2:751–2.
174. Renegar KJ, Small PA. Passive transfer of local immunity to influenza virus infection by IgA antibody. J Immunol 1991;146:1972–8.
175. Mazanec MB, Kaetzel CS, Lamm ME, Fletcher D, Nedrud JG. Intracellular neutralization of virus by immunoglobulin A antibodies. Proc Natl Acad Sci U S A 1992;89:6901–5.
176. Mazzoli S, Trabattoni D, Lo Caputo S, et al. HIV-specific mucosal and cellular immunity in HIV-seronegative partners of HIV-seropositive individuals. Nat Med 1997;3:1250–7.
177. Holmgren J, Lycke N, Czerkinsky C. Cholera toxin and cholera B subunit as oral-mucosal adjuvant and antigen vector systems. Vaccine 1993;11:1179–84.
178. Leong K, Ramsay AJ, Boyle D, Ramshaw IA. Selective induction of immune responses by cytokines coexpressed in recombinant fowlpox virus. J Virol 1994;68:8125–30.
179. Ramsay AJ, Leong KH, Ramshaw IA. DNA vaccination against virus infection and enhancement of antiviral immunity following consecutive immunization with DNA and viral vectors. Immunol Cell Biol 1997;75:382–8.
180. Ramsay AJ, Ramshaw IA. Cytokine enhancement of immune responses important for immunocontraception. Reprod Fertil Dev 1997;9:91–7.
181. Fynan EF, Webster RG, Fuller DH, et al. DNA vaccines: protective immunizations by parenteral, mucosal and gene-gun inoculations. Proc Natl Acad Sci U S A 1993;90:11478–82.
182. Okada E, Sasaki S, Ishii N, et al. Intranasal immunisation of a DNA vaccine with IL-12 and granulocyte-macrophage colony-stimulating factor (GM-CSF)–expressing plasmids in liposomes indues strong mucosal and cell-mediated immune responses against HIV-1 antigen. J Immunol 1997;159:3638–47.
183. Darji A, Guzman CA, Gerstel B, et al. Oral somatic transgene vaccination using attenuated *S. typhimurium*. Cell 1997;91:765–75.

184. Quiding-Jarbrink M, Granstrom G, Nordstrom I, et al. Induction of compartmentalized B-cell responses in human tonsils. Infect Immun 1995;63:853–7.
185. Lehner T, Wang Y, Cranage M, et al. Protective mucosal immunity elicited by a targeted iliac lymph node immunization with a subunit SIV envelope and core vaccine in macaques. Nat Med 1996;2:767–75.
186. Hirabayashi Y, Kurata H, Funato H, et al. Comparison of intranasal inoculation of influenza HA vaccine combined with cholera toxin B subunit with oral or parenteral vaccination. Vaccine 1990;8:243–8.
187. Pal S, Fielder TJ, Peterson EM, de la Maza LM. Protection against infertility in a BALB/c mouse salpingitis model by intranasal immunization with the mouse pneumonitis biovar of *Chlamydia trachomatis*. Infect Immun 1994;62:3354–62.
188. Elson CO, Zivny J. Oral tolerance: a commentary. In: Kagnoff MF, Kiyono H, editors. Essentials of mucosal immunology. San Diego: Academic Press; 1996. p. 543–54.
189. Holt PG. Immunoprophylaxis of atopy: light at the end of the tunnel? Immunol Today 1994;15:484–9.
190. McMenamin C, Pimm C, McKersey M, Holt PG. Regulation of IgE responses to inhaled antigen in mice by antigen-specific gamma delta T cells. Science 1994;265:1869–71.
191. Weiner HL, Friedman A, Miller A, et al. Oral tolerance: immunologic mechanisms and treatment of animal and human organ-specific autoimmune diseases by oral administration of autoantigens. Annu Rev Immunol 1994;12:809–37.
192. Miller SD, Hanson DG. Inhibition of specific immune responses by feeding protein antigens. IV. Evidence for tolerance and specific active suppression of cell-mediated immune responses to ovalbumin. J Immunol 1979;123:2344–50.
193. Burstein HJ, Shea CM, Abbas AK. Aqueous antigens induce in vivo tolerance selectively in IL-2- and IFN-gamma-producing (Th1) cells. J Immunol 1992;148:3687–91.
194. Melamed D, Friedman A. In vivo tolerization of Th1 lymphocytes following a single feeding with ovalbumin: anergy in the absence of suppression. Eur J Immunol 1994;24:1974–81.
195. Elson CO, Beagley KW, Sharmanov AT, et al. Hapten-induced model of murine inflammatory bowel disease: mucosa immune responses and protection by tolerance. J Immunol 1996;157:2174–85.
196. Mowat AM. Oral tolerance and regulation of immunity to dietary antigens. In: Ogra PL, Lamm ME, McGhee JR, editors. Handbook of mucosal immunology. San Diego: Academic Press; 1994. p. 185–201.
197. Titus RG, Chiller JM. Orally induced tolerance. Definition at the cellular level. Int Arch Allergy Appl Immunol 1981;65:323–38.
198. Melamed D, Friedman A. Modification of the immune response by oral tolerance: antigen requirements and interaction with immunogenic stimuli. Cell Immunol 1993;146:412–20.
199. Friedman A, Weiner HL. Induction of anergy or active suppression following oral tolerance is determined by antigen dosage. Proc Natl Acad Sci U S A 1994;91:6688–92.
200. Sanderson IR, Ouellette AJ, Carter EA, et al. Differential regulation of B7 mRNA in enterocytes and lymphoid cells. Immunology 1993;79:434–8.
201. Bland PW, Warren LG. Antigen presentation by epithelial cells of the rat small intestine. II. Selective induction of suppressor T cells. Immunology 1986;58:9–14.
202. Mayer L, Eisenhardt D, Shlien R. Selective induction of antigen nonspecific suppressor cells with normal gut epithelium as accessory cells. Monogr Allergy 1988;24:78–80.
203. Weiner HL. Oral tolerance for the treatment of autoimmune diseases. Annu Rev Med 1997;48:341–51.
204. Burrows PD, Cooper MD. IgA deficiency. Adv Immunol 1997;65:245–76.
205. Rosen FS, Cooper MD, Wedgwood RJ. The primary immunodeficiencies. N Engl J Med 1995;333:431–40.
206. Oxelius VA. IgG subclass pattern in primary immunodeficiency disorders. Monogr Allergy 1986;19:156–63.
207. Preud'homme JL, Hanson LA. IgG subclass deficiency. Immunodef Rev 1990;2:129–49.
208. Ammann AJ, Hong R. Selective IgA deficiency: presentation of 30 cases and a review of the literature. Medicine 1971;50:223–36.
209. Schaffer FM, Monteiro RC, Volanakis JE, Cooper MD. IgA deficiency. Immunodef Rev 1991;3:15–44.
210. Buckley RH, Dees SC. Correlation of milk precipitins with IgA deficiency. N Engl J Med 1969;281:465–9.
211. Buckley RH. Clinical and immunologic features of selective IgA deficiency. Birth Defects: Original Article Series 1975; 11:134–42.
212. Sandler SG, Eckrich R, Malamut D, Mallory D. Hemagglutination assays for the diagnosis and prevention of IgA anaphylactic transfusion reactions. Blood 1994;84:2031–5.
213. Conley ME, Cooper MD. Immature IgA B cells in IgA-deficient patients. N Engl J Med 1981;305:495–7.
214. Muller F, Aukrust P, Nilssen DE, Froland SS. Reduced serum level of transforming growth factor-beta in patients with IgA deficiency. Clin Immunol Immunopathol 1995;76:203–8.
215. Lebman DA, Nomura DY, Coffman RL, Lee FD. Molecular characterization of germ-line immunoglobulin A transcripts produced during transforming growth factor type beta-induced isotype switching. Proc Natl Acad Sci U S A 1990;87:3962–6.
216. Kagnoff MF. Celiac disease. A gastrointestinal disease with environmental, genetic, and immunologic components. Gastroenterol Clin North Am 1992;21:405–25.
217. Braegger CP, MacDonald TT. The immunologic basis for celiac disease and related disorders. Semin Gastrointest Dis 1996;7:124–33.
218. Maki M. The humoral immune system in coeliac disease. Baillieres Clin Gastroenterol 1995;9:231–49.
219. Schreiber S, Raedler A, Stenson WF, MacDermott RP. The role of the mucosal immune system in inflammatory bowel disease. Gastroenterol Clin North Am 1992;21:451–502.
220. Scott MG, Nahm MH, Macke K, et al. Spontaneous secretion of IgG subclasses by intestinal mononuclear cells: differences between ulcerative colitis, Crohn's disease, and controls. Clin Exp Immunol 1986;66:209–15.
221. MacDermott RP, Nahm MH. Expression of human immunoglobulin G subclasses in inflammatory bowel disease [editorial]. Gastroenterology 1987;93:1127–9.
222. MacDermott RP, Nash GS, Bertovich MJ, et al. Alterations of IgM, IgG, and IgA synthesis and secretion by peripheral blood and intestinal mononuclear cells from patients with ulcerative colitis and Crohn's disease. Gastroenterology 1981;81:844–52.
223. MacDermott RP, Nash GS, Bertovich MJ, et al. Altered patterns of secretion of monomeric IgA and IgA subclass 1 by intestinal mononuclear cells in inflammatory bowel disease. Gastroenterology 1986;91:379–85.
224. MacDermott RP. Altered secretion patterns of IgA and IgG subclasses by IBD intestinal mononuclear cells. In: Goevell H, Peskar BM, Malchow H, editors. Inflammatory bowel diseases—basic research and clinical implications. Lancaster, England: MTP Press; 1988. p. 105–11.
225. Kett K, Brandtzaeg P, Fausa O. J-chain expression is more prominent in immunoglobulin A2 than in immunoglobulin A1 colonic immunocytes and is decreased in both subclasses associated with inflammatory bowel disease. Gastroenterology 1988;94:1419–25.
226. Broberger O, Perlmann P. Autoantibodies in human ulcerative colitis. J Exp Med 1959;110:657–73.

227. Lagercrantz R, Hammarstrom S, Perlmann P, Gustafsson BE. Immunological studies in ulcerative colitis. 3. Incidence of antibodies to colon-antigen in ulcerative colitis and other gastro-intestinal diseases. Clin Exp Immunol 1966;1:263–76.
228. Broberger O, Perlmann P. In-vitro studies of ulcerative colitis. 1. Reactions of patients' serum with human fetal colonic cells in tissue culture. J Exp Med 1963;117:705–17.
229. Korsmeyer SJ, Williams RC Jr, Wilson ID, Strickland RG. Lymphocytotoxic antibody in inflammatory bowel disease. A family study. N Engl J Med 1975;293:1117–20.

CHAPTER 12

Development of the Enteric Nervous System

Dipa Natarajan, PhD

Vassilis Pachnis, MD, PhD

The enteric nervous system (ENS) of mammals is composed of a large number of interconnected ganglia, called the enteric ganglia, that are arranged as two concentric rings—the outer myenteric and the inner submucosal—throughout the gut wall.[1,2] The main function of the ENS is to control peristalsis of the wall of the gastrointestinal (GI) tract (by regulating the contractility of the smooth muscle) and the secretory activity of its glands. For many years, the enteric ganglia were considered as specialized parasympathetic ganglia,[3] but it is now clear that the ENS is an independent branch of the peripheral nervous system (PNS).[4] However, many features of the ENS set it apart from all other parts of the PNS. Among the unique characteristics of the ENS are the large number of neurons and glial cells, the diversity of neuronal phenotypes, and above all its functional independence from the central nervous system (CNS).[4] The mammalian ENS is the largest subdivision of the PNS, with the number of neurons in the gut of adult animals being comparable to the number of neurons present in the spinal cord.[4,5] In addition to the large number of cells, the ENS is characterized by a high degree of diversity in the phenotypic characteristics of its neuronal population. Individual types of neurons can be distinguished by the expression of unique combinations of neuroactive substances, such as neurotransmitters or neuropeptides. The combinatorial expression of such molecules generates a chemical code that has been used to define specific subpopulations of enteric neurons with unique physiologic properties.[6-10] Functionally, the neurons of the ENS are subdivided into three types: sensory neurons, which receive information regarding the state of the lumen of the gut; and interneurons, which process the sensory information and transmit it to motor neurons, the effector cells of the ENS that innervate the smooth muscle and the secretory glands of the gut wall.[2] In addition to their similar overall organization, brain and ENS neurons share many molecular and physiologic characteristics. Common features have also been identified between the glial cells of the bowel and the brain. For example, the glial cells of the ENS express glial fibrillary acidic protein (GFAP), a characteristic marker of CNS astrocytes.[11] The main feature, however, that distinguishes the ENS from the rest of the PNS is its ability to function independently of input from the brain or spinal cord. Thus, the function of the ENS is controlled mainly by local reflex circuits that integrate information relating to the state of the lumen and the gut wall and control muscle contractility and secretions.[2,4] It is evident from the above that anatomically and functionally the ENS of vertebrates have many similarities with the CNS, which has led to its characterization as the "second brain."[12]

ORIGIN AND FORMATION

Despite the high degree of complexity, the ENS of vertebrates is derived from the neural crest, the source of all other branches of the PNS.[13] The neural crest is a transient structure of vertebrate embryos that forms at the edges of the neural folds as they fuse in the dorsal midline to form the neural tube. Two features of the neural crest cells make them a unique cell type: (1) their highly migratory nature and (2) their ability to generate progeny of widely diverse phenotypes such as neurons and glia, melanocytes, endocrine cells, and most of the connective tissue, bone and cartilage of the head.[13,14] It is because of these properties that the neural crest has been used for many years as a model system for studies on cell migration and cell commitment and differentiation in vertebrate embryos. However, despite intensive investigation of the migratory behavior of neural crest cells, very little is known about the mechanisms that guide these cells to specific locations in the embryo. Also, although it is clear that the cellular phenotypes generated by neural crest cells depend to a large extent on local signals derived from the sites of final destination in the embryo,[14] the specific molecules that control the generation of cellular diversity in this cell population are largely unknown.

Studies on Avian Embryos

Most of the studies on the contribution of neural crest cells to the formation of specific structures in vertebrates have been conducted on avian embryos, which are easily accessible to experimental manipulation.[14] Mainly, two types of experiments have been performed. First, segments of dorsal neural tube have been ablated from early chick embryos and the defects in organogenesis that result from such manipulations have been recorded. The results of these studies have generally been confirmed and further refined by a second type of experiments involving the generation of neural chimeras in which small segments of chick neural crest are replaced, isotopically and isochronically, by the equivalent region from quail embryos. The ability to distinguish the donor cells from their host counterparts using histologic and immunocytochemical techniques has allowed several groups to study the derivatives of specific groups of quail neural crest in the resulting chick-quail chimeras. Using these experimental strategies, it has been demonstrated that the majority of neurons (with the exception of a subpopulation of cranial sensory neurons derived from placodal epithelium) and all glial cells of the PNS in vertebrates are derived from the neural crest.[13]

Yntema and Hammond were the first to suggest that the ENS of vertebrates is derived from the neural crest.[15] As part of their analysis of the origin of autonomic ganglia located in the walls of the thoracic and abdominal viscera, these authors removed systematically portions of the neural crest along the length of the neural tube. Analysis of the operated embryos several days later indicated that the development of the intrinsic ganglia of the GI tract depends on the presence of the cranial neural crest forming at the posterior hindbrain (the vagal neural crest). The pioneering studies of Yntema and Hammond were followed by the elegant experiments of Le Douarin and colleagues, who performed a systematic series of isotopic and isochronic grafts of small fragments of quail neural primordium into chick embryos.[16–18] These experiments confirmed the findings of Yntema and Hammond and demonstrated that the intrinsic nervous system of the chicken bowel arises mainly from two regions of the neural tube: the vagal region, corresponding to somites 1 to 7, and the sacral region, extending posterior to somite 28. No contribution to the ENS has been reported for trunk neural crest emigrating between the vagal and sacral regions of the neural tube.

Using as markers the prominent nucleoli of quail cells and quail-specific antibodies, several investigators have analyzed the pathway and timing of migration of enteric neural crest in chicken embryos.[17–19] The results of these experiments are consistent with similar studies performed on normal chick embryos using HNK-1 antibodies that specifically identify neural crest cells and their derivatives. Thus, presumptive enteric ganglioblasts emigrate from the dorsal aspect of the vagal neural tube and following a ventral migratory pathway enter the mesenchyme of the foregut wall via the posterior branchial arches. At stages Hamilton and Hamburger (HH) 16 to 17 (embryonic day E2; 51 to 56 hours of incubation), large numbers of neural crest cells are present in the cranial mesenchyme on their way to the developing pharyngeal gut. At stage HH20 (E3 to 3.5), the vagal-derived neural crest are present in the caudal branchial arches from where they enter the foregut mesenchyme. Between stages HH25 (E4.5 to 5) and HH30 (E6.5 to 7), vagal neural crest migrating along the long axis of the gut colonize progressively the esophagus, proventriculus, gizzard, and the pre- and postumbilical intestine up to the cecal region. Vagal neural crest cells enter the colorectal region at stage HH31 (E7 to 7.5), and by stage HH35 to 36 (E8.5 to 10.0), they colonize the entire colon. In general, the results of these experiments are in agreement with observations from other groups who have followed the progression of ENS precursors by transplanting defined segments of the gut of chick embryos into the chorioallantoic membrane and examining them for the appearance of mature neurons.[20,21]

Short-segment ablations have shown that neural crest emigrating from different regions of the vagal neural tube can differ in their ability to colonize specific regions of the bowel. Thus, innervation of the hindgut is specifically dependent on neural crest at the level of somites 3 to 5 whereas innervation of the midgut can be accomplished by all segments within the vagal neural crest. These studies have also suggested that in avian embryos a source of ENS cells lies outside the vagal region of the neural tube, since ablation of the entire vagal region resulted in apparently normal gangliogenesis in the foregut.[22,23]

In addition to the vagal region, neural crest emigrating from the sacral neural tube (posterior to somite 28) migrate into the gut and contribute to the formation of the postumbilical ENS.[17,24–26] Use of antibodies specific for quail cells on the appropriate chick-quail chimeras has allowed recently the detailed characterization of the contribution of the sacral neural crest to the avian ENS.[18] Sacral neural crest first migrate ventrally in close association with the dorsal aorta and accumulate within the dorsal wall of the developing rectum (at stage HH24). Initially, these cells migrate in a caudal-to-rostral direction and form the ganglion of Remak along the dorsal aspect of (and outside) the hindgut and midgut up to the opening of the bile and pancreatic ducts. Later on (stage HH31; E7.5), the first sacral neural crest cells enter the hindgut, and over the next 2 to 3 days their number increases significantly, reaching their maximum between days 10 to 12. The vast majority of the progeny of sacral-derived neural crest are found in the colo-rectum, whereas fewer cells are present in the ceca and in the postumbilical intestine. Sacral-derived neural crest cells were not observed in the region proximal to the umbilicus.

Although several studies have shown the contribution of the sacral neural crest to the postumbilical ENS, this view has been challenged by some investigators. Thus, by culturing segments of avian gut on the chick chorioallantoic membrane (CAM) and examining the appearance of mature neurons, Allan and Newgreen have suggested that enteric neuroblasts appear in the gut in a continuous rostrocaudal sequence and concluded that their data did not support contribution of the sacral neural crest to the hindgut.[20] In support of this hypothesis, the differentiation of enteric neurons in the hindgut can be prevented by severing the bowel proximal to this segment at 4 days of incubation.[20] In order to reconcile these apparently contradictory results, a recent study has suggested that correct migration and/or differentiation of sacral neural crest in the hindgut of avian (and mammalian) embryos is likely to require the presence of vagal neural crest.[18]

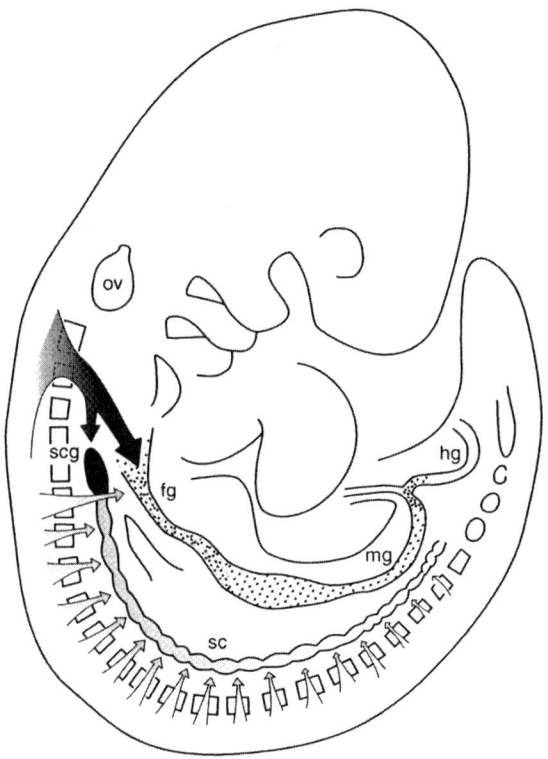

FIGURE 12–1. Schematic presentation of the derivatives of the sympathoenteric (SE) and sympathoadrenal (SA) lineages of the PNS. The c-RET-dependent SE lineage (shown in black) originates in the vagal neural crest of the hindbrain (corresponding to somites 1–5) and migrates ventrally to populate the entire gut and the superior cervical ganglion (shown in black in the anterior end of the sympathetic chain). The c-RET-independent SA lineage (shown in grey) originates in the trunk neural crest (somites 6 and 7) and populates the foregut as well as the ganglia of the sympathetic chain posterior to the SCG (in grey). The foregut is therefore populated by both SE and SA derivatives. fg = foregut; hg = hindgut; mg = midgut; ov = otic vesicle (Reproduced with permission from Durbec PL, Larsson-Blomberg LB, Schuchardt A, et al. Common origin and developmental dependence on c-ret of subsets of enteric and sympathetic neuroblasts. Development 1996;122:349.)

Studies on Mammalian Embryos

As is the case for avian embryos, the mammalian ENS is also derived from cranial (vagal) and sacral neural crest.[26,28] However, the direct analysis of the colonization of the mammalian bowel by neural crest cells and their derivatives has been hampered by the relative difficulty to access and experimentally manipulate these embryos. Thus, the first studies on mouse gut colonization by neural crest cells employed an organ culture system in which segments of fetal mouse gut were removed at various stages of embryogenesis and placed in culture under conditions capable of supporting development of enteric ganglia. The appearance of such ganglia at the end of the culture period, as identified by expression of various neuron-specific markers, indicated that at the time of removal this particular segment of gut had been colonized by the neural crest-derived progenitors. In contrast, failure to develop enteric ganglia indicated that a particular segment had not been colonized by neural crest at the time of removal. Using this approach, Gershon and his colleagues showed that the first neural crest cells invade the mesenchyme of the foregut at embryonic day E9.0 and that the terminal part of the colon is colonized at around embryonic day 12.5 to 13.5 of embryogenesis.[29,30] Although these experiments defined the time of colonization of the mouse fetal bowel by neural crest progenitors, they were unable to establish the temporal and spatial pattern of enteric crest migration.

Direct visualization of the migrating vagal neural crest in mice has been achieved by labeling the dorsal aspect of the postotic (vagal) hindbrain with the lipophilic dye DiI and then following the emigrating cells in embryos growing in culture. Using this approach, we have shown that neural crest cells emigrating from the postotic hindbrain of mouse embryos at E8.5 invade the mesenchyme of the foregut and, migrating in a rostrocaudal direction, colonize the entire gut.[28] In addition to the vagal neural crest, a small segment of the anterior trunk neural tube (corresponding to somites 6 to 7) also generates neural crest cells that find their way into the bowel.[28] These cells arise slightly later than the vagal neural crest and appear to be restricted mainly to the foregut of the embryos (esophagus and stomach). Our findings are consistent with studies on avian embryos in which ablation of the entire vagal region results in apparently normal innervation of the foregut and suggest that the anterior trunk neural tube of chicken embryos is also capable of generating neural crest progenitors that contribute to the formation of the foregut ENS. For a diagrammatic presentation of the vagal neural crest subpopulations colonizing the mammalian gut, see Figure 12–1.

Finally, the sacral neural crest of mammalian embryos also contributes to the formation of the ENS. To demonstrate such contribution Serbedzija and colleagues used DiI to trace neural crest emigrating from the dorsal neural tube posterior to somite 24.[26] These cells first colonized the dorsal side of the colorectum and subsequently appeared to extend to a more ventral region of the hindgut circumference.

Enteric Neural Crest Cell Migration

In mammalian embryos, no molecular marker has been identified that, like HNK1 in avian embryos, is unique to neural crest cells. Thus, to study in detail the migration of enteric neural crest cells in the gut of mammalian embryos, several laboratories have used a combination of molecular markers and approaches. A list of such molecular markers that have been used successfully to identify migrating precursors of the mammalian ENS are listed in Table 12–1.

TABLE 12–1 Molecular Markers Most Commonly Used in the Analysis of the Mammalian Enteric Nervous System

Molecular Marker	Study
TH	Baetge et al.[31,32]
c-RET	Pachnis et al.,[33] Tsuzuki et al.,[34] and Young et al.[35]
PHOX-2B	Young et al.[35] and Pattyn et al.[36]
MASH-1	Lo and Anderson[37] and Blaugrund et al.[38]
SOX-10	Southard-Smith et al.[39]
DβH-LacZ	Kapur et al.[40]
HNK-1	Young et al.[35] and Chalazonitis et al.[41]

One of the most complete studies of fetal gut colonization by neural crest emigres has been conducted by Kapur and his colleagues.[40] These investigators used as a reporter the DβH-nLacZ transgene, which is composed of the nuclearly localized β-galactosidase (nLacZ) under the control of the dopamine β-hydroxylase (DβH) promoter and is expressed widely in the PNS, including the progenitors of the ENS subsequent to invasion of the gut mesenchyme. In the fetal bowel, expression of the DβH-LacZ transgene is first detected in scattered cells in the foregut of E9.0 to 9.5 mouse embryos. Over the next few days (E9.5 to 13.5), expression is detected at progressively more caudal levels, indicating a rostrocaudal migration of the positive neural crest cells, until (by E13.5) the entire length of the gut is colonized by β-galactosidase(β-gal)-expressing cells. The timing and pattern of migration of enteric ganglioblasts in the gut of mouse embryos, as described by the expression of the DβH-nLacZ transgene, has been confirmed by the analysis of several endogenous markers expressed by these cells.[28,31–33,35,36] One such marker that has been used extensively over several years is the receptor tyrosine kinase (RTK) RET. RET is encoded by the c-RET proto-oncogene and is expressed widely in all lineages of the PNS of vertebrate embryos, including the ENS.[28,33,34,42–46] RET-expressing (RET+) cells first appear in the proximal foregut of mouse embryos at E9.0 to 9.5. These cells migrate isochronically with the DβH-nLacZ-expressing cells, and are found at progressively more caudal parts of the gut until they colonize the entire bowel by E12.5 to 13.5. Similar results have also been obtained by Young and colleagues, who used a combination of molecular markers (RET, PHOX-2B, p75) expressed in enteric neural crest during embryogenesis.[35]

Unlike several molecular markers expressed in enteric neural crest subsequent to invasion of the gut wall, expression of c-RET is induced in pre-enteric neural crest.[28] This allows the study of aspects of vagal neural crest cell migration prior to their entry into the foregut mesenchyme. Thus, in E9.0 mouse embryos prospective enteric crest cells (as identified by the expression of c-RET) accumulate in a region immediately posterior to the branchial arches and in close association with the ventral side of the cervical branches of the dorsal aorta (Figure 12–2). During the subsequent 12 hours of embryogenesis, this population of RET+ cells expands and eventually splits into two subpopulations, a ventrally migrating one that invades the foregut mesenchyme and a more dorsal group of cells that remains in close contact with the dorsal aorta. These two neural crest cell subpopulations eventually migrate into their final destination, the gut and the dorsal side of the dorsal aorta, thus contributing to the formation of the ENS and the superior cervical ganglia (SCG), respectively.[28] These studies have suggested that the precursors of the SCG and the ENS originate from a common pool of c-RET-expressing neuroectodermal cells and share a common progenitor (sympathoenteric progenitor) originating in the vagal neural crest. Additional support for this hypothesis is provided by the dependence of both ENS and SCG (but not the rest of the sympathetic chain) on the normal function of the RET RTK. Highlighting further the distinct lineal origin of the SCG relative to more posterior sympathetic ganglia, recent studies have shown that SCG neurons (sympathoenteric lineage) differ in their requirement for p21ras in the nerve growth factor (NGF)-mediated cell survival pathway when compared to the neurons derived from lumbar sympathetic ganglia (sympathoadrenal lineage).[47]

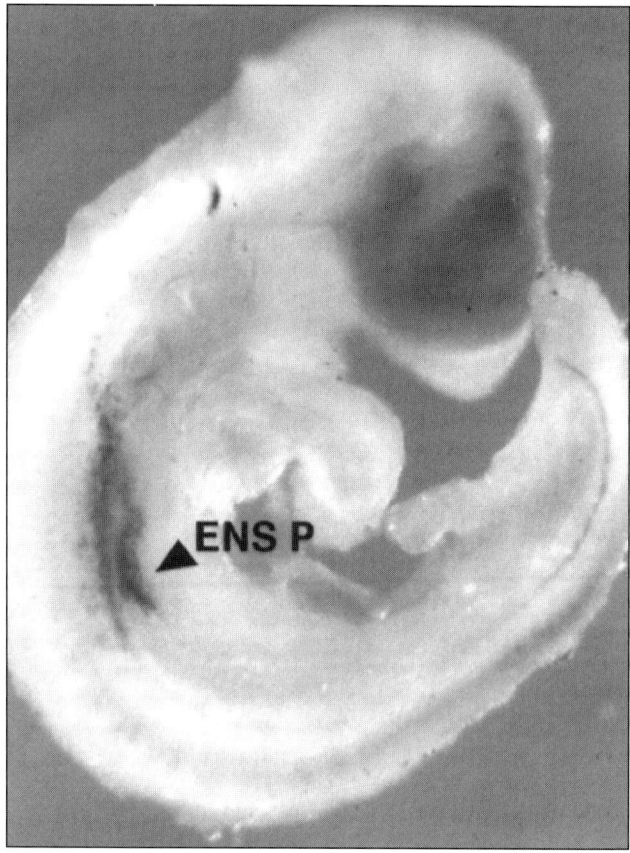

FIGURE 12–2. Expression of c-RET in the progenitors of the mammalian ENS. Whole-mount in situ hybridization of an E9.5 mouse embryo with a riboprobe specific for c-RET mRNA. The ventrally located enteric nervous system progenitors (ENS P) are derivatives from the vagal neural crest, and at this stage they are located at the anterior end of the foregut.

The pattern of migration of the enteric neural crest within the gut wall varies considerably depending on the origin of the cells and the particular segment of the gut they are populating. Throughout the foregut and the intestine, neural crest derivatives migrate as a loose group of individual cells dispersed radially and throughout the mesenchyme, extending from the innermost endodermal lining to the outermost serosa layer covering the gut wall.[35,40,48] However, the migration of enteric crest from the ileum into the proximal colon follows a different pattern when compared to the mode of migration of ganglioblasts through the mesenchyme of the small intestine. Here, stringlike groups of "pioneer" cells enter the colon at its mesenteric border and progress for a significant distance prior to invading the mesenchyme in a circumferential fashion. Eventually neural crest derivatives are arranged in intersecting linear groups of contiguous cells that are mainly located in the outermost part of the cecum and the proximal colon, forming the outer myenteric ganglia.[35,40]

Shortly after the front of migrating cells passes from a certain region of the intestine, the initially dispersed cell population that is left behind starts migrating outwards and they eventually form a tight ring of cells occupying the outermost region of the gut lying underneath the serosa[48] (Figure 12–3). Synchronously to these morphogenetic cell movements, cellular differentiation of the circular muscle layer is also occurring but at present it is not clear whether such differentiation is necessary for the radial migration of the enteric neural crest or is a consequence of it. On completion of the differentiation of the circular smooth muscle layer, the enteric neural crest cells are allocated into small cell groups that, being the precursors to the enteric ganglia, reside in the outer perimeter of the muscle layer. At later stages of embryogenesis, the longitudinal smooth muscle layer forms immediately under the serosa, resulting in the final embedding of the enteric ganglia between the two smooth muscle layers. Formation of the submucosal ganglia in the mammalian intestine is thought to form at later stages of embryogenesis by the inward migration of neural crest cells that initially reside in the outermost myenteric ganglia.[49] However, recent evidence has suggested that in the hindgut of chick embryos, the submucosal ganglia form first, and cells emigrating from these ganglia then reach the future (outer) region of myenteric ganglia formation by migrating along blood vessels connecting the inner and outer parts of the gut wall.[18]

The neural crest cells that invade the fetal gut retain their migratory capacity for a considerable period. Thus, postmigratory enteric crest present in the gut of older embryos is capable of re-initiating migration and colonizing various structures of the PNS on backtransplantation into the neural crest migratory pathway of younger embryos.[50,51]

Detailed analysis of the migration of enteric crest within the gut of mammalian embryos is currently restricted to the derivatives of vagal neural crest since no molecular markers are available that can uniquely identify the progeny of sacral crest in the fetal gut. However, it is clear that normal histogenesis of the ENS depends on complex morphogenetic movements of subpopulations of enteric crest (vagal, anterior trunk, and sacral), both along the anteroposterior axis of the gut as well as radially, at a given segment of the gut wall. Although it is likely that such cell movements are controlled by local or long-range signaling molecules, the identity and mechanism of action of such molecules are presently unknown. For example, it is unclear what controls the initial invasion of the gut by the vagal- and anterior spinal cord-derived neural crest cells. Are the RET-expressing pre-enteric neural crest attracted into the foregut by molecules secreted by its mesenchyme, or are they following pre-established migratory avenues? Once in the gut, what controls the caudal migration of the enteric neural crest? Do the cells respond to a caudally moving gradient of chemoattractants, or are they simply pushed posteriorly by cell division and the ensuing "population pressure?"[52] Also, what are the signals that control the radial migration of neural crest cells towards the outer limits of the gut wall? Finally, how do different subpopulations of enteric neural crest (vagal versus sacral) succeed in migrating in apparently opposite directions within the same microenvironment of the gut? These are some of the questions that require further experimentation using a variety of in vivo and in vitro approaches.

Enteric Neural Crest Cell Differentiation

A large number of neurotransmitters and neuropeptides have been identified in the mammalian ENS.[4] At present, no single molecular marker can identify uniquely neuronal subsets of the ENS. Instead, physiologically distinct subclasses of neurons can be identified by unique combinations of neuroactive substances that generate a chemical code.[6–10] However, such chemical coding is to a large extent species-specific, raising doubts as to the functional significance of the expression of a particular neurotransmitter or neuropeptide in a specific neuron. Nevertheless, the expression of various molecules in unique combinations provides the means to identify specific classes of ENS neurons during embryogenesis and thus study the mechanisms of enteric neuronal differentiation within a particular species.

Most of the studies on the differentiation of the mammalian ENS have focused so far on defining the time course of differentiation of neuronal and glial phenotypes during embryogenesis. The first "mature" cellular phenotype that can be recognized in the gut of mammalian (rodent) embryos is the one defined by the expression of tyrosine hydroxylase (TH). Tyrosine-hydroxylase-expressing (TH+) cells can be identified in the gut of E9.5 mouse (or E10.5 rat) embryos and are derived from the vagal neural crest.[31,32] However, the TH+ cells of the rodent gut are transient, as they eventually differentiate and give rise to the serotonergic lineage of the ENS.[38] Physiologic and molecular properties appropriate for terminally differentiated neurons first appear in the gut of mouse embryos on day E11.5 to 12.0. Among these properties are the specific uptake of (^{3}H)5-hydroxytryptamine ([^{3}H]5-HT) and (^{3}H)choline; the conversion of (^{3}H)choline to (^{3}H)acetylcholine; and the expression of neuropeptide Y (NPY). Later (E13.5) expression of substance P (SP) and vasoactive intestinal peptide (VIP) is detected while expression of calcitonin gene-related peptide (CGRP) has been detected from E15.5.[53] In mammalian gut, neuronal differentiation is not restricted to embryonic stages, but extends well into postnatal stages.[54]

In a very important study, Gershon and colleagues determined the birthdates of phenotypically distinct groups of neurons in the mouse gut. These experiments established that, consistently with the sequential appearance of the various neuronal phenotypes, enteric neurons do not withdraw from the cell cycle synchronously, but in sequential waves peaking at specific stages of gut organogenesis and generating specific types of neurons.[55] These findings indicate that the developing ENS in the gut of mammalian embryos is composed of a mixture of postmitotic terminally differentiated neurons alongside undifferentiated neuronal progenitors and suggest that the early differentiating neurons could play a role in inducing the differentiation of the late ones.[55] Although further experimental evidence is required, this hypothesis could provide an explanation for the sequential differentiation of various classes of neurons in enteric ganglia. Furthermore, this hypothesis suggests that, in addition to the gut mesenchyme,[56] another likely source of signals that promote neuronal differentiation in the mammalian ENS is the pre-existing population of postmitotic neurons.[55] The nature of the neuron-precursor interaction and the identity of the specific signals mediating such interactions are currently unknown.

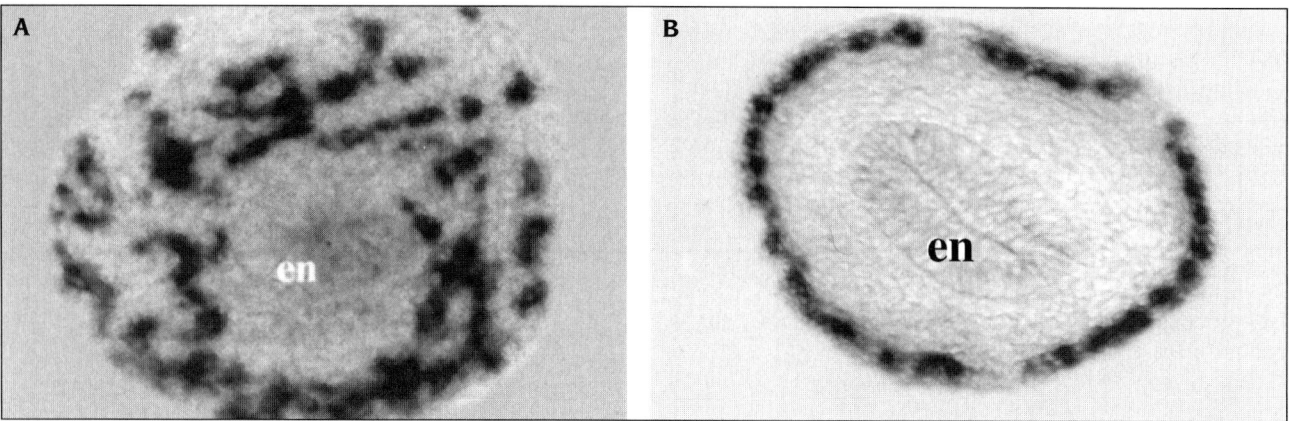

FIGURE 12–3. Shortly after their entry into the gut wall and during the early stages of migration (E9.0–11.5), the precursors of the ENS occupy the entire width of the gut wall (A). At later stages (E12.5), they are arranged as a tight ring of cells at the periphery of the gut wall (B). en = endoderm

What is the developmental potential of neural crest present in the gut mesenchyme? In vitro studies in which ENS progenitors were isolated from the gut of E14 rat embryos and plated at clonal cell densities have suggested that shortly after invasion of the gut mesenchyme, the developmental potential of enteric neural crest cells is restricted and they are irreversibly committed along specific differentiation pathways.[37] However, other studies have suggested that enteric neural crest cells remain in a multipotential state for a considerable time after invasion of the mammalian fetal gut. Thus, neural crest-derived cells isolated from the gut of rat embryos were capable of generating progeny expressing neuronal or glial phenotypes in mass cultures.[57] Furthermore, backtransplantation of gut segments into the neural crest migratory pathways of younger embryos has indicated that enteric crest cells retain their ability to migrate to distant sites and express neuronal and glial markers.[50,51] We have recently re-examined the developmental potential of enteric neural crest using a fetal gut organ culture system that preserves the three-dimensional organization of the organ and thus normal interactions between its various cell groups. Using such a system, we have shown that neural crest-derived cells isolated from the gut of E11.5 mouse embryos are multipotential. Thus, in all cases single enteric crest cells introduced by microinjection into the wall of gut in organ culture are capable of proliferating extensively and generating progeny with neuronal or glial phenotypic characteristics[48] (Figure 12–3). However, the developmental and proliferative capacity of the majority of the enteric neural crest is progressively restricted, since similar microinjection experiments have shown that cells isolated from the gut of later stage embryos generate progressively smaller clones that are restricted to the neuronal or glial cell lineage (our unpublished data). Despite this developmental restriction, it is very likely that a small but significant population of multipotential progenitors survives throughout embryogenesis and is present at postnatal stages or even in adult animals (our unpublished data). More important, it is possible that, under appropriate conditions, such cells can be stimulated to differentiate into mature neuronal and glial cells. Understanding the conditions and the mechanisms by which such dormant multipotential cells can differentiate could be critical in future attempts to reconstitute a functional ENS in gut segments lacking enteric ganglia.

Developmental Abnormalities of the Mammalian Enteric Nervous System: Congenital Megacolon (Hirschsprung's disease-HSCR)

It is evident from the previous description that the normal development of the ENS in vertebrates is dependent on the coordination and successful completion of several overlapping developmental processes in the gut of vertebrate embryos. Thus, neural crest cells must enter the gut and migrate along its rostrocaudal axis in order to colonize the entire length of a rapidly growing organ. These cells also need to migrate radially in order to occupy their characteristic positions in the periphery of the bowel. Survival of various embryonic groups of cells requires signaling by trophic factors, and it is likely that such factors are also necessary for the survival of subpopulations of neural crest cells including the progenitors of the mammalian ENS. Also, given the vast numbers of cells in the ENS of adult animals, the relatively small population of neural crest cells that enter the gut[28] needs to proliferate in order to generate the appropriate number of neuronal and glial progenitors that subsequently differentiate into mature neurons and glial cells. Finally, differentiation processes of such progenitors require accurate orchestration in order for the enteric ganglia to acquire the appropriate numbers and types of neuronal and glial cells. It is therefore not surprising that failure in any of the above developmental processes during gut organogenesis could have dramatic implications for ENS histogenesis, which are usually manifested as failure of enteric ganglia formation (aganglionosis). Indeed, several syndromes have been described that are associated with failure of enteric ganglia formation at varying lengths of the colon and the intestine (congenital megacolon, also called Hirschsprung's disease-HSCR).

Congenital megacolon was originally described in 1888[58] and has an incidence of approximately one in 4500 live births. It is characterized by severe constipation with abdominal distension, failure to thrive, and intestinal obstruction that becomes evident usually within the first year of life. The underlying histopathologic cause of the syndrome is absence of enteric ganglia (from both the myenteric and submucosal plexuses) from varying lengths of the hindgut (aganglionosis). Mild forms of HSCR are usually associated with aganglionosis in a relatively small part of the hindgut, while more severe cases are characterized by more extensive absence of enteric ganglia. Eighty percent of the cases of HSCR are sporadic with no obvious etiology, but the remaining 20% are inherited as an autosomal dominant trait with incomplete penetrance and variable expressivity.[59–63] Although Hirschsprung's disease is a congenital condition that can be found as part of a broader syndrome, most often it is the only abnormality encountered in otherwise healthy newborns. Similar conditions of congenital megacolon have been described in other mammalian species, such as rodents (mice and rats).[64] These animal models have provided extremely valuable tools for the understanding of the molecular and cellular mechanisms that underlie the development of Hirschsprung's disease in humans (see below).

NORMAL EXPRESSION AND FUNCTION OF MOLECULAR SIGNALS

The RET Tyrosine Kinase Receptor and its Functional Ligand Glial Cell Line-Derived Neurotrophic Factor

The RET protein is encoded by the c-RET proto-oncogene. c-RET was originally identified as an oncogene by transfection of T-cell lymphoma DNA into cultured NIH3T3 cells, but subsequent cloning and study of the endogenous gene revealed that it encodes a member of the RTK superfamily and that the transforming properties of RET in these transfection experiments were due to in vitro DNA rearrangements.[65–67] Similar to all other members of this family, RET is a cell surface molecule and contains an extracellular ligand-binding domain (including a cysteine-rich region), a transmembrane segment, a cytoplasmic kinase domain and a carboxy-terminal (COOH) tail. Following the identification and study of the human c-RET locus, several reports have shown that the gene is highly conserved in other mammalian species, such as mice,[68,69] as well as in all vertebrates that have been analyzed thus far, that is, chicken[42,43] and zebrafish.[45,46] Two major isoforms of RET, which differ in the COOH-tail, are produced by alternative splicing of the primary c-RET transcript: the RET51 isoform, which contains a 51-amino acid tail, and the RET9 isoform, in which the tail is replaced by an unrelated sequence of 9 amino acids.[70] In addition to the amino acid sequence, the generation of the RET9 and RET51 isoforms is a feature that is conserved in all vertebrates that have been studied thus far.[33,42,45,46,70] Finally, a gene homologous to the vertebrate c-RET locus is present and expressed in *Drosophila melanogaster*, suggesting a conservation of this signaling pathway in invertebrates.[71]

All classes of RTKs have been shown to play critical roles in a variety of developmental processes (in both invertebrate and vertebrate organisms), and some of them have been implicated in human disease (for review see Pawson[71a] and Hafen[71b]). The first indication of the potential function of the RET receptor came from expression studies. Thus, using in situ hybridization and whole-mount hybridization histochemistry several groups have shown that c-RET is expressed during vertebrate embryogenesis.[33,34,42–46,72] In mouse embryos, expression is initiated at E.8.5 with highly abundant c-RET transcripts present in various distinct lineages of the CNS and PNS and in the excretory system (pronephros, mesonephros, and eventually metanephros). Thus, during the early stages of neural crest cell migration c-RET expression is restricted to a subset of neural crest cells emigrating from the rhombencephalon and in the anlage of the facioacoustic ganglion. At later stages (E10.5 to 14.5), c-RET mRNA is observed in all cranial ganglia and in subsets of cells of the dorsal root ganglia. One of the main sites of expression of c-RET is the gut and in particular the developing ENS. c-RET transcripts are detected in enteric neural crest prior to invasion of the foregut mesenchyme and are maintained at high levels throughout their migration and colonization of the gut wall. In the CNS, c-RET is expressed in several regions, including the ventral spinal cord of E8.5 embryos, the midbrain dopaminergic neurons, and the motor neurons of brain and spinal cord, as well as various cell layers of the developing neuroretina.[33,34,44] Outside the nervous system, c-RET is expressed in the nephric (Wolffian) duct (pronephros and mesonephros) at E8.5 to 10.5, as well as the ureteric bud epithelium (E11.0 to 11.5) and the growing tips of the renal collecting ducts throughout nephrogenesis.[33,34,42,43,45,46] These studies clearly suggested that c-RET encodes for a receptor for a growth factor that is involved in the survival, proliferation, migration, and differentiation of various neuronal cell lineages as well as in inductive interactions underlying kidney organogenesis.[33] Furthermore, studies on chicken and zebrafish embryos have shown that, in addition to the conservation of its structure and sequence, the expression of the c-RET proto-oncogene is also highly conserved among higher and lower vertebrates.[42,43,45,46]

A combination of clinical and genetic studies have shown that mutations of c-RET are associated with several disease syndromes.[73] Thus, somatic rearrangements of chromosomal DNA, which result in juxtaposition of the transmembrane and kinase domains of RET to unrelated aminoterminal sequences, result in the generation of the PTC (papillary thyroid carcinoma) oncogenes, the cytosolic products of which are responsible for approximately 25% of PTCs.[74] In addition to such somatic mutations, germ-line mutations of c-RET have been detected in patients with multiple endocrine neoplasia (MEN) types 2A and B, inherited cancer syndromes characterized by medullary thyroid carcinomas.[75–78] The MEN2A syndrome, which in addition to medullary thyroid carcinoma is also associated with pheochromocytoma and hyperplasia of the parathyroid glands, results from point mutations that alter one of several cysteine (Cys) residues normally present in the juxtamembrane part of the extracellular domain of RET (usually Cys635). The MEN2B syndrome, which in addition to medullary thyroid carcinoma is characterized by gastrointestinal neurinomas and Marfanoid stature, results from a point mutation that alters threonine

(Thr) 918 into methionine (Met). Studies from several groups have shown that all mutations of c-RET that have been described so far—that is, the transforming in vitro rearrangements, the oncogenic somatic mutations, and the germ-line mutations responsible for MEN2A and 2B—are gain-of-function mutations that lead to constitutive activation of the kinase domain of RET, thus rendering it independent of binding of its cognate ligand(s).[65,79,80] Although the phenotypes associated with the gain-of-function MEN2A and MEN2B mutations do not automatically suggest a role of the RET receptor during organogenesis, it is interesting that the majority of cell types affected by these mutations are derivatives of the neural crest. This, together with the expression pattern of c-RET in mammalian and other vertebrate embryos, further suggested that the RET receptor has a role in the control of the survival, proliferation, and differentiation of neural crest cells and their derivatives.

The first indication that c-RET is indeed implicated in the development of the mammalian ENS and HSCR was derived from linkage studies that showed that an autosomal dominant gene for HSCR mapped on chromosome 10q11.2 in a region in which c-RET had been previously localized. This suggestion was subsequently confirmed by mutational analysis that showed that approximately 50% of patients with the inherited form of the disease carry mutations in c-RET.[81] To date, a variety of c-RET mutations have been identified in HSCR patients, ranging from deletions of the whole gene, small intragenic deletions or insertions, nonsense mutations, missense mutations, and splicing alterations.[73] In addition to these mutations that affect directly the coding capacity of the c-RET locus, it is possible that other mutations outside the coding region of c-RET (such as the promoter or other regulatory regions) might affect the levels of expression of this gene. The end result of all these types of mutations is a reduction or absence of signaling by the RET receptor that leads to abnormal behavior of the neural crest cells during ENS histogenesis and results in aganglionosis of the terminal colon.

The critical role of c-RET in the development of the mammalian ENS has been further confirmed from genetic studies in mice.[28,22] Using targeted mutagenesis in embryonic stem cells, we have generated a mutation (*Ret.k⁻*) which results in functional deletion of the intracellular tyrosine kinase domain of RET and absence of both (RET9 and RET51) isoforms.[82] Mice heterozygous for this mutation (+/*Ret.k⁻*) develop and behave normally in all respects. However, animals homozygous for this mutation (*Ret.k⁻/Ret.k⁻*), although they develop to term, die within 12 to 18 hours after birth. Consistent with the expression of c-RET in the developing excretory system, mutant mice have severe kidney hypodysplasia or agenesis. Furthermore, these animals have severe intestinal aganglionosis characterized by absence of enteric ganglia from the small and large intestine (severe intestinal aganglionosis).[82] However, a reduced number of apparently normal ganglia are present in the appropriate locations of the esophagus and the cardiac stomach.[28] It is likely that the surviving ganglia in the foregut of mutant (*Ret.k⁻/Ret.k⁻*) animals are derived from the component of the ENS contributed by the sympathoadrenal lineage that originates from the anterior neural tube at the level of somites 6 and 7. This would then indicate that, despite expression of c-RET in both the sympathoenteric and the sympathoadrenal lineages of the gut, RET function is only required in the sympathoenteric derivatives of the neural crest.[28] Analysis of RET-deficient mice during embryogenesis has shown that the effects of the c-RET mutation can be detected at early stages of ENS histogenesis, suggesting that RET controls the survival, migration, proliferation, or differentiation of the enteric neural crest.

Similar aganglionic phenotypes of variable severity have been observed in other natural or induced mutations in mice. Three of such targeted mutations, disrupting the gene encoding glial cell line–derived neurotrophic factor (GDNF), have been instrumental in establishing the functional relationship between this signaling molecule and the RET RTK.[83–85] The GDNF is a distant member of the transforming growth factor (TGF)-β superfamily and the most potent survival factor for dopaminergic and motor neurons of the CNS in culture.[86,87] This led to the suggestion that GDNF is a neurotrophic factor implicated in the etiology of Parkinson's disease or motor neuron degeneration. Consistent with this hypothesis, exogenous administration of GDNF has potent protective effects in vivo on motor neurons and ventral midbrain dopaminergic neurons compromised by axotomy or toxicity.[87–92] In addition to the CNS neurons, GDNF has neurotrophic effects on a wide range of neurons from the peripheral nervous system, such as autonomic, enteric, and subsets of sensory neurons of the dorsal root ganglia.[93]

Several studies have shown that GDNF is widely expressed during relatively late stages of mammalian embryogenesis.[94,95] Similar studies from our laboratory have shown that at the stage of somatogenesis in mouse embryos (E 8.0 to 12.5), GDNF mRNA is expressed mainly in the foregut and the kidney. Although these tissues also express high levels of c-RET mRNA, the products of the two genes are localized in distinct, albeit adjacent, cell types. Thus, in the embryonic gut, c-RET is expressed in the migrating neural crest cells while GDNF is expressed in the surrounding mesenchyme. In the developing kidney (metanephros), c-RET is expressed in the epithelial cells of the ureteric bud and its branches, and GDNF mRNA is localized in the mesenchymal cells that are in close proximity to the branching tips of the ureteric bud ([96] and our unpublished observations). Based on these studies, it was hypothesized that GDNF produced by mesenchymal cells in the foregut or kidney was capable of activating the RET RTK present on the cell surface of enteric neural crest cells or the epithelial cells of the ureteric bud, respectively. This hypothesis was further supported by genetic studies that showed that inactivating mutations of the GDNF locus in mice results in a phenotype remarkably similar to that of RET-deficient animals. Thus, mice homozygous for a null mutation at the GDNF locus die shortly after birth and are characterized by kidney agenesis and severe intestinal aganglionosis.[83–85] Simultaneously with these studies and in a parallel series of experiments, several groups established that GDNF is a functional ligand for RET capable of activating the catalytic tyrosine kinase domain of this cell surface receptor.[96–98] More recently, three novel polypeptides have been described (neurturin [NTN], persephin [PSP] and Artemin [ARTN]) that are closely related to GDNF and are capable of signaling through the RET RTK.[99–101] The interaction of all members of the GDNF family of neurotrophic factors with RET is not direct but is mediated by members of a subfamily of glycosyl phosphatidyl inositol (GPI)-linked cell surface molecules called GFRα (GFRα1-5). According to the prevailing model, GDNF, NTN, PSP, or ARTN bind (with different affinities) to the GFRα molecules, and the resulting complexes subsequently interact with RET, resulting in its dimerization, activation of its kinase domain, and receptor transphosphorylation.[100–113]

Further support for the hypothesis that GFRα1 is necessary for the in vivo interaction and activation of the RET RTK by GDNF comes from genetic studies. Thus, mice homozygous for a null mutation at the GFRα1 locus die at birth and have a phenotype identical to that of RET- and GDNF-deficient animals, that is, kidney agenesis and severe intestinal aganglionosis.[105,108] Mutations for the other members of the GFRα family of cell-surface molecules or the other members of the GDNF-related neurotrophic factors have not been described thus far. Therefore, the in vivo role(s) of these molecules is presently unknown.

It is clear from the findings described above that GDNF, GFRα1, and RET are components of a common signaling pathway that plays a critical role in the development of the ENS in mammalian embryos. But what is the mechanism(s) of action of these molecules? What are their cell targets? Which developmental process(es) and which aspect of cell function do they control? To address these questions several laboratories have used a variety of organ and cell culture model systems. Thus, to determine whether the effects of the *Ret.k-* mutation are cell-autonomous and thus begin to identify the cellular targets of its mutations, we have generated chimeric guts by transplanting RET-expressing (RET+) enteric neural crest cells isolated from the gut of wild-type embryos into aganglionic gut (derived from E11.5 *Ret.k--Ret.k-* mutant embryos) maintained in organ culture.[48] These experiments showed that the effects of the c-RET-null mutation are largely cell-autonomous and that the primary cell type in which RET function is normally required are the neural crest-derived progenitors of the ENS. In addition, these studies established that the failure of colonization of fetal gut by neural crest cells in *Ret.k--Ret.k-* embryos does not result from secondary effects of the mutation on the gut mesenchyme and that the aganglionic gut wall is capable of supporting the migration, proliferation, and differentiation of wild-type neural crest derivatives. This conclusion is of course of utmost importance in any future attempts to correct the aganglionic phenotype by transplantation of enteric neural progenitors.

The development of methods to isolate relatively pure populations of ENS progenitors from the mammalian and avian fetal gut[37,41,48,52,114] has allowed several groups to study the effects of several neurotrophic factors on these cells when cultured in vitro. Among the molecules that have been studied extensively are the functional ligands of RET, GDNF, and NTN and the neurotrophin NT3. These studies have shown that GDNF and NTN promote the survival, proliferation, and differentiation of multipotential ENS progenitors present in the gut of relatively young fetuses. However, the effects of these growth factors are stage-specific since similar cultures established from later-stage fetuses show markedly diminished response to GDNF and NTN but can survive efficiently in the presence of other neurotrophic fac-

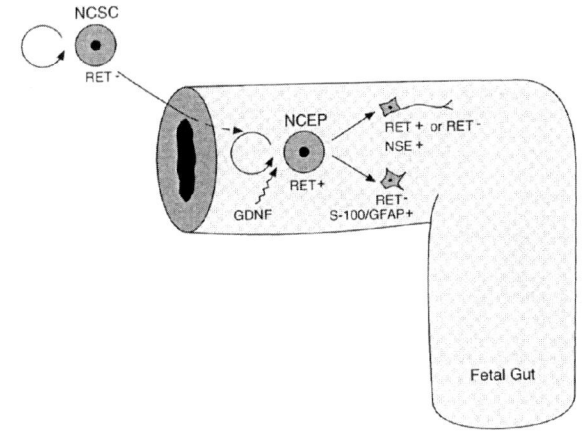

FIGURE 12–4. Potential role of the GDNF-RET signal transduction pathway during the early stages of ENS development. RET-vagal NC stem cells (NCSCs) emerge from the neural tube at the level of the postotic hindbrain and anterior spinal cord. A subpopulation of these cells initiate expression of c-RET prior to entry into the gut and form the RET+ NC-derived ENS progenitors (NCEP). Within the gut microenvironment and under the influence of GDNF, NCEP cells maintain their multipotential capacity, proliferate extensively, and colonize the entire bowel. Downregulation of c-RET expression is associated with differentiation of the glial cell lineage. Similarly, such downregulation might also be important for differentiation of a subset of enteric neurons. In addition to this early effect on NCEP cells, the RET RTK could function in the differentiation of the RET+ subpopulation of neuronal cells during later stages of ENS development. (Reproduced with permission from Natarajan D, Grigoriou M, Marcos-Gutierrez CV, et al. Multipotential progenitors of the mammalian enteric nervous system capable of colonising aganglionic bowel in organ culture. Development 1999;26:157.)

tors such as NT3 ([41,52,114] and our unpublished observations). It is therefore likely that GDNF/NTN and NT3 are components of two independent signaling systems that operate sequentially during embryogenesis to promote neurogenesis of the mammalian gut ([114] and our unpublished observations). That these in vitro studies reveal aspects of the in vivo function of the RET signaling pathway is strongly supported by analysis of the phenotype of c-RET knockout embryos, which shows that the ENS progenitors undergo apoptotic cell death prior to or during their invasion of the foregut mesenchyme (our own observations). Overall, studies on the c-RET and GDNF knockout animals and in vitro studies have clearly shown that the GDNF/RET signaling pathway is required in vivo for normal development of the mammalian ENS (Figure 12–4).

Endothelin-3 and the Endothelin Receptor B Signaling Pathway

Endothelins-1, -2, and -3 (ET1–3) constitute a small family of 21-amino acid peptides that activate G protein-coupled heptahelical receptors.[115,116] The original member of this family was identified as a product of endothelial cells, and the first recognized targets of endothelins were the smooth muscle cells of blood vessels that respond by vasoconstriction. Endothelins are encoded by separate genes that are now known to be expressed by a variety of vascular and nonvascular tissues.[115] Two types of receptors for endothelins have been identified, termed endothelin receptor-A and endothelin receptor-B (EDNRA and EDNRB), that are encoded by separate genes expressed in a variety of cells with partly overlapping distribution.[117–119] Endothelin receptor-B is capable of binding all three endothelins with equal affinity, but ET1 and ET2 are capable of activating only EDNRA. Mature endothelins are produced from large precursor forms called pre-proendothelins. These molecules are then cleaved enzymatically to produce 38- to 41-amino acid-long, biologically inactive intermediates, called big endothelins. The big endothelins are subsequently cleaved by endothelin-converting enzyme 1 (ECE1) to the biologically active 21-amino acid-long endothelins.[116]

Although the physiologic functions of endothelins have been studied extensively for many years, their developmental role is a relatively recent realization. Thus, a few years ago a series of reports showed that a number of naturally occurring and targeted mutations affecting the structure or expression of the genes encoding ET1 of EDNRB result in congenital megacolon in both humans and mice.[120–122] Several missense mutations in the EDNRB locus have been described in humans with Hirschsprung's disease. Also, mice homozygous for a severe allele of piebald (piebald-lethal; ls) are characterized by extensive white spotting of the coat and megacolon resulting from absence of enteric ganglia from the terminal colon. This phenotype, which is identical to that of mice homozygous for a targeted mutation of the EDNRB locus, is the result of a deletion of the entire gene from the mouse genome. A weaker piebald allele (s) is associated with a milder phenotype and results from a regulatory mutation affecting the levels of expression of the EDNRB locus. Aganglionic megacolon, identical to that observed in homozygous piebald-lethal animals, develops in mice homozygous for a targeted mutation of the ET-3 locus. Also, in mice homozygous for the lethal spotted mutation (ls/ls) big endothelin-3, an intermediate in endothelin-3 biosynthesis, cannot be converted to mature and biologically active ET-3. These genetic studies have clearly established that normal development of the mammalian ENS depends on normal processing and function of the ET-3 and its receptor EDNRB.

The effects of ET-3 on neural crest cells and their derivatives are dependent on the stage of differentiation of these cells. Thus, addition of ET-3 to cultures of neural crest that were established shortly after emigration from the neural tube results in dramatic increase in the rate of proliferation and the generation of large numbers of melanocytes.[123] However, the effects of ET-3 on enteric neural crest cells isolated from the gut of vertebrate embryos are quite different. In this case, activation of the ET-3-EDNRB signaling pathway appears to inhibit the differentiation of the neural crest cells into postmitotic neurons thus maintaining them in a proliferating and undifferentiated state.[52,124] This effect is independent of the cell cycle since ET-3 does not have an effect on cell proliferation. In addition to the effects of ET-3 on the neural crest cells and their derivatives, this molecule also affects the maturation and differentiation of the mesenchymal cells of the gut. Thus, ET-3 promotes in vitro the development of enteric smooth muscle cells and concomitantly inhibits the expression of laminin α1 by these cells.[124] It is therefore likely that in vivo ET-3 (which is exclusively produced by the non-neural crest cells of the gut) has multiple cellular targets, such as the mesenchymal smooth muscle cells of the fetal gut and the enteric crest, both of which express EDNRB.

The genetic and cell culture studies described here show clearly that the ET-3-EDNRB signaling pathway is required for normal development of the mammalian ENS. However, unlike the GDNF/RET signaling system, the absence of which leads to "catastrophic" elimination of almost the entire ENS, mutations of ET-3 or EDNRB affect specific subpopulations of enteric neural crest. Understanding the intracellular molecules that mediate the effects of both signaling systems and their potential interactions is a major challenge for the investigators of ENS development.

SOX-10

Another animal model of Hirschsprung's disease (Dominant Megacolon [Dom]) arose spontaneously in mice. Animals heterozygous for the Dom mutation (Dom-+) display regional deficiencies of the neural crest-derived enteric ganglia in the colon whereas animals homozygous for this mutation (Dom/Dom) die during embryogenesis and have severe defects of all neural crest derivatives of the PNS.[64] Positional cloning of the gene responsible for Dom has established that it encodes SOX-10, a member of the SRY-related family of HMG-containing transcriptional regulators.[39,125] In addition, patients with HSCR have been shown to carry various mutations likely to affect the function of SOX-10.[126,127]

SOX-10 is expressed in all migratory neural crest cells destined to contribute to the formation of the PNS, including the precursors of the enteric nervous system prior to invasion of the gut mesenchyme. The mechanism of action of the SOX-10 protein is not clear at present, but preliminary studies have shown that it has a critical role in the survival of several neural crest derivatives since absence of functional SOX-10 leads to apoptotic cell death of neural crest-derived peripheral ganglia.[39,128,129]

MASH-1

MASH-1 is encoded by the MASH-1 locus, the mammalian homolog of the *Drosophila melanogaster* achete-scute.[130] It is a member of the basic helix-loop-helix family of transcriptional regulators that is expressed and has a critical role in the differentiation of various lineages of the PNS and CNS.[131–133] Analysis of mice homozygous for a mutation at the MASH-1 locus has shown that it is required for the normal differentiation or survival of the majority of sympathetic neuroblasts, derivatives of the sympathoadrenal lineage of the PNS.[134] Although initial studies suggested that the ENS of MASH-1-null embryos shows only a delay in neuronal differentiation, subsequent detailed analysis showed that MASH-1 is required for the development of the serotonergic sublineage of the mammalian ENS. However, other neuronal cell groups, including those expressing peptidergic traits (such as calcitonin gene–related peptide [CGRP]) appear to develop normally.[38] This is the first report of a transcription factor that is required for the development of a phenotypically distinct group of neuronal cells in the mammalian ENS. To what extent additional transcription factors are necessary for the differentiation of other subclasses of neurons in the gut is an open question.

CONCLUSION

The number of molecules known to be important for the development of the mammalian ENS remained until relatively recently surprisingly low given the significance and the size of this branch of the PNS. However, during the last decade, in vitro and in vivo studies have identified several molecules that have a critical role in various aspects of ENS histogenesis. Furthermore, as the phenotypes of more mammalian genes are described and the effects of various signaling pathways are tested in vitro, the rate of identification of molecules important for mammalian ENS development will continue to increase. At present, the available information allows us to draw only a very general outline regarding the molecular and cellular interactions that govern formation of the enteric ganglia.

According to such a model, the majority of the ENS progenitors are generated by neural crest stem cells (NCSCs)[135] that emerge from the posterior hindbrain and anterior spinal cord and migrate ventrally to the cervical branches of the dorsal aorta and dorsally to the foregut. During this pre-enteric phase of migration, NCSCs destined to colonize the gut, express SOX-10 (a transcriptional modulator expressed and required in all neural crest derivatives) but are negative for expression of c-RET (SOX-10$^+$ RET$^-$). Prior to entry into the foregut and under the influence of local signals the neural crest-derived ENS progenitors (NCEP) induce expression of the RET RTK (SOX-10$^+$ RET$^+$). Within the gut wall microenvironment and under the influence of GDNF (and possibly other members of the GDNF-related family of neurotrophic factors), NCEP cells maintain their multipotential capacity, proliferate, and colonize the entire bowel (see Figure 12–4). "Assisting" the GDNF (NTN)-RET signaling pathway are other diffusible molecules such as ET-3 and its receptor EDNRB, activation of which prevents the terminal differentiation of NCEP cells and allows the proliferative signals to exert their maximal effect. In parallel with the proliferation of the majority of the cells, a fraction of NCEP cells differentiates and gives rise to mature (postmitotic) neuronal and, later, glial cells. It is likely that downregulation of c-RET expression is a prerequisite for glial cell differentiation. As the population of NCEP cells in the gut increases and significant numbers of differentiated cells accumulate (under the combined effect of GDNF and ET-3), the rate of cell number increase and differentiation is reduced in order for the appropriate number of mature cell types to aggregate and form functional enteric ganglia. This is likely to result from the reduction in the effective concentration of neurotrophic factors (such as GDNF?) produced by the gut wall and the reduced responsiveness of ENS progenitors to the activation of the cognate signaling receptors (such as RET). However, it is possible that a small number of NCEP cells survive in the gut throughout the animal's life and that under the appropriate conditions such cells are capable of differentiating additional neuronal and glial cells.

Despite filling up several spaces in the puzzle of ENS development, several critical questions remain unanswered; for example, What are the molecules and signals that control the entry into and subsequent rostrocaudal migration within the gut of NCEP cells? What mechanisms control the formation of enteric ganglia in the appropriate locations within the gut wall? What other molecules corroborate with the known ones to promote the proliferation and differentiation of NCEP cells, and what signals direct the differentiation of these cells along specific neuronal pathways?

REFERENCES

1. Langley J. The autonomic nervous system. Vol. 1. Cambridge: W Heffer; 1921.
2. Furness JB, Costa M. The enteric nervous system. New York: Churchill Livingstone; 1987.
3. Kuntz A. The autonomic nervous system. Philadelphia: Lea & Febiger; 1953.
4. Gershon MD, Kirchgessner AL, Wade PR. Functional anatomy of the enteric nervous system. In: Johson LR, editor. Physiology of the gastrointestinal tract. Vol. 1. New York: Raven Press; 1994. p. 381.
5. Gabella G. The number of neurons in the small intestine of mice, guinea-pigs and sheep. Neuroscience 1987;22:737.
6. Costa M, Brookes SJ, Steele PA, et al. Neurochemical classification of myenteric neurons in the guinea-pig ileum. Neuroscience 1996;75:949.
7. Sang Q, Young HM. Chemical coding of neurons in the myenteric plexus and external muscle of the small and large intestine of the mouse. Cell Tissue Res 1996;284:39.
8. Sang Q, Williamson S, Young HM. Projections of chemically identified myenteric neurons of the small and large intestine of the mouse. J Anat 1997;190:209.
9. Furness JB, Young HM, Pompolo S, et al. Plurichemical transmission and chemical coding of neurons in the digestive tract. Gastroenterology 1995;108:554.
10. Schemann M, Schaaf C, Mader M. Neurochemical coding of enteric neurons in the guinea pig stomach. J Comp Neurol 1995;353:161.
11. Jessen KR, Mirsky R. Glial cells in the enteric nervous system contain glial fibrillary acidic protein. Nature 1980;286:736.
12. Gershon MD. The second brain. New York: HarperCollins Publishers, Inc.; 1998.
13. Le Douarin N. The neural crest. Cambridge: Cambridge University Press; 1982.
14. Groves AK, Bronner-Fraser M. Neural crest diversification. Curr Top Dev Biol 1999;43:221.
15. Yntema CL, Hammond WS. The origin of intrinsic ganglia of trunk viscera from vagal neural crest in the chick embryo. J Comp Neurol 1954;101:515.
16. Le Douarin N, Teillet MA. Origin of intramural ganglionic system cells of the digestive tract of bird embryos. C R Acad Sci Hebd Seances Acad Sci D 1971;273:1411.
17. Le Douarin NM, Teillet MA. The migration of neural crest cells to the wall of the digestive tract in avian embryo. J Embryol Exp Morphol 1973;30:31.
18. Burns AJ, Douarin NM. The sacral neural crest contributes neurons and glia to the post-umbilical gut: spatiotemporal analysis of the development of the enteric nervous system. Development 1998;125:4335.

19. Tucker GC, Ciment G, Thiery JP. Pathways of avian neural crest cell migration in the developing gut. Dev Biol 1986;116:439.
20. Allan IJ, Newgreen DF. The origin and differentiation of enteric neurons of the intestine of the fowl embryo. Am J Anat 1980;157:137.
21. Newgreen DF, Jahnke I, Allan IJ, Gibbins IL. Differentiation of sympathetic and enteric neurons of the fowl embryo in grafts to the chorioallantoic membrane. Cell Tissue Res 1980;208:1.
22. Peters-van der Sanden MJ, Kirby ML, Gittenberger-de Groot A, et al. Ablation of various regions within the avian vagal neural crest has differential effects on ganglion formation in the fore-, mid- and hindgut. Dev Dyn 1993;196:183.
23. Peters-van der Sanden MJ, Luider TM, van der Kamp AW, et al. Regional differences between various axial segments of the avian neural crest regarding the formation of enteric ganglia. Differentiation 1993;53:17.
24. Pomeranz HD, Rothman TP, Gershon MD. Colonization of the post-umbilical bowel by cells derived from the sacral neural crest: direct tracing of cell migration using an intercalating probe and a replication-deficient retrovirus. Development 1991;111:647.
25. Pomeranz HD, Gershon MD. Colonization of the avian hindgut by cells derived from the sacral neural crest. Dev Biol 1990;137:378.
26. Serbedzija GN, Burgan S, Fraser SE, Bronner-Fraser M. Vital dye labelling demonstrates a sacral neural crest contribution to the enteric nervous system of chick and mouse embryos. Development 1991;111:857.
27. Meijers JH, Tibboel D, van der Kamp AW, et al. A model for aganglionosis in the chicken embryo. J Pediatr Surg 1989;24:557.
28. Durbec PL, Larsson-Blomberg LB, Schuchardt A, et al. Common origin and developmental dependence on c-ret of subsets of enteric and sympathetic neuroblasts. Development 1996;122:349.
29. Jacobs-Cohen RJ, Payette RF, Gershon MD, Rothman TP. Inability of neural crest cells to colonize the presumptive aganglionic bowel of ls/ls mutant mice: requirement for a permissive microenvironment. J Comp Neurol 1987;255:425.
30. Rothman TP, Nilaver G, Gershon MD. Colonization of the developing murine enteric nervous system and subsequent phenotypic expression by the precursors of peptidergic neurons. J Comp Neurol 1984;225:13.
31. Baetge G, Gershon MD. Transient catecholaminergic (TC) cells in the vagus nerves and bowel of fetal mice: relationship to the development of enteric neurons. Dev Biol 1989;132:189.
32. Baetge G, Pintar JE, Gershon MD. Transiently catecholaminergic (TC) cells in the bowel of the fetal rat: precursors of noncatecholaminergic enteric neurons. Dev Biol 1990;141:353.
33. Pachnis V, Mankoo B, Costantini F. Expression of the c-ret proto-oncogene during mouse embryogenesis. Development 1993;119:1005.
34. Tsuzuki T, Takahashi M, Asai N, et al. Spatial and temporal expression of the ret proto-oncogene product in embryonic infant and adult rat tissues. Oncogene 1995;10:191.
35. Young HM, Hearn CJ, Ciampoli D, et al. A single rostrocaudal colonization of the rodent intestine by enteric neuron precursors is revealed by the expression of phox2b, ret, and p75 and by explants grown under the kidney capsule or in organ culture. Dev Biol 1998;202:67.
36. Pattyn A, Morin X, Cremer H, et al. Expression and interactions of the two closely related homeobox genes Phox2a and Phox2b during neurogenesis. Development 1997;124:4065.
37. Lo L, Anderson DJ. Postmigratory neural crest cells expressing c-RET display restricted developmental and proliferative capacities. Neuron 1995;15:527.
38. Blaugrund E, Pham TD, Tennyson V, et al. Distinct subpopulations of enteric neuronal progenitors defined by time of development, sympathoadrenal lineage markers and Mash-1-dependence. Development 1996;122:309.
39. Southard-Smith EM, Kos L, Pavan WJ. Sox10 mutation disrupts neural crest development in Dom Hirschsprung mouse model. Nat Genet 1998;18:60.
40. Kapur RP, Yost C, Palmiter RD. A transgenic model for studying development of the enteric nervous system in normal and aganglionic mice. Development 1992;116:167.
41. Chalazonitis A, Rothman TP, Chen J, et al. Neurotrophin-3 induces neural crest-derived cells from fetal rat gut to develop in vitro as neurons or glia. J Neurosci 1994;14:6571.
42. Schuchardt A, Srinivas S, Pachnis V, Costantini F. Isolation and characterization of a chicken homolog of the c-ret proto-oncogene. Oncogene 1995;10:641.
43. Robertson K, Mason I. Expression of ret in the chicken embryo suggests roles in regionalisation of the vagal neural tube and somites and in development of multiple neural crest and placodal lineages. Mech Dev 1995;53:329.
44. Watanabe Y, Harada T, Ito T, et al. ret Proto-oncogene product is a useful marker of lineage determination in the development of the enteric nervous system in rats. J Pediatr Surg 1997;32:28.
45. Marcos-Gutierrez CV, Wilson SW, Holder N, Pachnis V. The zebrafish homologue of the ret receptor and its pattern of expression during embryogenesis. Oncogene 1997;14:879.
46. Bisgrove BW, Raible DW, Walter V, et al. Expression of c-ret in the zebrafish embryo: potential roles in motoneuronal development. J Neurobiol 1997;33:749.
47. Markus A, von Holst A, Rohrer H, Heumann R. NGF-mediated survival depends on p21ras in chick sympathetic neurons from the superior cervical but not from lumbosacral ganglia. Dev Biol 1997;191:306.
48. Natarajan D, Grigoriou M, Marcos-Gutierrez CV, et al. Multipotential progenitors of the mammalian enteric nervous system capable of colonising aganglionic bowel in organ culture. Development 1999;126:157.
49. Gershon MD, Chalazonitis A, Rothman TP. From neural crest to bowel: development of the enteric nervous system. J Neurobiol 1993;24:199.
50. Rothman TP, Le Douarin NM, Fontaine-Perus JC, Gershon MD. Developmental potential of neural crest-derived cells migrating from segments of developing quail bowel backgrafted into younger chick host embryos. Development 1990;109:411.
51. Rothman TP, Le Douarin NM, Fontaine-Perus JC, Gershon MD. Colonization of the bowel by neural crest-derived cells re-migrating from foregut backtransplanted to vagal or sacral regions of host embryos. Dev Dyn 1993;196:217.
52. Hearn CJ, Murphy M, Newgreen D. GDNF and ET-3 differentially modulate the numbers of avian enteric neural crest cells and enteric neurons in vitro. Dev Biol 1998;197:93.
53. Rothman TP, Gershon MD. Phenotypic expression in the developing murine enteric nervous system. J Neurosci 1982;2:381.
54. Matini P, Mayer B, Faussone-Pellegrini MS. Neurochemical differentiation of rat enteric neurons during pre- and postnatal life. Cell Tissue Res 1997;288:11.
55. Pham TD, Gershon MD, Rothman TP. Time of origin of neurons in the murine enteric nervous system: sequence in relation to phenotype. J Comp Neurol 1991;314:789.
56. Le Douarin NM, Dulac C. Influence of the environment on the development of the enteric nervous system from the neural crest. In: Advances in the innervation of the gastrointestinal tract. Amsterdam: Elsevier Science Publishers; 1992. p. 3.

57. Pomeranz HD, Rothman TP, Chalazonitis A, et al. Neural crest-derived cells isolated from the gut by immunoselection develop neuronal and glial phenotypes when cultured on laminin. Dev Biol 1993;156:341.
58. Hirschsprung H. Stuhltragheit Neugeborener in Folge von Dilatation und Hypertrophie des Colons. Jb Kinderheilk 1888;27:1.
59. Passarge E. The genetics of Hirschsprung's disease. Evidence for heterogeneous etiology and a study of sixty-three families. N Engl J Med 1967;276:138.
60. Badner JA, Sieber WK, Garver KL, Chakravarti A. A genetic study of Hirschsprung disease. Am J Hum Genet 1990; 46:568.
61. Kusafuka T, Puri P. Genetic aspects of Hirschsprung's disease. Semin Pediatr Surg 1998;7:148.
62. Puri P, Ohshiro K, Wester T. Hirschsprung's disease: a search for etiology. Semin Pediatr Surg 1998;7:140.
63. Puri P. Hirschsprung's disease and related disorders—recent progress. Semin Pediatr Surg 1998;7:137.
64. Lyon M, Rastan S, Brown SDM. Genetic variants and strains of the laboratory mouse. Oxford: Oxford University Press;1996.
65. Takahashi M, Ritz J, Cooper GM. Activation of a novel human transforming gene, ret, by DNA rearrangement. Cell 1985;42:581.
66. Takahashi M, Cooper GM. ret transforming gene encodes a fusion protein homologous to tyrosine kinases. Mol Cell Biol 1987;7:1378.
67. Takahashi M, Buma Y, Iwamoto T, et al. Cloning and expression of the ret proto-oncogene encoding a tyrosine kinase with two potential transmembrane domains. Oncogene 1988;3:571.
68. Pachnis V, Durbec P, Taraviras S, et al. Role of the RET signal transduction pathway in development of the mammalian enteric nervous system. Am J Physiol 1998;275:G183.
69. Iwamoto T, Taniguchi M, Asai N, et al. cDna cloning of mouse ret proto-oncogene and its sequence similarity to the cadherin superfamily. Oncogene 1993;8:1087.
70. Tahira T, Ishizaka Y, Itoh F, et al. Characterization of ret proto-oncogene mRNAs encoding two isoforms of the protein product in a human neuroblastoma cell line. Oncogene 1990;5:97.
71. Sugaya R, Ishimaru S, Hosoya T, et al. A *Drosophila* homolog of human proto-oncogene ret transiently expressed in embryonic neuronal precursor cells including neuroblasts and CNS cells. Mech Dev 1994;45:139.
71a. Pawson T, Bernstein A. Receptor tyrosine kinases: genetic evidence for their role in *Drosophila* and mouse development. Trends Genet 1990;6:350–6.
71b. Hafen E, Basler K. Role of receptor tyrosine kinases during *Drosophila* development. Ciba Found Symp 1990;150: 191–204, 204–211.
72. Attie-Bitach T, Abitbol M, Gerard M, et al. Expression of the RET proto-oncogene in human embryos. Am J Med Genet 1998;80:481.
73. Pasini B, Ceccherini I, Romeo G. RET mutations in human disease. Trends Genet 1996;12:138.
74. Takahashi M. Oncogenic activation of the ret protooncogene in thyroid cancer. Crit Rev Oncog 1995;6:35.
75. Mulligan LM, Kwok JB, Healey CS, et al. Germ-line mutations of the RET proto-oncogene in multiple endocrine neoplasia type 2A. Nature 1993;363:458.
76. Donis-Keller H, Dou S, Chi D, et al. Mutations in the RET proto-oncogene are associated with MEN 2A and FMTC. Hum Mol Genet 1993;2:851.
77. Hofstra RM, Landsvater RM, Ceccherini I, et al. A mutation in the RET proto-oncogene associated with multiple endocrine neoplasia type 2B and sporadic medullary thyroid carcinoma. Nature 1994;367:375.
78. Carlson KM, Dou S, Chi D, et al. Single missense mutation in the tyrosine kinase catalytic domain of the RET protooncogene is associated with multiple endocrine neoplasia type 2B. Proc Natl Acad Sci U S A 1994;91:1579.
79. Santoro M, Carlomagno F, Romano A, et al. Activation of RET as a dominant transforming gene by germline mutations of MEN2A and MEN2B. Science 1995;267:381.
80. Asai N, Iwashita T, Matsuyama M, Takahashi M. Mechanism of activation of the ret proto-oncogene by multiple endocrine neoplasia 2A mutations. Mol Cell Biol 1995;15:1613.
81. Romeo G, Ronchetto P, Luo Y, et al. Point mutations affecting the tyrosine kinase domain of the RET proto-oncogene in Hirschsprung's disease [comments]. Nature 1994;367:377.
82. Schuchardt A, D'Agati V, Larsson-Blomberg L, et al. Defects in the kidney and enteric nervous system of mice lacking the tyrosine kinase receptor Ret. Nature 1994;367:380.
83. Moore MW, Klein RD, Farinas I, et al. Renal and neuronal abnormalities in mice lacking GDNF. Nature 1996;382:76.
84. Pichel JG, Shen L, Sheng HZ, et al. Defects in enteric innervation and kidney development in mice lacking GDNF. Nature 1996;382:73.
85. Sanchez MP, Silos-Santiago I, Frisen J, et al. Renal agenesis and the absence of enteric neurons in mice lacking GDNF. Nature 1996;382:70.
86. Lin LF, Doherty DH, Lile JD, et al. GDNF: a glial cell line-derived neurotrophic factor for midbrain dopaminergic neurons. Science 1993;260:1130.
87. Henderson CE, Phillips HS, Pollock RA, et al. GDNF: a potent survival factor for motoneurons present in peripheral nerve and muscle. Science 1994;266:1062.
88. Beck KD, Valverde J, Alexi T, et al. Mesencephalic dopaminergic neurons protected by GDNF from axotomy-induced degeneration in the adult brain. Nature. 1995;373:339.
89. Tomac A, Lindqvist E, Lin LF, et al. Protection and repair of the nigrostriatal dopaminergic system by GDNF in vivo. Nature 1995;373:335.
90. Gash DM, Zhang Z, Ovadia A, et al. Functional recovery in parkinsonian monkeys treated with GDNF. Nature 1996;380:252.
91. Choi-Lundberg DL, Lin Q, Chang YN, et al. Dopaminergic neurons protected from degeneration by GDNF gene therapy. Science 1997;275:838.
92. Yan Q, Matheson C, Lopez OT. In vivo neurotrophic effects of GDNF on neonatal and adult facial motor neurons. Nature 1995;373:341.
93. Trupp M, Ryden M, Jornvall H, et al. Peripheral expression and biological activities of GDNF a new neurotrophic factor for avian and mammalian peripheral neurons. J Cell Biol 1995;130:137.
94. Hellmich HL, Kos L, Cho ES, et al. Embryonic expression of glial cell-line derived neurotrophic factor (GDNF) suggests multiple developmental roles in neural differentiation and epithelial-mesenchymal interactions. Mech Dev 1996;54:95.
95. Suvanto P, Hiltunen JO, Arumae U, et al. Localization of glial cell line-derived neurotrophic factor (GDNF) mRNA in embryonic rat by in situ hybridization. Eur J Neurosci 1996;8:816.
96. Durbec P, Marcos-Gutierrez CV, Kilkenny C, et al. GDNF signalling through the Ret receptor tyrosine kinase. Nature 1996;381:789.
97. Trupp M, Arenas E, Fainzilber M, et al. Functional receptor for GDNF encoded by the c-ret proto-oncogene. Nature 1996;381:785.
98. Vega QC, Worby CA, Lechner MS, et al. Glial cell line-derived neurotrophic factor activates the receptor tyrosine kinase RET and promotes kidney morphogenesis. Proc Natl Acad Sci U S A 1996;93:10657.

99. Kotzbauer PT, Lampe PA, Heuckeroth RO, et al. Neurturin a relative of glial-cell-line-derived neurotrophic factor. Nature 1996;384:467.
100. Milbrandt J, de Sauvage FJ, Fahrner TJ, et al. Persephin a novel neurotrophic factor related to GDNF and neurturin. Neuron 1998;20:245.
101. Baloh RH, Tansey MG, Lampe PA, et al. Artemin, a novel member of the GDNF ligand family supports peripheral and central neurons and signals through the GFRalpha3-RET receptor complex. Neuron 1998;21:1291.
102. Baloh RH, Tansey MG, Golden JP, et al. TrnR2, a novel receptor that mediates neurturin and GDNF signaling through Ret. Neuron 1997;18:793.
103. Baloh RH, Gorodinsky A, Golden JP, et al. GFRalpha3 is an orphan member of the GDNF/neurturin/persephin receptor family. Proc Natl Acad Sci U S A 1998;95:5801.
104. Buj-Bello A, Adu J, Pinon LG, et al. Neurturin responsiveness requires a GPI-linked receptor and the Ret receptor tyrosine kinase. Nature 1997;387:721.
105. Cacalano G, Farinas I, Wang LC, et al. GFRalpha1 is an essential receptor component for GDNF in the developing nervous system and kidney. Neuron 1998;21:53.
106. Creedon DJ, Tansey MG, Baloh RH, et al. Neurturin shares receptors and signal transduction pathways with glial cell line-derived neurotrophic factor in sympathetic neurons. Proc Natl Acad Sci U S A 1997;94:7018.
107. Enokido Y, de Sauvage F, Hongo JA, et al. GFR alpha-4 and the tyrosine kinase Ret form a functional receptor complex for persephin. Curr Biol 1998;8:1019.
108. Enomoto H, Araki T, Jackman A, et al. GFR alpha1-deficient mice have deficits in the enteric nervous system and kidneys. Neuron 1998;21:317.
109. Jing S, Yu Y, Fang M, et al. GFRalpha-2 and GFRalpha-3 are two new receptors for ligands of the GDNF family. J Biol Chem 1997;272:33111.
110. Klein RD, Sherman D, Ho WH, et al. A GPI-linked protein that interacts with Ret to form a candidate neurturin receptor. Nature 1997;387:717.
111. Naveilhan P, Baudet C, Mikaels A, et al. Expression and regulation of GFRalpha3, a glial cell line-derived neurotrophic factor family receptor. Proc Natl Acad Sci U S A 1998;95:1295.
112. Nomoto S, Ito S, Yang LX, Kiuchi K. Molecular cloning and expression analysis of GFR alpha-3, a novel cDNA related to GDNFR alpha and NTNR alpha. Biochem Biophys Res Commun 1998;244:849.
113. Worby CA, Vega QC, Chao HH, et al. Identification and characterization of GFRalpha-3, a novel Co-receptor belonging to the glial cell line-derived neurotrophic receptor family. J Biol Chem 1998;273:3502.
114. Chalazonitis A, Rothman TP, Chen J, Gershon MD. Age-dependent differences in the effects of GDNF and NT-3 on the development of neurons and glia from neural crest-derived precursors immunoselected from the fetal rat gut: expression of GFRalpha-1 in vitro and in vivo. Dev Biol 1998;204:385.
115. Inoue A, Yanagisawa M, Kimura S, et al. The human endothelin family: three structurally and pharmacologically distinct isopeptides predicted by three separate genes. Proc Natl Acad Sci U S A 1989;86:2863.
116. Rubanyi GM, Polokoff MA. Endothelins: molecular biology, biochemistry, pharmacology, physiology, and pathophysiology. Pharmacol Rev 1994;46:325.
117. Arai H, Hori S, Aramori I, et al. Cloning and expression of a cDNA encoding an endothelin receptor. Nature 1990;348:730.
118. Sakurai T, Yanagisawa M, Takuwa Y, et al. Cloning of a cDNA encoding a non-isopeptide-selective subtype of the endothelin receptor. Nature 1990;348:732.
119. Sakamoto A, Yanagisawa M, Sawamura T, et al. Distinct subdomains of human endothelin receptors determine their selectivity to endothelinA-selective antagonist and endothelinB-selective agonists. J Biol Chem 1993;268:8547.
120. Puffenberger EG, Hosoda K, Washington SS, et al. A missense mutation of the endothelin-B receptor gene in multigenic Hirschsprung's disease. Cell 1994;79:1257.
121. Hosoda K, Hammer RE, Richardson JA, et al. Targeted and natural (piebald-lethal) mutations of endothelin-B receptor gene produce megacolon associated with spotted coat color in mice. Cell 1994;79:1267.
122. Baynash AG, Hosoda K, Giaid A, et al. Interaction of endothelin-3 with endothelin-B receptor is essential for development of epidermal melanocytes and enteric neurons. Cell 1994;79:1277.
123. Lahav R, Dupin E, Lecoin L, et al. Endothelin 3 selectively promotes survival and proliferation of neural crest-derived glial and melanocytic precursors in vitro. Proc Natl Acad Sci U S A 1998;95:14214.
124. Wu JJ, Chen JX, Rothman TP, Gershon MD. Inhibition of in vitro enteric neuronal development by endothelin-3: mediation by endothelin B receptors. Development 1999;126:1161.
125. Herbarth B, Pingault V, Bondurand N, et al. Mutation of the Sry-related Sox10 gene in Dominant megacolon, a mouse model for human Hirschsprung disease. Proc Natl Acad Sci U S A 1998;95:5161.
126. Kuhlbrodt K, Schmidt C, Sock E, et al. Functional analysis of Sox10 mutations found in human Waardenburg-Hirschsprung patients. J Biol Chem 1998;273:23033.
127. Pingault V, Bondurand N, Kuhlbrodt K, et al. SOX10 mutations in patients with Waardenburg-Hirschsprung disease. Nat Genet 1998;18:171.
128. Pusch C, Hustert E, Pfeifer D, et al. The SOX10/Sox10 gene from human and mouse: sequence, expression, and transactivation by the encoded HMG domain transcription factor. Hum Genet 1998;103:115.
129. Bondurand N, Kobetz A, Pingault V, et al. Expression of the SOX10 gene during human development. FEBS Lett 1998;432:168.
130. Johnson JE, Birren SJ, Anderson DJ. Two rat homologues of Drosophila achaete-scute specifically expressed in neuronal precursors. Nature 1990;346:858.
131. Lo LC, Johnson JE, Wuenschell CW, et al. Mammalian achaete-scute homolog 1 is transiently expressed by spatially restricted subsets of early neuroepithelial and neural crest cells. Genes Dev 1991;5:1524.
132. Sommer L, Shah N, Rao M, Anderson DJ. The cellular function of MASH1 in autonomic neurogenesis. Neuron 1995;15:1245.
133. Casarosa S, Fode C, Guillemot F. Mash1 regulates neurogenesis in the ventral telencephalon. Development 1999;126:525.
134. Guillemot F, Lo LC, Johnson JE, et al. Mammalian achaete-scute homolog 1 is required for the early development of olfactory and autonomic neurons. Cell 1993;75:463.
135. Stemple DL, Anderson DJ. Isolation of a stem cell for neurons and glia from the mammalian neural crest. Cell 1992;71:973.

CHAPTER 13

Gastrointestinal Motor Activity in the Fetus and Newborn

W. Michael Bisset, MD, FRCPCH

David L. Wingate, DM, FRCP

Peter J. Milla, MSc, MBBS, FRCPCH

Expectations of survival for very small preterm infants have increased dramatically[1–5] as a result of major advances in neonatal intensive care over the past 30 years. Previously immaturity of the respiratory tract and of the gastrointestinal (GI) tract were major obstacles to the survival of these infants; but with the recent routine introduction of surfactant therapy[6] and improvements in neonatal care, death from respiratory distress syndrome is now less common. The focus has therefore moved to the GI tract and the ability to initiate early enteral nutrition. The preterm infant requires a steady, balanced input of nutrients to meet its own very rapid growth potential and the additional requirements imposed by thermal, infective, or metabolic stress. Where nutrition is inadequate growth and development fail, and morbidity and mortality from a wide range of neonatal insults increase.

Normally all nutritional requirements are met by the enteral route but in the preterm infant this is compromised by the immaturity of GI function. While absorption and secretion are moderately developed by the beginning of the third trimester, the development of adequate motor function is frequently immature, and this diminishes the efficacy of enteral feeding in these children[7] (Figure 13–1). Clinically, the premature introduction of feeds results in abdominal distension, with splinting of the diaphragm and vomiting; the latter may in turn result in aspiration that can further embarrass respiratory function.

The past two decades have seen major advances in our understanding of intestinal motor activity in the preterm infant. Advances in embryology, physiology, and molecular biology have given us some insight into how motor activity develops in the fetus and preterm infant, and how disturbances to these processes can lead to disorders of motility in the newborn infant.

NORMAL MOTOR FUNCTION

Food is moved, by the coordinated action of intestinal smooth muscle, from one specialized region of the gut to the next. The esophagus acts as a conduit for the transfer of food from the mouth to the stomach, where it is stored and mixed prior to its controlled passage into the small intestine. In the small intestine food is digested and absorbed, and subsequently passed into the large intestine, where salt and water are conserved prior to excretion. Propulsion within the gut is controlled primarily through a combination of neural and humoral mechanisms[3] that detect the presence of intraluminal nutrients and coordinate motor activity over the whole length of the intestine. This intrinsic activity is modulated by the brain stem, hypothalamus, and higher cerebral centers through the outflows of the parasympathetic and sympathetic nervous systems. The enteric nervous system,[8] which has as many neurons as the spinal cord,[9] is the "gut brain" that regulates not only motor activity but also mucosal transport, immune function, and blood flow. Most responses of the gut are programmed and controlled by the enteric nerves; and the number of autonomic neurons that link the intrinsic nerve plexuses of the gut with the central nervous system is small compared to the number of neurons

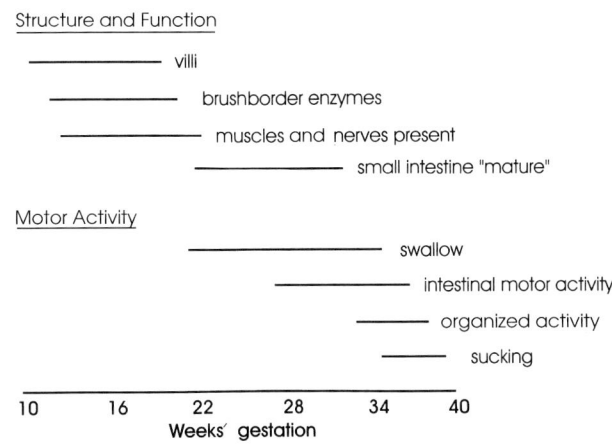

FIGURE 13–1. The developmental timetable for intestinal motor activity is delayed in comparison with most other structural and functional elements in the human intestine.

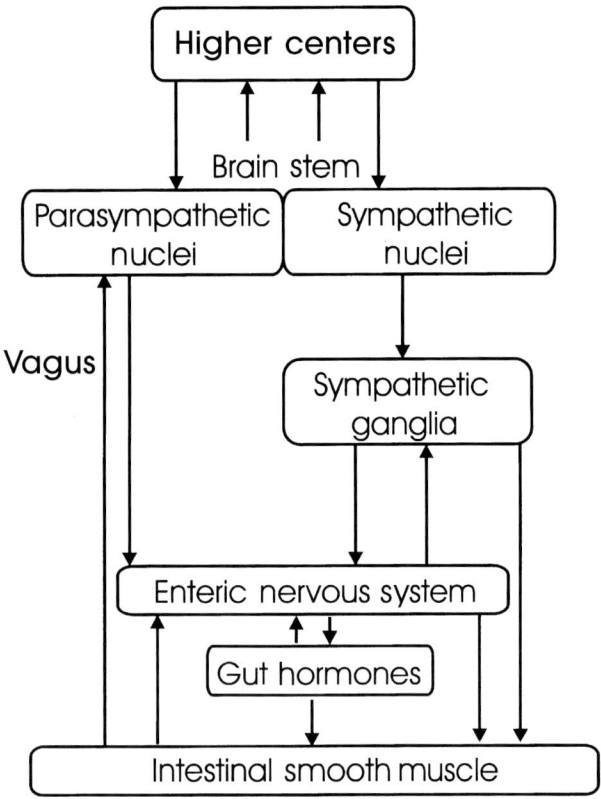

FIGURE 13–2. The hierarchy of controls involved in the maturation of intestinal motility.

within the gut wall. The vagus nerve,[10] which is the main connection to the central nervous system, contains 90% afferent fibers and is, therefore, primarily a sensory nerve, with only 10% of its fibers transmitting information that will modulate intestinal function (Figure 13–2).

DEVELOPMENT OF INTESTINAL MOTOR ACTIVITY

An understanding of the development of intestinal motility in the fetus and newborn infant requires a knowledge of the embryology of the GI tract and an appreciation of how the neural, muscular, and endocrine elements are integrated to produce a propulsive pattern of motor activity.

Gross Structure

The GI tract first appears at about 4 weeks' gestation as a hollow tube extending from the mouth to the cloaca. The non-neural elements of the gut—i.e., the endoderm lining, muscle, and loose connective tissue—are derived from endodermal and mesodermal cells. Bilateral infolding of these layers, forming an intestinal lumen surrounded by concentric endodermal and splanchnic epithelia, creates a tubular gut. Cells from the outer epithelium migrate outwards and form a loose mesenchyme, which later forms the muscle and connective tissue, while neural elements migrate from the neural crest at vagal and sacral levels to form the enteric nervous system. The most proximal part of the gut forms the esophagus, which is separated by the newly formed diaphragm from the developing abdominal cavity.[11] The stomach is formed, at 5 weeks' gestation, from a fusiform dilatation of the foregut, and by 7 weeks it has attained its final position in the upper abdomen. Rapid growth of the distal foregut and midgut exceeds the capacity of the abdominal cavity, resulting in the protrusion of this length of gut through the umbilicus. Before 10 weeks' gestation this loop undergoes 270° counter-clockwise rotation and returns to the abdomen. As early as 6 weeks' gestation the cloaca becomes flattened from side to side, and a septum forms, dividing the rectum posteriorly from the anterior urogenital sinus; and by 9 weeks hepatic and pancreatic tissue has appeared. Thus, by the end of the first trimester of pregnancy, the configuration of the intestinal tract within the abdominal cavity is almost identical to that found in the newborn infant.[12]

The Enteric Nervous System

The cells of the enteric nervous system are derived from the neural crest. Their pattern of migration has been clearly defined, initially through experiments with chicken, quail, chimera embryos[13] and, more recently, with monoclonal antibody studies[14] and transgenic animal models.[15] Vagal enteric neural crest cells arise from the neural crest at the level of somites 3 and 5, passing through branchial arches 4 and 6 to reach the foregut. The cells migrate caudally, lying in the mesenchyme close to the serosal surface. At all levels of the gut the migrating cells form a myenteric plexus prior to the later formation of a submucous plexus. Sacral neural crest cells also migrate among the mesenchyme cells of the hindgut near the stalk of the allantois. These neural precursor cells are present in the stomach and duodenum at 7 weeks' gestation in the human, and have reached the rectum by 12 weeks. The function of these cells at this stage, however, is very immature, and, as with the central nervous system, it is likely that maturation continues throughout fetal development into the first 12 to 18 months of life. Studies of intestinal motility show that even in the term infant, small-intestinal motor activity, in terms of fasting pattern, cycle length,[16] and degree of motor coordination, has not yet reached the level found in the adult. Similarly, studies of enteric neurons within the colon have shown that in the first month of life these cells are relatively hyperplastic and that their ability to take up silver stain only develops gradually over the first 6 months of life.[17]

Following colonization of the gut there is a prolonged period of maturation: the ultimate phenotypic expression of the developing cells is in part genetically programmed, but is also influenced by the cells with which the neurons are in contact, and by their neurohumoral environment.[18] Crest cells at the early stages of migration possess a remarkable heterogeneity, and most are pluripotent precursors that can become both adrenergic and nonadrenergic neurons. Subsequently these cells go through a period of oligopotency, until eventually they are differentiated into specific cell types.

Recent investigations have shown that regulatory homeobox (HOX) genes play an important role in the development of structures in the enteric nervous system.[19] Four clusters of genes on four chromosomes are expressed temporarily in a 3' to 5' linear order that corresponds to the spatiotemporal sequence of expression in the embryo. The importance of the HOX genes to normal enteric motor function is illustrated by the fact that overexpression of HOX A.4 leads to the development of megacolon,[20] while knockout of a HOX 11 L1 causes increased innervation of the hindgut.[21] Defects of these and other genes are likely to be causative in motility disorders of the newborn.

The extracellular matrix in the mesenchyme also provides important signals for crest-cell differentiation. In the transgenic lethal spotted mouse model, enteric nerves fail to migrate beyond the ileocecal valve.[15] Recent studies have shown that this abnormality is due to a defect in endothelin signaling, involving endothelin 3 (END3) and its receptor endothelin receptor B (ENDRB), which results in an alteration of the microenvironment of the neural crest cells. This defect curtails neural crest migration in the distal colon, and is associated with localized overexpression of extracellular matrix molecules.[22] A further mechanism that may lead to failure of neuronal migration occurs in individuals with Hirschsprung's disease, where it has been shown that mutations in the tyrosine kinase receptor RET are present in some individuals.[23] Growth or neurotrophic factors present in the mesenchyme ensure the survival of neurons. In mice with an absence of the gene coding for glial-derived neurotrophic factor (GDNF),[24] abnormalites in the development of the enteric nervous system similar to those found in Hirschsprung's disease have been described, and evidence has been presented that GDNF is the ligand for RET and ENDRB/END3.

Development of Gastrointestinal Smooth Muscle

The smooth muscle cells develop in the mesenchymal layer surrounding the gut lumen in a craniocaudal direction.[25] The outer circular muscle layer appears first in the esophagus at about 5 weeks' gestation in the human, and in the ileum by 8 weeks. Following this the outer longitudinal layer develops, as does the muscularis mucosa. With increasing gestation the muscle layers become thicker, which process continues well beyond birth.[26]

Most smooth muscle cells in the GI tract have an unstable cell membrane that regularly depolarizes and repolarizes; this property determines the rate and direction of muscular contractions in the GI tract. The recurring depolarization can be detected as the electrical slow wave: it occurs at 3 cycles per minute in the stomach, increases to 12 cycles per minute in the duodenum,[27] and then gradually slows along the length of the small intestine to a frequency of 9 cycles per minute in the ileum (Figure 13-3). It is not known when this cyclical activity begins in the human, although studies in preterm infants have clearly demonstrated cyclical electrical activity, both in the stomach and in the small intestine, prior to 30 weeks' gestation. There is also some evidence from studies in preterm infants that the slow-wave frequency in the duodenum increases by about 10% between 28 weeks' gestation and term.[16]

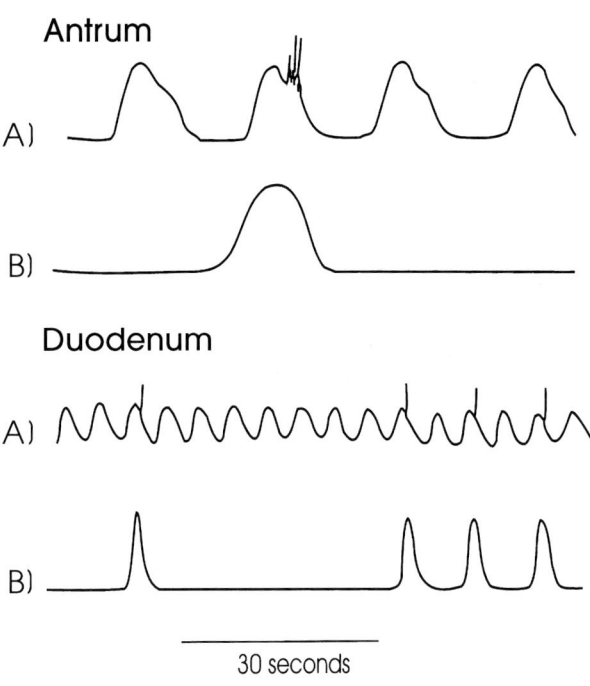

FIGURE 13-3. The (A) electrical slow wave and the associated (B) motor response for the human gastric antrum and duodenum (arbitrary units).

While smooth muscle cells undoubtedly have inherent rhythmicity, there is now compelling evidence that the pacemaker activity for the GI tract may not be primarily in these cells,[28] but in the intestinal cells of Cajal that are present in the smooth muscle layers of the gut. These cells also have intrinsic rhythmicity, and it has recently been shown that where they are absent spontaneous depolarization and repolarization of the smooth muscle cells fails to occur.[29] One of the many proteins present in the cell membrane of these cells is the KIT receptor, which is a member of the tyrosine kinase family of receptors, similar to the RET receptor that regulates enteric neuronal development. In the piebald mouse mutation of the KIT proto-oncogene not only leads to abnormalities of skin pigmentation, but has also been shown to reduce dramatically the number of intestinal cells of Cajal that develop in the muscle layers of the intestine. Electrical recording from the smooth muscle cells of affected mice shows that slow-wave activity is absent in the muscle layers of the small intestine. The affected mice develop megacolon, though no human equivalent has yet been described.

Development of Humoral Controls

Endocrine cells are first seen in the human fetal small intestine between 10 and 12 weeks' gestation, as the villi and crypts begin to form. These transitional cells contain two types of secretory granules: one characteristic of a very early precursor cell, and the other more typical of adult-type endocrine cells. With increasing gestation, the first type of secretory granules are lost, leaving a population of mature adult-type endocrine cells.[30]

Many different peptides are produced by these cells, including motilin and somatostatin, which are involved in the control of fasting motor activity, while cholecystokinin, gastrin, enteroglucagon, and peptide YY modulate postprandial motor activity.[31] These peptides are also neurotransmitters, and it is known that vasoactive intestinal peptide (VIP) and nitric oxide mediate the inhibitory responses of the lower esophageal sphincter, pylorus, and anus. Cholecystokinin is not only a potent inhibitor of fasting motor activity when secreted in response to a meal, but also produces a similar response when administered centrally. The level of gut peptides produced by these cells during the preterm period and their response to enteral nutrition has been studied in preterm infants less than 33 weeks. The first feed, whether given either as a bolus or as an infusion, fails to produce a significant change in circulating levels of insulin, growth hormone, or enteroglucagon when compared to the first feed in a term infant.[32] However, if feeding is continued in these preterm infants, after 3 weeks there is a marked postprandial response to motilin, enteroglucagon, and neurotensin.[33,34] This response is clearly dependent on the presence of nutrition in the gut, as it is absent in infants fed parenterally. Similarly, it has been shown that minimal luminal nutrition can also prime the gut to produce a larger humoral response to enteral nutrition.[35,36]

SUCKING

In order for an infant to be able to feed by mouth, sucking, swallowing, and respiration have to be appropriately coordinated. If one of these processes fails to develop or the coordination between them is lost, the infant will have major problems with feeding. In utero ultrasound studies have revealed mouthing and sucking movements as early as 15 weeks' gestation.[37] These mouthing patterns may persist until about 32 weeks' gestational age, and are eventually replaced after 34 weeks' gestation by more ordered rhythmic sucking movements that confer effective oral nutrition.[38,39]

Sucking involves the coordination of muscular activity in the lips, cheeks, jaw, tongue, and palate, and the sequence of muscular contraction is very important if the sucking is to be effective.[40] There are two main elements to sucking: the first is suction, which is the generation of negative pressure in the mouth that draws milk into it; and the second is expression, which leads to a positive pressure on the nipple. Where the infant is sucking against a dummy and no milk is being swallowed, the sucking is described as non-nutritive. This is characterized by short bursts and pauses of sucking, which occur at a frequency of approximately two per second. Non-nutritive sucking does not require the full development of coordination with swallowing and respiration, and has been observed as early as 26 to 30 weeks' gestation. The function of non-nutritive sucking is unclear, and it has been argued that it may enhance later nutrient tolerance and gastric emptying, although this has not been proven.[41,42] It may act as a stress reducer, since it has been shown that the behavior of infants is more relaxed during non-nutritive sucking.[43]

Nutritive sucking is characterized by bursts of sucks at a frequency of one per second, interspersed with short rest periods. In rat pups a period of prolonged fasting leads to more vigorous sucking movements,[44] while in human infants the efficiency of sucking improves over the first month of life.[45] Optimal sucking requires that sucking, swallowing, and breathing are synchronized in a ratio of 1:1:1 or 2:2:1, and this is present in most infants by 37 weeks' gestation.[46] In preterm infants, however, where this level of coordination may not have been achieved, effective sucking and swallowing still occurs, either by the infant having prolonged respiratory pauses during periods of vigorous sucking, or alternatively by controlling the flow of milk by blocking the nipple with their tongue. The coordination between sucking, swallowing, and breathing is in part brought about by the entrainment of the basal respiratory rhythms by the sucking center. Where this leads to ineffective respiration, with the development of either hypercapnia or hypoxia, sucking will be disrupted.[47] Similarly, central insult in the form of birth asphyxia is also likely to lead to delays in the development of effective sucking.

SWALLOWING

The movement of milk into the pharynx leads to elevation of the soft palate, closure of the larynx and propulsion of the bolus in an aboral direction through the pharynx toward the esophagus. With closure of the larynx inhibition of respiration occurs, and elevation of the soft palate prevents reflux into the nasopharynx. In the second esophageal phase of swallowing, the upper esophageal sphincter, which is formed by the thyropharyngeal muscle and the cricopharyngeal muscle, relaxes, and the bolus passes into the upper esophagus.[48]

Swallowing has been observed in utero as early as 16 to 17 weeks' gestation, and studies[51] with chromium tagged red blood cells administered into the amniotic fluid have shown that the volume of swallowed fluid increases from 13 to 16 mL per day at 20 weeks' gestation, up to 450 mL per day at term.[49] Fetal swallowing of amniotic fluid is important in the maintenance of amniotic fluid volume in later pregnancy, and may also supply nutrients to the developing intestine. As with sucking, swallowing is dependent on the complex interaction of many muscle groups under the control of the cranial nerves, and where this has yet to develop due to immaturity or been lost due to central insult, aspiration and respiratory embarrassment will inevitably occur. Fortunately these mechanisms are largely intact by the time the infant is able to suck effectively.

THE ESOPHAGUS

The esophagus is responsible for the controlled movement of food from the oropharynx to the stomach, where digestion and absorption can begin. Although the esophagus functions as a single unit, structurally the upper third is distinct inasmuch as the muscular coat is striated; and, unlike the smooth muscle elsewhere within the GI tract, it has no intrinsic excitability. The main extrinsic innervation of both striated and smooth muscle is inhibitory from the vagus nerves, and when the swallowing reflex is initiated the removal of the stimulus at a particular level results in muscular contraction, with the aboral propagation of the bolus down the esophagus. In the healthy infant and adult this wave of contraction that moves down the esophagus in response to swallowing is known as primary peristalsis. As the propulsive wave approaches the lower esophagus, the lower esophageal sphincter relaxes, and the bolus of food enters the stomach.

Inappropriate relaxation of the lower esophageal sphincter causes gastroesophageal reflux, and where secondary peristaltic waves fail to effectively clear refluxed food from the esophagus the risk of aspiration and esophagitis is greatly increased. Given that regurgitation of gastric contents commonly occurs in young babies, it seems likely that the maturation of esophageal peristalsis and effective lower esophageal sphincter function is still incomplete by term, and probably is not completed until well into the second year of life.

The Esophageal Body

The first studies of motility in the esophageal body were carried out with triple lumen-perfused manometric catheters to measure esophageal motility in both preterm and term infants.[50,51] In term infants who had been on feeds for a few days, there was well-propagated esophageal peristalsis, with pressures of 10 to 30 mm Hg generated in the esophageal body. In contrast, in newborn term infants and infants who were premature (2 to 2.4 kg), peristalsis was frequently not fully propagated, and biphasic peristaltic waves or simultaneous nonpropagated contractions were observed. It was suggested that these immature changes in the preterm and newborn infants are a reflection of the immaturity of the neural controls of the esophagus.

Recent studies have been performed with catheters that can record up to nine channels of pressure.[52] These purpose-built silicone rubber microassemblies have a central lumen for feeding, surrounded by nine perfused lumens, with the overall size of the tube being only 2 mm in diameter. A total of 27 preterm infants, ranging in age from 33 to 38 weeks' gestation, were studied on a total of 49 occasions, and the motor activity in the body of the esophagus was characterized as either peristaltic, synchronous, incomplete, or retrograde; the latter three classifications all represent nonperistaltic activity. In infants between 33 and 34 weeks' gestation, only 27% of motor activity was peristaltic, and surprisingly this percentage did not increase significantly as the infants became older. The percentage of retrograde contractions did, however, decrease significantly between 33 and 38 weeks. Nonperistaltic activity in the neonate is likely to lead to poor clearance of acid and reflux of food into the esophagus, consequently increasing the risk of aspiration and, through vagal reflexes, possible apnea or bronchospasm. This study clearly showed that, certainly by 38 weeks' gestation, the patterns of esophageal body motility were still immature, and suggests that the central integration of vagal efferent signals that is responsible for controlling peristaltic activity continues to develop well after term.

Disorders of the Esophageal Body

Disease of the esophageal body is relatively rare. In esophageal atresia, the esophagus is functionally transected and the muscular and neural controls of the upper and lower half are separate. Following surgery to restore continuity of the lumen, esophageal motility is abnormal, with decreased propagation and suboptimal function of the lower esophageal sphincter, leading to increased risk of gastroesophageal reflux and esophagitis. Abnormal motility of the esophageal body may be seen in intestinal pseudo-obstruction[53] and in some infants with severe gastroesophageal reflux.[54]

The Lower Esophageal Sphincter

It is known that the smooth muscle, along with its innervation and its response to neurohumoral control, is different in the lower esophageal sphincter from the remainder of the esophagus. The main neural mechanisms are: via cholinergic vagal neurons, which are partly responsible for generating the tone in the sphincter; and inhibition and relaxation, which are wholly neural, via vagal and nitrergic neurons. The length-tension characteristics of the smooth muscle are consistent with its function as a sphincter.[55,56]

The lower esophageal sphincter permits the passage of food from the esophagus to the stomach and prevents the regurgitation of gastric contents. Its function is complex and is not due solely to the contraction and relaxation of muscular tissue within the sphincter. In addition, the acute angle between the esophagus and the fundus of the stomach helps prevent reflux, as do the supporting structures of the diaphragm and the presence of an intra-abdominal esophagus. The mechanisms by which the sphincter function matures are only partly understood, but it is known that the length of the intra-abdominal esophagus increases from only a few millimetres in length at term to 15 mm by two years, at the same time as the angle between the fundus and oesophagus becomes more acute. Maturational changes take place within the muscles and nerves of the esophagus, and it is likely that the muscle bulk of the sphincter increases and that the innervation matures during the early years of life.[57,58]

Early studies of lower esophageal sphincter pressure relied on a pull-through technique that involved withdrawing a perfused catheter from the stomach into the esophagus; the pressure difference between the stomach and the lower esophageal sphincter represented the effective sphincter pressure.[59] One of the main limitations of this technique was that continuous measurement of sphincter pressure was not possible, and catheter withdrawal frequently disturbed the neonate, causing movement artefact. Using this pull-through technique, a longitudinal study of preterm infants between 28 weeks and term showed a steady rise in lower esophageal sphincter pressure from 4 mm Hg to 18 mm Hg at term. This rise was related to the postconceptional age of the infants, rather than their postnatal age, suggesting that the pressure rise was related to inherent maturational changes within the nerves and muscles of the sphincter, rather than acquired postnatal responses.

With the development of a miniaturized 2.5 cm-long sleeve that allows continuous measurement of both lower esophageal sphincter and esophageal body pressure without disturbing the infant, it has been possible to obtain more information not only about dynamic changes in sphincter pressure with time but also on how these changes are influenced by swallowing.[52,60] The lower esophageal pressure was shown to rise from 16.6 mm Hg at 33 to 34 weeks' gestation to 25.7 mm Hg between 37 and 38 weeks. Although this rise was not statistically significant, the range of ages studied and the amount of longitudinal data was less than earlier pull-through studies, and it does seem likely that there is a real increase in pressure with increasing postconceptional age. It was also noted that postprandially the sphincter pressure fell to between 12.9 and 14.9 mm Hg, with very little variation due to postconceptional age.

For many years it has been suggested that the increased reflux seen in young infants is due to the reduced level of the lower esophageal sphincter pressure. It is now known, however, that most episodes of gastroesophageal reflux are associated with transient relaxations of the lower esophageal sphincter.[61] The relationship of swallowing, reflux, and lower esophageal sphincter relaxation has been studied in the preterm infant using a miniaturized sleeve attached to a manometric assembly.[60] In a study of 13 preterm infants, with a mean postconceptional age of 35.7 weeks, a total of 511 separate lower esophageal sphincter relaxations were analyzed. Fifty-five percent of these relaxations occurred following a single swallow, with a mean onset time from swallowing to relaxation of 0.5 seconds, which is similar to that found in the adult. Twenty-three percent of relaxation episodes were related to multiple swallows, and a further 22% occurred more than 5 seconds either before or after the onset of a swallow and were classified as transient lower esophageal sphincter relaxations. These were observed in all 13 infants, with a frequency of between 0.5 and 6 occurring each hour. Although pH within the esophagus was not measured, reflux of gastric contents was implied by an abrupt, sustained increase in intraesophageal pressure occurring in the absence of any changes in intragastric pressure. A total of 34 such episodes were recorded, and of these 32 were associated with transient relaxation of the lower esophageal sphincter. Twenty-eight percent of transient lower esophageal sphincter relaxations were associated with reflux, compared to less than 1% associated with relaxations occurring at the time of swallowing. The similarity between the data found in preterm infants and in adults suggests that the integrated mechanism required to coordinate lower esophageal sphincter inhibition in swallowing is already present by 33 weeks' gestation, but it is not yet clear whether transient relaxation of the lower esophageal sphincter, which might be considered a nonphysiologic event, is more common in the more preterm infants (Figure 13–4).

Disorders of the Lower Esophageal Sphincter

Other than gastroesophageal reflux, abnormalities of the lower esophageal sphincter are very uncommon in preterm infants. Achalasia, a condition more normally associated with adults, has been reported in very young children.[62] Failure of relaxation of the lower esophageal sphincter is likely where there has been a defect in the development of the inhibitory innervation of the sphincter, and indeed absent or greatly reduced nitrergic innervation has been described in such cases.

THE STOMACH

From a functional point of view the stomach can be divided into two parts. The body and antrum are responsible for the storage of nutrients; and following the passage of food from

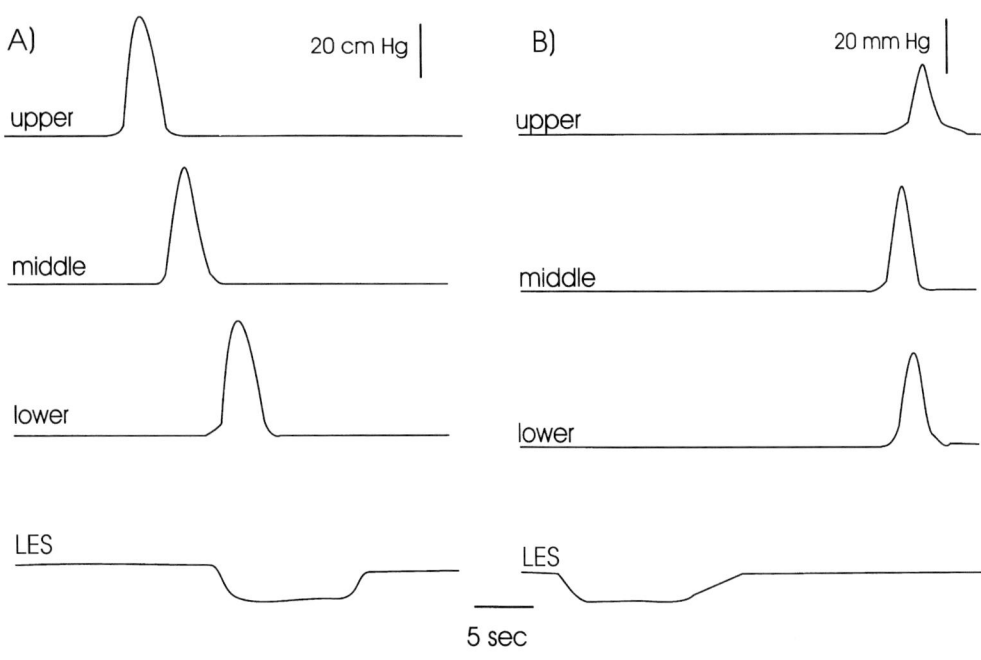

FIGURE 13–4. A schematic illustration of: A, A peristaltic esophageal contraction with synchronous relaxation of the lower esophageal sphincter (LES). B, Nonsynchronous relaxation of the lower esophageal sphincter followed by a nonpropagative esophageal contraction.

the esophagus, there is receptive relaxation of the proximal stomach that allows large volumes to be accommodated without a dramatic rise in intragastric pressure. Although the distal stomach—the antrum and pylorus—is responsible in older children for the grinding of food prior to emptying, in the preterm infant its role is less clear. The rate of emptying of liquids is determined largely by the pressure differences between the stomach and the duodenum, and is modulated by receptors in the duodenum that slow emptying when the calorie or volume load reaching the duodenum is excessive.[63]

From a clinical point of view, gastric emptying appears to be delayed in very preterm infants, and indeed, nasojejunal feeding may be required if enteral nutrition is to succeed.[64,65] This delayed gastric emptying may, in part, be developmental, but it is clear also that major insults, such as intracranial hemorrhage, sepsis or acidosis, that frequently occur in very small preterm infants will also compromise emptying.[66,67]

A characteristic feature of fasting motor activity in the older child and adult is the migrating motor complex (MMC), a highly-organized propagated sequence of contractions that migrates into the intestine from the stomach toward the ileum every 90 to 120 minutes in the fasting state.[68,69] The time of appearance of the gastric MMC has not been clearly defined, but it likely follows the same developmental timetable seen in the small intestine.[16] In the well-preterm infant normal gastric emptying may be present up to 6 weeks before MMC activity appears.

Gastric Electrical Slow Wave

Unlike the esophagus but like the smooth muscle of the small and large intestines, gastric smooth muscle is inherently excitable, with the cell membrane regularly depolarizing and repolarizing at a frequency of approximately three cycles per minute. An area high in the greater curve of the stomach that has the fastest rate of inherent rhythmicity acts as a pacemaker controlling the rate and direction of propagation of gastric electrical activity. The timing of depolarization appears to be determined by the intestinal cells of Cajal, and not, as was previously thought, by an intrinsic myogenic mechanism. If adequate neurohumoral stimuli are applied during the depolarization phase of the muscle cell, which corresponds to the extracellular slow wave, there will be complete depolarization of the smooth muscle cells, with associated contraction. Thus, the maximal rate of contractions is determined by the slow-wave frequency, but not every depolarization is associated with muscular activity. Disordered electrical activity takes the form of bradyarrhythmias or tachyarrhythmias,[70-72] although these are still of uncertain clinical significance. Tachyarrhythmias probably disrupt electromechanical coupling, leading to gastric atony with delayed emptying and intolerance to enteral feeding.

Gastric slow-wave activity can be measured noninvasively using the technique of electrogastrography.[73] Over a recording period of 30 to 60 minutes the dominant frequency of electrical slow-wave activity can be determined by the spectral analysis of overlapping segments of data, each lasting 5 to 10 minutes. In the older child and adult a clear

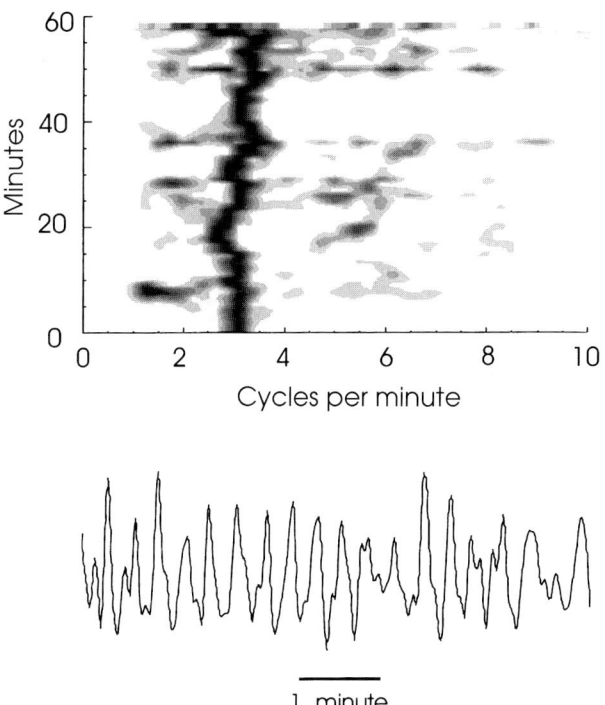

FIGURE 13–5. Normal gastric slow-wave activity, recorded by surface electrogastrography, showing a dominant frequency of three cycles per minute. The running spectral analysis of a 60 minute recording is shown above a short segment of the signal.

three-cycle-per-minute activity is seen for 70 to 90% of the recording in the fasting state (Figure 13–5). Postprandially the power of the three-cycle-per-minute activity and the dominant frequency both increase.

Studies of slow-wave frequency in preterm infants have suggested that the main frequency of activity is similar to that found in adults, but that this activity may only be present for about 30% of the time.[74,75] In addition, the postprandial response is often absent. The differences seen between preterm and term infants and infants of 2 to 6 months, who appear very similar to adults, indicate that the stability of gastric smooth-muscle electrical activity increases through the first year of life.[76]

Gastric Motor Activity

Manometric studies carried out in preterm infants have clearly shown that some contractile activity is present in the antrum of the stomach as early as 28 weeks' gestation.[16] Clearly in preterm infants the dominant frequency of this contractile activity remains at approximately three cycles per minute, and does not increase with increasing postconceptional age. One study has suggested that the pressure generated in the antrum of the stomach increases with increasing postconceptional age, whereas another has suggested there is little difference in pressures between preterm and term infants. Where antroduodenal coordination has been studied, this appears to increase as the preterm infant develops.[77]

Gastric Emptying

In the healthy fetus at 26 weeks' gestation, ultrasonography has shown contractile activity of the fetal stomach with a periodicity of approximately 45 minutes.[78] The ability to measure gastric emptying in the preterm infant has, however, been compromised by methodologic difficulties. There are clearly major ethical constraints in using isotopic techniques in preterm infants, and as a result dye dilution, ultrasonography, and impedance techniques have been attempted. In the preterm infant, half emptying time for breast milk of between 20 and 40 minutes has been reported, with breast milk emptying faster than formula feed.[66,79] This is slower than found in the full-term infant.

The rate at which food empties from the stomach also depends on the physical properties of the food, and it has been shown that as the calorie density of the feed increases from 0.2 to 0.66 kcal per mL, the rate of gastric emptying steadily decreases, indicating that the negative feedback processes that limit the excessive delivery of nutrients into the small intestine are active in the preterm infant.[63] This feedback is likely to be mediated by local, neural, and also humoral stimuli. It has also been shown that feeds containing glucose polymer empty more quickly than those containing glucose, and that feeds containing medium-chain triglyceride empty more quickly than long-chain triglyceride. Similarly, it has been shown that non-nutritive sucking and increasing feed osmolality have no effect on the rate of gastric emptying.[42,43,80]

Attempts have been made to increase the rate of gastric emptying to improve feed tolerance. Emptying has been increased by the use of metoclopramide, cisapride, and low-dose erythromycin, which have all been shown to stimulate increased gastric antral motor activity.[81–83]

Disorders of Gastric Motility

The majority of abnormalities of gastric function in the preterm infant relate to immaturity of the normal control mechanisms. Delayed emptying, however, is also present in children with intestinal pseudo-obstruction, where a more generalized abnormality of enteric nerves or smooth muscle may be present.[1,84,85] This is marked by disturbed slow-wave activity, which can be detected noninvasively using electrogastrography[70] (Figure 13–6). In infants with malrotation or with gastroschisis, upper GI motor function is frequently compromised by delayed gastric emptying.

Normal emptying of liquids from the stomach depends on the relaxation of the pylorus, which is, to a large extent, under the control of nitrergic nerves in a manner similar to that seen with the lower esophageal sphincter.[86] In children with hypertrophic pyloric stenosis, this nitrergic activity has been found to be absent in the hypertrophied circular muscle of the pylorus, where a persistently increased muscular tone results in gastric outflow obstruction.[87]

SMALL INTESTINAL-MOTILITY

Motor activity in the small intestine has to accommodate the passage of food from the stomach and promote its digestion and absorption by the small intestine and its movement at a controlled rate into the ileum and, thence, into the colon. Failure of these mechanisms results in either: delayed GI transit, with abdominal distension and vomiting; or, at the other extreme, the rapid passage of food into the colon, with resulting intestinal hurry. In the healthy infant and adult, the motor activity of the small intestine can be divided into two major types of activity. Between meals, a cyclical fasting or interdigestive pattern of motor activity is seen.[68,69] Following ingestion of food, the cyclical pattern is completely disrupted and replaced by the postprandial pattern of continuous, apparently random, segmenting and mixing activity. Following a normal meal, this may last for up to 3 or 4 hours in an adult, after which it is replaced again by the cyclical fasting pattern.

The length of disruption of the fasting pattern is determined by the caloric stimulus to the duodenum, which is a function of the content of the feed and the rate at which it is given. In herbivores, such as sheep, where there is a steady oral intake but the caloric content is low, the fasting pattern of activity is not interrupted. In carnivores, such as man, where meals are intermittent but of high nutrient value, disruption of fasting activity occurs with feeding.[88] The higher the calorie content of the feed, the longer postprandial activity is likely to endure. The postprandial pattern may be initiated following gastric distension by a vagally-mediated reflex, while the arrival of food in the small intestine leads to surges in levels of gut peptides such

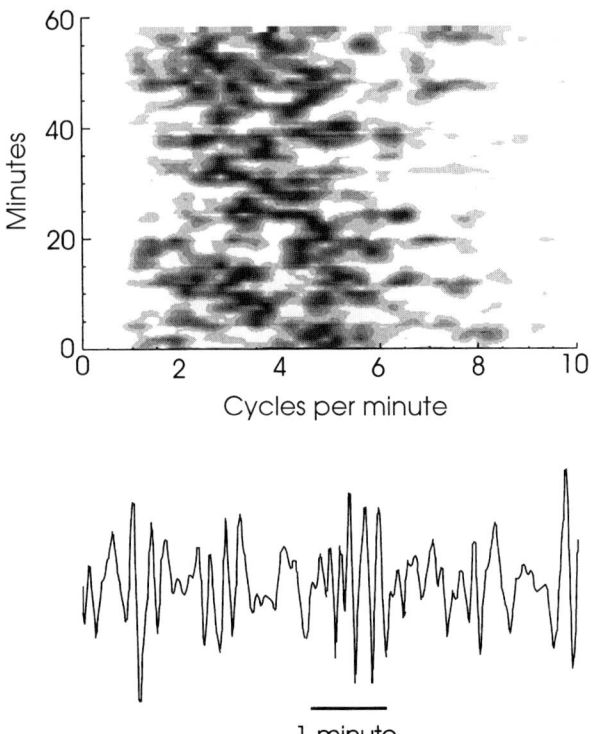

FIGURE 13–6. Gastric slow-wave activity, recorded by surface electrogastrography, in a child with neuropathic pseudo-obstruction. Compared to Figure 13–5, the running spectral analysis shows no dominant frequency and the signal shown below shows clear irregularity.

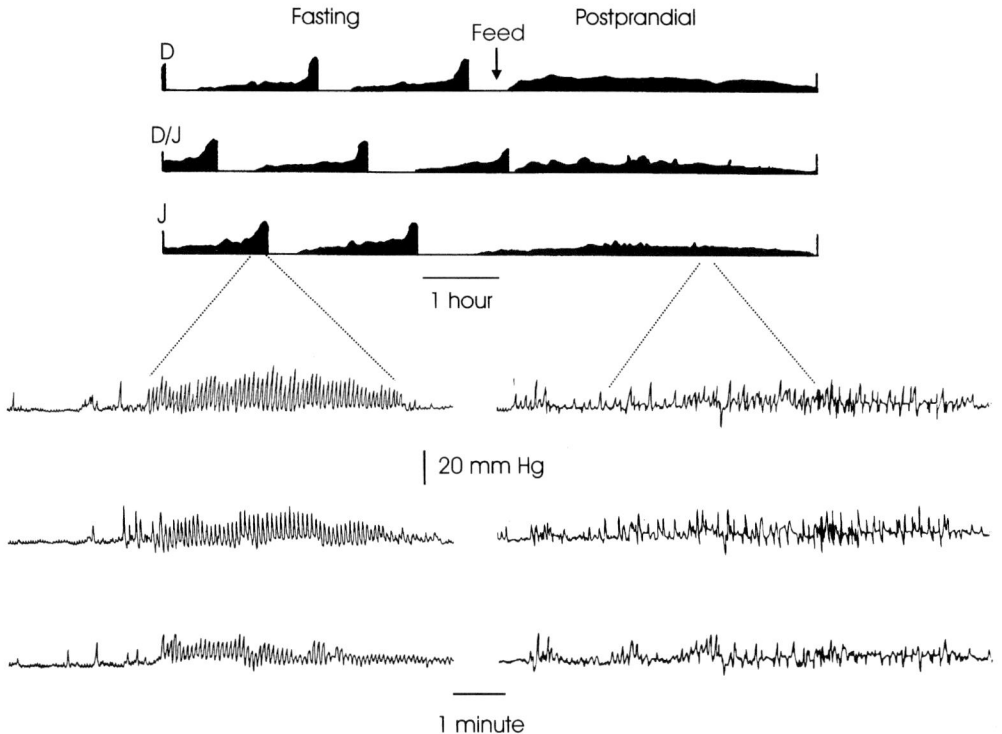

FIGURE 13–7. The normal pattern of fasting and postprandial motor activity in the small intestine of the mature human gut. The regular propagative activity of the MMC seen during fasting is contrasted to the "random" mixing activity seen in the postprandial phase. D = duodenum; J = jejunum.

as cholecystokinin, which help to maintain the postprandial pattern (Figure 13–7).

At any locus in the small bowel, mature fasting motor activity is characterized by three phases: a period of motor quiescence; a period of irregular activity; and a highly-organized propagated contractile sequence. This recurring or periodic sequence is the MMC, which in health migrates from the stomach through the small intestine for a variable distance toward the ileum approximately every 90 to 120 minutes. The presence of the MMC is an indication of the integrity of the enteric nervous system.[84,89] In the early preterm infant, where neural networks have yet to develop fully, or in disease processes that damage the nerves or muscles, MMC activity is frequently disrupted: this is associated with problems of feed tolerance, stasis of luminal contents, and bacterial overgrowth. The fasting motor response would appear to be hardwired into the nerves and muscles of the intestine; but this activity can be modulated by circulating gut peptides and from higher centers within the central nervous system via the extrinsic autonomic innervation of the gut.

Although a cyclical fasting variation of gastric motor activity and exocrine pancreatic secretions in the fasting dog was fully documented in 1905,[90] it was not until 1949[91] that multiple balloon kymography was used to record small-intestinal contractile activity. Although the different phases of MMC activity were recorded, their periodic nature was not recognized because of the relatively short recording period. Only in 1969[92] was the cyclical and migratory nature of small-intestinal activity fully explored by serosal electromyography in conscious dogs. In 1977[93] the fasting human MMC was described; since then it has become clear that the MMC is the pattern of fasting motor activity throughout vertebrate species.

Ontogeny of Small-Intestinal Motility

Studies of small-intestinal motor function in infants were limited for many years by ethical constraints and the lack of suitable recording techniques. In the early 1960s an amniographic technique, introduced to locate the placental position in pregnant women, was used to define the movement of injected radiographic contrast along the fetal GI tract.[94] Before 30 weeks' gestation there was little movement of contrast beyond the stomach, but with increasing gestational age the contrast moved into the small intestine, and by 34 weeks there was some movement into the colon. Studies of small-intestinal motor development have been carried out in fetal sheep and dogs using electromyography from chronically implanted serosal electrodes.[95,96] The fetuses were surgically delivered, electrodes were placed along the length of the intestine, and they were then returned to the uterus, allowing gestation to continue. This allowed the degree of organization of motor activity in the small intestine of these animals to be measured at intervals, both during pregnancy and immediately after delivery. In both of these species a clear timetable of motor activity was

Fasting Motor Activity

The first studies that clearly defined fasting motor activity in the human infant were published in 1988 and 1989, respectively.[16,99] The results of the studies were broadly similar. The first was a longitudinal study in which fasting small-intestinal motor activity was measured in 12 preterm infants on a total of 28 occasions. Recordings were made between 28 and 42 weeks, and the weight of the patients ranged from 650 to 3260 g. The second study was a largely cross-sectional study involving 31 infants ranging from 25 to 42 weeks' gestation. These infants ranged between 920 and 4260 g, and they had not received any enteral feed prior to the study.

Both studies showed that organization of fasting small-intestinal motor activity increased with postconceptional age. In the youngest preterm infants, between about 28 and 32 weeks' gestation, low-pressure motor activity was recorded that was without clear organization and with little evidence of propagation. The next level of organization was seen in infants between 28 and 35 weeks gestation, and was characterized by phasic clusters of motor activity similar to the "fetal" complexes described in the dog and sheep,[95] which lasted for 1 to 2 minutes. Between 34 and 36 weeks' gestation the phasic clusters became more prolonged, and in the most mature infants, between 37 and 42 weeks' gestation, MMC patterns could be seen. This evolution of motor patterns was seen in all the infants who were studied longitudinally, and was dependent primarily on the postconceptional age of the child rather than their chronologic age from birth (Figure 13–8).

It was also shown that fasting duodenal pressure increased from 5 to 30 mm of mercury with increasing postconceptional age, and that the propagation index of the clustered and MMC-like activity increased with postconceptional age. The maximal frequency of duodenal contractile activity, which is a function of the electrical pacemaking frequency, increased from just under 11 cycles per minute at 28 weeks to just over 12 cycles per minute at term. The periodicity of clustered or MMC activity was variable at any given gestational age, but there was a clear trend toward an increase in the period of cyclical activity, from 4 to 35 minutes in infants with clustered phasic activity, to 18 to 45 minutes in those with MMC activity. Since at one year of age the interval between fasting complexes is approximately 90 minutes, this was evidence that the maturation of small-intestinal motor activity continues well beyond birth.

If the developmental profile of small-intestinal motor activity is compared to that shown by in utero experiments in dog and sheep, it is evident that all three species follow a broadly similar pattern, with similarity between the human infant and the sheep when gestational ages are described as a proportion of term, while the dog, which is less mature and blind at birth lags[100] (Figure 13–9). The emergence of highly-organized propagated MMC activity is likely the result of the development of inhibitory networks within the enteric nervous system. In the sheep and dog there is evidence that with increasing gestation there is a threefold increase in the cycle length of fasting small-intestinal motor activity. It is thought that these changes may be due to the development of serotoninergic networks, and although little is known

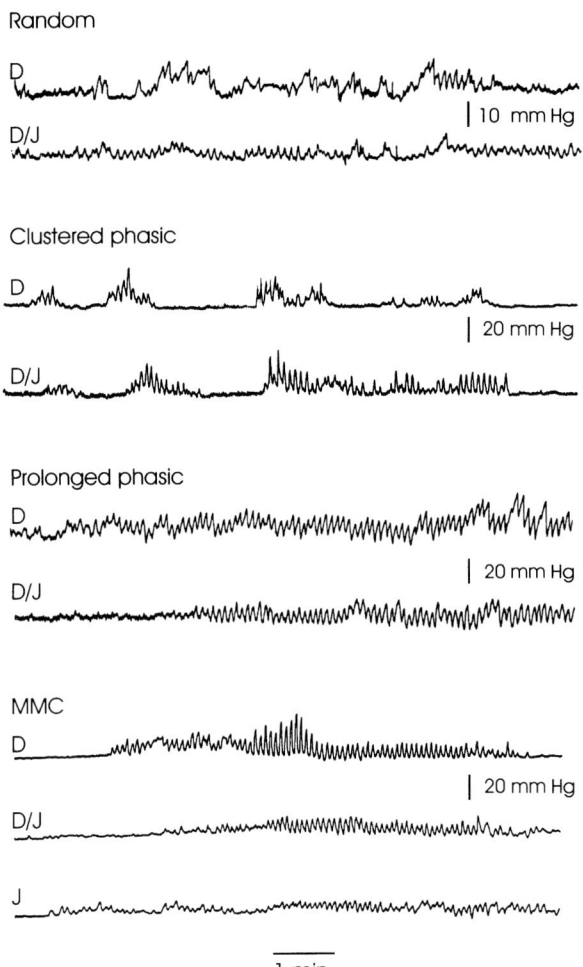

FIGURE 13–8. Patterns of developing small-intestinal motility in the preterm infant, showing a clear progression from low-pressure random activity before 30 weeks' gestation to the highly-organized MMC activity seen before term. D = duodenum; D/J = duodenal/jejunal flexure; J = jejunum (see text for full explanation).

defined, with irregular spiking activity developing into short "fetal" complexes, which then matured into more organized MMC activity that was seen at term in the sheep and 16 days past term in the dog. The relative delayed development in the dog reflected the neurologic immaturity seen in this animal at birth.

The first manometric studies in the human preterm infant were performed using single-lumen nasojejunal Silastic feeding tubes attached to a pressure transducer.[97] Although patterns similar to those that had been found in fetal dogs and sheep were visualized, the signals were attenuated, and the single recording site did not allow the measurement of contractile propagation. Major advances in the measurement of small-intestinal motor activity in the preterm infant came with the development of miniaturized multilumen catheter assemblies that allowed continuous pressure measurement, initially from three sites but subsequently from a larger number.[98]

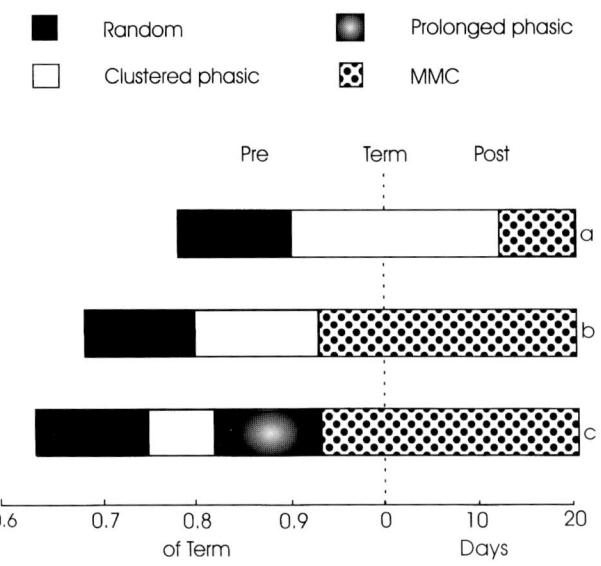

FIGURE 13-9. Comparison of the developmental profile of small-intestinal motility in the dog (a), sheep (b), and human (c). Timings before term are expressed as decimals. (Adapted from Bisset et al.,[16] Bueno et al.,[95] and Ruckebusch et al.[96])

about their development in the human gut, the fasting cycle length does become more prolonged as intestinal motor activity matures.[101]

Environmental Influences on Fasting Motor Activity

Although the program of development of fasting motor activity is preset, its timing can be altered slightly by environmental influences. For many years, authors have suggested that minimal enteral nutrition may allow developmental processes within the GI tract to advance without necessarily providing the infant with a significant nutritional load. In the very preterm infant a large enteral feed load might lead to aspiration and abdominal distension, which would compromise respiration and might increase the risk of developing necrotizing enterocolitis. Early studies looking at gut hormone levels clearly showed that withholding food from the preterm infant leads to lower fasting levels of gut hormones.[32,33] More recently the measurement of gut hormones and intestinal motor activity have been combined.[35,102] On entry, babies were randomly assigned to begin enteral feed supplements between days 3 and 5 (early) or postnatal days 10 and 14 (late). Initial motility studies in both groups of infants showed no significant difference in the state of development of fasting small-intestinal activity. After 10 days on this regimen, the infants were studied again, at which time the early feeding group had received enteral nutrition for over a week, while the late-fed group were only just starting enteral nutrition. Motility studies at this point showed that in the early-fed group of infants there was better organized activity, with longer periods of quiescence, and individual clusters were sustained for longer periods. The infants were studied again, for a third time, two weeks later, and the pattern of fasting motility for the two groups looked broadly similar.

Fasting levels of gastrin and gastric inhibitory polypeptide (GIP) were significantly higher in the early-fed group than in the late-fed group, although neurotensin and peptide YY were not significantly raised. More significantly, the early-fed infants were, on average, receiving full enteral nutrition by day 17 after birth, while late-fed infants did not achieve this goal until 31 days. The late-fed infants also took longer to establish nipple feeding, and on average were discharged from hospital two weeks later than the early-fed infants. Subsequent studies by the same author have also shown that this advancement of intestinal motility and feed tolerance resulted from the nutrients within the feed, as an equivalent volume of water delivered enterally fails to produce the same response.[36]

The development of fasting intestinal motor activity can be hindered by significant insult to the central nervous system, and it is known that infants who have suffered birth asphyxia or cerebral hemorrhage are far less likely to tolerate enteral feeds.[67,103] Motility studies of asphyxiated infants have shown that these infants have less migrating activity than nonasphyxiated neonates, and the episodes of quiescence and of clustered phasic activity are less well-organized. This less mature pattern of intestinal motility may result from an alteration in central modulation of enteric neural function, but it should be remembered that in the birth-asphyxiated infant the enteric nervous system will have also suffered an ischemic insult.

The presence of bacteria within the small intestine is important for the development of the normal patterns of fasting motor activity, and in studies where newborn animals have been reared in a germ-free environment the fasting motor activity is less mature and only emerges when a normal flora is established in the gut.[104]

A number of attempts have been made to use drugs to improve the maturation of intestinal motor activity and to improve feed tolerance. Administration of steroids[103] to the mother prior to delivery not only improves respiratory function in the preterm infant, but also appears to improve feed tolerance by advancing the maturation of intestinal motility. Drugs such as metoclopramide are known to increase gastric emptying in preterm infants, and cisapride and erythromycin, which mimic the action of motilin, have a "prokinetic" effect on the small intestine.[81–83] These drugs, however, may have significant adverse side effects, and their general use in the preterm infant is not recommended.

Postprandial Motor Response

In the older child and adult the fasting pattern of small-intestinal motor activity is abolished immediately following the ingestion of food, and it is only 3 or 4 hours later, once the meal has been fully digested and absorbed, that the fasting pattern of activity returns. This disruption of fasting activity depends on the calorie content of the food, and may be mediated, in part, by increased plasma levels of polypeptides such as gastrin, cholecystokinin, and peptide YY.[33,35]

Studies of the preterm infant have shown that the postprandial motor response, which normally leads to increased duodenal motor activity, may be attenuated in the very preterm infant.[105–107] While the fasting pattern of motor activity has a more distinct timetable of development, the postprandial motor response may develop in the preterm infant long before the mature fasting pattern of MMC has developed. Using a multiple regressional model to look at the factors that determine the length and the intensity of the postprandial motor response, it was shown that the length of time that the infants had been fed was a more important determinant than the postconceptional age of the infant.[108] This is consistent with the observation that the postprandial hormone response following the ingestion of enteral nutrition is boosted in children who have received regular enteral feeds and is attenuated where feeds have been withheld and the infants fed parenterally. It has also been shown that in infants in whom there is an immature pattern, with a poor postprandial response and an absence of quiescence in the fasting state, the tolerance of enteral feeding is likely to be poor.[109] It has, therefore, been suggested that small-bowel manometry might allow the prediction of feed tolerance prior to the infant's starting enteral nutrition, and thus allow problems of aspiration or abdominal distension to be avoided in those infants in whom tolerance is unlikely.

Disorders of Small-Intestinal Motility

Intestinal Pseudo-obstruction

The very preterm infant who is intolerant of enteral feeds has a functional pseudo-obstruction resulting from an immaturity of the control systems responsible for normal small-intestinal motor activity.[110] Where a primary disease process interferes with the development of the enteric nervous system, the smooth muscle of the gut, or the neurohumoral environment, normal patterns of small-intestinal motor activity will fail to develop and the infant will present with symptoms of vomiting, feed intolerance, abdominal distension, or constipation. This condition, which can affect any part of the intestine, may present in the neonatal period, although in some clinical presentation may be delayed for months or years.[1,85,111,112]

Neurologic disease may be limited entirely to the enteric nervous system, but in familial, peripheral, and autonomic neuropathies, other parts of the nervous system may also be involved. Although the clinical presentation may be similar, there is a wide range of conditions that may cause an enteric neuropathy, and it is only recently, with a clearer understanding of enteric neural development, that the mechanism of some of these disorders is becoming clearer. With the development of animal models of enteric neuropathies and an increased understanding of the role of HOX genes and genes controlling neuron membrane receptors such as the RET oncogene, it may soon be possible to characterize accurately the pathophysiology in many more cases.[20,21,113,114]

Primary disorders of enteric smooth muscle usually present as one of two syndromes; the pathogenesis of each is poorly understood. The first is the hollow visceral myopathy syndrome, which may be either sporadic or inherited. This condition can involve any level of the gut, but frequently involves the urinary tract, leading to the development of hydroureter, with resulting stasis and infection. The second syndrome is the megacystis-microcolon–intestinal hypoperistalsis syndrome, which is a disorder primarily affecting the colon and bladder.[115] Primary endocrine causes of pseudo-obstruction are very uncommon, and are unlikely to present in the neonatal period.

The diagnosis of these conditions is largely clinical, although manometric studies in children with pseudo-obstructive disorders have shown that where the enteric nerves are damaged the fasting cyclical pattern of motor activity is absent, and in particular the MMC may not be seen. In contrast, in myopathic pseudo-obstruction, the pressure generated by intestinal contraction is greatly reduced, although a cyclical pattern may still be discernible.[116] Diagnosis will be aided by full-thickness biopsy of the gut, with detailed histologic, histochemical, and electronmicrographic study. It is likely that genetic studies will be available in the near future to further characterize these conditions.

Studies in adults have clearly shown that absence of the MMC leads to overgrowth of bacteria in the small intestine, with consequent malabsorption and intestinal secretion. It is likely that in the very preterm infant, who has yet to develop mature patterns of fasting motor activity, a similar situation arises. Although many factors are responsible for necrotizing enterocolitis, excessive bacteria in the immature intestine might well predispose to bacterial translocation through the gut, leading to intramural inflammation and perforation.[117,118]

It is known that in infants with malrotation of the small intestine tolerance of enteral feed may be poor, even after any obstruction has been relieved. Manometric studies have shown a poorly developed pattern of fasting motor activity in these infants, with some features suggesting a mild pseudo-obstructive problem.[119] It is unclear whether these abnormalities are the consequence of the previous malrotation or whether some common factor may influence both the developing enteric nerves and the gross structure of the intestine.

COLONIC MOTILITY

Because of its relative inaccessibility, information about colonic motility in the preterm infant is limited. High-amplitude propagative contractions that are present in the colon following a meal are a marker of its neuromuscular integrity in much the same way as the MMC is a marker of small-intestinal integrity.[120] These high-pressure waves, which may be more than 60 mm Hg, decrease in frequency from four or more in the first 30 minutes after a meal in the young infant to only one or two per day in the adult. The overall motility index of the colon does, however, increase with age. No studies of colonic motility have been carried out in preterm human infants, although studies carried out in rhesus monkeys demonstrate an immature response in the preterm infant, whereas in the term infant high-amplitude propagative contractions are seen. This follows the pattern seen throughout the GI tract, with intestinal motility continuing to mature in the preterm infant well beyond term and into the first few years of life.

The presence of high-activity propagated contractions is not always associated with defecation, but the movement

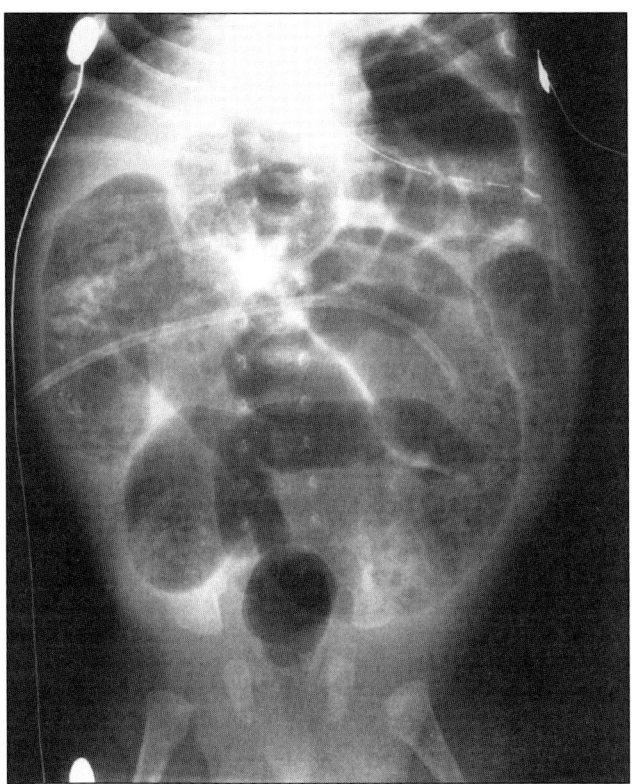

FIGURE 13–10. Abdominal radiograph of a neonate with intestinal pseudo-obstruction showing abdominal distension and fecal loading.

of a bolus of fecal material into the rectum will often lead to an increase in intraluminal rectal pressure, with associated relaxation of the anal sphincter and, consequently, defecation. Using anorectal manometry it has been shown that in the healthy term infant distension of a balloon in the rectum leads to relaxation of the internal anal sphincter. Studies in the preterm infant, using a fairly insensitive technique, suggested that this activity was not present before 39 weeks' gestation,[121,122] but with more sensitive techniques the reflex has been demonstrated in infants as young as 27 weeks' gestation.[123]

In healthy term infants, over 99% will pass their first meconium stool within 48 hours of birth.[124] In infants under 1000 g the median age that a motion is passed is 3 days, and 90% have their first stool by 12 days after birth.[125] In utero passage of meconium is frequently considered a sign of fetal distress, although it is occasionally found where fetal distress has not been apparent. It is not known whether this defecation in utero is due to activation of colonic motility or whether it is purely related to increased intra-abdominal pressure.

Disorders of Colonic Motility

Colonic motility can be disturbed in patients with intestinal pseudo-obstruction as part of a generalized problem affecting the whole intestine. In Hirschsprung's disease, a condition that affects up to 1:4500 live births, there is an absence of ganglion cells in the affected segment of the gut, which may extend a variable length from the anus, and levels of nitric oxide, an inhibitory neurotransmitter, are very low in the affected smooth muscle.[126] This leads to hypomotility and contraction of the affected segment of gut, with loss of the rectoanal inhibitory reflex, leading to failure of relaxation of the anal sphincter, with rectal distension.[127,128] In the majority of children this presents as a failure of defecation, abdominal distension, and symptoms of intestinal obstruction developing within the neonatal period, although in a small number the presentation may be delayed.

In intestinal neuronal dysplasia, both hypoganglionosis and hyperganglionosis can occur within the colon, and this may lead to symptoms that, at their worst, are similar to Hirschsprung's disease or pseudo-obstruction, while in others there may be much milder symptoms of constipation that present later in life (Figure 13–10). Some discussion of the genetic basis of these disorders is outlined in the earlier sections of this chapter and in Chapter 12. It is known that Hirschsprung's disease may recur in siblings with a frequency of 1:10, and an improved understanding of the etiology of these conditions should allow antenatal diagnosis and informative genetic counseling.[23,129,130]

CONCLUSION

Although the patterns of motor activity in and the function of each section of the GI tract are very different, there are similarities in the processes controlling the development of motility. At all levels, the integrity of the enteric nerves and muscles is essential before motor activity can occur. In many areas maturation of the enteric nerves leads to development of successively more mature patterns of motor activity, and it is likely that this process continues (as also occurs within the central nervous system) for at least a year or two after birth.

Maintenance of normal motor activity also depends on the general well being of the infant, and noxious stimuli such as sepsis, acidosis, or central nervous system insult may adversely affect the immature gut, leading to intolerance of feeding. This is of particular importance in the very preterm infant, where there is now very good evidence that the early introduction of enteral nutrition will not only promote the development of postprandial responses, but may also have a positive effect on the development of the enteric motor apparatus.

The majority of the advances outlined in this chapter have occurred over the past 15 years. This knowledge has not only led to improved care for and survival of the very preterm infant, but also offers a greater understanding of the mechanisms of GI disease that is relevant to individuals of all ages.

REFERENCES

1. Milla PJ. Intestinal motility during ontogeny and intestinal pseudo-obstruction in children. Pediatr Clin North Am 1996; 43:511–32.
2. Berseth CL. Gastrointestinal motility in the neonate. Clin Perinatol 1996;23:179–90.
3. Broussard DL. Gastrointestinal motility in the neonate. Clin Perinatol 1995;22:37–59.

4. Dumont RC, Rudolph CD. Development of gastrointestinal motility in the infant and child. Gastroenterol Clin North Am 1994;23:655–71.
5. Di Lorenzo C, Hyman PE. Gastrointestinal motility in neonatal and paediatric practice. Gastroenterol Clin North Am 1996;25:203–24.
6. Hellmann J. Surfactant replacement therapy in neonatal respiratory distress syndrome. Paediatr Anaesth 1995;5:81–8.
7. Milla PJ, Bisset WM. The gastrointestinal tract. Br Med Bull 1988;44:1010–24.
8. Goyal RK, Hirano I. The enteric nervous system. N Engl J Med 1996;334:1106–14.
9. Furness JB, Costa M. Types of nerves in the enteric nervous system. Neuroscience 1980;5:1–20.
10. Hoffman HH, Schnitzlein HN. The number of nerve fibres in the vagus nerve of man. Anat Rec 1961;139:429–35.
11. Grand RJ, Watkins JB, Torti FM. Development of the human gastrointestinal tract. Gastroenterology 1976;70:790–810.
12. Arey LB. Developmental anatomy. Philadelphia: Saunders; 1974.
13. Le Douarin NM. The ontogeny of the neural crest in avian embryo chimaeras. Nature 1980;286:663–9.
14. Tucker GC, Ciment G, Thiery JP. Pathways of avian neural crest development in the developing gut. Dev Biol 1986;116:439–50.
15. Kapur RP, Yost C, Palmiter RD. A transgenic model for studying development of the enteric nervous system in normal and aganglionic mice. Development 1992;116:167–75.
16. Bisset WM, Watt JB, Rivers RP, Milla PJ. Ontogeny of fasting small intestinal motor activity in the human infant. Gut 1988;29:483–8.
17. Smith VV, Milla PJ. Acquisition of argyrophilia in the human myenteric plexus. J Pediatr Gastroenterol Nutr 1994;19:361.
18. Le Douarin NM, Dupin E, Ziller C. Genetic and epigenetic control in neural crest development. Curr Opin Genet Dev 1994;4:685–95.
19. McGinnis W, Krumlauf R. Homeobox genes and axial patterning. Cell 1992;68:283–302.
20. Wolgemuth DJ, Beringer RR, Mostola MP, et al. Transgenic mice over expressing the mouse homeobox containing gene hox 1.4 exhibit abnormal gut development. Nature 1989;337:264–7.
21. Shirasawa S, Yunker AM, Roth KA, et al. Enx (Hox11L1)-deficient mice develop myenteric neuronal hyperplasia and megacolon. Nat Med 1997;3:646–50.
22. Payette RF, Tennyson VM, Pomeranz HD, et al. Accumulation of components of basal laminae: association with the failure of neural crest cells to colonise the presumptive aganglionic bowel of LS/LS mutant mice. Dev Biol 1988;125:341–60.
23. Romeo G, Ronchetto P, Luo Y, et al. Point mutations affecting the tyrosine kinase domain of the RET proto-oncogene in Hirschsprung's disease. Nature 1994;367:377–8.
24. Moore MW, Klein RD, Farinas I, et al. Renal and neuronal abormalities in mice lacking GDNF. Nature 1994;382:76–9.
25. Burnstock G. Development of smooth muscle and its innervation. In: Bulbring E, Brading AF, Jones AW, Tomita T, editors. Smooth muscle: an assesment of current knowledge. London: Edward Arnold; 1981. p. 431–57.
26. Hitchcock R, Pemble M, Bishop A. Quantative study of the development and maturation of human oesophageal innervation. J Anat 1992;180:175–83.
27. Sarna SK. Gastrointestinal electrical activity. Gastroenterology 1975;68:1631–5.
28. Hart Y, Kubota M, Szurszewski JH. Electrophysiology of smooth muscle of small intestine in of some mammals. J Physiol (Lond) 1986;372:501–20.
29. Huizinga JD, Thuneberg L, Kluppel M, et al. W/kit gene required for intestinal cells of Cajal and for intestinal pacemaker activity. Nature 1995;373:347–9.
30. Moxey PC, Trier JS. Endocrine cells in the human fetal small intestine. Cell Tissue Res 1977;183:33–50.
31. Holst JJ, Fahrenkrug J, Stadil F, Rehfeld JF. Gastrointestinal endocrinology. Scand J Gastroenterol Suppl 1996;216:27–38.
32. Lucas A, Bloom SR, Aynsley-Green A. Metabolic and endocrine events at the time of the first feed of human milk in preterm and term infants. Arch Dis Child 1978;53:731–6.
33. Lucas A, Adrian TE, Christofides N, et al. Plasma motilin, gastrin, and enteroglucagon and feeding in the human newborn. Arch Dis Child 1980;55:673–7.
34. Lucas A, Bloom SR, Aynsley-Green A. Development of gut hormone responses to feeding in neonates. Arch Dis Child 1980;55:678–82.
35. Berseth CL. Effect of early feeding on maturation of the preterm infant's small intestine. J Pediatr 1992;120:947–53.
36. Berseth CL, Nordyke C. Enteral nutrients promote postnatal maturation of intestinal motor activity in preterm infants. Am J Physiol 1993;264:G1046–51.
37. Hack M, Estabrook MM. Development of sucking rhythm in preterm infants. Early Hum Dev 1985;11:133–40.
38. Crump EP, Gore PM, Horton C. The sucking behavior of preterm infants. Hum Biol 1958;30:128–41.
39. Wolff PH. The serial organisation of sucking in the young infant. Pediatrics 1968;42:943.
40. Lau C, Schandler RJ. Oral motor function in the neonate. Clin Perinatol 1996;23:161–78.
41. Bernbaum JC, Pereira GR, Watkins JB, Peckham GJ. Nonnutritive sucking during gavage feeding enhances growth and maturation in premature infants. Pediatrics 1983;71:41–5.
42. Widstrom AM, Marchini G, Matthiesen AS, et al. Nonnutritive sucking in tube-fed preterm infants: effects on gastric motility and gastric contents of somatostatin. J Pediatr Gastroenterol Nutr 1988;7:517–23.
43. DiPietro JA, Cusson RM, Caughy MO. Behaviour and physiologic effect of nonnutritive sucking during gavage feeding in preterm infants. Pediatr Res 1994;36:207.
44. Brake SC, Sager DJ, Sullivan R. The role of intraoral and gastrointestinal cues in the control of sucking and milk consumption in rat pups. Dev Psychobiol 1990;15:529.
45. Pollit E, Consolazio B, Goodkin F. Changes in nutritive sucking during a feed in two day old and thirty day old infants. Early Hum Dev 1981;2:201–10.
46. Bu'Lock F, Woolridge WM, Baum JD. Development of co-ordination of sucking, swallowing and breathing: ultrasound study of term and preterm infants. Dev Med Child Neurol 1990;32:669–78.
47. Rosen CL, Glaze DG, Frost DJ. Hypoxia associated with feeding in the preterm infant and full term neonate. Am J Dis Child 1984;138:623–8.
48. Herbst JJ. Development of suck and swallow. J Pediatr Gastroenterol Nutr 1983;2 Suppl 1:S131–5.
49. Pritchard JA. Fetal swallowing and amniotic fluid volume. Obstet Gynecol 1966;28:606–10.
50. Gryboski JD. The swallowing mechanism of the neonate. 1. Esophageal and gastric motility. Pediatrics 1965;36:445–52.
51. Gryboski JD. Suck and swallow in the premature infant. Pediatrics 1969;43:96–101.
52. Omari TI, Miki K, Fraser R, et al. Esophageal body and lower esophageal sphincter function in healthy premature infants. Gastroenterology 1995;109:1757–64.
53. Euler AR, Ament ME. Esophageal motor dysfunction in idiopathic intestinal pseudoobstruction [letter]? Gastroenterology 1976;71:712.

54. Cucchiara S, Staiano A, Di Lorenzo C, et al. Esophageal motor abnormalities in children with gastroesophageal reflux and peptic esophagitis. J Pediatr 1986;108:907–10.
55. Goyal RK, Said S, Rattan S. Influence of VIP antiserum on lower esophageal sphincter relaxation; possible evidence for VIP as the inhibitory neurotransmitter. Gastroenterology 1979;76:1142.
56. Christensen J. Pharmacologic identification of the lower esophageal sphincter. J Clin Invest 1974;49:681–91.
57. Spedale SP, Weisbrodt W, Morriss JR. Ontogenic studies of gastrointestinal function II: lower esophageal sphincter maturation in neonatal beagle puppies. Pediatr Res 1982;16:851–5.
58. Boix-Ochoa J, Canals J. Maturation of the lower esophagus. J Pediatr Surg 1976;11:749–56.
59. Newell SJ, Sarkar PJ, Durbin GM, et al. Maturation of the lower oesophageal sphincter in the preterm baby. Gut 1988;29:167–72.
60. Omari TI, Miki K, Davidson G, et al. Characterisation of relaxation of the lower oesophageal sphincter in healthy premature infants. Gut 1997;40:370–5.
61. Mahoney MJ, Migliavacca M, Spitz L, Milla PJ. Motor disorders of the oesophagus in gastro-oesophageal reflux. Arch Dis Child 1988;63:1333–8.
62. Myers NA, Jolley SG, Taylor R. Achalasia of the cardia in children: a worldwide survey. J Pediatr Surg 1994;29:1375–9.
63. Siegal M, Lebenthal E, Krantz B. Effect of caloric density on gastric emptying in premature infants. J Pediatr 1984;104:118–22.
64. Kelly EJ, Newell SJ. Gastric ontogeny: clinical implications. Arch Dis Child 1994;71:F136–41.
65. Gupta M, Brans YW. Gastric retention in neonates. Pediatrics 1978;62:26–9.
66. Siegel M. Gastric emptying time in premature and compromised infants. J Pediatr Gastroenterol Nutr 1983;2 Suppl 1:S136–40.
67. Berseth CL, McCoy HH. Birth asphyxia alters neonatal intestinal motility in term neonates. Pediatrics 1992;90:669–73.
68. Wingate DL. Backward and forward with the migrating complex. Dig Dis Sci 1981;26:641–66.
69. Wingate DL. Complex clocks. Dig Dis Sci 1983;28:1133–40.
70. Devane SP, Ravelli AM, Bisset WM, et al. Gastric antral dysrhythmias in children with chronic idiopathic intestinal pseudoobstruction. Gut 1992;33:1477–81.
71. Yagi M, Homma S, Iwafuchi M, et al. Electrogastrography after operative repair of esophageal atresia. Pediatr Surg Int 1997;12:340–3.
72. Telander RL, Morgan KG, Kreulen DL, et al. Human gastric atony with tachygastria and gastric retention. Gastroenterology 1978;75:497–501.
73. Stern RM, Koch KL. Electrogastrography: methodology, validation and application. New York: Prager; 1985.
74. Tomomasa T, Miyazaki M, Nako Y, Kuroume T. Electrogastrography in neonates. J Perinatol 1994;14:417–21.
75. Koch KL, Tran TN, Stern RM, et al. Gastric myoelectric activity in premature and term infants. Gastrointest Motil 1993;4:41–7.
76. Chen JDZ, Co E, Liang J, et al. Patterns of gastric myoelectrical activity in human subjects of different ages. Am J Physiol 1997;272:G1022–8.
77. Ittmann PI, Amarnath R, Berseth CL. Maturation of antroduodenal motor activity in preterm and term infants. Dig Dis Sci 1992;37:14–9.
78. Devane SP, Soothill PW, Candy DCA. Temporal changes in gastric volume in the human fetus in late pregnancy. Early Hum Dev 1993;33:109–16.
79. Ewer AK, Durbin GM, Morgan MEI, Booth IW. Gastric emptying in preterm infants. Arch Dis Child 1994;71:F24–7.
80. Bernbaum JC, Gilberto RP, Watkins JB, Peckham GJ. Nonnutritive sucking during gavage feeding enhances growth and maturation in premature infants. Pediatrics 1983;71:41–5.
81. Blumenthal I, Costalos C. The effect of metoclopramide on neonatal gastric emptying. Br J Clin Pharmacol 1977;4:207–8.
82. Tomomasa T, Miyazaki M, Koizumi T, Kuroume T. Erythromycin increases gastric antral motility in human premature infants. Biol Neonate 1993;63:349–52.
83. Hyman PE. Absent postprandial duodenal motility in a child with cystic fibrosis. Correction of the symptoms and manometric abnormality with cisapride. Gastroenterology 1986;90:1274–9.
84. Hyman PE, McDiarmid SV, Napolitano J, et al. Antroduodenal motility in children with chronic intestinal pseudo-obstruction. J Pediatr 1988;112:899–905.
85. Cucchiara S, Annese V, Minella R, et al. Antroduodenojejunal manometry in the diagnosis of chronic idiopathic intestinal pseudoobstruction in children. J Pediatr Gastroenterol Nutr 1994;18:294–305.
86. Kawahara H, Imura K, Nishikawa M. The characteristic of the motor pattern of the pylorus in hypertrophic pyloric stenosis [abstract]. J Pediatr Gastroenterol Nutr 1997;25:S43.
87. Vanderwinden J, Mailleux P, Schiffmann SN, et al. Nitric oxide synthase activity in infantile hypertrophic pyloric stenosis. N Engl J Med 1992;327:511–5.
88. Ruckebusch Y, Bueno L. The effect of feeding on the motility of the stomach and small intestine in the pig. Br J Nutr 1976;35:397–405.
89. Summers RW, Anural S, Green J. Jejunal manometry patterns in health, partial intestinal obstruction and pseudo-obstruction. Gastroenterology 1983;85:1290–300.
90. Boldyreff WN. Le travail periodique de l'appareil digestif en dehors de la digestion. Arch Sci Biol 1905;11:1–157.
91. Chapman WP, Palazzo WL. Multiple balloon kymograph recording of intestinal motility in man with observations on the correlation of the tracing patterns with barium movement. J Clin Invest 1949;28:1517–25.
92. Szurszewski JH. A migrating electric complex of the canine small intestine. Am J Physiol 1969;217:1757–63.
93. Vantrappen G, Peeters TL, Hellemans J, Ghoos Y. The interdigestive motor complex of normal subjects and patients with bacterial overgrowth of the small intestine. J Clin Invest 1977;59:1158–66.
94. McLain CR. Amniography studies of the gastrointestinal motility of the human fetus. Am J Obstet Gynecol 1963;86:1079–87.
95. Bueno L, Ruckebusch Y. Perinatal development of intestinal myoelectrical activity in dogs and sheep. Am J Physiol 1979;237:E61–7.
96. Ruckebusch Y. Development of digestive motor patterns during perinal life. J Pediatr Gastroenterol Nutr 1986;5:523–36.
97. Milla PJ, Fenton TR. Small intestinal motility patterns in the perinatal period. J Pediatr Gastroenterol Nutr 1983;2 Suppl 1:S141–4.
98. Bisset WM, Watt JB, Rivers RP, Milla PJ. Measurement of small-intestinal motor activity in the preterm infant. J Biomed Eng 1988;10:155–8.
99. Berseth CL. Gestational evolution of small intestine motility in preterm and term infants. J Pediatr 1989;115:646–51.
100. Bisset WM. Development of intestinal motility. Arch Dis Child 1991;66:3–5.
101. Ruckebusch Y, Barton T. Involvement of serotoninergic mechanisms in initiation of small intestinal motor events. Dig Dis Sci 1984;29:520–7.
102. Berseth CL. Minimal enteral feedings. Clin Perinatol 1995;22:195–205.
103. Morriss FH Jr, Moore M, Weisbrodt NW, West MS. Ontogenic development of gastrointestinal motility. IV. Duodenal contractions in preterm infants. Pediatrics 1986;78:1106–13.

104. Abrams GD, Bishop JE. Effect of the normal microbial flora on gastrointestinal motility. Proc Soc Exp Biol Med 1967;126:301–4.
105. Berseth CL, Ittmann PI. Antral and duodenal motor responses to duodenal feeding in preterm and term infants. J Pediatr Gastroenterol Nutr 1992;14:182–6.
106. Berseth CL. Neonatal small intestinal motility: motor responses to feeding in term and preterm infants. J Pediatr 1990;117:777–82.
107. al Tawil Y, Berseth CL. Gestational and postnatal maturation of duodenal motor responses to intragastric feeding. J Pediatr 1996;129:374–81.
108. Bisset WM, Watt J, Rivers RPA, Mila PJ. Postprandial motor responses of the small intestine to enteral feed in preterm infants. Arch Dis Child 1989;64:1356–61.
109. Berseth CL, Nordyke CK. Manometry can predict feeding readiness in preterm infants. Gastroenterology 1992;103:1523–8.
110. Bagwell CE, Filler RM, Cutz E, et al. Neonatal intestinal pseudoobstruction. J Pediatr Surg 1984;19:732–9.
111. Peck SN, Altschuler SM. Pseudo-obstruction in children. Gastroenterol Nurs 1992;14:184–8.
112. Ament ME, Vargas J. Diagnosis and management of chronic intestinal pseudo-obstruction syndromes in infancy and childhood. Arq Gastroenterol 1988;25:157–65.
113. Robertson K, Mason I. The GDNF-RET signalling partnership. Trends Genet 1997;13:1–3.
114. Mak YF, Ponder BA. RET oncogene. Curr Opin Genet Dev 1996;6:82–6.
115. Berdon WI, Baker DH, Blane WA. Megacystis-microcolon-intestinal hypoperistalsis syndrome: a new cause of intestinal obstruction in the newborn. AJR Am J Roentgenol 1976;126:957–64.
116. Boige N, Faure C, Cargill G, et al. Manometrical evaluation in visceral neuropathies in children. J Pediatr Gastroenterol Nutr 1994;19:71–7.
117. Morriss FH Jr, Moore M, Gibson T, West MS. Motility of the small intestine in preterm infants who later have necrotizing enterocolitis. J Pediatr 1990;117:S20–3.
118. Berseth CL. Gut motility and the pathogenesis of necrotizing enterocolitis. Clin Perinatol 1994;21:263–70.
119. Devane SP, Coombes R, Smith VV, et al. Persistent gastrointestinal symptoms after correction of malrotation. Arch Dis Child 1992;67:218–21.
120. DiLorenzo C, Flores AF, Reddy SN. Colonic manometry differentiates causes of intractable constipation in children. J Pediatr 1992;120:690–5.
121. Howard ER, Nixon HH. Internal anal sphincter: observations on development and mechanism of inhibitory responses in premature infants and children with Hirschsprung's disease. Arch Dis Child 1968;43:569–78.
122. Ito Y, Donahoe P, Hendren W. Maturation of the rectoanal response in premature infants. J Paediatr Surg 1977;12:477–84.
123. Bowes K, Kling S. Anorectal manometry in premature infants. J Pediatr Surg 1979;14:533–5.
124. Clark D. Times of first void and first stool in 500 newborns. Pediatrics 1977;60:457–9.
125. Verma A, Dhanireddy R. Time of first stool in extremely low birth weight (<1000 gram) infants. J Pediatr 1993;122:626–9.
126. Tomita R, Munakata K, Kurosu Y, Tanjoh K. A role of nitric oxide in Hirschsprung's disease. J Pediatr Surg 1995;30:437–40.
127. Frenckner B. Ano-rectal manometry in the diagnosis of Hirschsprung's disease in infants. Acta Paediatr Scand 1978;67:187–92.
128. Faverdin C, Dornic C, Arhan P, et al. Quantitative analysis of anorectal pressures in Hirschsprung's disease. Dis Colon Rectum 1981;24:422–7.
129. Eng C, Mulligan LM. Mutations of the RET proto-oncogene in the multiple endocrine neoplasia type 2 syndromes, related sporadic tumours, and Hirschsprung's disease. Hum Mutat 1997;9:97–109.
130. Edery P, Lyonnet S, Mulligan LM, et al. Mutations of the RET proto-oncogene in Hirschsprung's disease. Nature 1994;367:378–80.

CHAPTER 14

Developmental Changes in Breast Milk Protein Composition during Lactation

Bo Lönnerdal, PhD

Yuriko Adkins, BS

Breast milk provides the newborn infant with a multitude of unique proteins. These proteins can aid the digestion of other nutrients (e.g., enzymes), bind and facilitate the absorption of micronutrients, kill or inhibit the attachment of microorganisms to the intestinal mucosa (e.g. antibodies and enzymes), stimulate the growth of the intestinal epithelium (e.g., growth factors), and modulate immune function. The biologic activities, however, for most of the proteins have been demonstrated in vitro, in cell systems or animal models, and solid evidence from clinical studies on human infants is rare. This lack of support is mainly due to difficulties in obtaining sufficient quantities of human milk proteins for large-scale, long-term studies on infants. Recent advances in genetic engineering are likely to remedy this problem; recombinant human milk proteins are now being produced in large quantities, which will allow studies to evaluate their physiologic significance. It is, though, quite possible that the biologic activity of breast milk components may only be present when fed in breast milk; if the component is added to a fundamentally different matrix, such as infant formula, its activity may be inhibited by other constituents in the formula, or by processing of the product.

When considering the physiologic activity of breast milk proteins, it is important to evaluate both the developmental changes that occur in the infant and the changes that occur in protein concentration and composition during lactation. During early infancy protein digestion is immature, and many milk proteins may retain their native structure and exert biologic functions. In late infancy protein digestion is considerably more efficient, and most proteins are likely to be digested and serve as a source of amino acids. Our knowledge about the timing and progression of these physiologic events is limited; for example, *how long* will there be sufficient quantities of a specific protein component to exert biologic activity, *when* will gastric acid secretion and digestive enzyme activities be high enough that a specific protein will be broken down into inactive fragments, and *how well* will the proteins in breast milk fulfill their dual roles as active components and supplier of amino acids for protein synthesis? A true developmental perspective is essential to assess these questions properly and it is apparent that, to date, collected information is inadequate for an in-depth understanding. This is an attempt to summarize the extent of our knowledge.

DEVELOPMENT OF MAMMARY GLAND FUNCTION

Milk Protein Gene Expression

Human milk contains proteins that not only provide the breastfed infant with amino acids but also help prevent infections (e.g., lactoferrin, lysozyme, secretory IgA) and facilitate digestion and absorption of other nutrients present in milk (e.g., lactoferrin, vitamin-binding proteins, bile-salt stimulated lipase, α-amylase). Previous studies have shown that concentrations of many human milk proteins do not stay constant throughout lactation (Table 14–1); there appears to be differential expression of casein and certain whey proteins throughout the course of lactation (Figure 14–1). Specific whey proteins, such as lactoferrin, secretory IgA, and α-lactalbumin are present in human colostrum at high concentrations with a gradual decrease over time.[1,2] Conversely, casein is present in human colostrum at low concentrations, but increases soon thereafter, followed by a gradual decrease throughout the rest of lactation.[3] Other human milk proteins, such as serum albumin, do not vary widely in concentration throughout lactation, possibly because they are not synthesized within the mammary gland but transported into the gland from the maternal circulation. Since the mammary gland is under the influence of steroid and peptide hormones during gestation and lactation, it is likely that hormones play a primary role in milk protein synthesis in the gland. Furthermore, the nutritional status of the mother may also affect milk protein gene expression. For instance, a deficiency in a specific nutrient, such as iron, which is known to have regulatory effects at the level of transcription, may influence the expression of genes encoding milk proteins within the mammary gland. Definite regulatory mechanisms explaining the different patterns of expression of

TABLE 14-1
Concentrations of Proteins in Human Milk

Protein	Reference	Stage of Lactation	
		Colostrum	Mature
Casein	3	2.5–5.5 mg/mL	3.3–4.5 mg/mL
α-Lactalbumin	2, 26, 60, 62	3–4 mg/mL	2–3 mg/mL
Lactoferrin	2, 26, 62, 63, 74	3–7 mg/mL	1–2 mg/mL
IgG	1, 2, 63, 81	0.3–0.7 mg/mL	0.03–0.1 mg/mL
IgM	1, 2, 81	0.1–0.6 mg/mL	0.02–0.2 mg/mL
sIgA	26, 43, 74	2–5 mg/mL	0.5–1.0 mg/mL
Serum albumin	2, 26, 43, 62, 63	0.4–1.0 mg/mL	0.4–1.0 mg/mL
Lysozyme	26, 62, 74, 81	0.07–0.3 mg/mL	0.07–0.2 mg/mL
α-Amylase	90	7920 U/L	1320 U/L
$α_1$-Antitrypsin	81, 90, 99	0.2–0.6 mg/mL	0.01–0.09 mg/mL
Bile salt-stimulated lipase	104, 108	NR	0.1 mg/mL
Myeloperoxidase	112	5–10 U/mL	NR
Lactoperoxidase	113	0–12.6 mU/mL	NR
Haptocorrin	126, 127	29–54 nmol/L*	15–43 nmol/L
Folate binding protein	133, 134	166–204 nmol/L†	119–179 nmol/L
IGF-I	136, 142	10 ng/mL	2–19 ng/mL
IGF-II	142	NR	2.7 ng/mL
EGF	144–146	25–40 ng/mL	5–12 ng/mL
IGF binding protein	148	85–245 ng/mL	27–167 ng/mL‡

NR = not reported
* Vitamin B_{12}-binding capacity
† Folate-binding capacity
‡ Only reported for 92 h

human milk proteins have yet to be elucidated. Studies on human milk proteins have been lacking; instead, the majority of the studies have been performed on rat or mouse milk. Animal models, organ explants, and cell culture systems have been developed to help understand the regulation of milk protein gene expression.

Previous animal and cell studies have shown that milk protein gene expression is regulated by cell-to-cell and cell-to-substratum interactions and by the synergistic interactions of steroid and peptide hormones, such as insulin, hydrocortisone, prolactin, and glucocorticoids at the transcriptional and post-transcriptional level.[4] Prolactin is necessary for the onset of milk secretion (lactogenesis) and for the continuation of milk secretion (lactation). Matusik et al.[5] showed that prolactin, when added to rat mammary gland explants, stimulated the synthesis of casein mRNA. In accordance with the observations by Matusik et al., studies using the COMMA-D mouse mammary epithelial cell line and explant cultures from transgenic mice carrying the β-casein promoter-chloramphenicol acetyltransferase (CAT) fusion genes demonstrated an increase in the rate of casein gene transcription by two- to fourfold upon prolactin addition.[6] Other peptide and steroid hormones, such as insulin, hydrocortisone, and glucocorticoids, have been found to work synergistically with prolactin. Poyet et al.[7] found that in COMMA-D cells, glucocorticoids, in the presence of prolactin, are capable of inducing β-casein mRNA accumulation. In a rat mammary gland organ culture experiment, both prolactin and hydrocortisone were found to be necessary for maximum induction of casein and whey acidic protein (WAP) mRNA.[8] Furthermore, Nishikawa and co-workers[9] found that β-casein mRNA levels in cultured mouse mammary epithelium increased in response to prolactin, insulin, and hydrocortisone. Regulation of milk protein gene expression by prolactin not only has been demonstrated at the level of transcription, but also

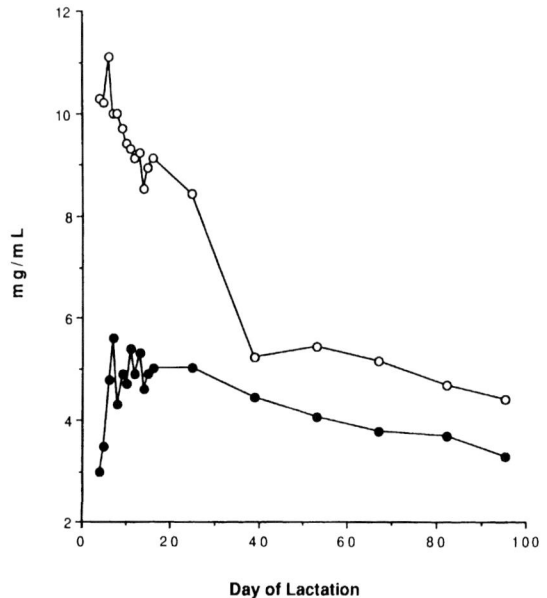

FIGURE 14-1. Developmental patterns for casein (*closed circles*) and whey proteins (*open circles*) during lactation. (Data from Kunz C, Lönnerdal B. Re-evaluation of the whey protein/casein ratio of human milk. Acta Paediatr 1992;81: 107–12.)

at the post-transcriptional level. Prolactin has been shown to have an effect on casein gene transcript stability in the nucleus.[10] It has also been suggested that glucocorticoids act indirectly on casein gene expression at the post-transcriptional level by regulating the expression of other gene products.[11] Furthermore, COMMA-D cells grown in the presence of insulin, glucocorticoids, and prolactin have been shown to synthesize proteins that exert an effect on β-casein mRNA stability.[7]

The temporal profile of changes in milk protein gene expression has been demonstrated across species. In the rat mammary gland, differential accumulation of α-, β-, and γ-casein and WAP mRNA has been observed; casein mRNA is high during early lactation, whereas WAP mRNA is low.[8] A similar casein mRNA pattern has also been observed in the mouse mammary gland.[12] κ-Casein mRNA in the mouse mammary gland has been shown to increase 2.5-fold from 4 hours after parturition to day 1 of lactation and then stays constant, while α-casein mRNA levels increase twofold from day 5 to day 15 of lactation. The level of α-casein mRNA is at least two times as high as that of κ-casein mRNA at all stages of lactation.[13] This pattern is unlike human milk, where casein concentration is low in early milk. On the other hand, rabbit casein synthesis is similar to human milk in early lactation. Concentrations of rabbit α_{S1}-, β-, and κ-casein mRNA were lower than that of WAP mRNA on day 3 of lactation, but increased to levels higher than WAP by day 25.[14]

Similar to human milk, whey protein synthesis in the rabbit is high in early lactation. Transferrin mRNA in the rabbit mammary gland is high on day 3 of lactation and remains relatively constant throughout, but decreases dramatically 8 days after weaning.[14] Puissant et al.[14] also showed that the concentration of WAP mRNA in the rabbit mammary gland was higher on day 3 of lactation than that of transferrin mRNA, but gradually decreased by day 25. In contrast, Grigor et al.[15] found that transferrin mRNA concentrations in the rat mammary gland were undetectable at days 5 through 10 of lactation, but increased thereafter. This observation is supported by McCracken et al.[16] who also demonstrated that rat transferrin gene expression was barely detectable at days 2 to 10 of lactation before increasing to higher levels in late lactation. It is thus apparent that gene expression of certain milk proteins differs across species. This may be attributed to different hormonal profiles in each species or different regulators of gene expression. Further studies are needed to understand the mechanisms involved in the regulation of gene expression of milk proteins throughout lactation.

Milk Volume

Lactation is the period defined as the continuing secretion of milk into the alveolar lumen, where it is stored until the infant removes the milk. The mechanisms regulating the volume of milk produced by the human mammary gland are not clearly understood; however, hormonal influences, as well as infant demand, seem to be involved. During lactation prolactin regulates the rate of synthesis and secretion of milk, and oxytocin stimulates the contraction of myoepithelial cells, allowing milk to flow from the alveoli into the ducts and sinuses. Tactile stimulation of the breast has been shown to increase serum prolactin levels.[17] However, whether or not serum prolactin levels correlate to the volume of milk produced is not clear. In the lactating mouse mammary gland, it has been demonstrated that the removal of milk by suckling pups increased prolactin receptor gene expression,[18] which may make cells more sensitive to serum prolactin. On the other hand, there is evidence that the volume of milk produced by the mammary gland may be under local control. Wilde et al.[19] recently isolated and characterized a protein that appears to inhibit milk production. This protein, termed FIL, or feedback inhibition of lactation, is a whey protein with a molecular weight of 7.6 kDa, and is secreted with other milk components into the alveolar lumen. It has been suggested that as milk accumulates in the lumen FIL also accumulates, and if milk is not removed FIL will interact with the alveolar cells by altering their sensitivity to prolactin, thus inhibiting milk synthesis.[19] Therefore, constant removal of milk from the mammary gland will bring on an increase in milk synthesis, and a decrease in emptying will decrease milk synthesis.

The milk volume produced by the mammary gland has been shown to be determined by infant demand.[20,21] A 1930s study by Macy et al.[22] reported wet nurses produced up to 3500 mL of milk per day. Also, mothers of multiple births are capable of producing adequate milk volumes to provide complete nutrition for their breastfed infants.[23] It has been shown that infants are capable of self-regulating their milk intake.[20,21] These studies demonstrate that infants do not empty the breast completely during a single feeding, nor do they empty the breast to the same degree at each feeding. Thus, it is important to realize that the amount of milk in the breast does not determine the amount of milk removed by the infant during a single feed.

CHANGES IN TOTAL PROTEIN AND NITROGEN DURING LACATION

Normal Changes in Generally Well-Nourished Women

Colostrum, or the milk produced by the mother the first few days of lactation, is very high in protein concentration. In part this is due to the low volumes of milk being produced: i.e., the milk is more "concentrated"; but it is also due to high levels of expression of several milk proteins, e.g., immunoglobulins, α-lactalbumin, and lactoferrin. It is also evident that passive transfer of serum proteins (such as serum albumin) is higher during this period; closure of tight junctions will later decrease the influx of these proteins into milk. The total protein concentration has been reported to be as high as 15 mg per mL, whereas mature human milk contains about 7 to 9 mg per mL (Figure 14–2).[2] Concentrations of secretory IgA have been measured to be 2 to 5 mg per mL, while α-lactalbumin and lactoferrin were present in concentrations of 3 to 4 and 3 to 7 mg per mL, respectively. Thus, colostrum levels of these proteins are about twofold higher than in mature milk. It should be noted, however, that gene transcription and translation varies considerably among the milk proteins; the caseins in human milk are absent or very low in concentration in colostrum, and their concentrations do not increase until after several days of lactation (see above). Thus, the developmental pattern for milk protein concentration during lactation is very different for whey proteins and caseins, and the whey-casein ratio, which sometimes is mimicked in infant formula, is not a setnumber (60:40), but varies throughout the lactation period (Figure 14–3).

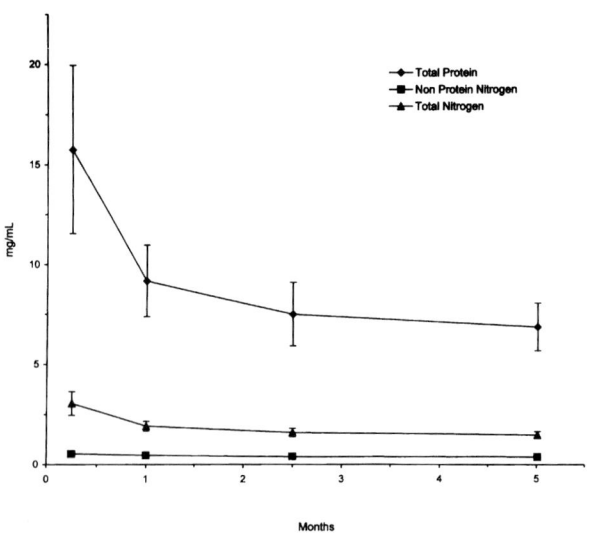

FIGURE 14–2. Concentrations of nitrogen and total protein in human milk during lactation. Data are means ± SD. (Adapted from Lönnerdal B, Forsum E, Hambraeus L. A longitudinal study of the protein, nitrogen, and lactose contents of human milk from Swedish well-nourished mothers. Am J Clin Nutr 1976;29:1127–33.)

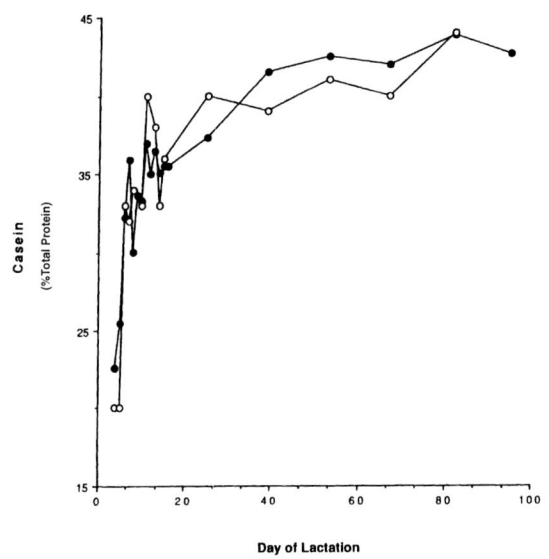

FIGURE 14–3. Changes in whey to casein ratio during lactation in two subjects. (Data from Kunz C, Lönnerdal B. Re-evaluation of the whey protein/casein ratio of human milk. Acta Paediatr 1992;81:107–12.)

The fraction of nonprotein nitrogen (NPN) in colostrum is lower than in mature milk: about 8 to 10% as compared to 20 to 25%. Concentrations of several NPN components (such as urea) are similar, although in colostrum and mature milk the fraction is smaller due to the high total nitrogen concentration of colostrum.

It has long been recognized that the prematurely born infant benefits from being fed breast milk, even if it may be advisable to fortify the milk with some nutrients, e.g., calcium and phosphorus. Many women therefore pump milk at the hospital to provide for their premature infants and then continue to breastfeed them. It has been found that such "preterm" milk contains very high concentrations of proteins; in fact, the concentration is frequently higher than in colostrum and early milk from women delivering at term.[24] The reasons for these high concentrations are not yet known, but a different hormonal profile from that at term, which then affects milk protein gene expression, may be an explanation. The issue of milk volume should also be evaluated. It is possible that the shortened pregnancy has affected mammary gland development, and therefore its capacity for milk synthesis and secretion, thereby affecting milk protein concentrations.

Effect of Maternal Nutrition and Various Conditions on Milk Protein Concentrations

Concern was raised early about the malnourished woman's ability to produce breast milk with adequate concentrations of nutrients to meet the infant's requirements. In particular, protein-calorie malnutrition was considered a risk factor for impaired nutritional quality of breast milk. When reviewing studies on milk protein concentration performed on women with varying degrees of malnutrition, it is often difficult to come to a unifying conclusion;[25] for example, the extent of malnutrition or dietary intake is often inadequately described, the volumes produced (or, rather, consumed by the infant) are rarely measured accurately, and the methods used to analyze protein vary considerably among investigators, all of which can have a pronounced effect on the results.[26] In spite of these shortcomings, it appears that maternal nutritional status and protein intake long-term has very limited or no effect on milk protein concentrations.[25,27] Support for this is obtained from studies on groups of women from similar ethnic backgrounds but with different nutritional status, and from studies on poorly nourished women given dietary supplements. In both types of studies, most investigators do not detect any significant differences in milk protein concentrations. As an example of the first type of study, Lönnerdal et al.[28] showed that concentrations of total nitrogen, NPN, and individual proteins were similar in milk from poorly nourished Ethiopian women and well-nourished women from both Sweden and Ethiopia. As an example of the second type of study, Prentice et al.[29] provided Gambian women with poor nutritional status a daily supplement containing protein and several micronutrients for an extended period, and found a slight increase in milk protein concentrations; however, this result may be attributed to an increase in NPN. Although many studies have supported the notion that protein concentration stays constant, others have observed an effect. From such studies it appears that the degree of malnutrition was quite severe, and that disease or dehydration, for example, may have affected the results. It is also possible that severe malnutrition per se may have a negative effect on milk production and protein synthesis. In such situations, not only a lack of substrate (amino acids), but impaired mammary gland function (transport mechanisms, etc.) may affect milk synthesis and secretion.

The apparent lack of effect of maternal malnutrition on milk volume and composition has raised questions about possible compensatory mechanisms. Lunn et al.[30] noted that poorly nourished Gambian women had significantly higher plasma prolactin concentrations than women in the U.K. When given food supplements, plasma prolactin decreased and became more similar to that of the well-nourished British women. The authors suggested that increased circulating prolactin levels might aid in channeling nutrients to the mammary gland and stimulating milk synthesis. Short-term caloric restriction during lactation does not appear to have any significant effect on milk volume or milk protein concentration.[31] Lactating women voluntarily restricted their food intake during 1 week to an average of 32% less than their regular intake, but not lower than 1500 kcal per day. Infant milk intake was not affected, nor was milk macronutrient composition. The majority of women in the experimental group had increased plasma prolactin concentrations, while most control women experienced a decrease in plasma prolactin, which normally occurs during lactation. Thus, even if this was a short-term study, the results support those of Lunn et al.[31] We have also explored the potential effects of a caloric deficit induced by exercise during lactation, and compared that with dietary restriction of caloric intake.[32,33] In affluent countries, many women are anxious to return to their pre-pregnancy weight, and often reduce their food intake voluntarily and/or start exercise programs. In our first study,[32] we found no effect of increased exercise (~400 kcal/day) during lactation on infant milk intake or milk composition, or on infant growth. The exercising women, however, increased their energy intake to a similar extent, thus compensating for the energy deficit. In a second study,[33] we compared the effects of short-term dietary energy restriction (35% energy deficit) to reduced caloric intake combined with increased energy expenditure through exercise (35% net energy deficit). Both the dietary and the dietary-exercise group lost weight, while the control women did not. There was no effect on milk volume or composition, milk energy output, or infant weight. It appears that short-term rapid weight loss during lactation does not compromise milk composition or yield.

It is important to distinguish between long-term effects on milk volume and composition and more acute effects. In a crossover design, we explored the effects of varying protein intakes on milk protein and nitrogen composition in healthy Swedish women during fully established lactation.[34] Subjects maintained the same energy intake during the study period, but the percentage of calories derived from protein was 8% during the low-protein period (4 days) and 22% during the high-protein period (4 days). Protein and nitrogen concentrations of the milk were significantly higher during the high-protein period than during the low-protein period. Similarly, blood urea nitrogen and milk urea concentrations were elevated in the high-protein group. Individual milk proteins, such as lactoferrin and α-lactalbumin, also increased during the high-protein period as compared to the low-protein period.[35] Although this study was performed on a limited number of subjects, and the difference in protein intake was substantial, it may be prudent for women not to alter their protein intake too dramatically during lactation. It further emphasizes the need to study adaptive mechanisms that regulate milk protein concentrations.

Oral contraceptive agents (OCAs) are commonly used by women during lactation to prevent a subsequent pregnancy. Recommendations regarding this use vary considerably, but generally there is no strict contraindication for use once lactation has been fully established. We investigated the effects of four different OCAs on milk volume and composition in healthy women.[36] Effects on milk volume were observed, and they varied among hormone concentrations or combinations used. Concentrations of several milk proteins were also dramatically affected, with no easily discernible pattern. It is possible that these hormones directly or indirectly affected milk protein gene expression (see above).

In affluent countries, lactating women may encounter an infection, and in developing countries infections are common. We explored the effects of maternal infection during the early postpartum period, as well as during fully-established lactation, in low-income Peruvian women.[37,38] We found no effect on milk volume consumed by the infants, and no effect on total milk protein or concentrations of individual milk proteins during either period, even though acute-phase plasma proteins and plasma trace element concentrations were significantly altered during the infection. Thus, it appears that mammary gland function and milk synthesis are unaffected by maternal acute infection, regardless of whether it occurs during initiation of lactation or after lactation has been fully established. However, the effects of chronic infection remain to be studied.

CHANGES IN INDIVIDUAL MILK PROTEINS DURING LACTATION

Breast milk is composed of vitamins, minerals, fat, carbohydrates, and proteins that provide optimum nutrition for breastfed infants. Proteins in milk are either synthesized by cells in the mammary gland or are transported directly from plasma to milk. The majority of the milk proteins are localized in the whey fraction (50 to 90%),[3] while somewhat lower amounts are found in the caseins; small amounts are bound to cells in the milk and in fat globule membranes (1 to 3%).[39] It has been found that concentrations of some human milk proteins vary considerably throughout lactation. In early lactation whey proteins predominate, while casein concentration is low; however, caseins become a larger part of mature milk, and as lactation progresses the whey-casein ratio approaches 50:50.[3] The varying concentrations of individual human milk proteins throughout lactation may either be a direct influence of hormones and/or maternal nutrition. The definite mechanisms regulating the temporal patterns remain to be elucidated. Such information will be useful when evaluating biologic functions of human milk proteins during infancy (Table 14–2).

Caseins

Human milk contains aggregates of casein protein subunits, calcium phosphate, and other ionic constituents in the form of micelles to give milk its characteristic white color. Caseins represent the major class of proteins in many species; however, this is not the case with human milk.

TABLE 14-2
Biologic Functions of Human Milk Proteins

Protein	Biologic Function
α-Casein	Inhibitor of angiotensin converting enzyme
β-Casein	Opioid activity; facilitates absorption of calcium
κ-Casein	Antibacterial properties
α-Lactalbumin	Lactose synthesis
Lactoferrin	Iron-binding protein; bacteriostatic/bactericidal properties; growth factor (?)
Immunoglobulins (sIgA, IgA, IgG, IgM)	Antibodies
Serum albumin	Source of amino acids
Lysozyme	Bactericidal properties
α-Amylase	Hydrolysis of poly- and oligosaccharides
$α_1$-Antitrypsin	Protection of milk proteins during digestion
Bile salt-stimulated lipase	Lipid digestion
Lacto- and myeloperoxidase	Bactericidal properties
Haptocorrin	Vitamin B_{12}-binding protein; facilitates absorption of B_{12} (?)
Folate-binding protein	Facilitates absorption of folate (?)
Insulin-like growth factors (IGF-I, IGF-II)	Growth factors; development of infant small intestine (?)
Epidermal growth factor (EGF)	
IGF-binding protein	Protects IGF (?)

Whereas cow's milk contains 80% caseins, caseins of human milk comprise 20 to 40% of the total protein. Based on their electrophoretic mobility, casein subunits are classified into α-, β-, and κ-casein.[40] In human milk, the major casein subunit is β-casein, while κ-casein is a minor component. Cow's milk contains both β-, and κ-casein, as well as α-casein, a subunit that was believed to be absent in human milk. Recently, however, $α_{S1}$-casein was isolated and characterized from human milk.[41] Its concentration is very low and is not more than 1 to 2% of total casein.

Casein micelles in human milk are smaller in size (30 to 75 nm) than bovine micelles (600 nm).[42] The differences in their size may be attributed to: a higher permeability of the lacteal ducts of the bovine mammary gland, allowing passage of larger micelles; the electrostatic forces within the micelle; or the composition of the casein micelle. In addition, post-translational modification is important in casein micelle formation.

The casein concentration is low in human colostrum, but increases markedly in early lactation, and then gradually decreases throughout the course of lactation. In mature milk, the concentration of casein is around 3.3 to 4.5 mg per mL.[3,43] Beta- and κ-casein subunits have different developmental patterns throughout lactation.[44] In early lactation, β-casein predominates (70 to 90% of all caseins is β-casein at this time); however, later in lactation, the concentration of κ-casein increases. This pattern may be due to changes in glycosylation and phosphorylation of the κ- and β-casein subunits, respectively, suggesting that not only are β- and κ-casein regulated differently at the transcription level, but also at the post-translational modification level.[44]

Beta-casein is a phosphorylated protein with a molecular weight of 24 kDa. Its amino acid sequence has been determined,[45] and the gene for the human β-casein,[46] as well as the β-casein genes of rats, mice, cows, goats, and sheep,[47] have been cloned and sequenced. There appear to be species differences in the β-casein gene; however, regions of conserved sequences have been found, particularly at the N-terminus, where the sites of phosphorylation are located. The phosphate groups in human β-casein are present as phosphothreonine and phosphoserine.

Human κ-casein is a glycoprotein with charged sialic acid residues. It has a molecular weight of 37 kDa, of which about 19 kDa is carbohydrate.[48] In comparison to bovine κ-casein, human κ-casein contains 40 to 60% carbohydrate, while bovine κ-casein contains only 10%.[49] Although the purification and characterization of κ-casein has proven a difficult task, largely due to its low concentration in human milk and its susceptibility to proteolysis, the human κ-casein cDNA has been cloned and sequenced, and the amino acid sequence has been deduced.[50]

Studies on the biologic function of human milk caseins have been limited due to difficulties in isolating and purifying sufficient quantities of the proteins. Caseins have been shown to provide a limited amount of calcium, phosphorus, and amino acids to the newborn infant in comparison to the total amount supplied. Therefore, caseins may have other physiologic functions. Peptides resulting from the proteolysis of human β-casein have been shown to contain N-terminal fragments containing phosphorylated amino acid residues, called casein phosphopeptides or CPP. Not only have CPP been shown to keep calcium in soluble form, but also to facilitate calcium uptake in the rat intestinal tract.[51] Other peptides resulting from the proteolytic degradation of human β-casein have been shown to possess opioid activities. These peptides have an affinity for opiate receptors and exhibit opiate-like effects.[52] Various casomorphins have been produced in vitro, and their effects have been demonstrated in isolated cells and experimental animals.[52–54] On the other hand, several peptides have demonstrated antiopioid characteristics. These peptides have been shown to disrupt sleeping and behavior patterns, modulate insulin and somatostatin activity, and affect pancreatic polypeptide release.[55] Another peptide has been identified that specifically inhibits angiotensin-converting enzyme activity, thus decreasing the production of angiotensin II in endothelial cells.[56]

It also appears likely that κ-casein can prevent attachment of bacteria to the mucosal lining by acting as a receptor analog.[57] The glycan of κ-casein has a structure similar to that of surface-exposed carbohydrates of cells in the GI tract, and it may therefore serve as a soluble "decoy" for pathogens. For example, we have been able to demonstrate that human milk κ-casein can inhibit the adhesion of *Helicobacter pylori* to human gastric mucosa.[58] Thus, κ-casein may be one component of the defense against infection provided by breast milk.

α-Lactalbumin

α-Lactalbumin is a major whey protein in milk of most species. In human milk, α-lactalbumin accounts for 10 to 20% of total protein and therefore supplies a significant amount of amino acids to the breastfed infant. It has a molecular weight of 14.1 kDa, and consists of a single polypeptide chain of 123 amino acids, with no carbohydrate moieties or phosphate groups.[59] It binds calcium in a 1:1 molar ratio, which changes its Stokes' radius, thus making the molecule more compact.[60] Although it is possible that α-lactalbumin performs its physiologic function in this compacted state, it is highly unlikely that it has any significant role in calcium transport or absorption, since only about 1% of human milk calcium is associated with the protein.[60]

The primary function of α-lactalbumin in human milk is its role in lactose synthesis in the mammary gland. The protein has been shown to be a part of lactose synthase, a Golgi enzyme complex that catalyzes the formation of lactose in the mammary gland. Lactose synthase consists of two proteins, α-lactalbumin and galactosyltransferase, that together catalyze the binding of glucose to UDP-galactose.[61] Since the K_m of galactosyltransferase for glucose is very high (~1M), α-lactalbumin increases the affinity of galactosyltransferase for glucose by reducing the K_m (~1mM), so that lactose synthesis can occur at physiologic conditions. Galactosyltransferase is found in many tissues, but it is the association of α-lactalbumin that makes this mammary enzyme unique.

The overall concentration of α-lactalbumin in human milk is around 2 to 4 mg per mL[2,26,60,62] (Figure 14–4). The concentration of α-lactalbumin in colostrum is around 4 mg per mL; then it decreases slightly in transitional milk to 3 mg per mL, and stays relatively constant at 2 to 3 mg per mL throughout lactation.[26,62,63] Since α-lactalbumin is involved in lactose synthesis, it has been proposed that lactose concentrations should be directly proportional to α-lactalbumin concentrations; however, an inverse relationship has been observed, suggesting that α-lactalbumin may not be a limiting factor in the synthesis of lactose.[63]

Lactoferrin

Lactoferrin, an iron-binding protein in human milk, was first described by Johansson.[64] It is an 80-kDa glycoprotein and consists of 703 amino acids. The protein consists of two separate globular lobes that are connected via an α-helix. Each lobe binds one iron atom, and the iron atoms are coordinated to four ligands: one histidine, one aspartate, and two tyrosines.

Lactoferrin is present in many body fluids, such as saliva, tears, and pancreatic juice; however, the concentration of the protein is much higher in human milk. Consequently, the potential biologic function of lactoferrin in milk has received much attention. One possible function of lactoferrin in human milk is in iron absorption, due to its high affinity for iron.[65] On a molar basis, there is much more lactoferrin than iron in human milk, but only 3 to 5% of the iron-binding capacity of lactoferrin is used.[66] Iron absorption from breast milk is considerably higher than from cow's milk or infant formula.[67] Cox et al.[65] suggested the presence of lactoferrin receptors in the jejunum, and Kawakami et al. found receptors in the infant small intestine that are specific for human lactoferrin.[68] The presence of receptors, as well as the presence of intact lactoferrin in the stool of breastfed infants,[69] support a physiologic role for human milk lactoferrin in the infant gut. Another potential function of lactoferrin is its antimicrobial effects. Since lactoferrin has a high affinity for iron, it may withhold iron from iron-requiring pathogens. It has also been shown that lactoferrin has bactericidal activity against several pathogens, and that this activity does not depend on its degree of iron saturation.[70,71] Several studies have shown these effects in vitro; however, in vivo studies have been lacking. Analysis of stool samples from infants fed formula with or without supplemental

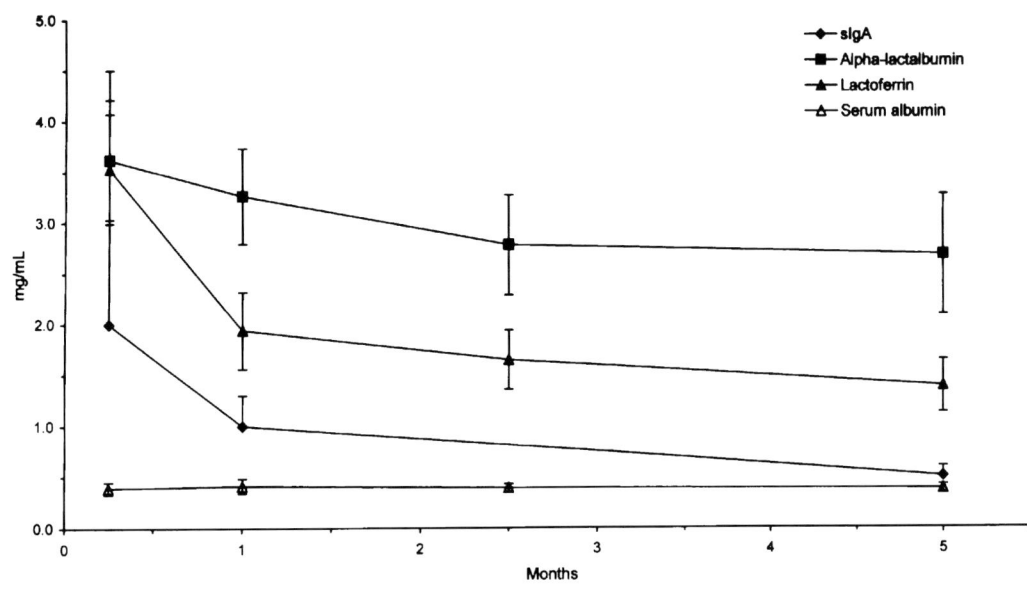

FIGURE 14–4. Concentrations of major whey proteins in human milk throughout lactation. Data are means ± SD. (Adapted from Goldman and Goldblum[1] and Lönnerdal et al.[2])

bovine lactoferrin did not show a significant effect on the gut microflora.[72] This may be due to the fact that bovine lactoferrin is not as efficient as human lactoferrin. However, Tomita et al.[73] showed a non-iron-containing fragment of bovine lactoferrin, called lactoferricin, that kills certain types of bacteria. A similar peptide has also been isolated from human lactoferrin. To what extent these peptides are formed in vivo remains to be elucidated.

The concentration of lactoferrin in colostrum ranges from 3 to 7 mg per mL; it then decreases during the first 12 weeks of lactation,[74] when it levels off to around 1 to 2 mg per mL[26,43,62,63,74] (Figure 14–4). Lactoferrin represents ~30% of total protein in colostrum, and decreases to ~20% in mature milk.[62]

Immunoglobulins

Human milk consists of many immunologic factors that protect the breastfed infant from infections. Human colostrum is rich in immunoglobulins[74] as well as immune cells, predominantly T cells.[75] The concentration of immunoglobulins decreases after the first day of lactation; however, they constitute a major part of the total protein throughout lactation. Approximately 90% of the total immunoglobulins in milk is secretory IgA (sIgA),[74] while other immunoglobulins, such as monomeric IgA, IgG, and IgM, are present, but in lower concentrations. Consequently most research efforts have concentrated on sIgA rather than on any of the other immunoglobulins.

Secretory IgA molecules in milk that are specific against bacterial and viral antigens arise from an enteromammary immune pathway. Briefly, antigens enter the mucosa of the maternal gut and are taken up by M cells on the surface of Peyer's patches. The antigens are passed on to underlying lymphoid tissue, where they stimulate lymphoblasts. The lymphoblasts enter the lymphatic system, and are then transported to the mammary gland, where they are transformed into plasma cells. These plasma cells synthesize sIgA by covalently linking two molecules of monomeric IgA with two other proteins: a joining chain (J chain) and a secretory component (SC).[76] The resulting molecular weight of the complete sIgA molecule is ~420 kDa. When the infant receives sIgA from breast milk, the infant will receive a portion of the maternal immune defense system. In addition, since sIgA in human milk is resistant to proteolytic degradation,[77] it survives the passage through the immunologically immature GI tract of the breastfed infant.[69] In the infant gut, the sIgA binds to the bacterial and viral antigens that the mother was once exposed to, thereby preventing the attachment of these microorganisms to the mucosal lining and inhibiting their colonization. Secretory IgA, together with lactoferrin, lysozyme, and other immune factors found in human milk, has been implicated to decrease the incidence of infections in breastfed infants.[78]

Similar to lactoferrin, the concentration of sIgA is fairly high in colostrum (2 to 5 mg per mL), but decreases rapidly during the first few days of lactation, and levels off to approximately 0.5 to 1.0 mg per mL[26,43,74] (see Figure 14–4). The initial high concentration of these host defense factors during the first days of lactation may reflect its importance during early neonatal life in preventing infections and maintaining a beneficial intestinal microflora.

Both IgG and IgM are present in mature human milk at very low concentrations.[2] Although the major immunoglobulin in human serum is IgG, the relative proportion of its subclass, IgG_4, is higher in human milk than in serum.[79] Therefore, it has been suggested that IgG_4 is either produced by the mammary gland or transported to it. Another explanation may be a more efficient exclusion of other IgG subclasses from human milk. In contrast to serum IgM, human milk IgM is complexed to the secretory component.[80] Both IgG and IgM concentrations are high in early lactation (0.3 to 0.7 mg per mL and 0.1 to 0.6 mg per mL, respectively) but they decrease rapidly to 0.03 to 0.1 mg/mL and 0.02 to 0.2 mg/mL, respectively, after the first month of lactation.[1,2,63,81]

Serum Albumin

Serum albumin is a major serum protein also found in human milk. Since serum albumin in milk is identical in properties to that in the blood, and its level is relatively constant throughout lactation, it has been proposed that the protein may not be synthesized by the mammary gland, but rather transferred from maternal circulation: either by an endocytotic mechanism or leaky junctions between the mammary epithelial cells. No significant physiologic function has been established for this protein besides being a source of amino acids for the breastfed infant. In blood, serum albumin has been found to bind many ligands, such as fatty acids, trace elements, calcium, hormones, and drugs. In milk, zinc, copper,[82] and thyroxine[83] have been found to be associated with serum albumin. However, the relative amount of this ligand-associated protein that is present in breast milk remains unknown. Therefore, it is not likely that serum albumin plays a major role as a nutrient binder or supplier of nutrients for the breastfed infant, since the association constants for many of these ligands are weak, and binding would not persist in the infant gut.[84]

Serum concentration is normally around 35 to 50 mg per mL; however, the concentration of serum albumin in colostrum ranges only from 0.4 to 1.0 mg per mL and stays relatively constant throughout lactation[2,26,43,62,63] (see Figure 14–4).

Lysozyme

Lysozyme is a 15-kDa protein present in human milk at concentrations higher than in milk of most other species.[85] Through N-terminal sequencing and immunochemical studies, human milk lysozyme appears identical to the lysozyme found in other body fluids, such as saliva, pancreatic juice, and leukocytes.[86] It is unclear whether lysozyme is synthesized by the mammary gland or transferred from the maternal circulation. Lysozyme has the capability of destroying the cell walls of bacteria by catalyzing the hydrolysis of β-1,4 linkages of N-acetylmuramic acid and 2-acetylamino-2-deoxy-D-glucose residues.[87] Lysozyme alone is capable of killing several gram-positive bacteria; however, recent findings show that lysozyme and lactoferrin can work synergistically to produce bactericidal effects on gram-negative bacteria.[88] By binding lipopolysaccharide (LPS), lactoferrin disrupts the outer bacterial membrane, thereby allowing lysozyme access to the inner proteoglycan matrix. Like other host defense factors, such as lactoferrin and sIgA, lysozyme is relatively resistant to proteolytic degradation. Therefore, it is possible that lysozyme can participate in the defense against bacterial colonization in the infant GI tract, and at the same time maintain a microbial flora native to the infant gut. Lysozyme in colostrum and mature milk ranges from 0.07 to 0.3 mg per mL.[26,62,74,81]

α-Amylase

Digestion of poly- and oligosaccharides not present in milk, such as starch and glycogen, is achieved by the action of α-amylase. α-Amylase, an enzyme with a molecular weight of ~60 kDa,[89] catalyzes the hydrolyses of carbohydrates by a random cleavage of α-D-1,4 glucan linkages to produce maltose, small-chain dextrins, and some glucose. The presence of amylase in human milk has long been recognized, and has been found identical to the salivary isozyme.[89,90] Little or no α-amylase activity has been detected in cow's milk compared to human milk.[91] It has been suggested that the mammary gland synthesizes α-amylase, since the pancreatic isozyme is present in plasma, but not in milk.[89] Not only does human milk α-amylase have a wide pH optimum of 4.5 to 7.5 and retains its activity even at pH 3.0, but it is also relatively stable to peptic degradation.[92] Therefore, α-amylase most likely survives passage through the stomach and remains active in the newborn intestine.[90] The presence of α-amylase in human milk may compensate for the low salivary and pancreatic amylase activity in the newborn infant and aid in carbohydrate digestion.[90] This may be of particular importance for premature infants, as preterm milk has an especially high activity of α-amylase.[91] In addition, infant formulas, which are often used as a supplemental food, contain starch and other oligosaccharides that may not be completely digested by the low concentration of endogenous amylase. Another biologic function of human milk α-amylase may be its potential antibacterial effect. *Neisseria gonorrhoeae* has been shown to be inhibited by salivary amylase in vivo,[93] and because milk amylase has been shown to be of the salivary-type isoamylases, it may inhibit the growth of other microorganisms by attacking the polysaccharides of the bacterial cell wall.

The α-amylase activity is highest in colostrum when the infant's salivary and pancreatic fluid amylase content is at its lowest; it then decreases throughout lactation.[89] The activity in colostrum is ~8000 U per L; it then decreases to 5800 U per L between days 15 and 90, and even lower beyond 90 days (1300 U per L).[90]

α₁-Antitrypsin

α₁-Antitrypsin has been identified in human milk[94] and has also been shown to be present in colostrum of pigs[95,96] and rats.[97] Its physiologic function is not clear, but it may act on the mammary gland as well as in the infant GI tract. α₁-Antitrypsin may protect the mammary gland from the proteolytic activity of leukocytic and lysosomal proteases during stages of differentiation of the mammary gland, and/or prevent the degradation of other enzymes and proteins in milk during mastitis.[98] Another proposed function is the protection of milk proteins from hydrolysis in the infant gut.[94,98] Since the gastric pH of newborns is high, milk α₁-antitrypsin can remain immunologically intact and biologically active in the infant intestine.[99] Also, the concentration of α₁-antitrypsin present in colostrum may inactivate the low amounts of pancreatic trypsin secreted by the newborn, thus preventing milk proteins from proteolytic degradation. The concentration of α₁-antitrypsin is around 0.2 to 0.6 mg per mL in colostrum, then rapidly decreases to 0.01 to 0.09 mg per mL in mature milk.[81,90,99]

Bile Salt–Stimulated Lipase

The high digestibility of lipids in breastfed infants has been documented.[100] The presence of a lipase in human milk that is stimulated by bile salts has been found to be part of this efficient lipid digestion.[101] Bile salt-stimulated lipase (BSSL), a glycoprotein with a molecular weight of 125 kDa, has been shown to be expressed by the human mammary gland,[102] and it has been cloned and sequenced.[103] This enzyme is identical to the pancreatic carboxylic ester hydrolase, and it therefore has been proposed that the two enzymes may be coded for by a common gene.[103] Its pH optimum is between 7.4 and 8.5, and it is stable at a pH as low as 3.0.[98]

Since endogenous lipid digestive function is immature in newborn infants, the biologic role of BSSL is of importance. Results from in vitro studies suggest that the enzyme remains active in the GI tract of infants, and that therefore BSSL contributes significantly to lipid digestion and absorption.[104,105] One reason for the high efficiency of BSSL in lipid digestion in human milk is that it has been found to have wide substrate specificity. When BSSL becomes activated by bile salts in the duodenum, it hydrolyzes mono-, di-, and triacylglycerols, cholesteryl esters, retinyl esters, and diacylphosphatidylglycerols, as well as micellar and water-soluble substrates.[104] Bile salt-stimulated lipase does not possess positional specificity; fatty acids esterified in *sn-1* and *sn-3* positions are hydrolyzed at the same rate, and fatty acids esterified in the *sn-2* position of triacylglycerols are also hydrolyzed. Also, BSSL does not discriminate between fatty acids with regard to the positioning of double bonds.[106]

The concentration of BSSL in human milk is approximately 0.1 mg per mL.[104] High activities of BSSL have been shown to be present in human milk,[107] and stay constant throughout lactation.[108] Preterm colostrum has a significantly higher activity than term colostrum, suggesting that preterm colostrum has a higher lipid digesting capability than colostrum from women delivering at term.[109]

Peroxidases

Gothefors and Marklund first demonstrated peroxidase activity in human milk.[110] They found that peroxidase activity is highest in colostrum, and then decreases during the first 2 weeks. Controversy has surrounded the source of peroxidase activity. Studies by Moldoveanu et al.[111] in 1982 showed that the peroxidase activity in human milk did not originate from a true secretory peroxidase (lactoperoxidase), but was derived from milk leukocytes (myeloperoxidase). In support of Moldoveanu's findings, the results of Hashinaka and Yamada in 1986[112] indicated that the peroxidase activity in human colostrum is identical to myeloperoxidase. On the other hand, in 1984, Langbakk and Flatmark[113] supported the presence of lactoperoxidase by partially purifying the enzyme from human colostrum. They also found that lactoperoxidase in human colostrum is quite stable at low pH (4.6) and at high ionic strengths (2M sodium acetate): characteristics similar to bovine lactoperoxidase, and conditions myeloperoxidase cannot tolerate. In 1989, Langbakk and Flatmark[114] confirmed that the peroxidase activity in human colostrum was indeed from lactoperoxidase. However, in 1991 Pruitt et al.[115] reported that colostrum contains peroxidase activity contributed by both lactoperoxidase and myeloperoxidase. It has been suggested that the reason for the conflicting reports is due to differences in the sensitivity and specificity of the techniques used.[115]

Lactoperoxidase, together with hydrogen peroxide, catalyzes the oxidation of thiocyanate ions to produce reactive products with antibacterial properties capable of destroying both gram-positive[116] and gram-negative bacteria[117] in vitro. Myeloperoxidase catalyzes the reaction of chloride ions, and like lactoperoxidase produces products with antibacterial activity. Also, it has been suggested that these peroxidases protect the mammary gland from the accumulation of hydrogen peroxide.[115] Variability in peroxidase activity between donors has been observed;[110,113] however, there is general agreement that peroxidase activity is highest in colostrum, and that it decreases to very low levels in mature milk. Although it is unclear whether the peroxidase activity originates from lactoperoxidase, myeloperoxidase, or both, lactoperoxidase activity has been detected in mature milk (Shin and Lönnerdal, unpublished observations). Myeloperoxidase in colostrum has been reported to have an activity of 5 to 10 U per mL,[112] and lactoperoxidase in colostrum was found to have 0 to 12.6 mU per mL.[113] Since the concentration of peroxidase in mature milk is very low,[115] perhaps the bactericidal properties are effective only in early lactation.[84]

Haptocorrin

Vitamin B_{12}, or cobalamin, is present in human milk bound to a vitamin B_{12}-binder, called haptocorrin (Hc).[118] Haptocorrin is a highly glycosylated protein; about 34% of its molecular weight consists of carbohydrates.[119] It has an approximate molecular weight of 63 kDa as determined by amino acid composition and carbohydrate residues, and in the range of 72 to 121 kDa and 120 to 150 kDa by SDS-polyacrylamide gel electrophoresis (SDS-PAGE) and gel filtration, respectively.[120] Transcobalamin II, another vitamin B_{12}-binding protein, is also present in human milk, but its concentration is negligible in comparison to haptocorrin.

Besides having a high affinity for vitamin B_{12}, the exact function of Hc in human milk is not well known. A bacteriostatic function has been proposed: it may withhold vitamin B_{12} from vitamin B_{12}-requiring microorganisms in the GI tract of breastfed infants, thereby regulating the growth of normal intestinal flora.[121] It has also been suggested that human milk Hc may facilitate the absorption of vitamin B_{12} during the neonatal period, when the GI tract of the newborn is immature.[122,123] In vitro experiments, using brushborder membrane vesicles prepared from piglet small intestine and Hc isolated from sow's milk, demonstrated a direct effect of milk Hc on vitamin B_{12} absorption.[122] In addition, Hc resisted proteolytic degradation in an in vivo study using suckling piglets.[124] Suckling piglets consistently absorbed and retained a higher dose of vitamin B_{12}-bound Hc than did piglets receiving a diet without Hc. Also, the amount of vitamin B_{12} absorbed in 21-day-old suckling piglets did not differ from early-weaned piglets, suggesting that intrinsic factor (another vitamin B_{12} binding protein secreted by the mature stomach) was being actively secreted by the 21-day-old piglets.[125] Human studies to describe similar effects of Hc are lacking.

The exact concentration of Hc in human milk remains to be determined due to a limitation of techniques; however, vitamin B_{12}-binding capacity in human milk has been determined. Human colostrum has a vitamin B_{12}-binding capacity of around 50 nmol per L. It then decreases to approximately 30 nmol per L in transitional milk, and then stays relatively constant throughout the rest of lactation.[126,127] Thus, vitamin B_{12}-binding capacity of human colostrum has been found to be highly unsaturated while it is less so in mature milk.[126] Similar results were obtained by Gullberg in a study of five samples.[121] In contrast, Trugo et al. in a longitudinal study showed an increase in vitamin B_{12}-binding capacity throughout lactation.[127] These conflicting results may be attributed to high variability between individual subjects as well as differences in assay methods.

Folate-Binding Protein

The folate-binding protein (FBP) was first identified in human milk by Ford et al.[128] Since then, human milk has been found to contain both particulate and soluble FBP. The soluble form, found in whey, has been purified and characterized, as well as the particulate (membrane-bound) form.[129] The soluble FBP has been shown to have a molecular weight of 40 kDa by SDS-PAGE and gel filtration and is glycosylated to about 22%. The solubilized membrane-bound form has a lower carbohydrate content (9%), and a similar molecular weight, of approximately 45 kDa, as judged by SDS-PAGE; however, analysis by gel filtration shows a molecular weight of 160 kDa.[129]

The physiologic significance of the FBPs in milk is that they may facilitate the uptake of folate in the gut. Folate-binding proteins have been shown to survive low gastric pH and resist proteolysis in newborn goats. In addition, Salter and Mowlem found functionally active FBPs present in small intestinal aspirates.[130] Experiments using rat intestinal cells found that uptake of folate was higher when it was complexed to FBP than in the free form.[131] On the other hand, Said et al.[132] suggested that the FBP may actually slow the release and uptake of folate in the small intestine to allow a gradual release and absorption of folate that may increase tissue use. Another function, proposed by Ford et al.,[128] is that the binding protein may "trap" folate from blood plasma in the mammary gland to ensure the transfer of the vitamin into milk. This hypothesis is supported by Selhub et al.,[133] who showed that human milk folate concentrations correlate with the concentration of FBP.

The concentration of FBP in human milk, expressed as folate-binding capacity, has been shown to vary considerably not only between individuals, but also between fore- and hindmilk.[133] Folate-binding capacity ranges from 170 to 200 nmol per L early in lactation, and decreases slightly to 120 to 180 nmol per L in mature milk.[133,134]

Growth Factors

Insulin-like growth factors I and II (IGF-I and IGF–II) and epidermal growth factor (EGF) are factors present in human milk that have been shown to promote the growth of various cells in culture and to stimulate DNA synthesis.[135–137] They have also been shown to promote the development of the neonatal GI tract.[138–140] The source of the growth factors in human milk has yet to be elucidated; they may either be synthesized by the mammary gland, or transferred from maternal circulation and subsequently secreted by the mammary gland. Insulin-like growth factors I and II are polypeptides with a molecular weight of approximately 7.5 kDa, and are functionally and structurally similar to insulin; they have a 70% and 50% overall amino acid homology to proinsulin, respectively.[141] The IGF-I concentration in human colostrum is approximately 10 ng per mL and between 2 and 20 ng per mL in mature milk.[136,142] The wide range in milk is attributed to differences in analytical methods used. Insulin-like growth factor II concentrations in colostrum have not been reported; however, mature milk (3 to 16 months) has been determined to contain an average of 3 ng per mL.[142]

Epidermal growth factor is a polypeptide that contains 53 amino acids with an approximate molecular weight of 6 kDa. The hypothesis that EGF stimulates gut proliferation and maturation of the neonate is supported by the fact that EGF receptors have been identified in the human fetal small intestine and colon.[143] Jansson et al.[144] found higher growth-promoting activity in colostrum than in mature milk. Human colostrum contains between 25 and 40 ng per mL of EGF,[144–146] and the concentration decreases to an average of 10 ng per mL in mature milk.

The IGFs in milk have been found to be associated with IGF-binding proteins (IGFBPs). Of the six known IGFBPs, three have been identified in human milk.[136,142] Insulin-like growth factor-binding protein-1 and IGFBP-2 are nonglycosylated, low molecular-weight proteins (25 kDa and 31 kDa, respectively).[142] Insulin-like growth factor-binding protein-3 has been cloned and sequenced, and has a core molecular weight of 29 kDa with three glycosylation sites.[147] The role of IGFBPs in milk has yet to be established. It is possible they have a function similar to serum IGFBP, which has been shown to protect circulating IGFs from degradation, thereby increasing their half-life. Insulin-like growth factor-binding proteins may also modulate the interaction of IGFs with their cellular receptors. Concentration of IGFBP-1 in human colostrum is between 90 and 245 ng per mL, but decreases to 30 to 170 ng per mL in mature milk.[148]

PROTEIN DIGESTIBILITY

Development of Digestive Function

During the first several months of life, pepsin secretion is considerably lower than in children and adults.[149] Further, gastric acid output is low, which results in a comparatively high pH in the stomach, further limiting pepsin activity. At 4 to 6 months of age, pepsin activity is considerably lower than during childhood, and much lower than in adult life. Further, gastric acid output is also much lower than later in life, which results in a comparatively high pH in the stomach, further limiting pepsin activity. It has been shown that the gastric pH of infants after a meal often is around 4 to 5, which will result in little or no pepsin activity. Less is known about pancreatic enzyme output in early life, but it appears that protein digestion is more effective in the duodenum than in the stomach. Also the transit time is very short during infancy, further limiting the capacity to break down proteins. It is therefore important to use infant animal models when assessing protein digestibility in vivo and realistic conditions (mimicking those in infants) in in vitro assay systems. Finally, human milk contains inhibitors of proteolytic enzymes (see above). For example, we have found substantial concentrations of α_1-antitrypsin in human milk;[99] thus, the presence of α_1-antitrypsin in the stool of healthy breastfed infants should not be viewed as an indicator of enteric protein loss, but rather as a remnant of undigested milk proteins (see below).

In Vitro versus In Vivo Digestibility

It is inherently difficult to directly assess protein digestibility in infants. Although qualitative information on the digestive fate of individual proteins may be obtainable from gastric, duodenal, and jejunal aspirates, it is difficult to perform such studies on a longitudinal basis in healthy newborns. Quantitative data are even more difficult to collect. We have used an indirect approach to circumvent this problem. Milk intake was registered, milk samples were analyzed, and fecal samples collected quantitatively from exclusively breastfed infants.[69] Similar studies were performed on preterm infants fed breast milk with or without "preterm formula."[150] Milk proteins and proteins extracted from the stool samples were assayed by immunologic methods. We found significant amounts of sIgA, lactoferrin, and α_1-antitrypsin in the fecal samples up to at least 4 to 5 months of age. In particular, high amounts of sIgA were detected: during the first week of life up to 1 g per day, while ~0.5 g per day was found thereafter. This corresponds to up to ~50% of the ingested sIgA. Smaller amounts of lactoferrin were found intact, but even at 4 months of age ~10 mg per day could be detected (Figure 14–5). This indicates that even if lactoferrin is relatively protected against proteolysis, it is not as stable as sIgA, and about 80 to 90% is digested by the time it is found in the stool. It is still possible, however, that lactoferrin exerts biologic function(s) in the upper gut and subsequently becomes digested. For example, we have shown that lactoferrin is taken up by CaCo-2 cells and then degraded intracellularly (unpublished observations). That the lactoferrin found in the stool is not of endogenous

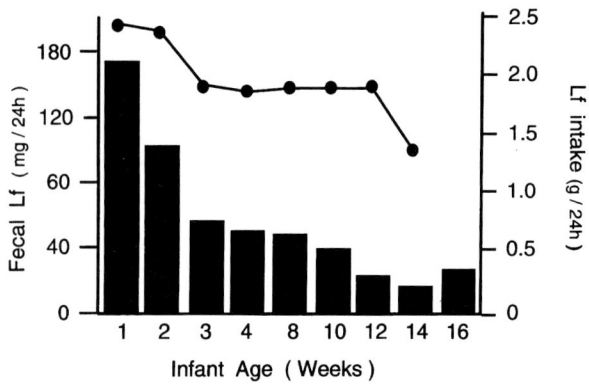

FIGURE 14–5. Lactoferrin intake and excretion by exclusively breastfed infants. (Data from Davidson LA, Lönnerdal B. Persistence of human milk protein in the breastfed infant. Acta Paediatr Scand 1987;76:733–40.)

origin (e.g., bile, pancreatic fluid) was demonstrated by Spik et al.[151] who only found very small amounts (0.5 mg per day) of human lactoferrin in the stool of formula-fed infants.

In a subsequent study on low-birth-weight infants,[150] we found that about 5% of ingested lactoferrin was found in the stool, whereas 24% of sIgA was intact. In these infants, it is possible that proteins are absorbed intact to some extent, possibly explaining the somewhat lower recovery of sIgA as compared to older term infants. That protein digestion is somewhat less effective is indicated by the finding of both lysozyme and serum albumin (which are present in human milk) in the stool of these infants; those proteins were not detected in the stool of term infants. Readily digested milk proteins, however, may be degraded more effectively. For instance, α-lactalbumin, which is a major milk protein, was not detected in the stool samples.

These studies on "survivability" of breast milk proteins do not provide quantitative information on protein digestibility. Darragh and Moughan[152] compared apparent fecal digestibility of proteins in milk formula in 3-month-old infants and compared it to 3-week-old piglets. They found that total nitrogen digestibility was high at this age and was about 94%. Similar results were found in the piglet, suggesting that this may be a good model for studying protein digestion in human infants of this age, but most likely not for newborn infants. This apparent nitrogen digestibility is higher than the 87 to 90% described in other studies.[153,154] The discrepancy may be due to different designs (outpatient versus inpatient), age of the infants, or methodologic differences. It should also be recognized that a considerable part of nitrogen in most infant formulas consists of NPN;[155] thus, protein digestibility may be substantially lower. Since breast milk contains several proteins that are relatively resistant against proteolysis, protein digestibility may, in fact, be lower than for formula proteins.

Most studies on digestibility of proteins in milk formula do not describe the composition of the protein and nitrogen (casein-whey ratio, NPN, etc.), or the extent of heat treatment the formula had been exposed to. We have shown in an in vitro study that these factors need to be considered carefully when assessing protein quality and digestibility.[156] The conditions for the in vitro were chosen to mimic protein digestion in infants.[157,158] Samples were digested with pepsin at pH 4.5 for 30 minutes and with pancreatic enzymes at pH 7.0 for 1 hour. Protein digestibility varied between 69% and 84%. When powdered and liquid "in-can" sterilized formulas of the same brand were compared, protein digestibility and available lysine were always higher for the powdered products. The highest digestibility was observed for a UHT (ultra-high temperature treatment for a very short time) formula. Thus, it appears that protein digestibility decreases with the extent of heat treatment.

We have also assessed protein digestibility of proteins in human milk, human milk fortifiers, and "preterm" formula.[159] Since gastric proteolysis is minimal in preterm infants, we subjected the samples to digestion with duodenal juice from healthy preterm infants. We found that casein was most rapidly degraded in all products. Human and bovine whey proteins were more slowly digested; as much as 68% of human lactoferrin was still immunoreactive after a 40 minute digestion, and 24 to 69% of bovine serum albumin, 20 to 40% of β-lactoglobulin, 20 to 50% of bovine α-lactalbumin, and 41% of human α-lactalbumin. Contrary to common belief, digestibility of bovine whey proteins decreased with the degree of denaturation of the proteins. These results suggest that preterm infants may have a limited capacity to digest bovine whey proteins and that the protein sources of human milk fortifiers may be improved to increase their use.

MILK PROTEIN INTAKE VERSUS PROTEIN REQUIREMENTS OF INFANTS

Breastfed Infants

When comparing the protein intake of breastfed infants to the estimated protein requirement of infants, it is evident that their protein intake is considerably lower (Table 14–3). This has led to the suggestion that the protein intake of breastfed infants may not be optimal,[160] and that, possibly, the differences in growth pattern observed between breastfed and formula-fed infants may be due to inadequate protein intake in breastfed infants. However, although the growth patterns of breastfed and formula-fed infants are different, there is little evidence of breastfed infants not meeting their protein requirements.[161] Outcomes such as immune function and behavioral development indicate that breastfed infants do better than formula-fed infants, despite lower protein intakes. Although it may be argued that there are many differences between breast milk and formula, it has been shown that even when functional measures such as morbidity and activity level are compared within a breastfed cohort, there is no evidence that lower protein intakes are associated with adverse outcomes.[162] In fact, higher protein intake at 6 to 9 months was significantly associated with greater morbidity. With respect to growth, the differences between breastfed and formula-fed infants are greater for weight than for length,[163] indicating that the level of fat differs more than does the rate of linear growth.[164] It does not appear that protein intake causes these differences; when controlling for energy intake,

TABLE 14-3
Protein Intake of Breastfed Infants and Revised Estimates of Protein Requirements

Age (Months)	Breast Milk Intake (g/d)	Weight (kg)	Total Nitrogen Intake		Adjusted Protein Intake		1985 Estimate (g prot/kg/d)	Revised Protein Requirement (g prot/kg/d)
			(mg/d)	(mg/kg/d)	(g/d)	(g/kg/d)		
0–1	—	—	—	—	—	—	—	1.99
1	794	4.76	1723	362	9.3–9.7	1.95–2.04	2.25	1.54
2	766	5.62	1486	264	7.9–8.3	1.41–1.48	1.82	1.19
3	812	6.24	1472	236	7.9–8.3	1.27–1.33	1.47	1.06
4	782	6.78	1408	208	7.5–7.8	1.11–1.16	1.34	0.98
6	881	7.54	1486	197	8.0–8.4	1.05–1.11	1.30	0.92

Adapted from Dewey KG, Beaton G, Fjeld C, et al. Protein requirements of infants and children. Eur J Clin Nutr 1996;63(Suppl 1):6225–6.

protein intake (i.e., protein density of the diet) was not associated with weight or length gain during any 3-month period of the first year of life within a breastfed cohort.[165] Had the protein concentration of breast milk been marginal, a positive association between protein and growth would have been expected. Thus, there appears to be little evidence for the amount of protein consumed by breastfed infants in the first 4 to 6 months being inadequate.[161]

A recent intervention study in Honduras addressed this issue.[161,166] Infants were randomly assigned to be exclusively breastfed for the first 6 months of life or to receive prepared solid foods (including egg yolk) in addition to breast milk, starting from 4 months. Neither weight gain nor length gain from 4 to 6 months differed between groups, despite a 20% higher protein intake in the second. When 20 infants with the highest protein intakes in the supplemented group were matched to 20 exclusively breastfed infants, on the basis of energy intake was 33% higher (1.46 ± 0.09 versus 1.19 ± 0.17 g per kg per day, respectively), but there was no difference in growth rate. Similarly, when the 20 infants with lowest protein intake in the exclusively breastfed group were matched (by energy intake) to 20 infants given the supplement, protein intake was very low in the former compared to the latter group (0.81 ± 0.13 versus 1.04 ± 0.20 g per kg per day), yet there was no difference in growth rate. These results also indicate that protein intake is not likely to be a limiting factor for growth of breastfed infants from 4 to 6 months of age. Similar studies need to be conducted in other age groups.

Formula-Fed Infants

Theoretical calculations, similar to those discussed above for breastfed infants, have also been used to assess the protein requirements of formula-fed infants. These calculations usually attempt to compensate for a somewhat lower digestibility of the proteins in formula. This is difficult, however, because there is limited knowledge about the digestibility of proteins from various infant formulas. Not only do the protein sources used in infant formulas (skim milk, whey protein concentrate, soy protein isolate, etc.) vary in composition and quality, but the formulas are also exposed to various degrees of heat treatment during processing. Formulas that have been exposed to in-can sterilization, spray-drying, or UHT are denatured to varying extents and as protein digestibility has been shown to be markedly different in vitro,[156] this is highly likely to occur in infants as well.

An indirect approach is often used to assess the adequacy of the amount and quality of protein provided from infant formula.[167] In clinical studies, infants are fed formula with different protein levels and composition (e.g., casein:whey ratio). Venous blood samples are drawn 3 to 4 hours post-feeding ("fasting" in this age group), and plasma amino acids and blood urea nitrogen (BUN) are analyzed. These parameters are then compared to the plasma amino acid pattern and BUN concentrations of exclusively breastfed infants.[168] Thus, the goal is to mimic the "performance" (i.e., clinical parameters) of breastfed infants rather than copying the protein concentration and composition of human milk.

Infant formulas have traditionally contained 15 to 18 g of protein per L. These values, however, represent "crude protein," and the true protein concentration will depend on the protein source used: i.e., its contents of NPN. Skim milk powder and soy isolate usually contain low concentrations of NPN, whereas whey protein concentrates prepared by different methods (ultrafiltration, electrodialysis, ion exchange) contain considerably higher amounts of NPN.[155] Studies by Räihä et al.[169] showed that the plasma amino acid pattern of infants fed formula with a protein concentration of 15 g per L was quite different from that of breastfed infants. Concentrations of several plasma amino acids in the formula-fed infants were substantially higher than in breastfed infants, while they were considerably closer when formula with a protein content of 13 g per L was fed. Since BUN concentrations also were considerably higher in infants fed formula with 15 g of protein per L than in breastfed infants and infants fed formula with the lower protein level, the authors suggested that a protein level of 15 g per L is excessive and may cause unnecessary stress on immature organs, such as liver and kidneys. This was supported by the finding of elevated concentrations of C-peptide in the urine, which may reflect increased plasma insulin concentrations caused by high plasma concentrations of branched-chain amino acids.[170] The same group subsequently showed that feeding term infants formula with a protein concentration of 11 g per L resulted in several plasma amino acids being significantly lower than in breastfed infants, suggesting that this protein level may not result in a protein intake that meets the infants' requirement.[171]

Other researchers found that feeding infants formula with a protein content of 13 g per L resulted in some amino acids being lower than in breastfed infants.[172,173] Since tryptophan, a known precursor of brain neurotransmitters, was one of the amino acids that was low, concern was raised that this protein level is inadequate; or, if it is to be used, that the formulas should be fortified with tryptophan. Not only did feeding infants formula with 13 g protein per L and additional tryptophan result in a plasma amino acid pattern similar to that of breastfed infants, but it also affected their sleeping behavior, which was claimed to be due to the tryptophan-serotonin connection. We found, however, no significant differences in plasma amino acid patterns between infants fed formula with 13 g of protein per L from birth and breastfed infants.[174] This is most likely due to the fact that this formula contained low amounts of NPN, and the true protein was therefore close to the "crude protein" concentration (see above). Since this formula was powdered, it is also possible that protein digestibility was high. It is thus obvious that if this approach to assessing the appropriate protein concentration in infant formula is to be used, the protein and nitrogen concentration and composition, as well as the extent of the heat processing to which the formula has been exposed, need to be given in some detail.

CONCLUSION

It is evident that proteins in breast milk have a pronounced effect on the GI development of the newborn. Milk proteins participate in the defense against infection by affecting the gut microflora either directly or indirectly, participate in nutrient digestion and absorption, and may also influence enterocyte growth, differentiation, and function. The rapid growth of the gut will involve an interplay between proteins (substrate), digestive enzymes, and the mucosal surface, and it appears that human milk provides a source of components that have uniquely developed to optimize this interplay. Further studies are needed, however, both on the function and biologic significance of milk proteins either alone or in combination. The availability of larger quantities of recombinant human milk proteins will greatly facilitate such studies.

REFERENCES

1. Goldman AS, Goldblum RM. Immunoglobulins in human milk. In: Atkinson SA, Lönnerdal B, editors. Protein and nonprotein nitrogen in human milk. Boca Raton: CRC Press; 1989. p. 43.
2. Lönnerdal B, Forsum E, Hambraeus L. A longitudinal study of the protein, nitrogen, and lactose contents of human milk from Swedish well-nourished mothers. Am J Clin Nutr 1976; 29:1127–33.
3. Kunz C, Lönnerdal B. Re-evaluation of the whey protein/casein ratio of human milk. Acta Paediatr 1992;81:107–12.
4. Rosen JM, Li S, Raught B, Hadsell D. The mammary gland as a bioreactor: factors regulating the efficient expression of milk protein-based transgenes. Am J Clin Nutr 1996;63:627S–32S.
5. Matusik RJ, Rosen JM. Prolactin induction of casein mRNA in organ culture. J Biol Chem 1978;253:2343–7.
6. Guyette WA, Matusik RJ, Rosen JM. Prolactin mediated transcriptional and post–transcriptional control of casein gene expression. Cell 1979;17:1013–23.
7. Poyet P, Henning SJ, Rosen JM. Hormone-dependent β-casein mRNA stabilization requires ongoing protein synthesis. Mol Endocrinol 1989;3:1961–8.
8. Hobbs AA, Kessler DJ, Rosen JM. Complex hormonal regulation of casein gene expression. J Biol Chem 1982;257: 3598–605.
9. Nishikawa S, Moore RC, Nonomura N, Oka T. Progesterone and EGF inhibit mammary gland prolactin receptor and β-casein gene expression. Am J Physiol 1994;267:C1467–72.
10. Houdebine LM, Devinoy E, Delouis C. Stabilization of casein mRNA by prolactin and glucocorticoids. Biochimie 1978; 60:57–63.
11. Eisenstein RS, Rosen JM. Both cell substratum regulation and hormonal regulation of milk protein gene expression are exerted primarily at the posttranscriptional level. Mol Cell Biol 1988;8:3183–90.
12. Takemoto T, Nagamatsu Y, Oka T. Casein and α-lactalbumin messenger RNAs during the development of mouse mammary gland. Dev Biol 1980;78:247–57.
13. Vonderhaar BK, Nakhasi HL. Bifunctional activity of epidermal growth factor on α- and κ-casein gene expression in rodent mammary glands in vitro. Endocrinology 1986; 119:1178–84.
14. Puissant C, Bayat-Sarmadi M, Devinoy E, Houdebine L-M. Variation of transferrin mRNA concentration in the rabbit mammary gland during the pregnancy-lactation-weaning cycle and in cultured mammary cells. A comparison with the other major milk protein mRNAs. Eur J Endocrinol 1994;130:522–9.
15. Grigor MR, McDonald FJ, Latta N, et al. Transferrin gene expression in the rat mammary gland. Biochem J 1990; 267:815–9.
16. McCracken JY, Molenaar AJ, Wilkins RJ. Spatial and temporal expression of transferrin gene in the rat mammary gland. J Dairy Sci 1994;77:1828–34.
17. Noel GL, Suh HK, Frantz AG. Prolactin release during nursing and breast stimulation in postpartum and non-postpartum subjects. J Clin Endocrinol Metab 1974;38:413–23.
18. Kim JY, Mizoguchi Y, Yamaguchi H, et al. Removal of milk by suckling acutely increases the prolactin receptor gene expression in the lactating mouse mammary gland. Mol Cell Endocrinol 1997;131:31–8.
19. Wilde CJ, Addey CVP, Boddy LM, Peaker M. Autocrine regulation of milk secretion by a protein in milk. Biochem J 1995;305:51–8.
20. Daly SEJ, Owens RA, Hartman PE. The short-term synthesis and infant-regulated removal of milk in lactating women. Exp Physiol 1993;78:209–20.
21. Dewey KG, Lönnerdal B. Infant self-regulation of breast milk intake. Acta Paediatr Scand 1986;75:893–8.
22. Macy IG, Hunscher HA, Donelson E, Nims B. Human milk flow. Am J Dis Child 1930;6:492–515.
23. Saint L, Maggiore P, Hartmann PE. Yield and nutrient content of milk in eight women breast-feeding twins and one woman breast-feeding triplets. Br J Nutr 1986;56:49–58.
24. Atkinson SA, Anderson GH, Bryan MH. Human milk: comparison of the nitrogen composition in milk from mothers of premature and full term infants. Am J Clin Nutr 1980;33:811–6.
25. Lönnerdal B. Effects of maternal dietary intake on human milk composition. J Nutr 1986;116:499–513.
26. Woodhouse LR, Lönnerdal B. Quantitation of the major whey proteins in human milk and development of a technique to isolate minor whey proteins. Nutr Res 1988;8:853–64.
27. Brown KH, Akhtar MA, Robertson AD, Ahmed MG. Lactational capacity of marginally nourished mothers: relationships between maternal nutritional status and quantity and proximate composition of milk. Pediatrics 1986;78:909–19.
28. Lönnerdal B, Forsum E, Gebre-Medhin M, Hambraeus L. Breast milk composition in Ethiopian and Swedish mothers. II. Lactose, nitrogen, and protein contents. Am J Clin Nutr 1976;29:1134–41.

29. Prentice AM, Roberts SB, Prentice A, et al. Dietary supplementation of lactating Gambian women. I. Effect on breast-milk volume and quality. Hum Nutr 1983;37C:53–64.
30. Lunn PG, Austin S, Prentice AM, Whitehead RG. The effect of improved nutrition on plasma prolactin concentrations and postpartum infertility in lactating Gambian women. Am J Clin Nutr 1984;39:227–35.
31. Strode MA, Dewey KG, Lönnerdal B. Effects of short-term caloric restriction on lactational performance of well-nourished women. Acta Paediatr Scand 1986;75:222–9.
32. Dewey KG, Lovelady CA, Nommsen-Rivers LA, et al. A randomized study of the effects of aerobic exercise by lactating women on breast-milk volume and composition. N Engl J Med 1994;330:449–53.
33. McCrory MA, Nommsen-Rivers LA, Mole PA, et al. A randomized trial of short-term effects of dieting with aerobic exercise on lactation performance. Am J Clin Nutr 1999;69.
34. Forsum E, Lönnerdal B. Effect of protein intake on protein and nitrogen composition of breast milk. Am J Clin Nutr 1980;33:1809–13.
35. Motil KJ, Thotathuchery M, Bahar A, Montandon CM. Marginal dietary protein restriction reduced nonprotein nitrogen, but not protein nitrogen, components of human milk. J Am Coll Nutr 1995;14:184–91.
36. Lönnerdal B, Forsum E, Hambraeus L. Effect of oral contraceptives on composition and volume of breast milk. Am J Clin Nutr 1980;33:816–24.
37. Zavaleta N, Lanata C, Butron B, et al. Effect of acute maternal infection on quantity and composition of breast milk. Am J Clin Nutr 1995;62:559–63.
38. Lönnerdal B, Zavaleta N, Kusunoki L, et al. Effect of postpartum infection on proteins and trace elements in colostrum and early milk. Acta Paediatr 1996;85:537–42.
39. Lönnerdal B, Woodhouse LR, Glazier C. Compartmentalization and quantitation of protein in human milk. J Nutr 1987;117:1385–95.
40. Jenness R. Biochemical and nutritional aspects of milk and colostrum. In: Larson BL, editor. Lactation. Ames: University of Iowa Press; 1985. p. 78–94.
41. Rasmussen LK, Due HA, Petersen TE. Human alpha (S1) casein—purification and characterization. Comp Biochem Physiol 1995;111:75–81.
42. Kunz C, Lönnerdal B. Casein micelles and casein subunits in human milk. In: Atkinson SA, Lönnerdal B, editors. Protein and non-protein nitrogen in human milk. Florida: CRC Press; 1989. p. 9.
43. Lönnerdal B, Forsum E. Casein content of human milk. Am J Clin Nutr 1985;41:113–20.
44. Kunz C, Lönnerdal B. Casein and casein subunits in preterm milk, colostrum, and mature human milk. J Pediatr Gastroenterol Nutr 1990;10:454–61.
45. Greenberg R, Groves ML. Human β-casein. Amino acid sequence and identification of phosphorylation sites. J Biol Chem 1984;259:5128–32.
46. Lönnerdal B, Bergström S, Andersson Y, et al. Cloning and sequencing of a cDNA encoding human milk β-casein. FEBS Lett 1990;269:153–6.
47. Bonsing J, Mackinlay AG. Recent studies on nucleotide sequences encoding the caseins. J Dairy Res 1987;54:447–61.
48. Brignon G, Chtourou A, Ribadeau-Dumas B. Preparation and amino acid sequence of human κ-casein. FEBS Lett 1985;188:48–54.
49. Azuma N, Kaminogawa S, Yamauchi K. Reconstitution of human casein micelle and its properties. Agric Biol Chem 1985;49:2655–60
50. Bergström S, Hansson L, Hernel O, et al. Cloning and sequencing of human κ-casein cDNA. DNA Seq 1992;3:245–6.
51. Sato R, Noguchi T, Naito H. Casein phosphopeptide (CPP) enhances calcium absorption from the ligated segment of rat small intestine. J Nutr Sci Vitaminol (Tokyo) 1986;32:67–76.
52. Brantl V. Novel opioid peptides derived from human β-casein. Eur J Pharmacol 1984;106:213–4.
53. Reymann KG, Chepkova AN, Schulzeck K, Ott T. Effects of β-casomorphin on dentate hippocampal field potentials in freely moving rats. Biomed Biochim Acta 1985;44:749–54.
54. Grecksch G, Schweigert C, Matthies H. Evidence for analgesic activity of β-casomorphin in rats. Neurosci Lett 1981;27:325–8.
55. Schusdziarra V, Holland A, Schick R, et al. Modulation of post-prandial insulin released by ingested opiate-like substances in dogs. Diabetologia 1983;24:113–6.
56. Murayama S, Nakagomi K, Tomizuka N, Suzuki H. Angiotensin-I-converting enzyme inhibitor derived from an enzymatic hydrolase of casein. II. Isolation and bradykinin-potentiating activity of the uterus and the ileum of rats. Agric Biol Chem 1985;49:1405–9.
57. Newburg DS. Do the binding properties of oligosaccharides in milk protect human infants from gastrointestinal bacteria? J Nutr 1997;127:980S–4S.
58. Strömquist M, Falk P, Bergström S, et al. Human milk κ-casein and inhibition of *Helicobacter pylori* adhesion to human gastric mucosa. J Pediatr Gastroenterol Nutr 1995;21:288–96.
59. Phillips NI, Jenness R. Isolation and properties of human α-lactalbumin. Biochim Biophys Acta 1971;229:407–10.
60. Lönnerdal B, Glazier C. Calcium-binding by α-lactalbumin in human milk. J Nutr 1985;115:1209–16.
61. Brew K, Hill RL. Lactose biosynthesis. Rev Physiol Biochem Pharmacol 1975;72:105–57.
62. Sanchez-Pozo A, Lopez J, Pita ML, et al. Changes in the protein fractions of human milk during lactation. Ann Nutr Metab 1986;30:15–20.
63. Kulski JK, Hartman PE. Changes in human milk composition during the initiation of lactation. Aust J Exp Biol Med Sci 1981;59:101–14.
64. Johansson BG. Isolation of an iron-containing red protein from human milk. Acta Chem Scand 1960;14:510–2.
65. Cox TM, Mazurier J, Spik G, et al. Iron binding proteins and influx of iron across the duodenal brush border. Evidence for specific lactotransferrin receptors in the human intestine. Biochim Biophys Acta 1979;588:120–8.
66. Fransson G-B, Lönnerdal B. Iron in human milk. J Pediatr 1980;96:380–4.
67. Saarinen UM, Siimes MA, Dallman PR. Iron absorption in infants: high bioavailability of breast milk iron as indicated by the extrinsic tag method of iron absorption and by the concentration of serum ferritin. J Pediatr 1977;91:36–9.
68. Kawakami H, Lönnerdal B. Isolation and function of a receptor for human lactoferrin in human fetal intestinal brush-border membranes. Am J Physiol 1991;261:G841–6.
69. Davidson LA, Lönnerdal B. Persistence of human milk proteins in the breastfed infant. Acta Paediatr Scand 1987;76:733–40.
70. Arnold RR, Cole MF, McGhee JR. A bactericidal effect for human milk lactoferrin. Science 1977;197:263–5.
71. Bullen JJ, Rogers HJ, Leigh L. Iron-binding proteins in milk and resistance to *Escherichia coli* infection in infants. BMJ 1972;1:69–75.
72. Balmer SE, Scott PH, Wharton BA. Diet and faecal flora in the newborn: lactoferrin. Arch Dis Child 1989;64:1685–90.
73. Tomita M, Bellamy W, Takase M, et al. Potent antibacterial peptides generated by pepsin digestion of bovine lactoferrin. J Dairy Sci 1991;74:4137–42.

74. Goldman AS, Garza C, Nichols BL, Goldblum RM. Immunologic factors in human milk during the first year of lactation. J Pediatr 1982;100:563–7.
75. Crago SS, Prince SJ, Pretlow TG, et al. Human colostral cells. I. Separation and characterization. Clin Exp Immunol 1979;38:585–597.
76. Weisz-Carrington P, Roux ME, McWilliams M. Hormonal induction of the secretory immune system in the mammary gland. Proc Natl Acad Sci U S A 1978;75:2928–32.
77. Lindh E. Increased resistance of immunoglobulin dimers to proteolytic degradation after binding of secretory component. J Immunol 1985;113:284–8.
78. Kovar MG, Serdula MK, Marks JS, Fraser DW. Review of the epidemiologic evidence for an association between infant feeding and infant health. Pediatrics 1984;74:615–38.
79. Keller MA, Heiner DC, Kidd RM, Myers AS. Local production of IgG4 in human colostrum. J Immunol 1983;130:1654–7.
80. Brandtzaeg P. Mucosal and glandular distribution of immunoglobulin components: differential localization of free and bound SC in secretory epithelial cells. J Immunol 1974;112:1553–9.
81. Lewis-Jones DI, Lewis-Jones MS, Connolly RC, et al. Sequential changes in the antimicrobial protein concentrations in human milk during lactation and its relevance to banked human milk. Pediatr Res 1985;19:561–5.
82. Lönnerdal B, Hoffman B, Hurley LS. Zinc and copper binding proteins in human milk. Am J Clin Nutr 1982;36:1170–6.
83. Etling N, Gehin-Fouque F. Iodinated compounds and thyroxine binding to albumin in human breast milk. Pediatr Res 1984;18:901–3.
84. Lönnerdal B. Biochemistry and physiological function of human milk proteins. Am J Clin Nutr 1985;42:1299–317.
85. Chandan RC, Parry RM, Shahani KM. Lysozyme, lipase, and ribonuclease in milk from various species. J Dairy Sci 1968;51:606–7.
86. Parry RM, Chandan RC, Shahani KM. Isolation and characterization of human milk lysozyme. Arch Biochem Biophys 1960;103:59–65.
87. Chipman DM, Sharon N. Mechanism of lysozyme action. Science 1969;165:454–65.
88. Ellison RTJ, Giehl TJ. Killing of Gram-negative bacteria by lactoferrin and lysozyme. J Clin Invest 1991;88:1080–91.
89. Fridhandler L, Berk JE, Montgomery KA, Wong D. Column-chromatographic studies of isoamylases in human serum, urine, and milk. Clin Chem 1974;20:547–52.
90. Lindberg T, Skude G. Amylase in human milk. Pediatrics 1982;70:235–8.
91. Jones JB, Mehta NR, Hamosh M. Alpha-amylase in preterm human milk. J Pediatr Gastroenterol Nutr 1982;1:43–8.
92. Heitlinger LA, Lee PC, Dillon WP, Lebenthal E. Mammary amylase: a possible alternate pathway of carbohydrate digestion in infancy. Pediatr Res 1983;17:15–8.
93. Mallersh A, Clark A, Hafiz S. Inhibition of *Neisseria gonorrhoeae* by normal human saliva. Br J Vener Dis 1979;55:20–3.
94. Lindberg T. Protease inhibitors in human milk. Pediatr Res 1979;13:969–72.
95. Kress LF, Martin SR, Laskowski M Sr. Isolation of isoinhibitors of trypsin from porcine colostrum. Biochim Biophys Acta 1971;229:836–44.
96. Carlsson LC, Bergelin IS, Karlsson BW. Trypsin inhibition in urine of developing neonatal pigs and in sow's colostrum. Enzyme 1974;18:176–88.
97. Weström BR, Carlsson LC. Trypsin inhibitors in serum of adult and suckling rats and in rat milk. Int J Biochem 1976;7:41–7.
98. Hamosh M. Enzymes in human milk. In: Jensen RG, editor. Handbook of milk composition. San Diego: Academic Press; 1995. p. 388–427.
99. Davidson LA, Lönnerdal B. Fecal alpha$_1$-antitrypsin in breast-fed infants is derived from human milk and is not indicative of enteric protein loss. Acta Paediatr Scand 1990;79:137–41.
100. Fredrikzon B, Hernell O, Bläckberg L, Olivecrona T. Bile salt-stimulated lipase in human milk: evidence of activity *in vivo* and of a role in the digestion of milk retinol esters. Pediatr Res 1978;12:1048–52.
101. Hernell O, Bläckberg L. Digestion of human milk lipids: physiologic significance of sn-2monoacylglycerol hydrolysis by bile salt-stimulated lipase. Pediatr Res 1983;16:882–5.
102. Bläckberg L, Angquist K-A, Hernell O. Bile salt-stimulated lipase in human milk: evidence for its synthesis in the lactating mammary gland. FEBS Lett 1987;217:37–42.
103. Nilsson J, Bläckberg L, Carlsson P, et al. cDNA cloning of human milk bile salt-stimulated lipase and evidence for its identity to pancreatic carboxylic ester hydrolase. Eur J Biochem 1990;192:543–50.
104. Hernell O, Bläckberg L, Lindberg T. Human milk enzymes with emphasis on the lipases. In: Lebenthal E, editor. Textbook of gastroenterology and nutrition in infancy. New York: Raven Press; 1989. p. 209.
105. Hamosh M. Lingual and breast milk lipases. Adv Pediatr 1982;29:33–67.
106. Hernell O, Bläckberg L, Chen Q, et al. Does the bile salt-stimulated lipase of human milk have a role in the use of the milk long-chain polyunsaturated fatty acids? J Pediatr Gastroenterol Nutr 1993;16:426–31.
107. Hernell O, Gebre-Medhin M, Olivecrona T. Breast milk composition in Ethiopian and Swedish mothers IV. Milk lipases. Am J Clin Nutr 1977;30:508–11.
108. Dupuy P, Saunièree JF, Vis HL, et al. Change in bile salt dependent lipase in human breast milk during extended lactation. Lipids 1991;26:134–8.
109. Pamblanco M, Ten A, Comin J. Bile salt-stimulated lipase activity in human colostrum from mothers of infants of different gestational age and birthweight. Acta Paediatr Scand 1987;76:328–31.
110. Gothefors L, Marklund S. Lactoperoxidase activity in human milk and in saliva of newborn infants. Infect Immun 1975;11:1210–5.
111. Moldoveanu Z, Tenovuo J, Mestecky J, Pruitt KM. Human milk peroxidase is derived from milk leukocytes. Biochim Biophys Acta 1982;718:103–8.
112. Hashinaka K, Yamada M. Identification of myeloperoxidase in human colostrum. Arch Biochem Biophys 1986;247:91–6.
113. Langbakk B, Flatmark T. Demonstration and partial purification of lactoperoxidase from human colostrum. FEBS Lett 1984;174:300–3.
114. Langbakk B, Flatmark T. Lactoperoxidase from human colostrum. Biochem J 1989;259:627–31.
115. Pruitt KM, Rahemtulla F, Månsson-Rahemtulla BM, et al. Peroxidases in human milk. Adv Exp Med Biol 1991;310:137–44.
116. Steele WF, Morrisons M. Antistreptococcal activity of lactoperoxidase. J Bacteriol 1969;97:635–9.
117. Bjorck L, Rosen CG, Marshall V, Reiter B. Antibacterial activity of lactoperoxidase system in milk against *Pseudomonas* and other gram-negative bacteria. Appl Microbiol 1975;30:199–204.
118. Sandberg DP, Begley JA, Hall CA. The content, binding, and forms of vitamin B_{12} in milk. Am J Clin Nutr 1981;34:1717–24.

119. Burger RL, Allen RH. Characterization of vitamin B_{12}-binding proteins isolated from human milk and saliva by affinity chromatography. J Biol Chem 1974;249:7220–7.
120. Allen RH. Human vitamin B_{12} transport proteins. Prog Hematol 1975;9:57–84.
121. Gullberg R. Possible influence of vitamin B_{12}-binding protein in milk on the intestinal flora in breast-fed infants. Scand J Gastroenterol 1973;8:497–503.
122. Trugo NMF, Ford JE, Salter DN. Vitamin B_{12} absorption in the neonatal piglet. 3. Influence of vitamin B_{12}-binding protein from sows' milk on uptake of vitamin B_{12} by microvillus membrane vesicles prepared from small intestine of the piglet. Br J Nutr 1985;54:269–83.
123. Ford JE. Some observations on the possible nutritional significance of vitamin B_{12}- and folate-binding proteins in milk. Br J Nutr 1974;31:243–57.
124. Trugo NMF, Newport MJ. Vitamin B_{12} absorption in the neonatal piglet. 2. Resistance of the vitamin B_{12} binding protein in sows' milk to proteolysis in vivo. Br J Nutr 1985;54:257–67.
125. Trugo NMF, Ford JE. Vitamin B_{12} absorption in the neonatal piglet. 1. Studies in vivo on the influence of the vitamin B_{12}-binding protein from sows' milk on the absorption of vitamin B_{12} and related compounds. Br J Nutr 1985;54:245–55.
126. Samson RR, McClelland DBL. Vitamin B_{12} in human colostrum and milk. Acta Paediatr Scand 1980;69:93–9.
127. Trugo NMF, Sardinha F. Cobalamin and cobalamin-binding capacity in human milk. Nutr Res 1994;14:23–33.
128. Ford JE, Salter DN, Scott KJ. The folate-binding protein in milk. J Dairy Res 1969;36:435–46.
129. Antony AC, Utley CS, Marcell PD, Kolhouse JF. Isolation, characterization, and comparison of the solubilized particulate and soluble folate binding proteins from human milk. J Biol Chem 1982;257:10081–9.
130. Salter DN, Mowlem A. Neonatal role of milk folate-binding protein: studies on the course of digestion of goat's milk folate binder in the 6-d old kid. Br J Nutr 1983;50:589–96.
131. Colman N, Hettiarachchy N, Herbert V. Detection of a milk factor that facilitates folate uptake by intestinal cells. Science 1981;211:1427–8.
132. Said HM, Horne DW, Wagner C. Effect of human milk folate binding protein on folate intestinal transport. Arch Biochem Biophys 1986;251:114–20.
133. Selhub J, Arnold R, Smith AM, Picciano MF. Milk folate binding protein (FBP): a secretory protein for folate? Nutr Res 1984;4:181–7.
134. Donangelo CM, Trugo NMF, Koury JC, et al. Iron, zinc, folate and vitamin B_{12} nutritional status and milk composition of low-income Brazilian mothers. Eur J Clin Nutr 1989;43:253–66.
135. Klagsbrun M. Human milk stimulates DNA synthesis and cellular proliferation in cultured fibroblasts. Proc Natl Acad Sci U S A 1978;75:5057–61.
136. Corps AN, Brown KD, Rees LH, et al. The insulin-like growth factor I content in human milk increases between early and full lactation. J Clin Endocrinol Metab 1988;67:25–9.
137. Corps AN, Blakeley DM, Carr J, et al. Synergistic stimulation of Swiss mouse 3T3 fibroblasts by epidermal growth factor and other factors in human milk. J Endocrinol 1987;112:151–9.
138. Corps AN, Brown KD. Stimulation of intestinal cell proliferation in culture by growth factors in human and ruminant mammary secretions. J Endocrinol 1987;113:285–90.
139. Berseth CL, Lichtenberger LM, Morriss FH. Comparison of the gastrointestinal growth-promoting effects of rat colostrum and mature milk in newborn rats in vivo. Am J Clin Nutr 1983;37:52–60.
140. Read LC, Upton FM, Francis GL, et al. Changes in the growth-promoting activity of human milk during lactation. Pediatr Res 1984;18:133–9.
141. Rosenfeld RG, Lamson G, Pham H, et al. Insulin-like growth factor-binding proteins. Recent Prog Horm Res 1990;46:99–159.
142. Donovan SM, Hintz RL, Rosenfeld RG. Insulin-like growth factors I and II and their binding proteins in human milk: effect of heat treatment on IGF and IGF binding protein stability. J Pediatr Gastroenterol Nutr 1991;13:242–53.
143. Menard D, Pothier P. Radioautographic localization of epidermal growth factor receptors in human fetal gut. Gastroenterology 1991;101:640–9.
144. Jansson L, Karlson FA, Westermark B. Mitogenic activity and epidermal growth factor content in human milk. Acta Paediatr Scand 1985;74:250–3.
145. Iacopetta BJ, Grieu F, Horisberger M, Sunahara GI. Epidermal growth factor in human and bovine milk. Acta Paediatr 1992;81:287–91.
146. Ichiba H, Kusuda S, Itagane Y, et al. Measurement of growth promoting activity in human milk using a fetal small intestinal cell line. Acta Paediatr 1992;61:47–53.
147. Wood WI, Cachianes G, Henzel WJ, et al. Cloning and expression of the growth hormone-dependent insulin-like growth factor binding protein. Mol Endocrinol 1989;2:1176–85.
148. Suikkari A-M. Insulin-like growth factor (IGF-I) and its low molecular weight binding protein in human milk. Eur J Obstet Gynaecol 1989;30:19–25.
149. Agunod M, Yamaguchi N, Lopez R, et al. Correlative study of hydrochloric acid, pepsin, and intrinsic factor secretion in newborns and infants. Am J Dig Dis 1969;14:401–14.
150. Donovan S, Atkinson S, Whyte R, Lönnerdal B. Partition of nitrogen intake and excretion in low-birth-weight infants. Am J Dis Child 1989;143:1485–91.
151. Spik G, Brunet B, Mazurier-Dehaine C, et al. Characterization and properties of the human and bovine lactotransferrins extracted from the feces of newborn infants. Acta Paediatr Scand 1982;71:979–85.
152. Darragh AJ, Moughan PJ. The three-week-old piglet as a model animal for studying protein digestion in human infants. J Pediatr Gastroenterol Nutr 1995;21:387–93.
153. Slater JE. Retention of nitrogen and minerals by babies of 1 week old. Br J Nutr 1961;15:83–98.
154. Fomon SJ. Nitrogen balance studies with normal full-term infants receiving high intakes of protein. Pediatrics 1961;28:347–61.
155. Donovan S, Lönnerdal B. Non-protein nitrogen and true protein in infant formulas. Acta Paediatr Scand 1989;78:497–504.
156. Rudloff S, Lönnerdal B. Solubility and digestibility of milk proteins in infant formulas exposed to different heat treatments. J Pediatr Gastroenterol Nutr 1992;15:25–33.
157. Adamson I, Esangbedo A, Okolo AA, Omene JA. Pepsin and its multiple forms in early life. Biol Neonate 1988;53:267–73.
158. Sondheimer JM, Clark DA, Gervaise EP. Continuous gastric pH measurement in young and older healthy preterm infants receiving formula and clear liquid feedings. J Pediatr Gastroenterol Nutr 1985;4:352–5.
159. Lindberg T, Engberg S, Sjöberg L-B, Lönnerdal B. In vitro digestion of proteins in human milk fortifiers and in preterm formula. J Pediatr Gastroenterol Nutr 1998;27:30–6.
160. Fomon SJ. Nutrition of normal infants. St. Louis: Mosby-Year Book; 1993. p. 121.
161. Dewey KG, Cohen RJ, Rivera LL, et al. Do exclusively breast-fed infants require extra protein? Pediatr Res 1996;39:303–7.

162. Heinig MJ, Nommsen LA, Peerson JM, et al. Intake and growth of breastfed and formula-fed infants in relation to the timing of introduction of complementary foods: the DARLING study. Davis Area Research on Lactation, Infant Nutrition, and Growth. Acta Paediatr 1993;82:999–1006.
163. Dewey KG, Heinig MJ, Nommsen LA, et al. Growth of breastfed and formula-fed infants from 0 to 18 months: the DARLING study. Pediatrics 1992;89:1035–41.
164. Dewey KG, Heinig MJ, Nommsen LA, et al. Breastfed infants are leaner than formula-fed infants at 1 y of age: the DARLING study. Am J Clin Nutr 1993;57:140–5.
165. Heinig MJ, Nommsen LA, Peerson JM, et al. Energy and protein intakes of breast-fed and formula-fed infants during the first year of life and their association with growth velocity: the DARLING study. Am J Clin Nutr 1993;58:152–61.
166. Cohen RJ, Brown KH, Canahuati J, et al. Effects of age of introduction of complementary foods on infant breast milk intake, total energy intake and growth: a randomized intervention study in Honduras. Lancet 1994;344:288–93.
167. Heird WC. Interpretation of the plasma amino acid pattern in low birth weight infants. Nutr Res 1989;5:145–6.
168. Lönnerdal B, Zetterström R. Protein content of infant formula—how much and from what age? Acta Paediatr Scand 1988;77:321–5.
169. Räihä NCR, Minoli I, Moro G, Bremer HJ. Milk protein intake in term infants. II. Effects on plasma amino acid concentrations. Acta Paediatr Scand 1986;75:887–92.
170. Axelsson IEM, Ivarsson SA, Räihä NCR. Protein intake in early infancy: effects on plasma amino acid concentrations, insulin metabolism and growth. Pediatr Res 1989;26:614–7.
171. Picone TA, Benson JD, Moro G, et al. Growth, serum biochemistries, and amino acids in term infants fed formulas with amino acid and protein concentrations similar to human milk. J Pediatr Gastroenterol Nutr 1989;9:351–60.
172. Steinberg LA, O'Connell NC, Hatch TF, et al. Tryptophan intake influences infants' sleep latency. J Nutr 1992;122:1781–91.
173. Hanning RM, Paes B, Atkinson SA. Protein metabolism and growth of term infants in response to a reduced-protein. Am J Clin Nutr 1992;56:1004–11.
174. Lönnerdal B, Chen C-L. Effects of formula protein level and ratio on infant growth, plasma, amino acids and serum trace elements. I. Cow's milk formula. Acta Paediatr Scand 1990;79:257–65.

CHAPTER 15

Role of the Intestinal Lumen in the Ontogeny of the Gastrointestinal Tract

Uzma Shah, MD

Ian R. Sanderson, MD, FRCPCH

ROLE OF THE INTESTINAL LUMEN ON THE ONTOGENY OF THE GASTROINTESTINAL TRACT

The major part of human gastrointestinal tract development occurs in utero. Information on the ontogeny of this system has, therefore, largely been derived from animal studies or from studies on abortuses and early neonatal deaths. Extrapolation of data from animal studies to humans may be open to question, since animals studied may be altricial, or relatively immature at birth. For example, the rat is less mature than the human neonate. While major functional and maturational changes in the rat gut occur after birth, the human fetus has a mature gut by 34 weeks of gestation. Nevertheless, the development of the intestine has a large degree of similarity in different mammals.

There are several phases in the development of the human gastrointestinal tract (see Chapter 1). The embryological phase of organogenesis starts soon after conception and is followed by the appearance of the primitive gut. Further differentiation and maturation occur as the fetus reaches term and prepares for changes at birth that include enteral nutrition with milk feeds. The final phase of development is the transition from milk feeds to weaning food or solids. The regulation of these gastrointestinal changes are thought to depend on a complex interaction between genetic factors and extrinsic, or environmental, factors. It is these factors, particularly the intraluminal contents of the intestinal tract, that are the subject of this chapter. The small intestine is constantly exposed to a changing intraluminal environment, and has the capacity to adapt its structure and function to variations in the diet. The lumen of the intestine is exposed to swallowed amniotic fluid in utero, and milk soon after birth. The contents of the intestinal lumen are not only composed of nutrients ingested, but also contain various growth factors, hormones, bacteria and their products. In order to understand the complex interactions between the developing gut and the intestinal milieu, we will provide an outline of the development of the gastrointestinal tract, emphasizing the role of the intestinal lumen.

CHANGES IN INTESTINAL MORPHOLOGY WITH ENTERAL NUTRITION

The human gut is formed from the endodermal layer of the embryo and is identifiable by 4 weeks of gestation. The third trimester is the period of maximum growth, during which the gut almost doubles in length. By the sixth week of gestation, the small intestinal mucosal epithelium is made by a single layer of cells,[1] and it is at 9 weeks that apical well-defined microvilli appear. The apical tubular system and lysozomes are best developed by 15 to 17 weeks. Differentiating Paneth's cells appear at the proximal and distal small intestine in the eleventh to twelfth week of gestation.[2] The presence of the M cell was noted in a 17-week-old fetus[3] and enteroendocrine cells at between 9 and 11 weeks of gestation.[4] Abundant deposits of epithelial glycogen prior to the appearance of hepatic glycogen suggests that the intestinal epithelium may serve as glycogen stores in early fetal development.

Birth brings about several challenges for the neonate, who has been moved from an environment of parenteral nutrition in utero to enteral nutrition. The demands on the gut now require effective sucking and swallowing, gastric emptying and secretions, hepatobiliary and pancreatic secretions and enterocyte function with the development of appropriate enzymes for the uptake and assimilation of nutrients. During the suckling period the neonate is exposed to breast milk and colostrum, which contain nutrients and factors that influence the neonate in this development.

Enteral feeding is a key environmental trigger to gastrointestinal development. Oral feeding stimulates marked structural changes and enhances enzyme activity and metabolism. During its intrauterine existence, amniotic fluid swallowed by the fetus provides nutrients that are effectively digested and absorbed and play an essential role in the development and maturation of the small intestine. Fetal swallowing of amniotic fluid has been documented in utero, with volumes as high as 750 mL per day at term.[5] Amniotic fluid contains amino acids and carbohydrates, and 10 to 15% of fetal nutrition requirements may be supplied through this enteric route[6,7]

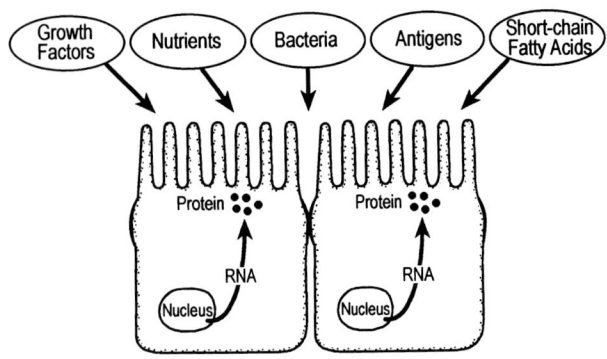

FIGURE 15–1. Luminal factors that influence gene expression in the enterocyte. Factors can affect individual genes, or they may influence enterocyte differentiation and new cell lineages. (With permission from Sanderson IR. Nutrition and gene expression. In: Walker WA, Watkins JB, editors. Nutrition in pediatrics. Basic science and clinical applications. Hamilton, Canada: BC Decker; 1997. p. 213–33.)

It contains small quantities of serum proteins, and several enzymes as well. The latter include lactase, sucrase-isomaltase, alkaline phophatase, and various lysosomal enzymes. Galactose, although not normally present in amniotic fluid, has prenatal absorption in the human that is maximal in the midjejunum.[8] Kinetic studies have demonstrated that maturation of galactose transport depends on changes in the distribution of the carrier rather than in the nature of the transporter itself.[8] In studies of the role of intra-amniotic nutrients on intestinal development involving rabbits, Buchmiller et al. demonstrated that intra-amniotic infusion of galactose induced mucosal hypertrophy and length, as well as an increase in specific mucosal transport of galactose and glucose along the intestine, suggesting that the developing fetal rabbit is capable of regulating intestinal mucosal transport in response to an intra-amniotic, and hence an intraluminal, infusion.[8] Restriction of nutrition during pregnancy retards fetal growth, particularly of the stomach and small intestine.[9]

With birth and the onset of milk feeds, the neonatal intestine is exposed to a variety of nutrients, hormones, and growth factors that modulate further development (Figure 15–1). The milk of mammals contains a large number of nutrients, hormones, and trophic factors.[10] The latter are discussed in greater detail later in this chapter and in Chapter 3. Intraluminal secretions also have an essential role to play in intestinal development, while a major contribution to postnatal development is by the endogenous secretion of regulatory peptides in response to food in the gut.

Intestinal growth and the rate of DNA synthesis is higher in rats fed colostrum than mature milk.[11] Suckled animals have a 75% greater mucosal mass than artificially-fed animals.[12] These data suggest that intestinal growth may be regulated by substances specifically present in natural milk. In some animals intestinal growth coincides with a maturational decline in brushborder hydrolases such as lactase. This ontogenic decline, although under hormonal control,[13] is also modulated by luminal factors.[14] Postnatal feeding is associated with major hormonal changes in the neonate, with increases in gastrin, insulin, growth hormone, and enteroglucagon.[15] These changes vary according to feed composition and method of feeding, so that an increase in enteroglucagon response was seen in term infants fed milk, but not with dextrose.[16] This difference can also be seen in the insulin response in formula- and breast-fed infants, with higher responses in the former.[17] In the preterm infant hormonal surges occur in response to feeding in the early postnatal days, and are marked by 24 days of life.[18] Preterm infants and, to some extent, term infants have much higher concentrations of peptides than the adult. Their significance remains unclear, but it is possible that they are needed for the induction of receptor activity, and hence function of target tissue in the developing newborn.

Weaning is accompanied by increases in circulating hormones that influence intestinal maturation and brushborder enzyme activity in preparation for adult-type food. Early weaning and exposure to antigens have been implicated in the development of food allergies and delayed small intestinal maturation.[19] However, intestinal maturation is also impaired if weaning is delayed or if animals are weaned to milk-like food.[20] The timing of weaning plays an important role in cellular proliferation and differentiation of the intestine. Premature weaning is associated with stress-induced release of steroids and an enhancement of sucrase activity in the jejunum.[21,22] Delayed weaning, in contrast, decreases crypt cell population and production rate. Dietary protein at weaning may modulate cellular DNA synthesis.[23]

To demonstrate whether it is enteral stimulation itself that is required for development, or whether the composition of nutrients involved is important, Castillo et al. used an animal model with chronic exclusion of intraluminal nutrients to look at the importance of nutrients on the maturing rat small intestine. Litters of infant Wistar rats were fed a diet of weaning chow or received an elemental diet composed of dextrose-amino acid and lipid intraluminally or intravenously. During weaning, an increase in mucosal DNA and protein content was higher in rats fed normally and intraluminally than in rats fed parenterally. Longitudinal growth of the small intestine was also severely diminished in the parenterally-fed infant rats, suggesting that intraluminal nutrients are essential for appropriate mucosal growth during weaning. The enzymatic development as studied in this experiment was less affected by the lack of intraluminal nutrition. No effect was noted on the maturational decline of lactase and maltase-glucoamylase. Their data suggested that while intraluminal nutrients were extremely important for mucosal growth, their absence slowed but did not prevent maturation. A similar pattern of development occurred in rats fed the milk-chow diets and those that received the dextrose-amino acid lipid composition, although they were vastly different diets; which suggests that a common mechanism was used by intraluminal nutrients to influence gastrointestinal maturation.[24]

Malnutrition causes a profound reduction in mucosal mass and villus height.[25] In an experiment demonstrating the importance of nutrition in development, intrauterine growth-retarded pups, control and preterm rats were studied at birth under conditions of low- or normal protein feeds using foster dams. With chronic malnutrition a delayed decline in ileal lactase activity and a delayed rise in sucrase activity occurs, suggesting that nutrient deprivation leads to delayed maturation of brushborder enzymes.[26]

LUMINAL EFFECTS ON THE BIOCHEMICAL MATURATION OF THE GASTROINTESTINAL TRACT

Data derived from experiments on laboratory animals suggest that brushborder proteins, mucus and membrane lipids undergo change during development of the small intestine. Fluorescence polarization spectrometry and electron spin resonance have demonstrated that there is greater membrane fluidity in the newborn than in the adult, which may in part be explained by altered lipid-protein and cholesterol-phospholipid ratios.[27,28] Such developmental changes may not only influence antigenic transport by the epithelium, but enterocyte transport as well.[29,30] A full description of brushborder enzyme development is given in Chapter 7, but we will review this area with particular attention to luminal molecules.

Polysaccharidases

Salivary and pancreatic amylase activity has been found as early as in 22-week-gestation fetuses, with an increase in 27-week-old fetuses to levels that are only 30% of that reached in newborns.[31] During the postnatal period the activity of salivary amylases rises earlier than that of pancreatic amylase. Carbohydrate tolerance and balance studies of the newborn indicate that rises in blood glucose levels are slower with a starch than with a glucose meal.[32,33] Maltose and maltodextrin feeds achieved an intermediate value. Amylopectin hydrolysis into glucose, maltose, and dextrins was rapid and complete in 1-year-olds but incomplete in 6-month-old infants. It has been shown that early administration of a starch feed to premature babies for 1 month increases the activity of alpha amylase in the duodenal juice obtained after pancreozymin-secretin stimulation.[34] However, another report showed feeding milk- and soy-based formula had no effect on pancreatic amylase.[35] The dichotomy can be explained if amylase induction requires complex starches that are lacking in soy-based formulas.

Present as early as 13 weeks of gestation, glucoamylase activity is potentially very important in starch digestion in early infancy, with levels increasing from the duodenum to the ileum. In the preterm infant, during a period of pancreatic amylase insufficiency, salivary amylase and intestinal glucoamylase provide an alternate pathway for the digestion of glucose polymers.[36,37] To determine whether intestinal enzyme maturation is dependent on hormones, brushborder enzyme activity was studied in response to insulin and dexamethasone stimulation. Except for lactase levels, there was no increase in enzyme activity.

Disaccharidases

At birth, most mammals have glucoamylase and the betaglucosidase complexes in their intestinal epithelium. While sucrase, trehalase, maltase, and isomaltase activity is present in fetal intestine by 10 weeks, it reaches 70 to 100% of adult levels by 14 weeks.[38]

During development, changes in the structure of brushborder enzymes may occur. In the rat, a decrease of sialylation of intestinal dissacharidases has been noted at weaning.[39] In humans too there are structural differences between fetal and adult disaccharidases.[40,41] The human fetal sucrase differs in its electrophoretic mobility from the adult form, and the binding of crude enzyme to lectins also differs from that in adults.[42] In fetuses younger than 30 weeks of gestation, it is present as one large molecule, while in adults it is split into sucrase and isomaltase.[42] Variations in post-translational processing may contribute to this diversity. The intestinal mucosa is under a complex system of genetic expression and control, and luminal factors may have a marked effect on enzyme expression. Animal experiments have shown that early feeding with sucrose will induce precocious sucrase induction in rodents, while a reduction in carbohydrate intake reduces sucrase activity.[43,44] Feeding with glucose instead of sucrose reduces brushborder hydrolase activity, with a resumption when sucrose is reintroduced.[45,46] Examination of the molecular biology of sucrase expression has shown that sucrase activity depends primarily on the sucrase promoter: as seen in the expression of growth hormone in transgenic animals containing a sucrase-growth hormone promotor construct.[47] Regulation of sucrase-isomaltase activity seems to be controlled at the transcriptional level in both humans and rabbits. A high correlation of activity was found between the enzyme and sucrase-isomaltase mRNA. Sucrase activity is present in fetal colon, and disappears before birth.[48] In organ culture experiments on human fetal colon, addition of EGF to fetal colon from 14 to 17-week-old fetuses induces a significant decrease in sucrase activity, while increasing lactase activity. At the time of weaning in mammals there is an increase in intestinal sucrase and a decrease in lactase, as well as a decrease in enterocyte life span.[49,50]

Lactase appears by 10 weeks of gestation, with levels at term that reach two to four times values obtained in normal infants of 2 to 11 months of age. Lactase phlorizin hydrolase mRNA accumulation correlates with lactase activity.[51] As with sucrase and maltase, maximal activity is in the proximal jejunum and occurs at birth. After birth, lactase activity in children of European origin drops slightly, reaching adult values after the first years of life.[52] In some populations, however, there is a slower decline over a period of 2 to 20 years after birth.[53] Newborn term and preterm babies have a limited capacity to absorb lactose, with lactose malabsorption occurring more commonly in breastfed rather than formula-fed babies, even if the lactose concentration in milk is similar.[54,55] In term babies the absorption capacity increases in the first few days of life, this increase being slower in preterm babies.[56-59] Small-for-dates infants of birth weight less than 1500 grams also show decreased lactose absorption.[58] The intestine of the 28 to 30-week-old preterm neonate is functionally and morphologically immature.[60,61] However, within the first week of life an accelerated rise of lactase activity is seen on enteral feeding.[61,62] This accelerated maturation of the intestinal tract may be under hormonal rather than nutrient control. Data derived from the addition of hydrocortisone to fetal jejunal explants in culture indicate that there is a complex developmental regulation of lactase, with post-transcriptional modification by hydrocortisone. Simultaneous application of EGF and hydrocortisone led to an increase in lactase alone.[63-65] Post-translational modification of rat intestinal lactase, with changes in glycosylation, have been correlated to the postweaning decline of rat lactase.[66] Analyses of the distribution of lactase-phlorizin hydrolase mRNA in the intestine with changes in the intraluminal contents before and after weaning have shown that preweaned rats, force-fed an artificial diet, had a high amount of lactase activity in the jejunum, with a precocious decline in lactase levels in the distal ileum. Prolonged nursing, in contrast, delayed this ontogenetic enzyme decline in the distal segment. It is likely that the longitudinal distribution of lactase-phlorizin hydrolase mRNA in the intestine is preprogrammed, with dietary changes acting as regulators in development.[14]

Monosaccharide Transport

Monosaccharides—glucose, galactose, and fructose—form important sources of energy. Active transport of glucose in the human fetal intestine was demonstrated by the "everted sac" in vitro technique, and was found to commence by 10 weeks of gestation (Chapter 8). Using small intestinal brushborder vesicles, active glucose transport in 17 to 20 week fetuses was found to be higher in the proximal than the distal small intestine.[67] Malo and Berteloot demonstrated a sodium dependent D-glucose cotransport system with a proximodistal gradient of activity. It was later demonstrated that there were, in fact, two distinct cotransport systems that could be distinguished on the basis of kinetic properties and substrate and inhibitor specificity.[67-69] The development and expression of mRNA-encoding, sodium-dependent-and-facilitated glucose transport were studied in human fetal and adult intestine, and it was found that the mRNA encoding the Na+glucose-transporter isoform SGLT1 and the facilitative glucose-transporter isoforms GLUT2 and GLUT5 exhibited highest levels in the adult small intestine, with GLUT1 higher in fetal intestine. The Na+-dependent glucose-transporter expression was also found in the fetal colon with levels lower than adult colon.[70] Postnatal glucose absorption is less efficient than in adults and reaches adult values between 4 and 8 years. In premature infants, the retention of glucose increases with age, with maturation involving increased proximal intestinal absorption.[71]

While earlier transport studies had indicated that glucose uptake increased with glucose feeding, Diamond, Ferraris, et al. have demonstrated an increase in nutrient transporters in response to an increase in substrate in the diet.[72-76] Sequential elution of various fractions of epithelial cells were used to distinguish different cells along the crypt-villus axis in mice to show that changes in expression of the glucose transporter varied along the crypt-villus axis.[77,78] Increases in carbohydrate intake resulted in enhanced expression of the glucose transporter, with changes in the crypts before they were seen in the villi. Similarly, when carbohydrates were stopped, changes were detected in the crypt before being observed in the villi. It is the stem cell in the crypt that must, therefore, be capable of detecting the change in carbohydrate, with expression of this change in the cell population that ascends the crypt-villus axis. Hence, carbohydrate detection differs temporally and spatially from glucose-transporter expression. The exact molecular mechanisms underlying these events are unknown, and it is unclear whether changes in the glucose transporter are transcriptional or translational events.[79]

Gastrin

First discovered in 1905, gastrin is responsible for a variety of actions, including secretion of gastric acid and stimulation of mucosal and pancreatic growth. In the human fetus gastrin-secreting G cells have been detected in the duodenum at 11 weeks of gestation[80] and at 19 to 20 weeks in the antrum. Hormone levels rise sharply toward the end of gestation. Duodenal gastrin was found to be higher than antral gastrin in fetal life.[81] Larrson et al. have determined that component -111 (G17) predominates in antrum and component -11 (G340) in the duodenum. Dietary factors, such as the high protein and calcium content of milk, stimulate gastrin release.[82] Dietary deprivation in early postnatal life may, on the other hand, affect the subsequent development of G cells in the antrum: as shown by Majumdar et al., with a report that undernutrition of rats from birth to 14 days caused a 40% reduction in antral gastrin levels compared to controls.[83] Glucocorticoids may also regulate gastrin cell development. In an experiment with 7 to 10-day-old suckling rats injected with hydrocortisone, there was a significant enhancement in antral gastrin levels and a decrease in pancreatic gastrin levels compared to controls. Duodenal gastrin levels remained unchanged. The pH of gastric fluid is initially neutral in newborns, with acidity increasing rapidly in a few hours after birth.[84] The gastric acidity of the newborn may thus be more favorable than the action of pepsins for the survival of other enzymes.

Development of Pepsinogens

Proteolytic activity has been described as present in fetuses at 16 weeks of gestation.[85] Pepsin, important in protein digestion, also acts as a milk clotting factor in neonates. A functional chymosin, however, like human neonatal protease has not been identified.[86] Immunohistological studies using antisera specific for pepsinogen A (PGA) and pepsinogen C (PGC) have shown that PGA is produced by chief cells and mucus neck cells in fundic gland mucosa, whereas PGC is produced by these cells and cardiac glands in the gastric cardia, pyloric glands, and Brunner's glands in the duodenum. In 1976 Hirsch-Marie et al. published a study on the ontogeny of human pepsinogens.[87] They found SMP (slow-moving proteases, or fetal pepsinogen) in significant amounts in fetal stomach with low levels of PGA and PGC by the eighth to ninth week in rudimentary glands near the superficial epithelium. After 20 weeks of gestation PGA appears in amniotic fluid, and its presence is concomitant with a sharp increase in peptic activity. Peptic activity in the newborn corresponds to the level of maturity, and increases in the fundus fourfold after food intake by the second day of life.[85]

Premature infants weighing 1000 grams have half the peptic activity of term infants.[88]

Pancreatic Enzymes

Pancreatic enzyme production starts at the third month of gestation, with secretion by the fifth month (Chapter 16). Immunoreactive trypsin 1 and chymotrypsin A were detected in amniotic fluid taken at 17 to 18 weeks of pregnancy.[89] Using the NBT-PABA test, low activity of chymotrypsin was demonstrated, that increased by 6 months of age.[90] Although developmental changes may be preprogrammed, however, some are inducible by diet. For example, feeding a high-starch diet to preterm infants increases amylase, while feeding a high-protein diet enhances secretion of lipase and trypsin.[34] In this experiment feeding a high-fat diet had no effect on lipase secretion.

Peptidases

Lindberg demonstrated that peptidases are present by 11 weeks of gestation. Glyceryltripeptide hydrolysis is equally active over different parts of the intestine and remains the same, while the activity of leucine aminopeptidase increases with age and exhibits a proximal-to-distal gradient with higher distal values. Gamma-glutamyl transpeptidase activity follows a similar gradient.[91] Alkaline phosphatase is detectable by 11 weeks, and reaches high levels by 23 weeks of gestation. However, only 50% of the activity of epithelial origin occurs in the proximal intestine, in contrast to other brushborder enzymes.

Undetectable prior to 26 weeks, enterokinase activity increases between 26 and 40 weeks, with highest activity in the duodenum.[92] In the rat enterokinase activity appears at 20 days of gestation, with an increase to adult levels by postnatal day 2. In the mouse, enterokinase activity is present soon after birth, reaching adult levels by 3 weeks of life. The appearance of enterokinase activity at birth coincides with major morphological changes in the intestinal epithelium. The gradual increase to adult levels also coincides with a change to a weaning, and then an adult diet.[93] The dependence of enterokinase activity on contact with pancreatic secretions has been demonstrated in rats, guinea pigs, and dogs. In a mouse model of exocrine pancreatic insufficiency, enterokinase activity, previously absent, was induced to normal levels on feeding trypsinogen. Additional studies will be needed to determine if luminal contents regulate enterokinase expression at transcription, translation, or zymogen activation.

Brushborder enzyme activity is also found in the colon at 13 weeks of gestation. Subsequent development leads to the disappearance of these enzymes from the colon. Activities of aminopeptidases and alkaline phosphatase remain high until term, and persist in the adult stage but at lower levels.[60]

Glutamine Synthetase Activity

Glutamine is the principal metabolic fuel for small intestinal mucosal cells, and an important precursor for nucleotide biosynthesis.[94–96] Glutamine synthetase (GS) activity has been reported in rat small intestine in fetal life and infancy.[97] Glutamine synthetase protein has been localized to crypt epithelial cells of the adult rat small intestine,[98] while it has also been detected in the full thickness of fetal mice villi.[99] During transition from fetal to postnatal life, amniotic fluid is replaced with the more nutritional milk diet, and during early infancy there is also a massive increase in intestinal absorptive capacity, with increased crypt mitotic activity and, most likely, an increased requirement for GS. Glutamine synthetase activity in the rat small intestine increases from late fetal life to 32 days postnatally, and then declines in adulthood.[100] Steady-state mRNA measurements revealed highest concentrations in the fetus and 19-day-old preweanling rat small intestine.[100]

Lipases and Bile Acid Secretion

Lipase activity, first found in the fundus of the stomach, is detected in fetuses at 10 weeks of gestation.[101,102] Pancreatic lipase appears later at 21 weeks of gestation. Other lipolytic enzymes include bile salt-stimulated lipase (BSSL), lipoprotein lipase, and preduodenal lipases. Bile salt-stimulated lipase is present in colostrum in term and preterm milk, and increases in concentration in mature milk during feeding.[103,104] At low bile salt concentrations in the infant duodenum, BSSL survives and facilitates fat absorption.[105,106] It hydrolyzes triglycerides into free fatty acids.[107] Bile salts activate the enzyme and protect it from proteolytic digestion. Milk also contains a serum-activated lipoprotein lipase (LPL),[103,108] the activity of which increases during lactation, with a peak at 3 weeks of life.[103] Other lipases, including gastric and lingual lipase, have been demonstrated in humans.[109,110] Release is stimulated by feeding, and these lipases reduce milk triglycerides to diglycerides and fatty acids.[111] Lipase activity is present in gastric aspirates as early as 6 months of gestation, and increases by 8 to 9 months.[112] Gastric lipase activity does not change when long-chain triglycerides are fed, but decreases considerably when medium-chain triglycerides are present.[113] Lipase activity in gastric aspirates from premature infants was lower at 26 gestational weeks, peaked at 32 weeks and declined to lower levels at term. Lipase activity was promoted by continuous feeding.[114] Pancreatic lipase activity is low at birth and increases by 6 months of age. Premature infants have lower values of pancreatic lipase activity than term infants.[115] Gastric lipase activity responds more avidly than pancreatic lipase to changes in dietary lipids. Increasing dietary fat in rabbits from 2.7 to 6% was associated with a 100 percent increase in gastric lipase, while a modest (12%) rise was seen in pancreatic lipase.[116] Studies in adult human volunteers also showed an increase in gastric lipase with an increase in dietary fat.[117] The exact mechanisms involved in this augmented gene expression are presently unclear, but elucidation would undoubtedly have potential therapeutic implications where manipulation of gene expression is important, such as in patients with cystic fibrosis.

Infants during the first few days of life have very low levels of duodenal bile acids. Fetal gallbladder contains cholic and chenodeoxycholic acid.[118,119] The cholic:chenodeoxycholic ratio is higher postnatally and decreases later. In early infancy bile acids are conjugated, mostly with taurine, and with glycine later in life.[120] The pattern of conjugation depends on the diet, and a deficiency of taurine in the diet did not seem to influence the formation of taurine conjugates in the first month of life.[121] Feeding evokes an increase in serum bile acids in normal infants and children.[122] Preterm infants show more fecal excretion of bile acids than term infants.[123] The type of feeds also determined bile acid output, with greater excretion in preterm infants fed cow's milk than in those fed human milk,[124] and greater excretion in term infants on soy milk versus cow's milk.

In term infants absorption of fat increases over the first month and reaches almost 90%. In preterm infants absorption is lower, and reaches 80% by 10 weeks.[125] Studies of Signer and Jarvenpaa show that the absorption of human milk fat is less dependent on bile acids than is the absorption of fat from cow's milk. Using cultured jejunal explants from human fetuses, it was shown that fetuses have the ability to produce lipoprotein fractions to transport lipids.[126-128] Enzymes involved in intracellular lipid synthesis include monoacylglycerol acyltransferase (MGAT), 3-hydroxy-3-methyl-glutaryl CoA (HMG CoA) reductase and CoA cholesterol acyltransferase (ACAT). Monoacylglycerol acyltransferase activity was mostly detected in the proximal small intestine, with a distal-to-proximal gradient by 10 to 20 weeks of gestation. 3-Hydroxy-3-methyl-glutaryl reductase activity was proximal at 18 to 20 weeks, while ACAT activity was dominant over the proximal segment by 10 to 14 weeks of gestation. Using organ culture it was possible to demonstrate that addition of EGF increased apolipoprotein B48 production and decreased apolipoprotein B100.[127,128] Apolipoprotein mRNA appears at 10 weeks of gestation and reaches a level of 80% by the end of the second trimester of gestation,[129] suggesting a potential role of apolipoprotein B48 in prenatal lipid metabolism.[130]

Although there are data on the complex luminal phase of lipid digestion and absorption, the mechanisms involved in the intracellular processing of lipids remain undefined. Additional studies are needed to further elucidate the role of HMG-CoA reductase, ACAT, and MGAT in intracellular lipid handling.

ROLE OF HUMAN MILK IN THE ONTOGENY OF THE GASTROINTESTINAL TRACT

Soon after birth the newborn's intestine is exposed to milk that contains essential nutrients and various other factors that modulate intestinal maturation and further development. Human milk provides several immunological and nonimmune factors that serve to provide the newborn protection against dietary antigens and microbial pathogens. While proteins and phosphates provide acid buffering, prostaglandins provide cytoprotection, increase intestinal peristalsis, and release brushborder enzymes.[131] Other protective factors include phospholipids, EGF, glucocorticoids, and corticosteroid-binding proteins. Antimicrobial substances include bile salt-stimulated lipases that bind to microbes;[132] lactoferrin, lyzozymes, and lactoperoxidase control intraluminal

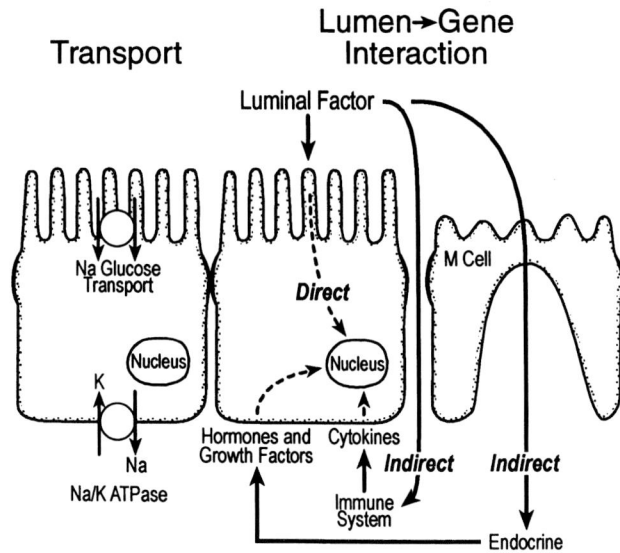

FIGURE 15–2. Dietary changes may affect gene expression directly (being mediated through the apical membrane) or indirectly (through the basolateral membrane). (With permission from Sanderson IR. Nutrition and gene expression. In: Walker WA, Watkins JB, editors. Nutrition in pediatrics. Basic science and clinical applications. Hamilton, Canada: BC Decker; 1997. p. 213–33.)

replication of bacteria; while oligosaccharides, glycolipids, and mucin-like glycoproteins serve as soluble receptors for bacterial adhesins and enterotoxins.[133,134] The feeding of natural milk has been shown to decrease intestinal permeability in newborn humans and guinea pigs, an effect that has been attributed to maturation of the mucosal barrier. A number of factors present in human milk are capable of regulating intestinal epithelial gene expression and, hence, differentiation. Included are growth factors such as EGF and substances such as nucleotides. We will review the effects of some of the factors present in human milk on the developing gastrointestinal tract (Figure 15–2).

Epidermal Growth Factor

Epidermal growth factor, a polypeptide, was first isolated from the submaxillary gland of the mouse by Carpenter and Cohen.[135] Epidermal growth factor, present in many body fluids—breast milk, bile, gastric juice, and saliva—may play an important role in epithelial proliferation and development of the intestinal tract (see Chapter 3). It acts by binding to a protein kinase receptor on the cell membrane to stimulate ornithine decarboxylase and DNA synthesis and prostaglandin release. Using pure isolated cell preparations derived from fetuses 12 to 17 weeks old, the presence of specific EGF receptors was established in human small intestine and colon.[136] Epidermal growth factor binding was found to be higher in younger fetuses, with greatest binding between 8 and 12 weeks, the period of major morphological changes in the intestine. Epidermal growth factor enhances the differentiation of human fetal small intestine in organ culture as well as in serially-passaged normal fetal colonic epithelial cells.[136] It enhances development of the rough endoplasmic reticulum and of fetal colonic epithelial cells in vitro, and appears to regulate synthesis and secretion of cellular macromolecules rather than cell proliferation.[64] It binds to apical membranes of distal fetal rat intestine, and is transported through the tubulocis-ternae. Binding, internalization, and processing of the EGF in vitro change during the postnatal period,[136,137] and in the fetal rat some EGF is transported via lysosomes, while some reaches the basolateral surface directly. There are controversial reports, however, on enterocyte expression of the EGF receptor, with some indicating luminal expression and others a basolateral location.[138–140]

The route of administration may have a key role in the trophic effects of EGF on the intestine. In neonatal rabbits given either oral or parenteral EGF, an increase in mucosal growth, glucose, and electrolyte transport was documented. Orogastric administration of EGF stimulated cellular proliferation at the ileal, antral, and fundic mucosa.[141] Both trophic changes and induction of transport systems may account for these alterations. Parenteral administration into 3-day piglets increased sucrase and maltase activities measured 3 days later in the mid- and distal small intestine.[142]

To assess survival of EGF in the gastric milieu, gastric aspirate from preterm infants was used to study the hydrolysis of ^{125}I-human recombinant EGF in vitro. The gastric survival of dietary EGF in a potentially active form has several possible implications for the preterm infant, in whom gastric acid secretion is low in the first 4 weeks postnatally. Its secretion may be inhibited by EGF.[143] Gastric survival of EGF in term infants and with increasing postnatal age remains to be determined. Epidermal growth factor hydrolysis was also studied in suckling and weanling rats. Results indicated that intraluminal survival of EGF was more likely in the stomach and proximal small intestine than distally, and was lower in the suckling rat, increasing the availability of active growth factor in the developing intestine.[144,145] Recently, quantitative autoradiography and indirect immunofluorescence using an antibody for human EGF receptor was performed using fetal gastric tissue (12 to 20 weeks' gestation). Epidermal growth factor receptors present as early as 12 weeks were localized on basolateral membranes of all gastric epithelial cells. On culture with EGF, an increase in DNA and glycoprotein synthesis was noted after 24 hours, but decreased after 5 days in culture. Epidermal growth factor also decreased lipase activity without affecting pepsin activity after 5 days in culture.

In contrast to other species, such as the rat, in humans EGF stimulates gastric mucosal cell proliferation and functional development. It is an important growth factor, with myriad effects on the gastrointestinal tract. An understanding of underlying molecular mechanisms is awaited.

Insulin-Like Growth Factor

It was in 1978 that Klagsburn discovered that human milk stimulated the growth of cultured fibroblasts. Insulin-like growth factor-I was first demonstrated in human milk by Baxter in 1984. Growth factors were present in higher concentrations in colostrum, and decreased with lactation.[146] Various forms of IGF-I have been detected, including des-IGF-I, an additional, truncated form of IGF-I that has reduced affinity for IGF-binding proteins (IGFBP) and greater bioavailability.[147] Six IGFBP have been demonstrated, and four (BP-1, -2, -3, and -4) have been found in milk. It is still unclear if these binding proteins serve to facilitate attachment of IGF to the enterocyte or protect from proteolytic digestion. Apart from IGF-I present in milk and colostrum, IGF-I is also derived endogenously from pancreatic juice, saliva, and bile.[148] IGF-ImRNA and peptides have been detected throughout the intestinal tract, with greater localization to the mesenchymal cells of the submucosa and lamina propria of the stomach and small intestine.[149] A greater concentration of IGF-I receptors were found in crypt versus villus enterocytes, suggesting that, along with circulating IGF, local stimulation for mucosal growth may be an important function. The cellular localization and function of the binding proteins is still poorly understood.

While several studies have demonstrated that parenteral administration of IGF-I may promote mucosal proliferation and protein synthesis,[150] there has been little information on the use of enteral IGF-I. Intraluminal IGF-I increases mucosal growth in rats, neonatal pigs, and calves;[151–153] Baumrucker et al. have shown that oral IGF-I at physiologic doses had little effect on intestinal growth. However, use of pharmacologic doses of IGF-I, greater than that normally present in colostrum or milk, induced an increase in mucosal thickness and small intestinal growth in neonatal pigs.[154] Burrin et al. later demonstrated the effects of oral IGF-I in suckling mice, using a transgenic mouse model with targeted overexpression of the des(1-3) human IGF-I, with the IGF-I delivered to the offspring 1000-fold greater than in wild-type mouse milk. An increase in protein synthesis and villus height was demonstrated in mice suckled on the transgenic dams. Hence, IGF-I at pharmacologic doses may promote intestinal growth. The mechanism postulated includes IGF-I's effect on DNA synthesis or on enterocyte life span.[154] Fasting leads to mucosal atrophy in the rat, and is associated with a decrease in both serum and IGF-I and intestinal IGF-ImRNA. Rapid restoration on refeeding suggests that intraluminal nutrients are important regulators of IGF-I expression in the gut.[155]

Insulin-like growth factor-I may also have a role to play in intestinal maturation and development. Houle et al. demonstrated that in neonatal pigs, IGF-I given orally induced a dose-dependent increase in lactase activity and a decrease in leucine aminopeptidase activity. In contrast to the effect of physiologic doses of IGF-I, a similar response was not demonstrated at pharmacologic doses.[154] It has been suggested that IGF-I exerts its effect on lactase ontogeny by means of its influence on enterocyte maturation. It is unclear whether IGF-I acts via apical receptors or via those on the basolateral membrane. There is some evidence that receptors are present on the brushborder membrane in small intestine in piglets, and that their density decreases with age.[156] Insulin-like growth factor-I may also exert inhibitory effects on chloride secretion in intestinal epithelial cell lines.[156] It remains to be seen if oral IGF-I has the same response, since use in the neonatal diet may have a potential therapeutic role in decreasing chloride secretion in response to bacterial toxins and other secretagogues.

For IGF-I to be an effective growth factor, it must survive luminal digestion. The low gastric acidity in neonates, along with the protective action of milk protein, prevents luminal degradation.[157] However, although almost 30% of orally-administered IGF-I may be recovered in the intestine, there is very little systemic absorption. It is possible that in premature and ill neonates with increased intestinal permeability, significant amounts of IGF-I may pass into the systemic circulation to support growth.[154]

The regulation of IGF-I, its receptors and binding proteins in response to development and intestinal luminal contents remains to be elucidated. Insulin-like growth factor-I has been demonstrated to have local anabolic effects in the intestine. Determination of cellular mechanisms explaining the latter, as well as its role in intestinal enzyme development, remain quests for future researchers.

Lactoferrin

Lactoferrin is an iron-binding glycoprotein that was first isolated in 1960 by Johanson.[158] It has a molecular weight of approximately 80,000, is structurally similar to transferrin, and is present in high concentrations in breast milk and colostrum.[159,160] Lactoferrin is considered to survive proteolytic digestion and act on the surface intestinal epithelium via binding to specific sites in intestinal brushborder membrane vesicles.[161-165] It may have a role in the regulation of iron absorption. In cultured epithelial cells depleted of iron, an increase in lactoferrin binding sites, and hence an increase in iron transport, has been documented.[166] Recent studies have also indicated that lactoferrin may act as a proliferative factor in several cell types, such as human lymphocytes, the HT-29 human colon cancer cell line, and adult rat crypt cells.[167,168] It may also affect brushborder enzyme activity, a feature that seems to depend on iron saturation.[169] It has been reported that lactoferrin stimulated thymidine incorporation into DNA in crypt cells in vitro, and in fact may act as a growth factor.[168] He and Furmanski determined the nucleotide sequences of DNA that binds to lactoferrin, and also showed greater binding with iron-saturated lactoferrin. Gene transfection of leukemia cells, with sequences attached to a reporter gene, showed an upregulation of the reporter gene with the addition of lactoferrin, and greater upregulation with the addition of iron-saturated lactoferrin to the culture media. A role for lactoferrin as an iron scavenger rather than as a transporter has been postulated. In that capacity lactoferrin would function as an antioxidant, binding excess iron and preventing free radical damage to the intestinal epithelium.

Lactoferrin has antibacterial properties, and has been shown to bind to lipopolysaccharide and hence alter its effect on the epithelium. It has anti-inflammatory properties, and inhibits leukocyte activation and recruitment.[170] Experiments on germ-free, colostrum-deprived piglets were used to evaluate the ability of lactoferrin to protect against lethal shock induced by intravenously administered endotoxin. Prefeeding with lactoferrin resulted in a significantly decreased piglet mortality compared to feeding with bovine serum albumin. In vitro studies using flow cytometric assays demonstrated that lipopolysaccharide binding to porcine monocytes was inhibited by lactoferrin in a dose-dependent manner.[171] It is suggested that the action of lactoferrin in vivo may be due to binding and inhibition of monocytes and the release of inflammatory cytokines.

It is postulated that any direct effects of lactoferrin on gene expression should be transmitted through a receptor. The lactoferrin receptor has now been isolated from human fetal and infant small intestine, and the receptor cloned. It is hoped that manipulation of lactoferrin DNA in transfected cell lines will show whether the receptor signals information to the molecular machinery of the enterocyte.

Lactoferrin's role in enterocyte gene expression is being studied, with recent work demonstrating an effect on the proliferation and differentiation of intestinal epithelial cells.[169] Lactoferrin derived from maternal milk may act via receptors on the enterocyte to alter epithelial cell programming. How this is achieved, and what benefits this would provide the developing infant, are questions that remain to be answered.

Polymeric IgA, IgG, IgM

Polymeric IgA (pIgA) accounts for 90% of the immuno-globulin in human milk, and may represent as much as 80% of the total protein content of colostrum.[172] At least 30% of IgA from breast milk survives transport through the small intestine.[173] The main role of pIgA is to block the adhesion of microbial pathogens to the enterocyte. IgA may also cross the mucosal barrier into the systemic circulation.[174] Such absorption may particularly occur in preterm low-birth-weight infants. IgG and IgM antibodies are also present in human milk, and play a significant role in defense. The percentage of

TABLE 15–1
Functions of Antimicrobial Agents in Human Milk

Agents	Primary Functions	Synergy
Proteins		
Lactoferrin	Fe^{+++} chelation	SIgA
Lysozyme	Degrade peptidoglycans	SIgA
Fibronectin	Opsonins	?
Secretory IgA	Antigen binding	LF-LZ
C3	Fragments are opsonins	SIgA-LZ
Mucins	Antirotavirus; receptor analogs	
Oligosaccharides	Receptor analogs	
Lipids	Dirsrupt enveloped viruses	

With permission from Goldman AS. The immune system of human milk: antimicrobial, anti-inflammatory and immuno-modulating properties. Pediatr Infect Dis J 1993;12:664–71.

TABLE 15–2
Anti-inflammatory Factors in Human Milk

Categories	Examples
Cytoprotectives	Prostaglandins E2, F2α
Epithelial growth factors	EGF, lactoferrin
Maturational factors	Cortisol
Enzymes that degrade mediators	PAF-acetylhydrolase
Binders of enzymes	α1-antichymotrypsin
Modulators of leukocytes	Lysozyme, SIgA
Antioxidants	Uric acid, α-tocopherol, β-carotene, ascorbate

With permission from Goldman AS. The immune system of human milk: antimicrobial, anti-inflammatory and immuno-modulating properties. Pediatr Infect Dis J 1993;12:664–671.

IgG2 and IgG4 subclasses in human milk and saliva are significantly greater than in human serum.[175] The mechanism responsible is currently unknown. Possible explanations include an increase in IgG2 and IgG4 plasma cells, or preferential transfer across selective Fc receptors on cell membranes to mucosal glands. The expression of these two antibodies is delayed in newborns.[176] Passive transfer via milk and colostrum would augment neonatal host mucosal defense.

Almost 90 major milk oligosaccharides have been isolated and function to inhibit binding of pathogens to cell-surface glycoproteins. They bear structural homology to cell surface glycoconjugates used as receptors by pathogens. The oligosaccharide fraction is the third-largest solid fraction of milk, after fat and lactose, and forms over 12g per L of mature milk and 22g per L of colostrum. Many of the oligosaccharides are fucosylated and have been found to inhibit the binding of invasive strains of *Campylobacter jejuni* to its host cell, and to inhibit the toxicity of *E. coli* in vivo. Many aspects of oligosaccharides, such as their relation to maternal genetics, stages of lactation, and cellular mechanisms of pathogen inhibition, require further study.

Lysozyme

Lysozyme is an enzyme that cleaves peptidoglycans from bacterial cell walls, and is present in high concentrations in human milk throughout the different stages of lactation, with concentrations increasing as lactation progresses. Its major role is in host defense against intestinal pathogens by bacterial cell wall lysis. Lysozyme lyses bacteria by hydrolyzing β-1,1 linkages between N-acetylmuramic acid and 2-acetyl-amino-2-deoxy-D-glucose residues in bacterial cell walls. Human milk-fed infants have higher fecal levels of lysozyme than infants fed cow's milk. Lysozyme in conjunction with lactoferrin has bactericidal properties that may be important in mucosal defense.

Nucleotides

Studies over the past several years have highlighted the importance of nucleotides in infant development, intestinal colonization, and intestinal maturation and repair after injury.[178–180] Nucleotides are reported to account for 2 to 5% of human milk nonprotein nitrogen, and may contribute to more efficient use of protein in human milk-fed infants, who receive a lower protein intake than formula-fed infants. Increases in mucosal protein, DNA, villus height, and disaccharidase activity were found in the intestines of weanling rats fed a diet supplemented with nucleotides. Supplementation with adenosine monophosphate alone increased jejunal wall thickness and protein and cell number. In the supplemented rats an increase in maltase activity was also noted as lactase declined, suggesting a possible role of nucleotides in gut maturation.[181] Intestinal epithelial cell-line studies suggest that nucleotides enhance the expression of brushborder enzymes, sucrase, lactase, and alkaline phophatase when the cells are stressed by glutamine deprivation. Dietary nucleotides have been reported to have significant effects on intestinal, lymphoid, and hepatic tissue. The nutritional role of nucleotides remains controversial, and the mechanisms involved in its various functions unknown (Figures 15–3, 15–4).

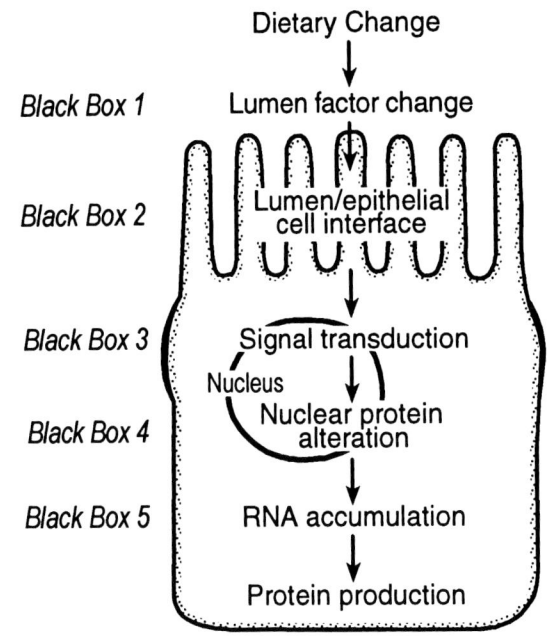

FIGURE 15–3. The pathway connecting dietary alterations to changes in gene expression is not well understood. It is likely that the pathway is mediated by a series of steps that at present we can only regard as black boxes. Different luminal events will influence gene expression through different series of black boxes. (With permission from Sanderson IR. Nutrition and gene expression. In: Walker WA, Watkins JB, editors. Nutrition in pediatrics. Basic science and clinical applications. Hamilton, Canada: BC Decker; 1997. p. 213–33.)

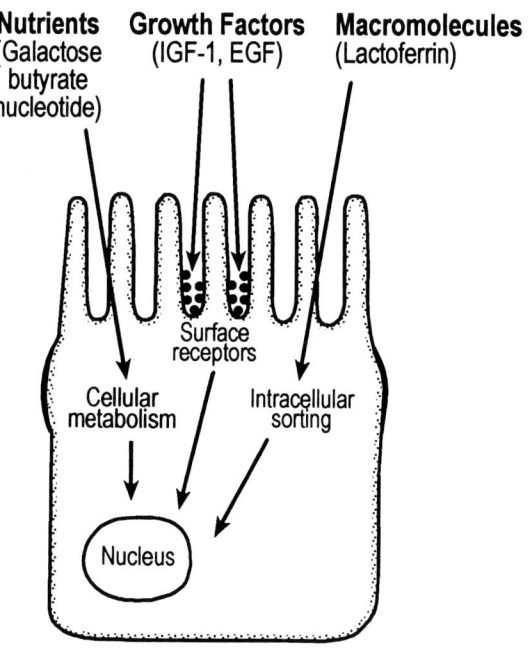

FIGURE 15–4. Crosstalk through the apical membrane will depend on the particular signal involved. (With permission from Sanderson IR. Nutrition and gene expression. In: Walker WA, Watkins JB, editors. Nutrition in pediatrics. Basic science and clinical applications. Hamilton, Canada: BC Decker; 1997. p. 213–33.)

MACROMOLECULAR TRANSPORT AND INTESTINAL MATURATION

In humans, maturation of intestinal epithelial cells occurs much earlier than in ruminants and rodents. Changes occur in epithelial uptake as the newborn moves from an intrauterine life and exposure to amniotic fluid to an extrauterine existence and a diet of milk feeds and weaning food. After the neonatal period there is a decline in intestinal permeability, called gut closure. The time and pattern of gut closure vary among species. In humans, the exact time is unknown, but intrinsic factors, as well as growth factors, hormones, and breast milk constituents, are thought to play roles (Figure 15–5). Despite early morphologic changes in the epithelium suggesting closure, as seen by the disappearance of the apical tubular system in the third week of gestation, an increased permeability exists at birth, particularly in the preterm infant. Many studies have tried to assess the uptake of immunologically-intact proteins in the human infant's intestinal tract. Jakobsson et al. used human alpha lactalbumin as marker to show that macromolecular uptake was related to postconceptual and postnatal age.[182] Robertson et al. showed that the concentration of serum beta lactoglobulin was higher in preterm infants than in term infants receiving this milk protein,[183] suggesting an increased epithelial permeability. Ivanger and Selvaraj found high concentrations of immunoglobulins in neonates fed colostrum rather than artificial or natural milk,[184] and Vukavic et al. suggested that spontaneous closure may be delayed if breastfeeding is postponed beyond the first 30 hours of life.[185] Breast milk constituents that may have an important role in macromolecular transport in the intestine include immunoglobulins, growth factors, EGF, IGF, hormones such as insulin, cortisol, thyroxine, and amino acids. While steroids may play a role in the normal ontogenetic closure of neonatal rat intestine, it remains to be seen whether steroids or other factors present in milk are involved in intestinal maturation and closure in humans. Prenatal cortisone treatment has been shown to decrease the incidence of necrotizing enterocolitis in neonatal rats,[186] while jejunal uptake of horse radish peroxidase was found to be higher in pups fed the artificial formula than in those fed maternal milk and similar to maternal milk when they were fed steroids as well.[191] The authors suggest that cortisol may work in conjunction with other hormones to affect gut closure, and may have surface stabilizing effects in the gut.

Uptake of immunoglobulins at the epithelial surface is facilitated by Fc receptors at the microvillus membrane. This receptor-mediated endocytosis is energy-dependent and saturable.[187] Uptake of macromolecules by nonspecific bulk transfer has also been documented in fetal rat intestine.[188] Specialized M cells preferentially take up antigenic material, which is then transferred to lymphoid cells, with which they are in immediate contact.[189] During human fetal development among the major changes that occur in the gastrointestinal tract are morphologic changes in the mucosal epithelial cells and the development of a crypt-villus axis. Once mature, there is continuous epithelial renewal from a common progenitor cell. The role of the mucus gel layer with intestinal permeability was examined in neonatal rats using FTC-dextran and N-acetyl-cysteine, a mucolytic agent. There was a significant increase in absorption of FTC-dextran in suckling rats over the weaned rats. On morphology an increase in intervillus mucus gel was found in the weaned rats, suggesting that an increase in the mucus gel layer with weaning may explain a decline in intestinal permeability.[190]

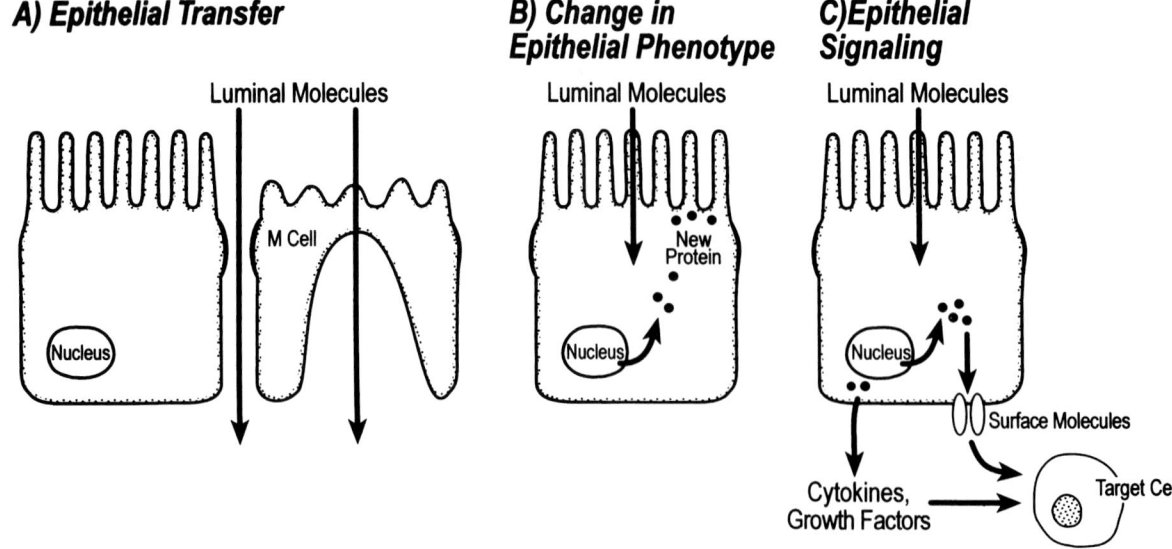

FIGURE 15–5. Possible interactions of molecules from the intestinal lumen with the epithelium. Traditionally the epithelium has been seen as a selective barrier to molecules, admitting those required for energy intake or immunosurveillance, and excluding others (A). However, nutrients can alter the phenotype of the epithelium to adapt to changing nutritional needs (B). When changes in the intestinal lumen induce new proteins that interact with mucosal immune cells, the epithelium can act as a membrane signaling information from the lumen to the immune system (C). (With permission from Sanderson IR. Nutrition and gene expression. In: Walker WA, Watkins JB, editors. Nutrition in pediatrics. Basic science and clinical applications. Hamilton, Canada: BC Decker; 1997. p. 213–33.)

Paneth's cells located at the base of crypts have an important role in the synthesis of host defense-effector molecules such as lysozyme, phospholipase A_2, and antimicrobial peptides.[191,192]

INTESTINAL FLORA

The gastrointestinal tract is sterile in the normal neonate, with colonization in early postnatal life (Chapter 17). Initial colonization in the first 2 weeks of life is independent of the type of feeding. In breastfed babies *Bifidobacterium* reaches 1010 to 1011 organisms per g of feces by 4 to 7 days. In contrast, enterobacteria are the predominant organisms in formula-fed infants. Presence of organisms such as *Bifidobacterium* and *Lactobacilli* appears to promote resistance against enteric infections.[193] This effect may be due to an inhibition of pathogenic strains or occupancy of receptors required for mucosal colonization.[194] Their presence is associated with the production of volatile fatty acids and a decrease in stool pH to 5 to 5.5. There is a predominance of coliform organisms in formula-fed neonates. The introduction of solids changes the bacterial flora in the breastfed infant to resemble that of the formula-fed infant, with an increase in coliform and anaerobic organisms that then provide the major antipathogenic effect. Commensal bacterial flora may also produce other differences in enteroendocrine function between breast- and formula-fed infants: for example, differences in motilin, gastrin, pancreatic polypeptide, and enteroglucagon responses.[195] In studies done on germ-free rats, an increase in the size of gastrin and somatostatin cells was produced, and it appears that alteration in luminal microflora may effect gut hormone secretion and motility as well. Volatile fatty acids produced by fermentation may facilitate better absorption of other nutrients by increasing intestinal blood flow. These volatile fatty acids may also be an energy source. Elemental diets reduce fecal steroid concentration, bile acid excretion, and volatile fatty acid production.[196] A large percentage of mono- and disaccharides reaching the colon undergo bacterial fermentation into short-chain fatty acids that are then absorbed, so that there is a reduction in the amount of osmotically active carbohydrates reaching the colon. Dietary nutrients provide substrates for microbial processes and yield products that can then be used by the host. Bacteria also use mucus, desquamated cells, and proteins provided by the host.

EFFECT OF LUMINAL MOLECULES ON IMMUNOLOGICAL GENES IN THE EPITHELIUM

The small intestine forms an important part of the mucosal immune system. It not only contributes to direct antigen presentation to T cells, but also secretes cytokines, which modulate immune responses, growth factors, and binding proteins that affect the proliferation of immune cells. The intestinal luminal contents are able to alter this immune response via epithelial signaling. A brief outline of examples of immunologically relevant genes follows.

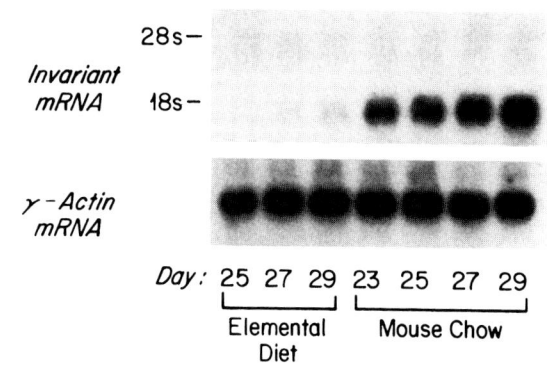

FIGURE 15–6. Dietary factors alter the expression of class II MHC and invariant chain expression in intestinal epithelial cells. Northern blot of RNA from epithelial cells taken from individual mice of a single split litter weaned at day 17 onto elemental diet or Purina mouse chow. The blot was probed with invariant chain cDNA and autoradiographed for 48 hours. Mice were examined at days 23, 25, 27, and 29. Blots were also probed with -actin cDNA to verify uniformity of enterocyte extraction. (From Sanderson IR, Ouellette AJ, Carter EA, Harmatz PR, et al. Ontogeny of Ia messenger RNA in the mouse intestinal epithelium is modulated by age of weaning and diet. Gastroenterology 1993;105:974–80, with permission.)

Cytokines

IL-8 is secreted by the intestinal epithelium and is a potent cytokine active in the recruitment of immunological cells into the epithelium. It is also a potent chemotactic factor for T cells and neutrophils; invasion by the latter is a hallmark of Crohn's disease, in which IL-8 is also elevated. It increases vascular permeability, increases superoxide generation, and promotes tissue edema. There is now evidence that its expression may be altered by dietary factors. N butyrate is a short-chain fatty acid produced by the normal metabolism of intestinal microbial flora. The latter vary according to diet. For example, infants fed a casein formula produce large amounts of butyric acid and propionic acid in the stool, while the predominant fatty acid in breastfed infants is acetic acid.[197,198] Butyrate increases the production of IL-8 in enterocytes and simultaneously down-regulates another chemotactic cytokine, macrophage chemotactic protein-1 (MCP-1). In contrast to IL-8, which promotes recruitment of neutrophils, MCP-1 attracts monocytes and macrophages and is constitutively expressed by the intestinal epithelium. Thus, dietary substances such as butyrate may alter the inflammatory response at the intestinal epithelium through changes in chemokine production.[157]

Class II MHC and Invariant Gene Expresssion

Class II MHC heterodimers are the molecules responsible for the presentation of antigen to T cells. Intestinal epithelial cells express MHC class II antigens, and hence may act as antigen-presenting cells (APC). Processing and presentation require an additional protein, the invariant chain. Diet has a marked effect on the intestinal epithelial expression of Class II MHC and its associated invariant chain in the mouse.

Although the expression is developmentally regulated, the timing of expression can be altered by delaying weaning from maternal milk to chow feeds.[199,200] However, this expression is only evident on weaning to chow, and not on weaning to an elemental diet, suggesting that gene expression in the intestinal epithelium could be altered by dietary manipulation (Figure 15-6).[199]

The mechanisms by which a nutrient or its metabolite alters RNA transcription, and hence gene expression, are not clearly understood. It is likely that epithelial signaling by manipulation of the luminal environment may have important therapeutic roles in gastrointestinal disease in the future.

CONCLUSION

An intrinsic timing or genetic determinants have been known to be responsible for specific developmental changes that occur in the gut. It is increasingly being realized that diet and luminal contents may modulate this development. The intestinal epithelium acts as an active membrane that responds to varying nutrients with changes in signal transduction and enzyme expression, and also acts as an effective barrier by modulating the activity of the mucosal immune system according to the intestinal environment. Extensive research is needed to understand nutrient-gene interaction and the role of the enterocyte in epithelial signaling. This understanding would have important therapeutic implications, allowing dietary manipulation of the intestinal environment in the management of gastrointestinal disease.

REFERENCES

1. Varkonyi T, Gergely G, Varro V. The ultrastructure of the intestinal mucosa in the developing human fetus. Scand J Gastroenterol 1974;9:495–500.
2. Coloney Moxey P, Trier JS. Specialized cell types in the human fetal small intestine. Anat Rec 1978;191:269–86.
3. Colony PC. Successive phases of human fetal intestinal development. In: Kretchmer N, Minkowski A, editors. Nutritional adaptation of the gastrointestinal tract of the newborn. Vevey-New York: Nestle-Raven Press; 1983. p. 3–28.
4. Menard D. Growth promoting factors and the development of the human gut. In: Lebebenthal E, editor. Human gastrointestinal development. New York: Raven Press; 1989. p. 123–50.
5. Pritchard JA. Fetal swallowing and amniotic fluid volumes. Obstet Gynecol 1966;28:606.
6. Lind T. The biochemistry of amniotic fluid. In: DVI Fairweather, TKAB Eskes, editors. Amniotic fluid research and clinical application. 2nd ed. Amsterdam, The Netherlands: Excerpts Medica; 1978. p. 73–80.
7. Pitkins RM, Reynolds WA. Fetal ingestion and metabolism of amniotic fluid protein. Am J Obstet Gynecol 1975;123:356–63.
8. Buchmiller TL, Fonkalsrud EW, et al. Upregulation of fetal transport in fetal rabbit intestine by transamniotic substrate administration. J Surg Res 1992;52:443–7.
9. Shrader RE, Ferlatte MI, Zeman FJ. Early postnatal development of the intestine in progeny of protein deprived rats. Biol Neonate 1977;31:181–98.
10. Koldovsky O, Thornburg W. Hormones in milk. J Pediatr Gastroenterol Nutr 1987;6:172–96.
11. Berseth CL, Lichtengerger LM, Morris FH. Comparison of the growth promoting effects of rat colostrum and mature milk in newborn rats in vivo. Am J Clin Nutr 1983;37:52–60.
12. Heird WC, Schwarz SM, Hansen IH. Colostrum induced enteric mucosal growth in beagle puppies. Pediatr Res 1984;18:512–5.
13. Henning SJ. Functional development of the gastrointestinal tract. In: Johnson LR, editor. Physiology of the gastrointestinal tract. New York: Raven Press; 1987. p. 285–300.
14. Duluc I, Galluser M, et al. Dietary control of the lactase mRNA distribution along the rat small intestine. Am J Physiol, 1992; 262 (Gastrointest Liver Physiol):G954–57.
15. Aynsley Green A, et al. Endocrine and metabolic response in the human newborn to first feed of breast milk. Arch Dis Child 1977;52:291–5.
16. Aynsley Green A, Lucas A, Bloom SR. The effect of feeds of different composition on entero-insular hormone secretion in the first hours of life in human neonates. Acta Pediatr Scand 1979;68:265–70.
17. Lucas A, Boyes S, Bloom SR, et al. Metabolic and endocrine responses to a milk feed in six day old term infants: differences between breast milk and cow's milk formula feeding. Acta Pediatr Scand 1981;70:201–6.
18. Lucas A, Adrian TE, Bloom SR, et al. Plasma pancreatic polypeptides in the human neonate. Acta Pediatr Scand 1980;69:211–4.
19. Arvola T, Rantala I, Martinen A, Isolauri E. Early dietary antigens delay the development of the gut mucosal barrier in preweaning rats. Pediatr Res 1992;32:301–5.
20. Attaix D, Meslin JC. Changes in intestinal mucosa morphology and cell renewal in suckling, prolonged suckling and weaned lambs. Am J Physiol 1991;261:R811–8.
21. Raul F, Kedinger M, Simon PM, et al. Comparative in vitro and in vivo effects of mono and dissaccharides on intestinal brush border enzyme activities in suckling rats. Biol Neonate 1981;39: 200–7.
22. Lee PC, Lebenthal E. Early weaning and precocious development of small intestine in rats: genetic, dietary or hormonal control. Pediatr Res 1983;17:645–70.
23. Buts JP, Nyakabosa M. Role of dietary protein adaptation at weaning in the development of the rat gastrointestinal tract. Pediatr Res 1985;19:857–62.
24. Castillo RC, Feng JJ, Stevenson JJ, et al. Regulation of intestinal ontogeny by intraluminal nutrients. J Pediatr Gastroenterol Nutr 1990; 10:199–205.
25. Decker BJ, Gall G. Impact of protein calorie malnutrition on the developing small intestine. A model in young rabbits. Biol Neonate 1988;54:151–9.
26. Butzner JD, Gall DG. Impact of refeeding on intestinal development and function in infant rabbits subjected to protein energy malnutrition. Pediatr Res 1990;27:245–51.
27. Chu SHW, Walker WA. Development of the gastrointestinal mucosal barrier: changes in phospholipid head groups and fatty acid composition of intestinal microvillus membranes from newborn and adult rats. Pediatr Res 1988;23:439–42.
28. Pang KY, Bresson JL, Walker WA. Development of the gastrointestinal mucosal barrier. Comparative effects of calcium binding on microvillus membrane structure in newborn and adult rats. Pediatr Res 1983;17:856–61.
29. Walker WA, Isselbacher KJ. Uptake and transport of macromolecules by the intestine. Possible role in clinical disorders. Gastroenterology 1974;67:531–50.
30. Hayashi K, Kawasaki T. The characteristic changes of amino acid transport during development in brush border membrane vesicles of the guinea pig ileum. Biochim Biophys Acta 1984;778:341–8.

31. Skude G. Sources of serum isoamylases and their normal range of variation with age. Scand J Gastroenterol 1975; 10:577–84.
32. Anderson TA, Fomon SJ, Filer LJ. Carbohydrate tolerance studies with 3 day old infants. J Lab Clin Med 1972;79:31–7.
33. Husband J, Husband P, Mallinson CN. Gastric emptying of starch meals of the newborn. Lancet 1970;2:290–2.
34. Zoppi G, Andreotti G, Pajno-Ferrara F, et al. Exocrine pancreas function in premature and full term neonates. Pediatr Res 1972;6:880–6.
35. Lebenthal E, Choi TS, Lee PC. The development of pancreatic function in premature infants after milk based and soy based formulas. Pediatr Res 1981;15:1240–4.
36. Borgstrom B, Lindquist B, Lund G. Digestive studies in children. Am J Dis Child 1961;100:454–66.
37. Madey S, Dancis J. Proteolytic enzymes of the premature infant. Pediatrics 1949;4:177–82.
38. Grand RJ, Watkins JB, Torti FM. Development of the human gastrointestinal tract. A review. Gastroenterology 1976;70: 790–810.
39. Kraml J, Kolinska J, Kadlecova L, et al. Analytical isoelectric focusing of rat intestinal brush border enzymes: postnatal changes and effects of neura-minidase in vitro. FEBS Lett 1985;151:193–6.
40. Aurrichio S, Caporale C, Santamaria F, et al. Fetal forms of oligoaminopeptidase, dipeptidylaminopeptidase and sucrase in human intestine and meconium. J Pediatr Gastroenterol Nutr 1984; 3:28–36.
41. Hauri H, Sterchi EE, Bienz D, et al. Expression and intracellular transport of microvillus membrane hydrolases in human intestinal epithelial cells. J Cell Biol 1985;101:838–51.
42. Triadou N, Zweibaum A. Maturation of sucrase-isomaltase complex in human fetal small and large intestine during gestation. Pediatr Res 1985;19:136–8.
43. Goda T, Bustamante S, Edmond J, et al. Precocious increase of sucrase activity by carbohydrates in the small intestine of suckling rats. Significance of the stress effect of sugar induced diarrhea. J Pediatr Gastroenterol Nutr 1985;4: 468–75.
44. Rosamond WD, Savaiano DA. Maintenance of sucrase activity in rat small intestine: influence of diet and age. Dig Dis Sci 1988;33:1397–402.
45. Alpers DH, Gerber JE. Monosaccharide inhibition of human intestinal lactase. J Lab Clin Med 1971;78:265–74.
46. Castillo RO, Feng JJ, Stevenson DK, et al. Altered maturation of small intestinal function in the absence of intraluminal nutrients: rapid normalization with refeeding. Am J Clin Nutr 1991; 53:558–61.
47. Markowitz A, Birkenmeier E, Traber PG. The 5' flank of the human sucrase isomaltase gene directs intestine specific transcription in transgenic mice. Gastroenterology 1991; 102:A285.
48. Menard D, Pothier P. Differential distribution of digestive enzymes in isolated epithelial cells from developing human fetal small intestine and colon. J Pediatr Gastroenterol Nutr 1987;6:509–16.
49. Tsuboi KK, Kwong LK, Harlingue AE, et al. The nature of maturational decline of intestinal lactase activity. Biochim Biophys Acta 1985;840:69–78.
50. Jonas MM, Montgomery RK, Grand RJ. Intestinal lactase synthesis during postnatal development in the rat. Pediatr Res 1985;19:956–62.
51. Villa M, Menard D, Semenza G, Mantei N. The expression of human lactase enzymatic activity and mRNA in human fetal jejunum. Effect of organ culture and treatment with hydrocortisone. FEBS Lett 1992;301:202–6.
52. Welsh JD, Poley JR, Bhatia M, et al. Intestinal disaccharidase activities in relation to age, race and mucosal damage. Gastroenterology 1978; 74:847–55.
53. Simoons FJ. Primary adult lactose intolerance and the milking habit: a problem in biological and cultural interrelations. Review of the medical research. Am J Dig Dis 1969;14: 819–36.
54. Whyte RK, Homer R, Pennock CA. Fecal excretion of oligosaccharides and other carbohydrates in normal neonates. Arch Dis Child 1978;53:913–5.
55. Heine W, Zunft HJ, Muller-Beuthow W, et al. Lactose and protein absorption from breast milk and cow's milk preparations and its influence on intestinal flora. Acta Pediatrica Scand 1977;66:699–703.
56. Jones DV, Latham MC. Lactose intolerance in young children and their parents. Am J Clin Nutr 1974;27:547–9.
57. MacLean WC, Fink BB. Lactose malabsorption by premature infants: magnitude and clinical significance. J Pediatr 1980; 97:383–8.
58. Fekete M, Galfi L, Soltesz G, et al. Lactose absorption in growth retarded newborn infants. Acta Pediatr Acad Sci (Hungary) 1969; 10:303–13.
59. Weaver LT, Laker MF, Nelson R. Neonatal intestinal lactase activity. Arch Dis Child 1986;61:896–9.
60. Raul F, Lacroix B, Aprahamian M. Longitudinal distribution of brush border hydrolases and morphological maturation in the intestine of the preterm infant. Early Human Dev 1986; 13:225–34.
61. Aurrichio S, Rubino A, Murset G. Intestinal glycosidase activity in the human embryo, fetus and the newborn. Pediatrics 1965;35:944–54.
62. Mayne A, Hughes CA, Sule D, et al. Development of intestinal disaccharidases in preterm infants. Lancet 1983;2:622–3.
63. Menard D, Corriveau L, Arsenault P. Differential effect of epidermal growth factor and hydrocortisone on human fetal colon. J Pediatr Gastroenterol Nutr 1990;10:13–20.
64. Menard D, Arsenault P, Pothier P. Biological effects of epidermal growth factor in human fetal jejunum. Gastroenterology 1988;94:656–63.
65. Arsenault P, Menard D. Influence of hydrocortisone on human fetal small intestine in organ culture. J Pediatr Gastroenterol Nutr 1985;4:893–901.
66. Nsi-Emvo E, Launay JF, Raul F. Is adult type hypolactasia in the intestine of mammals related to changes in intracellular processing of lactase? Cell Mol Biol (Noisy-le-grand) 1987; 33:335–44.
67. Malo C, Berteloot A. Proximodistal gradient of Na+ dependent D-glucose co-transport systems in the normal human fetal small intestine. FEBS Lett 1987;220:201–5.
68. Malo C. Kinetic evidence of heterogeneity in Na+ D-glucose transport systems in the human fetal small intestine. Biochim Biophys Acta 1988;938:181–8.
69. Malo C. Separation of two distinct Na+ D-glucose co-transport systems in the human fetal jejunum by means of their differential specificity for 3-O-methylglucose. Biochim Biophys Acta 1990;1022:8–16.
70. Davidson NO, Hausman AM, Ifkovits CA, et al. Human intestinal glucose transporter expression and localization of GLUT 5. Am J Physiol 1992;262:C795–800.
71. Murray RD, Bouton TW, Klein PD, et al. Comparative absorption of 13C glucose and 13C lactose by premature infants. Am J Clin Nutr 1990;51:59–66.
72. Kotler DP, Levine GM, Shiau YF. Effects of nutrients, endogenous secretions and fasting on in vivo glucose uptake. Am J Physiol 1980;238:G219–27.
73. Diamond JM, Karasov WH. Effect of dietary carbohydrate on monosaccharide uptake by mouse small intestine in vitro. J Physiol (Lond) 1984;349:419–40.

74. Diamond JM, Karasov WH. Adaptive regulation of intestinal nutrient transporters. Proc Natl Acad Sci U S A 1987;84:2242–5.
75. Ferraris RP, Diamond JM. Specific regulation of intestinal nutrient transporters by their dietary substrates. Annu Rev Physiol 1989;51:125–41.
76. Solberg DH, Diamond JM. Comparison of different dietary sugars as inducers of intestinal sugar transporters. Am J Physiol 1987;252:G574–84.
77. Ferraris R, Villenas SA, Hirayama BA, et al. Effect of diet on glucose transporter site density along the intestinal crypt-villus axis. Am J Physiol 1992;262:G1060–8.
78. Weiser MM, Quill H. Intestinal villus and crypt cell response to cholera toxin. Gastroenterology 1975;69:479–82.
79. Lescale-Matys L, Dyer J, Freeman TC, et al. Regulation of the ovine intestinal Na+/glucose co-transporter (SGLT1) is dissociated from mRNA abundance. Biochem J 1993;291:435–40.
80. Larrsson LI, Hakanson R, et al. Fluoroscence histochemistry of the gastrin cell in fetal adult man. Gastroenterology 1975;68:1152–9.
81. Larrsson LI, Rehfeld JF, Goltermann N. Gastrin in the human fetus. Distribution and molecular forms of gastrin in the antropyloric gland area, duodenum and pancreas. Scand J Gastroenterol 1977;12:869–72.
82. Lichtenberger L. A search for the origin of neonatal hypergastrinemia. J Pediatr Gastroenterol Nutr 1984;3:161–6.
83. Majumdar APN. Postnatal undernutrition: effect on gastrin levels at a later age. Experientia 1984;40:751–2.
84. Wolman IJ. Gastric phase of milk digestion in childhood. Am J Dis Child 1946;71:394–422.
85. Wagner H. The development to full functional maturity of the gastric mucosa and the kidneys in the fetus and the newborn. Biol Neonate 1961;3:257–74.
86. Foltmann B. Chymosin: a short review on fetal and neonatal gastric proteases. Scand J Clin Lab Invest 1992;210 Suppl:65–79.
87. Hirsch-Marie H, Liosilier F, Touboul JP, et al. Immunochemical study and cellular localization of human pepsinogens during ontogenesis and in gastric cancer. Lab Invest 1976;34:623–32.
88. Adamson I, Esangbedo A, Okol AA, et al. Pepsin and its multiple forms in early life. Biol Neonate 1988;53:267–73.
89. Carrere J, Figarella-Branger D, Senegas-Balas F, et al. Immunohistochemical study of secretory proteins in the developing human exocrine pancreas. Differentiation 1992;51:55–60.
90. Bujanover Y, Harel A, et al. The development of chymotryptic activity during postnatal life using the bentiromide test. Int J Pancreatol 1988;3:53–8.
91. Aurrichio C, Ciccimarra F, Vegnente A, et al. Enzymatic activity hydrolyzing γ-glutamyl-β-napthylamide in human intestine during adult and fetal life. Pediatr Res 1973;7:95–9.
92. Antonowicz I, Lebenthal E. Developmental pattern of small intestinal enterokinase and dissaccharidase activities in the human fetal. Gastroenterology 1977;72:1299–303.
93. Yuan X, Zheng X, et al. Structure of murine enterokinase and expression in small intestine during development. Am J Physiol 1998;274:G342–9.
94. Windmueller HG, Spaeth AW. Intestinal metabolism of glutamine and glutamate from the lumen as compared to glutamine from blood. Arch Biochem Biophys 1975;171:662–72.
95. Windmueller HG. Glutamine utilization by the small intestine. Adv Enzymol 1982;53:202–37.
96. Frisell WR. Synthesis and catabolism of nucleotides. In: Frisell WR, editor. Human biochemistry. New York: Macmillan; 1982. p. 292–304.
97. Meetze W, Shenoy V, Martin G, et al. Ontogeny of the small intestinal glutaminase and glutamine synthetase in the rat: response to dexamethasone. Biol Neonate 1993;64:6368–75.
98. Sarantos P, Chakrabarti R, Copeland EM, et al. Dexamethasone increases jejunal glutamine synthetase expression via translational regulation. Am J Surg 1994;167:8–13.
99. Kuo FC, Hwu WL, et al. Co-localization in pericentral hepatocytes and similarity in developmental expression pattern of ornithine aminotransferase and glutamine synthetase mRNA. Proc Natl Acad Sci U S A 1991;88:9468–72.
100. Shenoy V, Roig JC, Chakrabarti R, et al. Ontogeny of glutamine synthetase in rat small intestine. Pediatr Res 1996;39:643–8.
101. Sales J, Moreau H, Verger R. Human gastric lipase: ontogeny and variations in children. Acta Paediatr 1992;81:511–3.
102. Menard D, Monfils S, Trembley RE. Ontogeny of human gastric lipase and pepsin activities. Gastroenterology 1995;108:1650–6.
103. Mehta NR, Jones JB, Hamosh M. Lipases in preterm human milk, ontogeny and physiological significance. J Pediatr Gastroenterol Nutr 1982;1:317–26.
104. Hernell O, Gebre-Medhin M, Olivecrona D, et al. Breast milk composition in Ethiopian and Swedish mothers: IV. Milk lipases. Am J Clin Nutr 1977;30:508–11.
105. Hall B, Muller DPR. Studies on the bile salt stimulated lipolytic activity of human milk using whole milk as source of both substrate and enzyme. Nutritional implications. Pediatr Res 1982;16:251–5.
106. Hernell O. Human milk lipases. III. Physiological implications of the bile salt stimulated lipase. Eur J Clin Invest 1975;5:267–72.
107. Hernell O, Blackberg L. Digestion of human milk lipids: physiological significance of sn-2-monoacylglycerol hydrolysis by bile salt stimulated lipase. Pediatr Res 1982;16:882–5.
108. Luzeau R, Odievre M, Levillian P, et al. Activite de la lipoproteine lipase dans les laits de femm inhibiteurs in vitro de la conjugaison de la bilirubine. Clin Chim Acta 1975;59:133–8.
109. Hamosh M, Burns WA. Lipolytic activity of human lingual glands. (Ebner) Lab Invest 1977;37:603–8.
110. Moreau H, Laugier R, Gargouri Y, et al. Human preduodenal lipase is entirely of gastric fundal origin. Gastroenterology 1988;95: 1221–6.
111. Fredrikzon B, Hernell O. Role of feeding on lipase activity in gastric contents. Acta Pediatr Scand 1977;66:479–84.
112. Hamosh M, Scanlon JW, Ganot D, et al. Fat digestion in the newborn: characterization of lipase in gastric aspirates of premature and term infants. J Clin Invest 1981;66:836–46.
113. Hamosh M. Fat digestion in the newborn: role of lingual lipase and preduodenal digestion. Pediatr Res 1979;13:615–22.
114. Lee PC, Borysewicz R, Struve M, et al. Development of lipolytic activity in gastric aspirates from premature infants. J Pediatr Gastroenterol Nutr 1993;17:291–7.
115. Katz L, Hamilton JR. Fat absorption in infants of birth weight less than 1300 gm. J Pediatr 1974;85:608–14.
116. Borel P, Armand M, Senft M, et al. Gastric lipase: evidence of an adaptive response to dietary fat in the rabbit. Gastroenterology 1991;100:1582–9.
117. Armand M, Hamosh M, et al. Human gastric lipase expression is affected by dietary fat. Pediatr Res 1995;37:119A.
118. Poley JR, Dower JC, et al. Bile acids in infants and children. J Lab Clin Med 1964;63:838–40.
119. Sharp HL, Peller J, et al. Primary and secondary bile acids in meconium. Pediatr Res 1971;5:274–9.
120. Brueton MJ, Berger HM, Brown GA, et al. Duodenal bile acid conjugation patterns and dietary sulfur amino acids in the newborn. Gut 1978;19:95–8.

121. Wahlen E, Strandvik B. Effects of different formula feeds on the development pattern of urinary bile acid excretion in infants. J Pediatr Gastroenterol Nutr 1994;18:9–19.
122. Barbara L, Lazarri R, Roda A, et al. Serum bile acids in newborns and children. Pediatr Res 1980;14:1222–5.
123. Potter JM, Nestel PJ. Greater bile acid excretion with soy bean than with cow milk in infants. Am J Clin Nutr 1976; 29:546–51.
124. Signer E, Murphy GM, Edkins S, et al. Role of bile salts in fat malabsorption of premature infants. Arch Dis Child 1974;49: 174–80.
125. Jarvenpaa AL. Feeding the low birth weight infant. Fat absorption as a function of diet and duodenal bile acids. Pediatrics 1983;72:684–9.
126. Loirdighi N, Menard D, Levy E. Insulin decreases chylomicron production in human fetal small intestine. Biochim Biophys Acta 1992;1175:100–6.
127. Thibault L, Menard D, Loirdighi N, Levy E. Ontogeny of intestinal lipid and lipoprotein synthesis. Biol Neonate 1992; 62:100–7.
128. Levy E, Thibault L, Delvin E, Menard D. Apolipoprotein synthesis in human fetal intestine: regulation by epidermal growth factor. Biochem Biophys Res Commun 1994;204:1340–5.
129. Patterson AP, Tennyson GE, Hoeg JM, et al. Ontogenic regulation of apolipoprotein B mRNA editing during human and rat development in vivo. Arterioscler Thromb 1992;12: 468–73.
130. Mishom R, Eloy R, et al. Prostaglandin E1 and E2 stimulate release of intestinal brush border enzymes. Prostaglandins 1977;14:463–75.
131. Reiner DS, Wang CS, Gillin FD, et al. Human milk kills *Giardia lamblia* by generating toxic lipolytic products. J Infect Dis 1986; 154:825–32.
132. Newburg DS, Pickering LK, McCluer RH, et al. Fucosylated oligosaccharides of human milk protect suckling mice from heat stable enterotoxin of *Escherichia coli*. J Infect Dis 1990;162:1075–80.
133. Cravioto A, Tello A, Villafan H, et al. Inhibition of localized adhesion of enteropathogenic *Escherichia coli* to Hep2 cells by immuno-globulin and oligosaccharide fractions of human colostrum and breast milk. J Infect Dis 1991;163:1247–55.
134. Schroten H, Lethen A, Hanisch PG, et al. Inhibition of adhesion of S-fimbriated *Escherichia coli* to epithelial cells by meconium and feces of breast fed and formula fed newborns, mucins are the major inhibitory component. J Pediatr Gastroenterol Nutr 1992; 15:150–8.
135. Carpenter G, Cohen S. Epidermal growth factor. Annu Rev Biochem. 1979;48:193–216.
136. Rao RK, Thornburg W, Kore M, et al. Processing of epidermal growth factor by suckling and adult rat intestinal cells. Am J Physiol 1987;250:C850–5.
137. Thornburg W, Rao RK, Martisian LM, et al. Effect of maturation on gastrointestinal absorption of epidermal growth factor in rats. Am J Physiol 1987;235:G68–71.
138. Thompson JF. Specific receptors for epidermal growth factor in rat intestinal microvillus membranes. Am J Physiol 1988; 254:G429–36.
139. Sheving LA, et al. Epidermal growth factor receptor of the intestinal enterocyte: localization to latero-basal but not brush border membrane. J Biol Chem 1989;264:1735–41.
140. Menard D, Pothier P. Radioautographic localization of epidermal growth factor receptor in human fetal gut. Gastroenterology 1991;1:640–9.
141. Pucio F, Lehy T. Oral administration of epidermal growth factor in suckling rats stimulates cell DNA synthesis in fundic and antral gastric mucosae as well as in intestinal mucosa and pancreas. Regul Pept 1988;20:53–64.
142. James PS, Smith MW, Tivey DR. Epidermal growth factor selectively increases sucrase and maltase activities in neonatal piglet intestine. J Physiol 1987;393:583–94.
143. Bower JM, Camble R, Gregory H, et al. The inhibition of gastric acid secretion by epidermal growth factor. Experientia 1975;31:825–6.
144. Berseth CL. Enhancement of intestinal growth in neonatal rats by epidermal growth factor in milk. Am J Physiol 1987; 253:G662–5.
145. Berseth CL, Go VLW. Enhancement of neonatal somatic and hepatic growth by orally administered epidermal growth factor in rats. J Pediatr Gastroenterol Nutr 1988;789–893.
146. Donovan SM, Hintz RL, Rosenfeld RG, et al. Insulin like growth factors I and II and their binding proteins in rat milk. Pediatr Res 1991; 29:50–5.
147. Francis GL, Read LC, Ballard FJ, et al. Purification and partial sequence analysis of insulin-like growth factor 1 from bovine colostrum. Biochem J 1986;233:207–13.
148. Chaurasia OP, Marcuard SP, Seidel SR. Insulin like growth factor 1 in human gastrointestinal exocrine secretions. Regul Pept 1994;50:113–9.
149. Lund PK, Moata-Staats BM, Hynes MA, et al. Somatomedin C/insulin-like growth factor I and insulin-like growth factor II mRNAs in rat fetal and adult tissue. J Biol Chem 1986; 261:14539–44.
150. Potten CS, Owen G, Hewitt D, et al. Stimulation and inhibition of proliferation in the small intestinal crypts of the mouse after in vivo administration of growth factors. Gut 1995;36:864–73.
151. Olanrewaju H, Patel L, Siedel ER. Trophic action of local intraileal infusion of insulin-like growth factor 1: polyamine dependence. Am J Physiol 1992;263:E282–6.
152. Houle EM, Schroeder EA, Odle J, et al. Small intestinal disaccharidase activities are upregulated whereas peptidase activities is decreased by orally administered insulin-like growth factor 1 in the neonatal piglet. FASEB J 1996;10:A728.
153. Lo HC, Benevenga N, Ney DM. Insulin-like growth factor 1 (IGF-1)increases the fractional rate of protein synthesis (K_S) in jejunal mucosa and growth hormone (GH) increases K_S in skeletal muscle during total parenteral nutrition. FASEB J 1996;A728.
154. Burrin DG. Is milk-borne insulin-like growth factor 1 essential for neonatal development. J Nutr 1997;127:975S–9S.
155. Ulshen MH, et al. Effect of fasting and refeeding on IGF-1 expression in small bowel. Gastroenterology 1993;104:A651.
156. Burrin DG, Wester TJ, Davis TA, et al. Orally administered IGF-1 increases intestinal mucosal growth in formula fed neonatal pigs. Am J Physiol 1996;270:R1085–91.
157. Sanderson IR. Nutrition and gene expression. In: Walker WA, Watkins JB, editors. Nutrition in pediatrics. Basic science and clinical application. Hamilton, Canada: BC Decker; 1997. p.213–33.
158. Johanson BG. Isolation of an iron-containing red protein from human milk. Acta Chem Scand 1960;14:510–12.
159. Metz-Boutigue MH, Jolles J, Mazurier J, et al. Human lactoferrin: amino acid sequence and structural comparisons with other transferrins. Eur J Biochem 1984;145:659–76.
160. Masson PL, Heremans JF. Lactoferrin in milk from different species. Comp Biochem Physiol 1971;39B:119–29.
161. Kawakami H, Lonnerdal B. Isolation and function of a receptor for human lactoferrin in human fetal intestinal brush border membrane. Am J Physiol 1991;261:G841–6.
162. Davidson LA, Lonnerdal B. Specific binding of lactoferrin to brush border membrane: ontogeny and effect of glycan chain. Am J Physiol 1988;254:G580–5.
163. Mazurier J, Montreuil J, Spik G. Visualization of lactoferrin brush border receptor by ligand blotting. Biochim Biophys Acta 1985;821:453–60.

164. Davidson LA, Lonnerdal B. Persistence of human milk proteins in the breast fed infant. Acta Pediatr Scand 1987; 76:733–40.
165. Britton JR, Koldovsky O. Gastric luminal digestion of lactoferrin and transferrin by preterm infants. Early Hum Dev 1989;19:127–35.
166. Cox TM, Mazurier J, Spik G. Iron binding proteins and influx of iron across the duodenal brush border. Evidence for specific lactoferrin receptors in the human intestine. Biochim Biophys Acta 1979;588:120–8.
167. Amouric M, Marvaldi J, Pichon J, et al. Effect of lactoferrin on the growth of a human colon adenocarcinoma cell line-comparison with transferrin. In Vitro 1984;20:543–8.
168. Nichols BL, McKee KS, et al. Human lactoferrin stimulates thymidine incorporation into DNA of rat crypt cells. Pediatr Res 1987;21:563–7.
169. Oguchi S, Walker WA, Sanderson IR. Iron saturation alters the effect of lactoferrin on the proliferation and differentiation of human enterocytes (Caco-2 cells). Biol Neonate 1995;67:330–9.
170. Crouch SRM, Slater KY, Fletcher Y. Regulation of cytokine release from mononuclear cells by the iron binding protein lactoferrin. Blood 1992;90:235–40.
171. Lee WJ, Farmer J, Hilty M, et al. The protective effects of lactoferrin feeding against endotoxin lethal shock in germfree piglets. Infect Immun 1998;66:1421–6.
172. Goldman AC, Garza C, Nichols BL, et al. Immunological factors in human milk during the first year of lactation. J Pediatr 1982; 100:563–7.
173. Prentice A, McCarthy A, Stirling DM, et al. Breast milk IgA and lactoferrin survival in the gastrointestinal tract. A study in rural Gambian children. Acta Pediatr Scand 1989;78:505–12.
174. Ogra PL. Ontogeny of the local immune system. Pediatrics 1979;64 Suppl:765–74.
175. Keller MA, Gemdreau-Ried L, Hehner DC, et al. IgG4 in human colostrum and human milk. Continued local production of selective transport from serum. Acta Pediatr Scand 1988;77:24–9.
176. Kim K, Keller MA, Heiner DC. Immunoglobulin G subclasses in human colostrum, milk and saliva. Acta Paediatr 1992; 91:113–8.
177. Leyva-Cobian F, Clements J. Phenotype characterization and functional activity of human milk macrophages. Immunol Cell 1984;8:249.
178. Kulkarni AD, Rudolph FB, Van Buren CT. The role of dietary sources of nucelotides in immune function: a review. J Nutr 1994;124:1442S–6S.
179. Gil A, Coval E, Martinez A, Molina JA. Effect of dietary nucleotides on the microbial pattern of feces at term newborn infants. J Clin Nutr Gastroenterol 1986;1:34–8.
180. Carver JD. Dietary nucleotides: cellular immune; intestinal and hepatic system effects. J Nutr 1994;124:144S–8S.
181. Uuay R, Quan R, Gil A. Role of nucleotides on intestinal development and immune function. J Nutr 1994;124:1436S–41S.
182. Jakobsson I, Lindberg T, Lothe L, et al. Human alpha-lactalbumin as a marker of macromolecular absorption. Gut 1986; 27:1029–34.
183. Robertson DM, Paganelli R, Dinwiddie R, et al. Milk antigen absorption in the preterm and term neonate. Arch Dis Child 1982;57:369–72.
184. Ivengar L, Selvaraj RJ. Intestinal absorption of immunoglobulins by newborn infants. Arch Dis Child 1972;47:411–4.
185. Vukavic T. Timing of gut closure. J Pediatr Gastroenterol Nutr 1984;3:700–3.
186. Lucas A, Cole JJ. Breast milk and neonatal necrotizing enterocolitis. Lancet 1990;336:1519–25.
187. Wileman T, Harding C, Stahl P. Receptor mediated endocytosis. Biochem J 1985;232:1–14.
188. Orlic D, Lev R. Fetal rat intestinal absorption of horseradish peroxidase from swallowed amniotic fluid. J Cell Biol 1973; 56:106–19.
189. Owen RL. Sequential uptake of horseradish peroxidase by lymphoid follicle epithelium of Peyer's patches in the neonatal unobstructed mouse intestine: an ultrastructural study. Gastroenterology 1977;72:440–51.
190. Iboshi Y, Nezu R, Khan J, et al. Developmental changes in distribution of the mucus gel layer and intestinal permeability in the rat small intestine. J Parenteral Enteral Nutr 1996; 20:406–11.
191. Teichberg S, Wapnir R, Moyse J, Lifshitz F. Development of the neonatal rat small intestinal barrier to nonspecific macromolecular absorption. Role of dietary corticosterone. Pediatr Res 1992;32:50–7.
192. Mallow EB, Harris A, Salzman N, et al. Human enteric defensins. J Biol Chem 1996;271:4038–45.
193. Midtvedt AC, Carlstedt-Duke B, Norin KE, et al. Development of five metabolic activities associated with the intestinal microflora of healthy infants. J Pediatr Gastroenterol Nutr 1988;7:559–67.
194. Kennedy MJ, Volz PA. Ecology of *Candida albicans* gut colonization: inhibition of *Candida* adhesion, colonization and dissemination from the gastrointestinal tract by bacterial antagonism. Infect Immun 1985;49:654–63.
195. Lucas A, Sarson DL, Blackburn AM, et al. Breast vs bottle: endocrine responses are different with formula feeding. Lancet 1980;1:1267–9.
196. Hudson MJ, Boriello SP, Hill MJ. Elemental diets and the bacterial flora of the gastrointestinal tract. In: Russell RI, editor. Elemental diets. Boca Raton: CRC Press; 1981. p. 105–25.
197. Bullen CL, Tearle PV, Stewart MG. The effect of 'humanized" milk and supplemental feeding on the fecal flora of infants. J Med Microbiol 1977;10:403–13.
198. Weaver GA, Krause JA, Miller TL, et al. Cornstarch fermentation by colonic microbial community yields more butyrate than does cabbage fiber fermentation. Am J Clin Nutr 1992; 55:70–7.
199. Sanderson IR, Ouelette AJ, Carter EA, Harmatz PR. Ontogeny of Ia messenger RNA in the mouse intestinal epithelium is modulated by age of weaning and diet. Gastroenterology 1993;105:974–80.
200. Sanderson IR, Ouelette AJ, Carter EA, Harmatz PR. Ontogeny of class II MHC mRNA in the mouse small intestinal epithelium. Mol Immunol 1992;29:1257–63.

CHAPTER 16

Development of Digestive Enzyme Secretion

Margit Hamosh, PhD

Paul Hamosh, MD

This chapter will review recent developments in the biology of secreted digestive enzymes. The emphasis will be on the ontogeny of these enzymes and examples will be given from research in the human and, where appropriate, in other species. Because of the slow development of several major digestive enzymes, such as pancreatic colipase-dependent lipase and amylase, the compensatory function in the newborn of similar enzymes in milk will be discussed. Many aspects of these topics have been reviewed recently.[1–6] We will discuss the digestive enzymes that act in the stomach and in the intestine: that is, enzymes secreted in the stomach or acting in the stomach and enzymes secreted by the pancreas.

DIGESTIVE ENZYMES SECRETED OR ACTIVE IN THE STOMACH

The digestion of all major nutrients—carbohydrate, protein, and lipid—could start in the stomach through the action of salivary amylase, pepsin, and gastric lipase. In fact, however, only fat digestion is of major consequence.

Salivary Amylase

The food of newborns of all species is mother's milk, which does not contain starch; and therefore amylase activity is not important until weaning. The human infant is often fed formula that contains glucose polymers in addition to lactose, and is often given supplements (beikost) rich in starch during the neonatal period. Amylase, which cleaves internal α1-4 bonds to maltose, maltotriose, limit dextrin, and glucose, is the only enzyme that hydrolyzes starch. Because synthesis and secretion of pancreatic lipase in the newborn is very low,[7,8] salivary and breastmilk amylase are quantitatively much more important at this age.

In the human, pancreatic and salivary amylase are different isozymes; the structure of the latter is almost identical (94% homology) to that predicted for the former.[9,10] Salivary amylase is present in glycosylated and nonglycosylated forms that are degraded differently in the liver.[9] Free salivary amylase is inactivated at low pH but is protected by short-chain substrates (polymers of three to eight glucose residues).[11] In the newborn, such polymers in the formula and the high gastric pH[12–14] might protect salivary amylase from inactivation. Indeed, there is good evidence that salivary amylase remains active in the stomach.[15] The extent of polysaccharide digestion by salivary amylase could be significant.[16] Salivary, but not pancreatic, amylase was detected in amniotic fluid of 16-week fetuses.[17,18] Although salivary amylase levels are lower in children than in adults,[19–21] it is the only form of amylase detected in serum and urine of infants and children.[18,22–24] Three salivary amylase genes have been isolated from the human amylase gene cluster, which contains also two pancreatic amylase genes and two truncated pseudogenes.[25] The human amylase gene cluster has been localized to chromosome band Ip21.[26]

Pepsin

The structure and function of pepsins have recently been reviewed.[27] The gastric mucosa produces several pepsinogens.[27] Based on immunoactivity, they are pepsinogens A and C. The genes for these enzymes have been localized to different chromosomes in humans: pepsin A genes on chromosome 11[28,29] and pepsin C on chromosome 6.[30] Two additional proteinases are produced by the gastric mucosa: chymosin (rennin) and cathepsin E.[31] Chymosin is secreted primarily by the newborn of many species[32] and is highly effective in the digestion of milk proteins, whereas adults secrete mainly pepsins A and C. These enzymes are known as aspartic proteinases because of two aspartic residues that participate in the catalytic process. The general structure of aspartic proteinases appears to be well conserved. With the exception of cathepsin E, a homodimer that is probably an intracellular proteinase, the aspartic proteinases are single polypeptide chains averaging 35 kD (excluding the activation segments). These enzymes are synthesized as inactive preproenzymes that consist of a signal sequence (pre), an activation peptide (the pro region), and the active enzyme region. Pepsinogens are converted to active enzymes (pepsins) in an acid milieu (pH less than 4) by the cleavage of a 44-amino acid N-terminal peptide. The latter probably has a stabilizing effect, because the proenzymes are stable at a pH greater than 9.0 and at high temperature, contrary to pepsins, which are denatured.

Secretion of pepsinogens is stimulated or inhibited by a variety of natural and pharmacologic agents,[27,33] and their intracellular second messengers have been identified. These are either cyclic adenosine monophosphate (cAMP) or calcium, secretin, vasoactive intestinal peptide (VIP), adrenergic agents (cAMP) cholecystokinin (CCK), carbachol. The principal mechanism for release of pepsinogens has been identified as compound exocytosis,[27] the exocytotic mechanism being regulated by a feedback mechanism independent of secretagogues.[27] The ontogeny of pepsin has been investigated[34,35] and gastric proteolytic activity has been described in fetuses older than 16 weeks.[36,37] Cathepsin C seems to be the predominant proteinase from 12 weeks' gestation, whereas the other proteinases could be detected only at 17 to 18 weeks' gestation.[38] Development of gastric proteolytic enzymes may be affected by glucocorticoids[39] and thyroxin[40] and could also be affected by factors that are involved in the development of the stomach.[41–44] In a recent study, Menard et al.[37] have used fetal gastric explants cultured in a chemically-defined medium to assess tissue levels as well as pepsin secretion. Pepsin secretion could be detected at 16 weeks' gestation; however, its distribution, mainly in the antrum, was different from that in infants[45] or adults (gastric body and antrum).[45–47] Furthermore, the secretory mechanism for pepsin did not seem well developed at this stage of fetal development. Examination of pepsin activity in biopsy specimens from infants, children, and adults showed similar activity and distribution, suggesting that pepsin expression is fully developed in full-term infants at 3 to 8 months of age.[45] Pepsin secretion is, however, much lower in preterm infants than in full-term infants[35,48–51] or adults.[14,50] Diet—that is, formula or human milk—does not affect pepsin secretion.[14] It seems, however, that only limited proteolysis occurs in the stomach of the newborn. This might be the result of lower pepsin activity and output as well as of lower hydrochloric acid output.[12–14,52–60] The latter would maintain the postprandial gastric environment at a higher pH than that needed for optimal peptic activity.[27,33] Indeed, studies that have been carried out to assess the in vitro hydrolysis of human or bovine milk proteins by gastric[61] or duodenal juice[62] of preterm or full-term infants show only minimal digestion at conditions that simulate the gastric or intestinal environment. Indeed, bioactive human milk proteins, such as lactoferrin and immunoglobulin A, are present in the stools of human milk-fed infants,[63,64] suggesting impaired milk protein digestion in the stomach as well as in the intestine. Recent studies that have quantified protein digestion in vivo show that it amounts to only 15% of either formula protein or the proteins in human milk.[65] These in vivo studies in preterm infants show that protein digestion starts in the stomach and that previous in vitro studies do not accurately reflect the in vivo situation. There was a great difference

TABLE 16–1
Pepsin and Lipase Activity and Output in the Human Stomach: Comparison Between Newborn and Adult

	Enzyme Activity*		Enzyme Output**	
	Pepsin	Lipase	Pepsin	Lipase
Infant	125	10.0	597	25.0
Adult	600	5.7	3352	23.0

* Units per mL gastric aspirate; ** units × vol/kg body weight.
Data from Armand et al.[14,67]

TABLE 16–2
Nonparallel Development of Gastric Digestive Enzymes: Pepsin and Lipase

	Human		Ferret	
Age	Pepsin	Lipase	Pepsin	Lipase
Early fetal 10–20 wk	2.0	4.0–5.0	ND	ND
Late fetal 25–35 wk human, 5 weeks ferret	ND	60–100	0	2.0
Newborn 1 week	ND	100	0.3	20
4 weeks	18	100	30.0	153

Data are % of adult activity.
ND=not determined.
Data from Armand et al.,[14,67] Menard et al.,[37] and Hamosh et al.[71]

between the extent of gastric protein digestion and fat digestion. The latter was markedly affected by the nature of the meal, the fat in human milk being hydrolyzed to a greater extent than that in formula.[14] Thus, while the nature of the substrate (milk fat globules or formula fat particles)[14] greatly affects the extent of lipolysis, the extensive glycosylation of the proteins in human milk does not appear to have a protective function against hydrolysis when compared to formula proteins.[65]

There are also marked differences in the ontogeny of the two main enzymes secreted by the gastric mucosa. Although in the human pepsin and gastric lipase are located at the same site, in the chief cells of the gastric mucosa,[66] the enzymes do not develop in parallel fashion. Thus, whereas pepsin activity and output are much lower in infants[14] than in adults,[67] gastric lipase activity and output are equal in infants and adults[14,67] (Table 16–1).

A recent survey of the ontogeny of pepsin and lipase in the ferret, a species very similar to the human in its digestion of fat (gastric lipase is the principal preduodenal lipase,[68] pancreatic lipase activity is low in the newborn,[69] and milk bile salt dependent lipase [BSDL] is high in the jill's milk),[69,70] shows a similar nonparallel development of gastric proteolytic and lipolytic enzymes.[71] Indeed, in the newborn, pepsin amounts to only 0.3% of adult activity, as compared with 20% for gastric lipase.[71] Furthermore, at the end of the nursing period (4 weeks of age) pepsin amounts to only 30% of adult activity, whereas lipase is at a level higher than in the adult (153%).[71] A similar picture is seen in the human, where at 4 weeks of age pepsin amounts to only 18% of adult activity, but lipase activity is equal to the adult.

Table 16–2 summarizes the nonparallel development of pepsin and gastric lipase in these two species.

Gastric Lipase

Gastric lipolysis is catalyzed by three enzymes of similar structure and characteristics but, depending on species, of different origin.[72-77] The enzymes originate either in the lingual serous glands (lingual lipase), the glossoepiglottic area (pregastric esterase), or the gastric mucosa (gastric lipase).

Rat lingual lipase[78] and human gastric lipase[79] have been cloned and expressed in *Escherichia coli* or yeast. They are glycoproteins of an approximate molecular weight of 5 kD and consist of 277 and 279 amino acid residues with an unglycosylated molecular weight of 42.56 kD and 43.16 kD for lingual and gastric lipase, respectively.[78,79] The amino acid sequence of the two enzymes has an overall homology of 78%.[80,81] Deglycosylation does not reduce catalytic activity; however, the terminal tetrapeptide, in particular lysine-4, is essential for enzyme binding to lipid-water interfaces.[82] Rabbit and human gastric lipases have been crystallized recently.[80]

Low pH optimum (2.5 to 6.5), absence of requirements for specific cofactors or bile salts, and stability to pepsin enable these enzymes to act in the stomach, and in certain diseases associated with pancreatic insufficiency (cystic fibrosis and chronic alcoholism),[83,84] also in the intestine.

Substrate selectivity is relevant to specific aspects of neonatal digestion. Fatty acid and site selectivity (that is, position of the fatty acid on the triglyceride molecule) of gastric lipase result in release of the fatty acids at the Sn3 position.[85–87] Long-chain polyunsaturated fatty acids (LC-PUFA) of milk are located mainly in this position and are efficiently released by gastric lipase.[88] Similar location of medium-chain fatty acids (MCFA) in milk fat[89] leads also to their preferential release in the stomach,[90] an observation that started the erroneous belief that gastric lipase is specific for MCFA. This site specificity indicates that fatty acids essential for infant development, such as LC-PUFA, necessary for optimal brain and retinal development (docosahexaenoic acid, C22:6 n3) and infant growth (arachidonic acid, C20:4 n6) as well as MCFA, an easily available energy source, are preferentially released.

In vitro studies that simulate the gastric milieu have shown strong product inhibition that limits lipolysis to 10 to 20%;[1,2] however, in vivo studies that have actually measured the extent of lipolysis show that this process is extensive.[91–96]

The extent of gastric digestion of fat has been studied most extensively with mother's milk as the substrate. Depending on species, fat digestion in the stomach can account for 25 to 60% of total lipid digestion.[90] In the human, although gastric function and expression of gastric lipase are unaffected by diet, the extent of fat digestion is significantly greater in preterm infants fed mother's milk (25%) than formula (14%).[14] This difference is probably due to the structural differences in substrate presentation, that is, triglyceride in the milk fat globules or in formula fat particles.

The accessibility of triglyceride, the main energy source of the newborn, to the other lipases that affect lipid digestion, has been examined. Earlier in vitro studies have shown that pancreatic colipase-dependent lipase cannot penetrate milk fat globules and, therefore, is unable to hydrolyze the core triglyceride.[97,98] These studies have also shown that gastric lipase[97] and lingual lipase[98] can hydrolyze the triglyceride in milk fat globules. Access to the core triglyceride is probably facilitated by the hydrophobic nature of lingual and gastric lipases, as well as by the fact that these enzymes do not hydrolyze the acyl bond of phospholipids[99] (major components of the milk fat globule membrane[100]) or cholesteryl ester.[99]

More recently, it became apparent that the milk BSDL is also unable to penetrate milk fat globules[17,47] and that its activity in the hydrolysis of milk fat depends on initial partial hydrolysis by gastric lipase.[90,101] One can conclude that the phospholipid-protein membrane of milk fat globules is not an obstacle to the action of preduodenal lipases. Phospholipids are a major barrier to triglyceride hydrolysis by milk BSDL[102,103] and a mixture of proteins and phospholipids prevents triglyceride hydrolysis by pancreatic colipase-dependent lipase.[97] Indeed, the hydrolysis of milk fat globule triglyceride by either of these enzymes depends on the initial predigestion by gastric lipase.[90,97]

Recent electron microscopy studies of milk fat globules at the end of 50 minutes of gastric digestion in infants show that the globules maintain their initial shape, and that the products of lipolysis are contained in the particles.[14] Similar milk fat globule-contained lipolysis products were previously reported during in vitro incubation of milk fat globules with lingual lipase and visualization by phase contrast or freeze etching techniques.[104] The free fatty acids and monoglycerides produced are more polar than the globule core triglyceride and migrate to the polar membrane. At this site, they might destabilize the membrane, which facilitates its breakdown in the intestine and subsequent action by pancreatic and milk lipases. Breaking of the fat globule membrane is also aided by bile salts, even at very low concentrations.[105] Thus, contrary to the limited contribution of the stomach to protein digestion, the stomach is essential to fat digestion not only because (depending on the species) 30 to 60% of milk fat is digested at this site in the newborn, but also because partial hydrolysis in the stomach is a prerequisite for the subsequent intestinal digestion of fat. Furthermore, recent studies show that lipase activity and output in preterm infants is equal to that of healthy adults kept on a high-fat diet (23±1.3 U per kg).[67] The regulation of gastric lipase expression by dietary fat[67,106–110] combined with the high fat consumption in infancy might explain the high gastric lipase activity even in very preterm infants. Gastric lipolysis might also be of considerable importance during the transition from total parenteral nutrition (TPN) to gavaging because, contrary to intestinal and pancreatic digestive enzymes whose activity decreases during TPN,[111–117] gastric lipase activity is unaffected by mode of feeding.[118]

FACTORS THAT AFFECT ENZYME SYNTHESIS AND SECRETION

In vivo and in vitro studies have shown that cholinergic and α-adrenergic agonists stimulate lipase secretion from lingual serous glands.[106,119] Cholinergic agonists act more rapidly than β-adrenergic agonists; α-adrenergic agonists do not affect the secretion of enzymes (lipase or amylase) from lingual serous glands. Thus, neurotransmitter regulation of protein secretion from lingual serous glands appears to be principally cholinergic[120] in contrast to the β-adrenergic stimulation of protein secretion by the parotid gland.[121] Stimulation of the secretion of lingual lipase in vivo and in vitro by CCK-8 was also reported.[122] Denervation, that is bilateral resection of the glossopharyngeal nerves or of the sympathetic ganglia,[123] leads to marked decrease in the lipase content of lingual serous glands,[106] suggesting that the structure and function of these glands, as previously shown for taste buds, depend on the trophic influence of the gustatory nerves. The secretion of lipase from isolated human or rabbit gastric glands is stimulated by carbachol (100 µM) and CCK-8 (10 µM), while histamine has no effect.[74,124] The secretory process is energy-dependent and is completely inhibited by carbonyl m-chlorophenyhydrazone (30 µM), an inhibitor of mitochondrial oxidative energy production. The inhibitor, however, did not affect basal lipase secretion.[61,124] Histamine did not stimulate lipase secretion from isolated gastric glands, a finding similar to that reported earlier for pepsinogen secretion from similar preparations.[125] Several secretagogues have recently been reported to stimulate gastric lipase secretion in the dog: urecholine, pentagastrin, secretin, dimethyl prostaglandin E_2, and to a lesser extent histamine.[126] Based on this study and on earlier studies of gastric lipase secretion in the dog,[127] it may be that in this species lipase is synthesized and secreted from mucous cells of gastric glands. Earlier studies may have underestimated the secretory response because of inactivation of the lipase at low (less than 1.5) gastric pH.[128,129] Human studies have previously shown the coupled secretion of lipase and pepsin in response to pentagastrin stimulation.[130]

Recent studies indicate that in the human postprandial gastric lipase and acid secretion are under positive cholinergic but negative CCK control, whereas pancreatic lipase secretion is stimulated by both cholinergic and CCK-dependent mechanisms.[131]

Although it is not known what affects the activity of gastric lipase during development, a precocious response to secretagogue-stimulated pepsin release in the rat stomach (not present at birth or the following day)[132] can be induced by hydrocortisone, which also stimulates pepsin synthesis.[132] Corticosteroids and thyroxine have been shown to affect the ontogeny of lingual lipase in the rat.[133]

A recent study reports that epidermal growth factor (EGF) decreases lipase activity in fetal gastric tissue maintained in organ culture.[134] Epidermal growth factor receptors appear early in human development and at 12 weeks' gestation are widely distributed in the developing gastric surface and glandular epithelia.[135] However, although EGF decreases lipase activity it does not affect pepsin activity, suggesting that (as discussed on pp. 261–2) not only do these two gastric digestive enzymes develop at different rates,[14,71] they are also under different regulatory mechanisms during development.[134]

Gastric lipase can be detected earlier in the human fetal stomach than pepsin: that is, at 10 to 13 weeks as compared to 16 weeks, respectively.[37] Furthermore, localization—that is, mostly in the body—was already as in the adult. Contrary to pepsin, secretion of lipase from cultured human fetal stomach was well developed during early fetal development.[37]

Gastric lipase activity levels quantitated in biopsy specimens from the stomach of infants, children, and adults[45] were similar in all age groups and were in the range of 1.8 to 5.3 U per mg protein (1 unit of lipase activity = 1 µmol of oleic acid released from triolein per minute). Lipase activity was present in the body of the stomach and was low or undetectable in the antrum at all ages.[45]

Lipase activity in gastric aspirates could be detected already in premature infants born at 25 weeks' gestation,[136] and did not differ in several groups of very low birth-weight infants (26 to 34 weeks' gestation), but was 40% lower than in infants of 35 to 40 weeks' gestation. Activity was slightly lower in full-term infants than in the gestational age ranges 35 to 37 weeks. Lipase activity was higher in gastric aspirates obtained at birth[136] than at several days to several weeks after birth.[137] This could be due to accumulation of enzyme with little loss to the duodenum before birth, as compared to passage of enzyme with each meal from the stomach to the duodenum after feeding.

Lingual lipase might contribute relatively more to total preduodenal lipase activity in the newborn than in the adult.[138] This is based on observations of infants with congenital esophageal atresia in whom oral secretions can be collected from the esophageal pouch. In these infants esophageal aspirates contained slightly higher lipase activity than the gastric aspirates.[138] High gastric lipase levels are present in the newborn dog,[91,139] ferret,[71] and rabbit,[140] where this lipase contributes significantly to the digestion of milk fat.[91,93]

Whether gastric lipase compensates for low or absent pancreatic lipase activity in diseases such as cystic fibrosis, and pancreatic insufficiency secondary to chronic alcoholism is still open to debate. While fat malabsorption is evident in these conditions, considerable amounts of dietary fat are absorbed.[141,142] Preduodenal lipase activity in gastric aspirates of infants, children, and adults with cystic fibrosis was found to be similar,[83,84,143] higher,[144,145] or lower[146] than normal. The possible reason for this variability may be the qualitative nature of study design (that is, lack of a specific marker for quantitation of secretion rates),[147] different ages of patients, and differences in lipase assay techniques.

A comparison of our data[83,84] on preduodenal lipases in pancreatic-insufficient patients with data[148] reported for pancreatic lipase in healthy subjects show that the total amount of unstimulated lingual and gastric lipases delivered to the ligament of Treitz, during the first and second postprandial hours, amounts to 25 to 40% of the maximal amount of pancreatic lipase released in response to cholecystokinin-pancreozymin stimulation in healthy adults. The low postprandial pH in the upper small intestine might be associated with higher activity of lingual and gastric lipases, enzymes active at pH 3.0 to 6.5. There was a relationship between preduodenal lipase levels and fat absorption in individual patients, and high lipase activity was associated with low fat excretion.[83]

Deficient gastric lipase secretion in pancreatic insufficiency associated with chronic pancreatitis was recently reported and attributed to failure of gastrin stimulation of gastric secretion.[149]

PANCREATIC SECRETORY ENZYMES

Amylase

Studies in several species, including the human, have shown no or only very limited pancreatic amylase. In the human no amylase could be detected for the first two months after birth in duodenal aspirates from full-term or preterm infants.[8] Similar observations have been made in mice,[150] piglets,[151,152] and kid goats.[153,154] Only in the guinea pig is amylase well developed at birth.[155] Studies in fetal pigs have shown that the pancreas contained mainly chymotrypsinogen and barely detectable amounts of amylase, trypsin, lipase, and elastase.[151] Furthermore, GP-2, a sulfated glycoprotein of the pancreas localized to the luminal surface of the granule membrane and thought to be involved in granule biogenesis,[156] is not expressed until weaning. Recent studies[151] have shown that GP-2 and amylase evolve in parallel during pig development. Under acidic conditions similar to those in the sorting compartment of the secretory pathway, GP-2 binds exclusively to amylase.[157] Zymogen granules in fetal pancreas have a very light appearance, which could be due to the fact that they contain almost exclusively chymotrypsinogen, rather than adult granules, which contain three times as much amylase as chymotrypsinogen.[154] Studies in developing pigs[151] and mice[150] suggest that the expression of both GP-2 and amylase is required for the formation of zymogen granules of normal appearance. While the other enzymes, such as elastase, trypsin, and lipase may also be required for the production of normal secondary granules, they may not have a crucial role in zymogen condensation.[151] The evolution of chymotrypsinogen is in total opposition to all other zymogens, the latter rising substantially after weaning, concomitant with a decrease in chymotrypsinogen granule content.[158]

A glucocorticoid response element (GRE) linked with binding of the glucocorticoid receptor and subsequent activation of transcription[159] is associated with human pancreatic and salivary amylase genes,[25] and may explain the effects of these hormones on amylase expression.[160] The structure of human pancreatic α-amylase has recently been determined at a 1.8A resolution using x-ray diffraction techniques.[160a] The enzyme has three domains: domain A is the largest, and contains the active site; domain B is the smallest; and domain C is only loosely associated with the other two domains.[161] Several differences between human pancreatic and salivary amylase have been localized to the vicinity of the active site.

Proteases

The structure and function of pancreatic enzymes were recently reviewed.[3] All pancreatic proteases are secreted as inactive enzymes. Trypsinogen is activated by the action of enteropeptidase (enterokinase), an enzyme originating from the intestinal mucosa[162] to yield active trypsin.

Enteropeptidase initiates the activation cascade of pancreatic digestive enzymes by the cleavage of trypsinogen to trypsin, which in turn activates the other pancreatic zymogens.[162] Purified human enterokinase (molecular weight 296 kD) is composed of three subunits, each heavily glycosylated[163] with a total carbohydrate content of 57%. Because of its central role in initiating the activation of pancreatic digestive enzymes, the ontogeny of enteropeptidase has been investigated in many species, including the human.[164] The enzyme can be detected in human intestinal mucosa at 24 weeks' gestation.[164] Activity at birth is about 25% of that in 1-year-old infants.[164] Activity is highest in the duodenum; the gradient between duodenum and jejunum increases postnatally. Enteropeptidase differs from other intestinal enzymes, such as the disaccharidases, by its relatively late appearance during fetal development.

Congenital enteropeptidase deficiency, first reported in 1969,[165] leads to impaired digestion, and the affected infants require special formulas or pancreatic enzymes.

After activation, trypsin in turn activates the proteases by cleaving their activation peptides to produce active enzymes. This activation produces a conformational change in the enzyme protein.[166]

Trypsin is probably the most important digestive protease, and accounts for 20% of the protein in pancreatic fluid. Trypsinogen 3, the most cationic form, is present in twice the quantity of the most anionic form, trypsinogen 1.[167] A minor form, trypsinogen 2, is also present in human pancreatic juice. This form is antigenically different from trypsinogens 1 and 3, although the molecular weight is in the same range (25 kD) as for trypsinogen 1 and 2 (25 kD and 23.5 kD, respectively). A multigene family of at least 10 trypsin-like genes probably includes also trypsinogen 2. Site-directed mutagenesis is being used to elucidate the mechanism of catalysis.[3]

Chymotrypsin has been extensively studied.[168] In human pancreatic juice there are two chymotrypsins: a major form (24 kD) and a minor form of only 7% of total chymotrypsin (27 kD) that could actually be a product of proteolysis.

Elastase 1 (26.6 kD) and the more prevalent elastase 2 (33 kD) are secreted by the human pancreas.[167] Whereas the cDNA for elastase 2 has been reported,[3,169] there is no such information for elastase 1. Recent evidence suggests that human elastase 1 is a different gene product from elastase 1 of pig and rat.[170] After cleavage, the activation peptides of elastase and chymosin remain bound to the enzyme proteins.[3] Protease E is a pancreatic enzyme similar to elastase, but its substrate is not elastin.[171] A minor component of pancreatic secretions (0.4% of total protein) is kallikrein, a glycoprotein (35 to 48 kD) whose function is not well known.[172]

The carboxypeptidases are exopeptidases, contrary to the preceding enzymes (trypsin, chymotrypsin, and elastase), which are endopeptidases. Carboxypeptidases are metalloenzymes; the metal ion is zinc. There are two main forms, carboxypeptidases A and B, each containing several isoforms. Molecular weights after trypsin activation are similar for both groups: 33 kD and 35 kD for A and B, respectively. Contrary to many of the animal studies, which show low activity of all pancreatic exocrine digestive enzymes (except chymotrypsinogen) (Figure 16–1)[150–154] in the human, these enzymes can be detected in the fetal pancreas at 3 months' gestation, and their secretion was reported to start in the fifth month of gestation. Contrary to the other pancreatic enzymes, such as lipase and amylase,[7,8] proteolytic activity increases rapidly after birth in premature and full-term infants[7,8,173] (Figure 16–2). Elastase, however, is low in early infancy. Its development parallels that of pancreatic amylase; that is, adult activity levels are reached only at 2 years of age.[8] Different patterns of development of trypsin and elastase I and II were recently reported in several species.[174]

The development patterns of trypsinogen and lipase have recently been examined in the human fetal pancreas from the thirteenth gestational week. Fetal mRNA levels for both

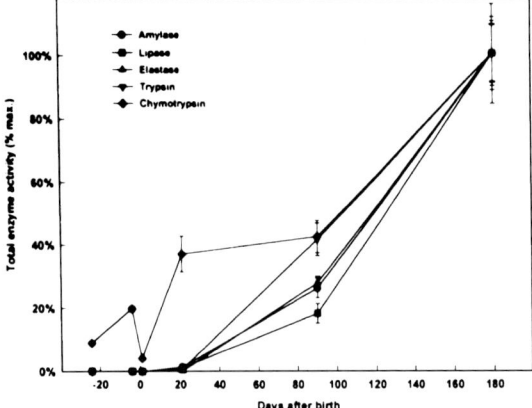

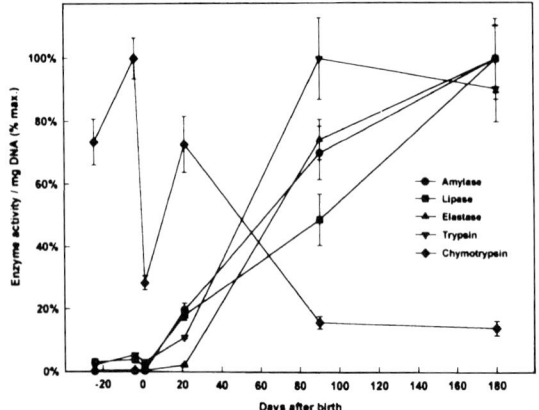

FIGURE 16–1. Development in the pig of five pancreatic zymogens from day 90 of fetal life to full maturity. U*pper panel,* Activity expressed as units/pancreas except for chymotrypsin, all other zymogens are almost absent until weaning (day 21 of age). L*ower panel,* Zymogen activity expressed as units/mg DNA. The number of animals studied at each time point varied from 12 to 33. (With permission from Laine J, Pellestier G, Grondin G, et al. Development of GP-2 and five zymogens in the fetal and young pig: biochemical and immunochemical evidence of an atypical zymogen granule composition in the fetus. J Histochem Cytochem 1996;44:481–99.)

enzymes remained low during fetal development.[175] No correlation was found between trypsinogen and lipase gene expression in the fetal pancreas, whereas such a correlation was present in the adult pancreas.[175]

Recent studies indicate that trypsin-catalyzed proteolysis is essential for the subsequent lytic effect of lysozyme on bacteria.[176] The concerted action of lysozyme and trypsin on bifidobacteria and lactobacilli could explain the release of microbial nitrogen and its colonic absorption and retention in the breast-fed infant.[177]

Pancreatic Lipases

Several lipases can participate in the intestinal digestion of dietary fat: pancreatic colipase-dependent lipase (CDL), carboxyl ester lipase (CEL), and in the breast-fed infant, milk BSDL. The latter two lipases are identical and are expressed in the pancreas (CEL) and in the mammary gland (BSDL). We will describe briefly the characteristics of CDL and will discuss BSDL (identical to CEL) in greater detail in the section on milk enzymes.

Numerous investigators have reported the very slow development of CDL in the newborn [7,8] and have suggested that the efficient digestion of fat is probably accomplished by other lipases.[1] The "classical" CDL has a molecular weight of 48 kD, is glycosylated, has a serine at the catalytic site, and has a signal peptide that comprises the first 16 amino acids.[3] The preferred substrates of CDL are emulsions of triglycerides or insoluble micelles.[3,6] Water-soluble esters are hydrolyzed at much lower rates. Colipase-dependent lipase is inhibited by bile salts in concentrations found in the duodenum. This inhibition is reversed by pancreatic colipase, a 10-kD, 86-amino acid protein that is secreted as procolipase and is activated to colipase by trypsin through the cleavage of a pentapeptide activation peptide.[178] Pancreatic lipase (which has no activation peptide) activity might be regulated by the balance between colipase and procolipase.[3] The three-dimensional structure of pancreatic lipase has been determined and shows the presence of two domains: an amino terminal domain (residues 1–336) containing the active site, and a carboxyl-terminal domain (337–449).[179] Procolipase binds to the C-terminal domain of the lipase.[179] Recent studies show that lipase activity is regulated by a "lid," a surface helix covering the catalytic triad that moves, and thereby changes the hydrophobicity around the active site. This explains the interfacial activation of pancreatic lipase: that is, the increase in activity in the presence of a water-lipid interface. Site-specific mutagenesis has recently been used to clarify further the function of colipase. These studies have established that colipase has a function in lipolysis in addition to anchoring lipase to an interface: namely, to stabilize the lid domain of lipase in the open conformation, thereby facilitating lipolysis.[180] Pancreatic lipase has lower activity on triglycerides containing LC-PUFA probably because of the proximity of the double bond to the carboxyl end of the fatty acid,[181,182] but is still able to hydrolyze manhaden oil, rich in LC-PUFA.[183] There is a six-fold difference between the best (oleic acid) and worst (docosahexaenoic acid) substrates.[184]

Lower lipase activity as compared with trypsin activity in small-for-gestational age (SGA) than in appropriate-for-gestational age (AGA) premature infants,[185] suggests that pancreatic lipase might be more susceptible to nutrient deprivation in utero than are proteolytic enzymes.

Another lipase, the carboxylester lipase, a 100-kD glycoprotein, amounts to 4% of total protein in adult pancreatic juice.[186] As indicated above, this lipase is identical to the milk BSDL; however, whereas the latter is assumed to contribute to fat digestion in the breastfed infant, little is known about the contribution of pancreatic carboxylester lipase at this age in the human. The enzyme is, however, well represented among other species; it is the only pancreatic lipase in the shark,[187] and is the main pancreatic lipase in the suckling rat[188] before the development of CDL.

The pancreas also secretes a group of pancreatic lipase-related proteins (PLRP1 and PLRP2),[189] whose characteristics differ from those of CDL by exhibiting high phospholipase activity, absence of interfacial activation, and absence

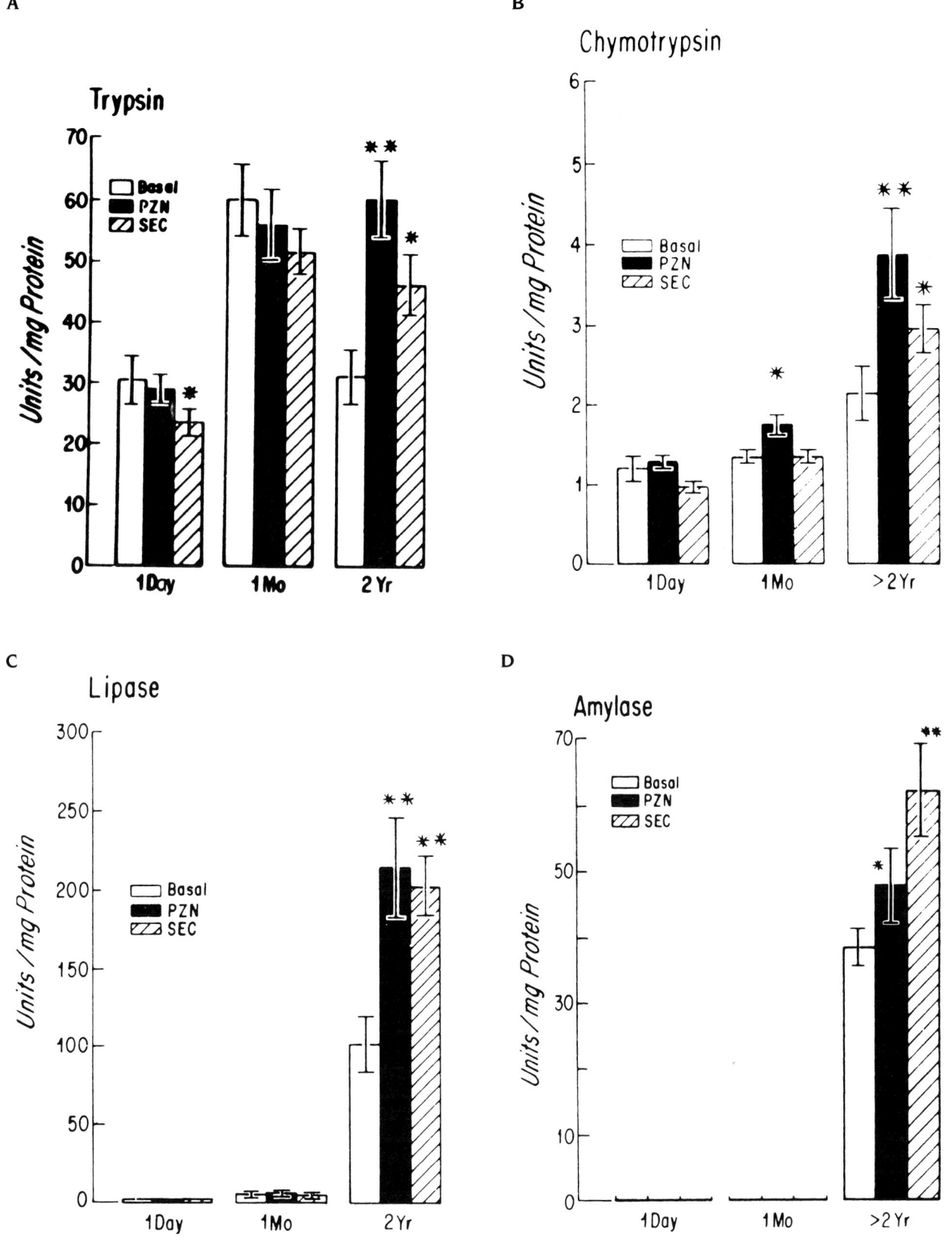

FIGURE 16–2. Development of pancreatic digestive enzymes in the human. (With permission from Lebenthal E, Lee PC. Development and funtional response in human exocrine pancreas. Pediatrics 1980;66:556–60.)

of colipase effect in maintaining activity at high bile salt concentrations.[189] These pancreatic lipase-related proteins are under investigation in the human,[189] as well as in several animal species.[190–192] There is high homology between PLRP1 and PLRP2, and still remarkable but somewhat lower homology between these pancreatic proteins and CDL. Because of their high phospholipase activity and inhibition by bile salts (that cannot be overcome by colipase), it has recently been suggested that they function mainly as phospholipases.[192] The potential role of these additional members of the lipase gene family, especially PLRP1, which is present in high amounts only during the suckling period, in neonatal fat digestion is currently unknown.

Although the similarities between these proteins and CDL (65% and 68% amino acid identity with CDL) suggest that the three proteins are related, the differences prove that the proteins are encoded by different genes of the growing lipase gene family.[192] There are differences among PLRP of different species.[192] Thus, the inactivation by bile salts and procolipase dependence of rat PLRP2 are in contrast to the properties reported for human and mouse PLRP2.[192] Rat PLRP1 has little activity against triolein, and could act on other substrates, possibly phospholipids, cholesterol esters, or vitamin esters.[193] There are also marked developmental differences between PLRP1 and PLRP2 (Figure 16–3). Rat PLRP1 and PLRP2 mRNA is abundant before birth, contrary to rat CDL mRNA. Pancreatic lipase-related protein 1 mRNA, however, remains high until weaning, whereas PLRP2 mRNA decreases sharply after birth.[193] Payne et al. suggest that the genes for the rat PLRPs are under different regulatory controls during development than is the rat CDL gene. Procolipase mRNA differs from that of CDL mRNA; the former is present during fetal and neonatal development contrary to the absence of the latter until the weaning period,[193] (see Figure 16–3). Payne et al.[193] suggest that PLRP1 and 2 may be important in the digestion of colostrum and milk in the absence of CDL. Whereas a substrate has not yet been identified for PLRP1, the significant activity of PLRP1 against triglycerides, phospholipids, and galactolipids suggests that it could be important in the hydrolysis of milk fat globules, which contain a phospholipid-rich membrane in addition to the triglyceride core.[193] The tight association of PLRP2 and the pancreatic zymogen granule,[161] suggests it may also be active in the release of zymogen granule contents.

Hormonal Regulation of Secretory Enzyme Development

Epidermal growth factor (EGF) has been shown to decrease lipase expression in cultured human fetal stomach; there was no effect, however, on pepsin activity.[44] It has also been shown to inhibit gastric acid secretion.[194] There are ontogenic differences in the potency and efficacy of this inhibitory action of EGF in the rat.[195] Corticosteroids have been shown to affect the ontogeny of lingual lipase[196] and of gastric proteolytic enzymes[197] in several species.

Pancreatic enzyme ontogeny is also affected by corticosteroids in many species studied.[198–201] Discordant effects on the expression of pancreatic CDL, PLRP1, and PLRP2[201] have recently been reported in studies conducted in AR42J cells used as a model system for pancreatic acinar cells.[202] Thyroid hormones have also been shown to affect the development of pancreatic digestive enzymes.[203,204]

Diet, especially components in mother's milk (probably growth factors) also affect the development of digestive enzymes,[205] as does the transition from the high-fat milk diet to the high post-weaning carbohydrate diet.[175,199,206,207]

DIGESTIVE ENZYMES IN HUMAN MILK

Human milk contains high activity of amylase and BSDL.[5]

Bile Salt–Dependent Lipase

There is indirect evidence that the milk bile salt–dependent lipase (BSDL) improves fat absorption in the newborn,[208,209]

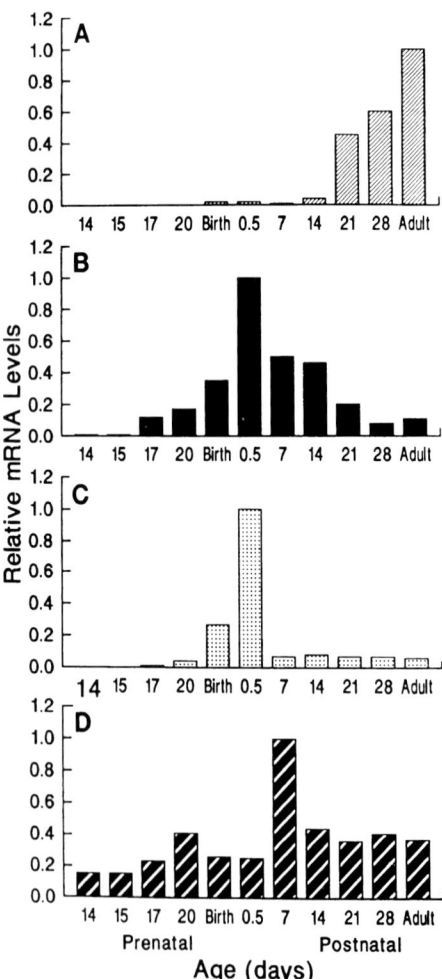

FIGURE 16–3. Developmental patterns of pancreatic lipase (A), PLRP1 (B), PLRP2 (C), and colipase (D) mRNA in the rat. Data are average of 2–3 separate determinations. (With permission from Payne RM, Sims HF, Jennens ML, Lowe ME. Rat pancreatic lipase and two related proteins: enzymatic properties and mRNA expression during development. Am J Physiol 1994;266:G914–21.)

and a greater body of evidence gathered from in vitro studies that the enzyme remains active in the infant's gastrointestinal tract and, therefore, might contribute significantly to fat digestion.[209-213] Milk lipolytic activity was discovered early[214] and has been extensively studied.[213]

Great progress has been made recently in our understanding of this enzyme's origin, structure, enzymology and species distribution, and possible function. The enzyme is identical to carboxylester hydrolase, a pancreatic enzyme of wide species distribution that is involved in the intestinal absorption of dietary cholesteryl esters and fat soluble vitamins.[215,216] In human and carnivore species this enzyme is also expressed in the mammary gland.[69,70,217,218] The BSDL cDNA sequence has been cloned from several species: human,[219] rat,[220,221] cow,[222] rabbit,[223] salmon,[224] and mouse.[225,226] In all species except mouse and human the BSDL cDNA has been cloned from pancreas only. The enzyme has recently been cloned from ferret lactating mammary gland.[227] The characterization of this enzyme as distinct from lipoprotein lipase (an enzyme present in the milk of many species, but with no function in the process of fat digestion),[228-231] first in human[232] and then in gorilla[233] milk, led to the assumption that this enzyme is a "newcomer" present only in the milk of high primates.[234]

In mature human milk BSDL activity is higher than in colostrum[230,231,235] and is present in prepartum mammary secretions collected during the last 2 months of pregnancy as well.[236] Other milk enzymes, including lipoprotein lipase, appear first only during the colostral phase.[236]

There is good evidence that BSDL may be a constitutive enzyme of the mammary gland because it is independent of milk volume, activity being similar before the onset of lactation[236] and during weaning.[237] This assumption is also supported by the high concentration of this lipase protein (1% of total milk protein) in human and carnivore milk.[69,217] Although activity varies among women, it seems to remain constant within each woman,[230,231] a characteristic shared with the other milk digestive enzyme, amylase.[238] During the first 3 months of lactation, activity levels are similar irrespective of length of gestation,[230,231] although it has been reported that in the initial colostrum stage lipase activity is higher in the milk of mothers of premature infants.[235]

Recently two variants of the cDNA[239] as well as the existence of two active forms of the enzyme with molecular masses of 97 and 120 kD[240] have been reported. Some women produce two forms of this enzyme in approximately equal amounts.[239] It remains to be established whether differences in activity levels associated with handling of certain milk specimens[210,241] are the result of different forms of the enzyme or of interaction between lactoferrin, previously shown to increase lipase activity,[242] and this lipase.

Enzyme characteristics are identical in milk from mothers of preterm and full-term infants.[243] Activity in milk is constant and does not change diurnally or within a feeding.[244] Bile salt–dependent lipase activity is also remarkably stable during prolonged storage (1 to 2 years) at either −20°C or −70°C[245] and during short-term storage (at least 24 hours) at higher temperatures (15° to 38°C).[246] Thus, banked human milk stored frozen maintains its fat-digesting capacity for long periods, as does the milk of working women or of mothers of sick or low-birth-weight infants who might have to keep the milk at suboptimal conditions for short periods after collection and during transport.

Bile salt–dependent lipase acts at a pH optimum of 7.5 to 9.0 and has an absolute dependence on primary bile salts.[230,247] Thus, the enzyme's action is limited to the intestine, where it continues the digestive process started in the stomach by gastric lipase. Indeed, as discussed earlier in this chapter, partial digestion by gastric lipase is a prerequisite for the subsequent hydrolysis of milk fat by BSDL.[90,91]

Bile salt–dependent lipase has no positional or fatty acid specificity and, therefore, can catalyze the complete hydrolysis of milk triglyceride. This is an important aspect of this enzyme's function, because neither gastric nor pancreatic lipase completely hydrolyzes triglycerides; the former produces mainly diglycerides, and the latter monoglycerides.[1] It is of great physiologic importance that BSDL hydrolyzes diglyceride (the product of gastric lipolysis) at higher rates than triglyceride,[248] whereas monoglyceride (the product of intestinal lipolysis by pancreatic lipase) hydrolysis does not require the presence of bile salts.[249] The lipolysis product of BSDL, free fatty acids, is more readily absorbed than monoglycerides[250] at the low-bile salt concentrations found in the newborn.[251] Indeed, fat absorption in breastfed, contrary to formula-fed, infants is not correlated with bile salt levels.[251] The low substrate specificity of milk lipase is probably the reason for hydrolysis of retinyl palmitate.[252,253]

The high extent of intragastric lipolysis indicates that the combined action of gastric lipase and BSDL could accomplish the process of milk fat digestion in the presence of very little or even in the absence of pancreatic lipase.[254] There may be distinct advantages for the newborn in having digestion at this stage depend mainly on gastric and milk lipases. Pancreatic lipase release of LC-PUFA, especially docosahexaenoic acid (22:6n3), is inefficient because of the proximity of the double bond to the carboxyl group, which interferes with the hydrolytic activity of this enzyme.[181-183] As discussed previously, gastric lipase readily releases these fatty acids from milk lipids,[88] as does BSDL.[255] The sequential release of fatty acids from milk triglyceride as well as the complete hydrolysis of the triglyceride molecule, catalyzed only by BSDL, probably explain the excellent fat absorption in breastfed preterm infants.[14]

Data are conflicting with regard to the effect of maternal nutrition on the activity of BSDL. Although an earlier study reported similar activity levels in the milk of well-nourished and undernourished women,[256] two recent studies indicate that the milk of malnourished women has lower digestive lipase levels,[257,258] which decrease by 80 to 90% during the first 4 months of lactation,[258] contrary to the constant activity levels in the milk of well-nourished women,[258] even after prolonged lactation.[237] This low lipase activity could adversely affect infants in undernourished areas or during periods of malnutrition. Not only would mother's milk provide insufficient digestive lipase, which might be needed even more than during normal conditions because of the malnutrition-induced decrease in pancreatic digestive function, but it could also affect the infant's resistance to infection, since free fatty acids and monoglycerides (the products of fat digestion) have anti-infective properties.[259-263]

Amylase

No disaccharidase activity has been reported in human milk; however, amylase activity was identified more than a century ago.[264] Only recently have its properties and possible functions in the newborn been studied. Contrary to the wealth of information on the BSDL, relatively little is known about the structure and the function of milk amylase. Milk amylase is identical to the salivary amylase,[265–267] and digests polysaccharides that are not present in milk, such as starch and glycogen, by hydrolyzing the 1,4-glucan bonds. Amylase may be more important to the infant after initiation of starch supplements, or when formula (which contains oligosaccharides hydrolyzed by amylase) is fed to partially breastfed infants.

Studies of amylase in milk of mothers of preterm and term infants have shown similar levels of activity in both groups.[265,267] Activity varies among women, but is constant in individual women beyond the initial phase of lactation, when activity is higher. Amylase activity is present in milk even after prolonged lactation of up to 27 months.[237] Activity is unchanged during feeding or at different times during the day. Amylase is stable during storage at −20°C and −70°C for months,[236] and there is no loss of activity even during storage of milk at higher temperatures (15°, 25°, and 38°C) for 24 hours.[246] Furthermore, recent studies show that only 15% of amylase activity is lost during Holder pasteurization of human milk, contrary to the complete loss of BSDL activity.[268]

Human milk α-amylase has a broad pH optimum range of 4.5 to 7.5 and loses little activity during incubation for 2 hours at pH 3.0 and above.[265] Thus, hydrolysis of polysaccharide could start in the stomach. (The postprandial pH of milk-fed or formula-fed infants is in the range of 5.0 to 6.0.) The milk enzyme is relatively stable to peptic degradation,[11,15,269] and remains active in the newborn's intestine.

The level of α-amylase activity is 10 to 60 times higher in milk than in normal human serum.[212,265] Little or no α-amylase activity is detected in fresh milk from cows, sheep, goats, or swine.[265] High-parity (10 or more children) women produce milk with only half the amylase activity of primiparous women.[238] Breast feeding can provide infants with a continuing supply of amylase, which may be even more important in malnourished infants and toddlers during the first 2 years of life than in healthy, well-nourished children. Supplementation with starch might be better tolerated in breastfed infants because of high intestinal levels of amylase provided by human milk, as has been reported from Egypt.[270] A direct antibacterial effect of amylase has also been described; *Neisseria gonorrhoeae* is inhibited by salivary amylase.[271] Because milk amylase is of the same isozyme group as salivary amylase, it might also inhibit the growth of certain microorganisms.

Proteolytic Activity of Human Milk

Although a number of proteases are present in human milk,[272,273] the high level of antiprotease activity probably prevents their action.[274]

It has been suggested that the antitryptic and antichymotryptic activity of human milk may prevent the absorption of endogenous and bacterial proteases in infants and thereby contribute to the passive protection of extraintestinal organs such as the liver.[275] The high concentration of antiproteases in colostrum coincides with the period of greatest transfer of nonimmunoglobulin protein from the intestine to the systemic circulation of the newborn.[276] In the human, who acquires maternal antibodies mainly in utero,[277] additional antibody is provided when breast milk immunoglobulins are transported across the intestine into the circulation of the newborn infant.

Estimates of the trypsin-inhibitory activities in human milk suggest that 90% of the pancreatic trypsin secreted by the infant in the first 50 minutes after eating could be inactivated if all the milk α_1-antitrypsin was biologically active when entering the intestine.[274] Although in the adult α_1-antitrypsin is denatured in the stomach, it might remain active in the newborn because of the buffering capacity of human milk. Alpha$_1$-antitrypsin remains functionally and immunologically intact in the intestine.[278] The severe liver disease often seen in α_1-antitrypsin-deficient infants is significantly diminished in such infants if fed breast milk.[275,279,280]

The interaction between milk-secretory digestive enzymes and the infant's endogenous digestive enzymes ensures optimal nutrient digestion and absorption, even where the latter have not yet reached their full expression.

REFERENCES

1. Hamosh M. Lingual and gastric lipases: their role in fat digestion. Boca Raton: CRC Press; 1990.
2. Hamosh M. Gastric and lingual lipases. In: Johnson LR, editor. Physiology of the gastrointestinal tract. 3rd ed. New York: Raven Press; 1994. p. 1239–53.
3. Lowe ME. The structure and function of pancreatic enzymes. In: Johnson LR, editor. Physiology of the gastrointestinal tract. 3rd ed. New York: Raven Press; 1994. p. 1531–42.
4. Hamosh M. Digestion in the newborn. Clin Perinatol 1996;23:191–209.
5. Hamosh M. Digestion in the premature infant: the effects of human milk. Semin Perinatol 1994;18:485–94.
6. Lowe ME. Structure and function of pancreatic lipase and colipase. Annu Rev Nutr 1997;17:141–58.
7. Zoppy G, Andreotti G, Payno-Ferrara F, et al. Exocrine pancreatic function in premature and full-term neonates. Pediatr Res 1997;6:880–4.
8. Lebenthal E, Lee PC. Development and functional response in human exocrine pancreas. Pediatrics 1980;66:556–60.
9. Alpers DH. Digestion and absorption of carbohydrates and protein. In: Johnson LR, editor. Physiology of the gastrointestinal tract. 3rd ed. New York: Raven Press; 1994. p. 1723–43.
10. Nishide T, Emim M, Nakamura Y. Sequence of cDNA for human salivary and pancreatic alpha amylase. Gene 1984;28:263–9.
11. Rosenblum JL, Irwin CL, Alpers DH. Starch and glucose oligosaccharides protect salivary-type amylase activity at acid pH. Am J Physiol 1988;254:G775–80.
12. Mason S. Some aspects of gastric function in the newborn. Arch Dis Child 1962;37:387–91.
13. Koldovsky O. Digestion and absorption. In: Stave U, editor. Perinatal physiology. New York: Plenum Press; 1978. p. 317–28.
14. Armand M, Hamosh M, Mehta NR, et al. Effect of human milk or formula on gastric function and fat digestion in the premature infant. Pediatr Res 1996;40:429–37.

15. Hodge C, Lehenthal E, Lee PC, Topper W. Amylase in the saliva and in the gastric aspirates of premature infants: its potential role in glucose polymer hydrolysis. Pediatr Res 1983;17:998–1002.
16. Keen CL, Heitlinger LA, Li BU, Murray RD. Digestion, absorption and fermentation of carbohydrates. Semin Perinatol 1989;13:78–87.
17. Wolf RO, Taussig L. Human amniotic fluid isoamylases: functional development of fetal pancreas and salivary glands. Obstet Gynecol 1973;41:337–42.
18. Skude G. Sources of serum isoamylases and their normal range of variation with age. Scand J Gastroenterol 1975;10:577–84.
19. Mayer WB. Comparison of amylase concentration in saliva of infants and adults. Bull Johns Hopkins Hosp 1929;44:246–7.
20. Nicory C. Salivary secretion in infants. Biochem J 1922; 6:387–91.
21. Rossiter MA, Barrowman JA, Dand A, Wharton BA. Amylase content of mixed saliva in children. Acta Paediatr Scand 1974;63:389–92.
22. Kamaryt VJ, Fintajslova O. Die Entwicklung der Speichel und Pankreas-Amylase bei Kindern in laufe des ersten Lebensjahres. Z Klin Chem Klin Biochem 1970;8:564–68.
23. Laxova R. Antenatal development of amylase isoenzymes. J Med Genet 1972;9:321–3.
24. Tye JG, Karn RC, Merritt AD. Differential expression of salivary (AMY 1) and pancreatic (AMY 2) human amylase loci in prenatal and postnatal development. J Med Genet 1976;13:96–102.
25. Gumucio DL, Wiebauer K, Caldwell RM, et al. Concerted evolution of human amylase genes. Mol Cell Biol 1988; 8:1197–205.
26. Zabel BU, Naylor SL, Sakaguchi AY, et al. High-resolution chromosomal localization of human genes for amylase, proopiomelanocortin, somatostatin and a DNA fragment (D3S1) by in situ hybridization. Proc Natl Acad Sci U S A 1983; 80:6932–6.
27. Hersey SJ. Gastric secretion of pepsins. In: Johnson LC, editor. Physiology of the gastrointestinal tract. 3rd ed. New York: Raven Press; 1994. p. 1227–38.
28. Taggard RT, Mohandas TK, Shows TB, Bell GM. Variable numbers of pepsinogen genes are located in the centromeric region of human chromosome 11 and determine the high frequency electrophoretic polymorphism. Proc Natl Acad Sci U S A 1985;82:6240–4.
29. Zelle B, Geurts Van Kessel A, de Witt J. Assignment of human pepsinogen A locus on the q12 pter region of chromosome 11. Hum Genet 1985;70:337–43.
30. Taggart RT, Cass LG, Mohandas TK, et al. Human pepsinogen G (progastricsin). J Biol Chem 1989;264:375–79.
31. Kageyama T, Ichinose M, Tsukada S, et al. Gastric procathepsin E and progastricsin from guinea pig. J Biol Chem 1992; 267:16450–9.
32. Kageyama T, Tanabe K, Koiwai O. Structure and development of rabbit pepsinogens. J Biol Chem 1990;265:17031–8.
33. Defize J. Development of pepsinogens. In: Lebenthal E, editor. Human gastrointestinal development. New York: Raven Press; 1989. p. 299–324.
34. Hirsch-Marie H, Loisilier F, Touboul JP, Burtin R. Immunohistochemical study and cellular localization of human pepsinogens during ontogenesis and in gastric cancer. Lab Invest 1976;34:623–32.
35. Wagner H. The development to full functional maturity of the gastric mucosa and the kidneys in the fetus and newborn. Biol Neonate 1961;3:257–62.
36. Foltman B, Axelsen NH. Gastric proteinases and their zymogens: phylogenetic and developmental aspects. In: Mildner P, Ries B, editors. Enzyme regulation and mechanism of action. Oxford: Pergamon Press; 1980. p. 271–80.
37. Menard D, Monfils E, Tremblay E. Ontogeny of human gastric lipase and pepsin activities. Gastroenterology 1995; 108:1650–6.
38. Reid WA. Immunolocalization of aspartic proteinases in the developing human stomach. J Dev Physiol 1989;11:299–305.
39. Sanglid PT, Silver M, Fowden AL, et al. Adrenocortical stimulation of stomach development in the prenatal pig. Biol Neonate 1994;65:378–89.
40. Kumegawa M, Takuma T, Hosoda S, et al. Precocious induction of pepsinogen in the stomach of suckling mice by hormones. Biochim Biophys Acta 1978;543:243–50.
41. Xu R-J, Mellor DJ, Birtles MJ, et al. Effects of oral IGF-I or IGF-II on digestive organ growth in newborn piglets. Biol Neonate 1994;66:280–7.
42. Xu R-J, Mao Y-L, Tso M-YW. Stability of gastrin in the gastrointestinal lumen of suckling, weanling and adult pigs. Biol Neonate 1996;70:60–8.
43. Tremblay E, Menard D. Differential expression of extracellular matrix components during the morphogenesis of human gastric mucosa. Anat Rec 1996;245:668–76.
44. Tremblay E, Monfils S, Menard D. Epidermal growth factor influences cell proliferation, glycoproteins and lipase activity in human fetal stomach. Gastroenterology 1997;112:1188–96.
45. DiPalma JS, Kirk C, Hamosh M, et al. Lipase and pepsin activity in the gastric mucosa of infants, children and adults. Gastroenterology 1991;101:116–21.
46. Abrams CK, Hamosh M, Lee TC, et al. Gastric lipase: localization in the human stomach. Gastroenterology 1988;95: 1460–4.
47. Moreau H, Laugier R, Gargouri Y, et al. Human preduodenal lipase is entirely of fundic gastric origin. Gastroenterology 1988;95:1221–6.
48. Adamson I, Esangbedo A, Okolo AA, Omene TA. Pepsin and its multiple forms in early life. Biol Neonate 1988;53:267–73.
49. Agunod M, Yamaguchi R, Lopez A, et al. Correlative study of hydrochloric acid, pepsin and intrinsic factor secretion in newborns and infants. Am J Dig Dis 1969;19:400–14.
50. Weisselberg B, Yahav J, Reichman B, Jones B. Basal and meal-stimulated pepsinogen secretion in preterm infants: a longitudinal study. J Pediatr Gastroenterol Nutr 1992;15:58–62.
51. Yahav J, Carrion V, Lee PC, Lebenthal L. Meal stimulated pepsinogen secretion in premature infants. J Pediatr 1987;110:949–51.
52. Harries JT, Frazer AJ. The acidity of the gastric contents of premature babies during the first fourteen days of life. Biol Neonate 1968;12:186–93.
53. Miller RA. Observations on the gastric acidity during the first month of life. Arch Dis Child 1941;16:22–5.
54. Avery GB, Randolph JG, Weaver T. Gastric acidity in the first day of life. Pediatrics 1966;37:1005–7.
55. Euler AR, Byrne WJ, Meis PJ, et al. Basal and pentagastrin-stimulated acid secretion in newborn human infants. Pediatr Res 1979;13:36–7.
56. Rodbro P, Krasilnikoff PA, Christiansen PM. Parietal cell secretory function in early childhood. Scand J Gastroenterol 1967;2:209–13.
57. Kelly EJ. Gastric secretory function in the developing human stomach. Early Hum Dev 1992;31:163–6.
58. Kelly EJ, Brownlee KJ. When is the fetus first capable of gastric acid, intrinsic factor and gastrin secretion? Biol Neonate 1993;63:153–6.
59. Kelly EJ, Lagopoulos M, Primrose JN. Immunocytochemical localization of parietal cells and G cells in the developing human stomach. Gut 1993;34:1057–9.
60. Kelly EJ, Newell SJ, Brownlee KG, et al. Gastric acid secretion in preterm infants. Early Hum Dev 1993;35: 215–20.

61. Britton JR, Koldovsky O. Gastric luminal digestion of lactoferrin and transferrin by preterm infants. Early Hum Dev 1989;19:127–35.
62. Lindberg T, Borulf S, Jakobsson I. Digestion of milk proteins in infancy. Acta Paediatr Scand 1989;351:29–33.
63. Schanler RJ, Goldblum RM, Garza C, Goldman AS. Enhanced fecal excretion of selected immune factors in very low birth weight infants fed fortified human milk. Pediatr Res 1986;20:711–5.
64. Davidson LA, Lonnerdal B. Persistence of human milk proteins in the breast-fed infant. Acta Paediatr Scand 1988;76:733–40.
65. Henderson TR, Hamosh M, Armand M, et al. Gastric proteolysis in preterm infants fed mother's milk or formula. In: Newburg DS, editor. Bioactive components of human milk. New York: Plenum Press; 1998. [In press]
66. Moreau H, Bernadac A, Gargouri Y, et al. Immunocytolocalization of human gastric lipase in chief cells of the fundic mucosa. Histochemistry 1989;91:419–23.
67. Armand M, Hamosh M, DiPalma JS, et al. Dietary fat modulates gastric lipase activity in healthy humans. Am J Clin Nutr 1995;62:74–80.
68. Hamosh M, Henderson TR, Hamosh P. What is the quantitative contribution of milk bile salt dependent lipase to the fat digestion ability of the newborn [abstract]. FASEB J 1995;9:A735.
69. Ellis LA, Hamosh M. Bile salt stimulated lipase: comparative studies in ferret milk and lactating mammary gland. Lipids 1992;27:917–22.
70. Sbarra J, Mas E, Henderson TR, et al. Digestive lipases of the newborn ferret: compensatory role of milk bile salt dependent lipase. Pediatr Res 1996;40:263–8.
71. Hamosh M, Henderson TR, Hamosh P. Gastric lipase and pepsin activities in the developing ferret: non-parallel development of the two gastric digestive enzymes. J Pediatr Gastroenterol Nutr 1998;26:162–6.
72. Hamosh M, Scow RO. Lingual lipase and its role in the digestion of dietary lipid. J Clin Invest 1973;52:88–95.
73. Ramsey HA, Wise GH, Tove SB. Esterolytic activity of certain alimentary and related tissues from cattle in different age group. J Dairy Sci 1956;39:1312–21.
74. De Nigris SJ, Hamosh M, Kasbekar DK, et al. Lingual and gastric lipases: species differences in the origin of prepancreatic digestive lipases and in localization of gastric lipase. Biochim Biophys Acta 1988;959:39–45.
75. Moreau H, Gargouri Y, Lecat D, et al. Screening of preduodenal lipases in several mammals. Biochim Biophys Acta 1988;959:247–52.
76. Sweet BJ, Matthews LC, Richardson T. Purification and characterization of pregastric esterase of calf. Arch Biochem Biophys 1984;234:144–50.
77. Bernback S, Hernell O, Blackberg L. Purification and molecular characterization of bovine pregastric esterase. Eur J Biochem 1985;148:233–8.
78. Docherty AJP, Bodmer MW, Angal S, et al. Molecular cloning and nucleotide sequences of rat lingual lipase cDNA. Nucleic Acids Res 1985;13:1891–903.
79. Bodmer MW, Angal S, Yarraton GT, et al. Molecular cloning of a human gastric lipase and expression of the enzyme in yeast. Biochim Biophys Acta 1987;902:237–44.
80. Moreau H, Abergel C, Carriere F, et al. Isoform purification of gastric lipase. J Mol Biol 1992;225:147–53.
81. Moreau H, Gargouri Y, Lecat D, et al. Purification, characterization and kinetic properties of the rabbit gastric lipase. Biochim Biophys Acta 1988;960:286–93.
82. Bernback S, Blackberg L. Human gastric lipase. The N-terminal peptide is essential for lipid binding and lipase activity. Eur J Biochem 1989;182:495–9.
83. Abrams CK, Hamosh M, Dutta SK, et al. Lingual lipase in cystic fibrosis. Quantitation of enzyme activity in the upper small intestine of patients with exocrine pancreatic insufficiency. J Clin Invest 1984;73:374–82.
84. Abrams CK, Hamosh M, Dutta SK, Hamosh P. Role of nonpancreatic lipolytic activity in exocrine pancreatic insufficiency. Gastroenterology 1987;92:125–9.
85. Paltauf R, Esfandi F, Holasek A. Stereospecificity of lipases. Enzymatic hydrolysis of enantiomeric alkayldiacylglycerols by lipoprotein lipase, lingual and pancreatic lipases. FEBS Lett 1974;40:119–23.
86. Jensen RG, de Jong FA, Clark RM, et al. Stereospecificity of premature human lingual lipase. Lipids 1982;17:570–2.
87. Rogalska E, Ransac S, Verger R. Stereospecificity of lipases. II. Stereoselective hydrolysis of triglycerides by gastric and pancreatic lipases. J Biol Chem 1990;265:20271–6.
88. Iverson SJ, Sampugna J, Oftedal OT. Positional specificity of gastric hydrolysis of long-chain n-3 polyunsaturated fatty acids of seal milk triglycerides. Lipids 1992;27:870–8.
89. Parodi PW. Positional distribution of fatty acids in triglycerides from milk of several species of mammals. Lipids 1982;17:437–42.
90. Hamosh M, Iverson SJ, Kirk CL, Hamosh P. Milk lipids and neonatal fat digestion: relationships between fatty acid composition and endogenous and exogenous digestive enzymes and digestion of milk fat. World Rev Nutr Diet 1994;75:86–91.
91. Iverson SJ, Kirk CL, Hamosh M, Newsome J. Milk lipid digestion in the neonatal dog: the combined actions of gastric and bile salt stimulated lipases. Biochim Biophys Acta 1991;1083:109–19.
92. Aw TY, Grigor MR. Digestion and absorption of triacylglycerol in 14 day old suckling rats. J Nutr 1980;110:2133–40.
93. Perret JP. Lipolyse gastrique des triglycerides du lait maternel et absorption gastrique des acids gras a chaine moyenne chez le lapereau. J Physiol (Lond) 1980;76:159–66.
94. Staggers JE, Fernando-Warnakulasuriya GJP, Wells MA. Studies on fat digestion and transport in the suckling rat. II. Triacylglycerols, molecular species, stereospecific analysis and specificity of hydrolysis by lingual lipase. J Lipid Res 1981;22:675–9.
95. Douglas GR, Reinauer AJ, Brooks WC, Pratt JH. The effect on digestion and absorption of excluding the pancreatic juice from the intestine. Gastroenterology 1953;23:452–9.
96. Chiang SH, Pettigrew J, Clarke SD, Cornelius SG. Digestion and absorption of fish oil by neonatal piglets. J Nutr 1989;119:1741–3.
97. Cohen J, Morgan GRH, Hofmann AF. Lipolytic activity of human gastric and duodenal juice against medium and long-chain triglycerides. Gastroenterology 1971;60:1–15.
98. Plucinski TM, Hamosh M, Hamosh P. Fat digestion in the rat: role of lingual lipase. Am J Physiol 1979;237:E541–7.
99. Liao TH, Hamosh M, Hamosh P. Fat digestion by lingual lipase; mechanism of lipolysis in the stomach and upper small intestine. Pediatr Res 1984;18:402–9.
100. Reugg M, Blanc B. Structure and properties of the particulate constituents of human milk. A review. Food Microstructure 1982;1:25–40.
101. Bernback S, Blackberg L, Hernell O. The complete digestion of human milk triacylglycerol in vitro requires gastric lipase, pancreatic colipase dependent lipase and bile salt stimulated lipase. J Clin Invest 1990;85:1221–6.
102. Lindstrom MB, Persson J, Thurn L, Borgstrom B. Effect of pancreatic phospholipase A2 and gastric lipase on the action of pancreatic carboxylester lipase against lipid substrates in vitro. Biochim Biophys Acta 1991;1084:194–7.

103. Lindstrom MB, Stenrby B, Borgstrom B. Concerted action of human carboxyl ester lipase and pancreatic lipase during lipid digestion in vitro: importance of the physicochemical state of the substrate. Biochim Biophys Acta 1988;959:178–84.
104. Patton JS, Rigler MW, Liao TH, et al. Hydrolysis of triacylglycerol emulsions by lingual lipase—a microscopic study. Biochim Biophys Acta 1982;712:400–7.
105. Patton S, Borgstrom B, Stemberger BH, Welsch U. Release of membrane from milk fat globules by conjugated bile salts. J Pediatr Gastroenterol Nutr 1986;5:262–7.
106. Hamosh M. Rat lingual lipase: factors affecting enzyme activity and secretion. Am J Physiol 1978;235:E416–21.
107. Lairon D, Borel P. La regulation nutritionnelle des enzymes de la digestion des lipides. Cah Nutr Diet 1989;24:413–23.
108. Armand M, Borel P, Cara L, et al. Adaptation of lingual lipase to dietary fat in the rat. J Nutr 1990;120:1148–56.
109. Borel P, Armand M, Senft M, et al. Gastric lipase: evidence of an adaptive response to dietary fat in the rabbit. Gastroenterology 1991;100:1582–9.
110. Roberts IM, Seidner DL, Solomon S, et al. High fat diet induces lingual lipase mRNA [abstract]. Clin Res 1990; 38:386A.
111. Levine GM, Deren JJ, Steiger E, Zinno R. Role of oral intake in maintenance of gut mass and disaccharidase activity. Gastroenterology 1974;67:975–82.
112. Eastwood GL. Small bowel morphology and epithelial proliferation in intravenously alimented rabbits. Surgery 1977;82: 613–20.
113. Hughes CA, Dowling RH. Speed of onset of adaptive mucosal hypofunction in the intestine of parenterally fed rats. Clin Sci (Colch) 1980;59:317–27.
114. Johnson L, Copeland EM, Dudrick JJ, et al. Structural and hormonal alterations in the gastrointestinal tract of parenterally fed rats. Gastroenterology 1975;68:1177–83.
115. Rossi TM, Lee PC, Lebenthal E. Total parenteral nutrition in infancy affects amylase and lipase but not trypsin secretion. Pediatr Res 1987;21:276A.
116. Rossi TM. Effect of total parenteral nutrition on the digestive organs. In: Lebenthal E, editor. Total parenteral nutrition: indications, utilization, complications, and pathophysiological considerations. New York: Raven Press; 1986. p. 173–84.
117. Hughes CA. Intestinal adaptation. In: Tanner MS, Stocks RJ, editors. Neonatal gastroenterology, contemporary issues. Newcastle-Upon-Tyne, England: Intercept; 1984. p. 69–91.
118. Mehta NR, Liao TH, Hamosh M, et al. Effect of total parenteral nutrition on lipase activity in the stomach of very low birth weight infants. Biol Neonate 1988;53:261–6.
119. Hand AR. The fine structure of von Ebner's gland of the rat. Cell Biol 1970;44:340–53.
120. Field RB, Hand AR. Secretion of lingual lipase and amylase from rat lingual serous glands. Am J Physiol 1987;253:G217–25.
121. Amsterdam A, Ohad Y, Schramm M. Dynamic changes in the ultrastructure of the acinar cell of the rat parotid gland during the secretory cycle. J Cell Biol 1969;41:753–73.
122. Roberts IM, Solomon S, Brusco O. CCK-octapeptide stimulates lingual lipase release in vivo and in vitro. [abstract] Gastroenterology 1989;96:A419.
123. Guth L. The effects of glossopharyngeal nerve transection on the circumvallate papilla of the rat. Anat Rec 1957;128:715–32.
124. Fink CS, Hamosh M, Hamosh P, et al. Lipase secretion from dispersed rabbit gastric glands. Am J Physiol 1985;248:G68–72.
125. Kasbekar DK, Jensen RT, Gardner JD. Pepsinogen secretion from dispersed glands from rabbit stomach. Am J Physiol 1983;244:G392–6.
126. Carriere F, Ralphel V, Moreau H, et al. Dog gastric lipase: stimulation of its secretion in vivo and cytolocalization in mucous pit cells. Gastroenterology 1992;102:1535–45.
127. Gerard A, Lev R, Jerzy Glass GB. Histochemical study of the mucosubstances in the canine stomach. II. The effect of histamine, gastrin, urecholine, and food. Lab Invest 1968;19: 29–39.
128. Blum AL, Linscheer WG. Lipase in canine gastric juice. Proc Soc Exp Biol Med 1970;135:565–8.
129. Clementi A, Urbano A, Cambria A. Sede della secrezione della gastrolipasi nel sistema ghiandolare della mucosa gastrica del cane. Boll Soc Ital Biol Sper 1969;44:802–4.
130. Szafran Z, Szafran H, Popiela T, Tromperter G. Coupled secretion of gastric lipase and pepsin in man following pentagastrin stimulation. Digestion 1978;18:310–8.
131. Borovicka J, Schwizer W, Mettraux C, et al. Regulation of gastric and pancreatic lipase secretion by CCK and cholinergic mechanisms in humans. Am J Physiol 1997;273;G374–80.
132. Yahav J, Lee PC, Lebenthal E. Ontogeny of pepsin secretory response in isolated rat gastric glands. Am J Physiol 1986; 250:G200–4.
133. Lee PC, Struve MF, Werlin SL. Modulation of lingual lipase development by glucocorticoids in the rat. Pediatr Res 1991; 29:46–9.
134. Tremblay E, Monfils S, Menard D. Epidermal growth factor influences cell proliferation, glycoproteins and lipase activity in human fetal stomach. Gastroenterology 1997;112:1188–96.
135. Hormi K, Lehy T. Developmental expression of transforming growth factor-α and epidermal growth factor receptor protein in the human pancreas and digestive tract. Cell Tissue Res 1994;278:439–50.
136. Hamosh M, Scanlon JW, Ganot D, et al. Fat digestion in the newborn: characterization of lipase in gastric aspirates of premature and term infants. J Clin Invest 1981;67:838–46.
137. Hamosh M, Sivasubramanian KN, Salzman-Mann C, Hamosh P. Fat digestion in the stomach of premature infants. Characteristics of lipase activity. J Pediatr 1978;93:674–82.
138. Salzman-Mann C, Hamosh M, Sivasubramanian KN, et al. Congenital esophageal atresia: lipase activity is present in the esophageal pouch and in the stomach. Dig Dis Sci 1982;27: 124–8.
139. Kirk CL, Iverson SJ, Hamosh M. Lipase and pepsin activities in the stomach mucosa of the suckling dog. Biol Neonate 1991;59:78–85.
140. Perret JP. Lipolyse gastrique chez le lapereau. Origine et importance physiologique de la lipase. J Physiol (Lond) 1982: 78:221–30.
141. Ross CAC. Fat absorption studies in the diagnosis and treatment of pancreatic fibrosis. Arch Dis Child. 1955;30:316–21.
142. Lapey A, Kattwinkel J, diSant Agnese PA, Laster L. Steatorrhea and azotorrhea and their relation to growth and nutrition in adolescents and young adults with cystic fibrosis. J Pediatr 1974;84:328–34.
143. Fredrikzon B, Blackberg L. Lingual lipase: an important enzyme in the digestion of dietary lipids in cystic fibrosis? Pediatr Res 1980;14:1387–90.
144. Roulet M, Weber AM, Paradis Y, et al. Gastric emptying and lingual lipase activity in cystic fibrosis. Pediatr Res 1980; 14:1360–2.
145. Balasubramanian K, Zentler-Munro PL, Batten JC, Northfield TC. Increased intragastric acid-resistant lipase activity and lipolysis in pancreatic steatorrhea due to cystic fibrosis. Pancreas 1992;7:305–10.
146. Moreau H, Saunier JF, Gargouri Y, et al. Human gastric lipase: variations induced by gastrointestinal hormones and by pathology. Scand J Gastroenterol 1988;23:1044–8.
147. Malagelada JR, Longstreth GF, Summerskill WHJ, Go VLW. Measurement of gastric function during digestion of ordinary solid meals in man. Gastroenterology 1976;70: 203–10.

148. DiMagno EP, Go VLW, Summerskill WHJ. Relations between pancreatic enzyme outputs and malabsorption in severe pancreatic insufficiency. N Engl J Med 1973;288:813–5.
149. Wojdemann M, Olsen O, Larsen S, et al. Deficient gastric lipase secretion in pancreatic insufficiency. Scand J Gastroenterol 1997;32:268–72.
150. DeLisle RC, Isom KS. Expression of sulfated GP300 and changes in glycosylation during pancreatic development. J Histochem Cytochem 1996;44:57–66.
151. Laine J, Pellestier G, Grondin G, et al. Development of GP-2 and five zymogens in the fetal and young pig: biochemical and immunochemical evidence of an atypical zymogen granule composition in the fetus. J Histochem Cytochem 1996; 44:481–99.
152. Pierzynowski SG, Westrom BR, Svendsen J, et al. Development and regulation of porcine pancreatic function. Int J Pancreatol 1995;18:81–94.
153. Lopez V, Martinez-Victoria E, Yago MD, et al. Postnatal development of the exocrine pancreas in suckling goat kids. Arch Physiol Biochem 1997;105:210–5.
154. Naranjo JA, Martinez-Victoria E, Valverde A, et al. Effect of age on the exocrine pancreatic secretion in the preruminant milk-fed goat. Arch Physiol Biochem 1997;105:144–50.
155. Pierzynowski SG, Westrom BR, Erlanson-Albertsson C, et al. Induction of pancreas maturation at weaning in young developing pigs. J Pediatr Gastroenterol Nutr 1993;16:287–93.
156. DeLisle RC. Characterization of the major sulfated protein of mouse pancreatic acinar cells: a high molecular weight peripheral membrane glycoprotein of zymogen granules. J Cell Biochem 1994;56:385–92.
157. Jacob M, Laine J, LeBel D. Specific interactions of pancreatic amylase at acidic pH. Amylase and the major protein of the zymogen granule membrane (GP-2) bind to purified amylase when immobilized or polymerized. Biochem Cell Biol 1992; 70:1105–14.
158. Bendayan M. Protein A-gold and protein G-gold postembedding microscopy. In: Hayat MA, editor. Colliodal gold: principles, methods and applications. Vol 1. New York: Academic Press; 1989. p. 33–42.
159. Sanders TG, Rutter WJ. The developmental regulation of amylolytic and proteolytic enzymes in the embryonic rat pancreas. J Biol Chem 1974;249:3500–6.
160. Yamamoto KR. Steroid receptor regulated transcription of specific genes and gene networks. Annu Rev Genet 1985; 19:209–52.
160a. Brayer GD, Luo Y, Withers SG. The structure of human pancreatic alpha-amylase at 1.8A resolution and comparison with related enzymes. Protein Sci 1994;4:1730–42.
161. Wishart MJ, Andrews PC, Nichols R, et al. Identification and cloning of GP-3 from rat pancreatic acinar zymogen granules as a glycosylated membrane-associated lipase. J Biol Chem 1993;268:10303–11.
162. Light A, Janska H. Enterokinase (enteropeptidase): comparative aspects. Trends Biochem Sci 1989;14:1101–7.
163. Grant DAW, Hermon-Taylor J. The purification of human enterokinase by affinity chromatography and immunoadsorption. Biochem J 1976;155:243–54.
164. Antonowicz I. The role of enteropeptidase in the digestion of protein and its development in human fetal intestine. In: Harries JT, editor. Development of mammalian absorptive processes. Amsterdam: Excerpta Medica; 1979. p. 169–87.
165. Hadorn B, Tarlow MJ, Lloyd JK, Wolff OH. Intestinal enterokinse deficiency. Lancet 1969;1:812–3.
166. Brunger AT, Huber R, Karplus M. Trypsinogen-trypsin transition: a molecular dynamics study of induced conformational change in the activation domain. Biochemistry 1987; 26:5153–62.
167. Largman C, Brodrick JW, Geokas MC. Purification and characterization of two human pancreatic elastases. Biochemistry 1976;5:2491–500.
168. Appel W. Chymotrypsin: molecular and catalytic properties. Clin Biochem 1986;19:317–22.
169. Fletcher TS, Wei-Fang S, Largman C. Primary structure of human pancreatic elastase 2 determined by sequence analysis of the cloned mRNA. Biochemistry 1987;26:7256–61.
170. Tani T, Kawashima I, Furukawa H, et al. Characterization of a silent gene for human pancreatic elastase I: structure of the 5'-flanking region. J Biochem (Tokyo) 1987;101:591–9.
171. Shen W, Fletcher TS, Largman C. Primary structure of human pancreatic protease E determined by sequence analysis of the cloned mRNA. Biochemistry 1987;26:3447–52.
172. Amouric M, Figarella C. Some properties of human pancreatic kallikrein and comparison with human trypsins and porcine kallikrein. Hoppe-Seyler s Z Physiol Chem 1980;361:85–90.
173. Boehm G, Bierbach U, Del Santo A, et al. Activities of trypsin and lipase in duodenal aspirates of healthy preterm infants: effects of gestational age and postnatal age. Biol Neonate 1996;67:248–53.
174. Gestin M, Le Hueron-Luron I, Peiniau C, et al. Method of measurement of pancreatic elastase II activity and postnatal development of proteases in human duodenal juice and bovine and porcine pancreatic tissue. Dig Dis Sci 1997;42:1302–11.
175. Moriscot C, Renaud W, Carrere J, et al. Developmental gene expression of trypsinogen and lipase in human fetal pancreas. J Pediatr Gastroenterol Nutr 1997;24:63–7.
176. Heine W, Braun OH, Mohr C, Leitzmann P. Enhancement of lysozyme-trypsin-mediated decay of intestinal bifidobacteria and lactobacilli. J Pediatr Gasteroenterol Nutr 1995;21:54–8.
177. Heine W, Mohr C, Wutzke KD, Radke M. Symbiotic interactions between colonic microflora and protein metabolism in infants. Acta Paediatr Scand 1991;80:7–12.
178. Erlanson-Albertson C. Pancreatic colipase. Structural and physiological aspects. Biochim Biophys Acta 1992;1125:1–7.
179. Van Tilbeurgh H, Sarda L, Verger R, Cambillau C. Structure of the pancreatic lipase-procolipase complex. Nature 1992;359:159–62.
180. Lowe ME. Colipase stabilizes the lid domain of pancreatic triglyceride lipase. J Biol Chem 1997;272:9–12.
181. Brockerhoff H. Substrate specificity of pancreatic lipase: influence of the structure of fatty acids on the reactivity of esters. Biochim Biophys Acta. 1979;212:92–101.
182. Savary P. The action of pure pancreatic lipase upon esters of long-chain fatty acids and short chain primary alcohols. Biochim Biophys Acta 1971;159:296–303.
183. Yang L-Y, Kuksis A, Myher JJ. Lipolysis of menhaden oil triacylglycerols and the corresponding fatty acid alkyl esters by pancreatic lipase in vitro: a reexamination. J Lipid Res 1990; 31:137–48.
184. Lowe ME. Molecular mechanisms of rat and human pancreatic triglyceride lipases. J Nutr 1997;127:549–57.
185. Boehm G, Bierback U, Senger H, et al. Activities of lipase and trypsin in duodenal juice of infants small for gestational age. J Pediatr Gastroenterol Nutr 1991;12:324–7.
186. Lombardo D, Guy O, Figarella C. Purification and characterization of a carboxyl ester hydrolase from human pancreatic juice. Biochim Biophys Acta 1978;527:142–9.
187. Patton JS, Warner TG, Benson AA. Partial characterization of the bile salt-dependent triacylglycerol lipase from the leopard shark pancreas. Biochim Biophys Acta 1977;486:322–30.
188. Bradshaw WS, Rutter WJ. Multiple pancreatic lipases. Tissue distribution and pattern of accumulation during embryological development. Biochemistry 1972;11:1517–28.
189. Giller T, Buchwald P, Blum-Kaelin D, Hunziker W. Two novel human pancreatic lipase related proteins, h PLRP 1 and h PLRP2. J Biol Chem 1992;267:16509–16.

190. Thirstrup K, Verger R, Carriere F. Evidence for a pancreatic lipase subfamily with new kinetic properties. Biochemistry 1994;33:2748–56.
191. Carriere F, Thirstrup K, Hjiorth S, Boel E. Cloning of the classical guinea pig pancreatic lipase and comparison with the lipase related protein 2. FEBS Lett 1994;338:63–8.
192. Cygler M, Schrog JD, Sussman JL, et al. Relationship between sequence conservation and three-dimensional structure in a large family of esterases, lipases and related proteins. Protein Sci 1993;2:366–82.
193. Payne RM, Sims HF, Jennens ML, Lowe ME. Rat pancreatic lipase and two related proteins: enzymatic properties and mRNA expression during development. Am J Physiol 1994; 266:G914–21.
194. Bower JM, Gamble R, Gregory H, et al. The inhibition of gastric acid secretion by epidermal growth factor. Experientia 1975;31:825–6.
195. Rao RK, Chang H-H, Levenson S, et al. Ontogenic differences in the inhibition of gastric acid secretion by epidermal growth factor. J Pharmacol Exp Ther 1993;266:647–54.
196. Lee PC, Struve MF, Werlin SL. Modulation of lingual lipase development by glucocorticoids in the rat. Pediatr Res 1991; 29:46–9.
197. Sanglid PT, Westrom BR, Silver M, Fowden AL. Maturational effects of cortisol on the exocrine abomasum and pancreas in fetal sheep. Reprod Fertil Dev 1995;7:655–8.
198. Sanglid PT, Westrom BR, Fowden AL, Silver M. Developmental regulation of porcine exocrine pancreas by glucocorticoids. J Pediatr Gastroenterol Nutr 1994;19:204–12.
199. Deschodt-Lankman M, Robberech P, Camus J, et al. Hormonal and dietary adaptation of pancreatic hydrolases before and after weaning. Am J Physiol 1974;226:39–44.
200. Puccio F, Chariot J, Lehy T. Influence of hydrocortisone on the development of pancreas in suckling rats. Biol Neonate 1988;54:35–44.
201. Kuhlman J, Gisi C, Lowe ME. Dexamethasone regulated expression of pancreatic lipase and two related proteins in AR42J cells. Am J Physiol 1996;270:G746–51.
202. Christophe J. The pancreatic tumoral cell line AR42J: an amphicrine model. Am J Physiol 1994;266:G963–71.
203. Lee P-C, Mao X-C. Thyroxine control of pancreatic amylase gene expression: modulation of PTF1 binding activity. Moll Cell Endocrinol 1994;101:287–93.
204. Lin CH, Moshier JA, Luk GD, et al. Effect of thyroxine on pancreatic digestive enzymes and ornithine dicarboxylase gene expression in neonatal rats. J Pediatr Gastroenterol Nutr 1997;24:18–24.
205. Muribu JN, Xu RJ. Growth and development of the exocrine pancreas in newborn pigs: the effect of colostrum feeding. Biol Neonate 1997;71:317–26.
206. Joekel CS, Herrington MK, Vanderhoof JA, Adrian TE. Postnatal development of circulating cholecystokinin and secretin, pancreatic growth and exocrine function in guinea pigs. Int J Pancreatol 1993;13:1–13.
207. Mokkink CA, Negulescu GP, Qin G, Verstegen MW. Effect of dietary protein source on food intake, growth, pancreatic enzyme activities and jejunal morphology in newly-weaned piglets. Br J Nutr 1994;73:353–68.
208. Williamson S, Finucane E, Ellis H, Gamsu H. Effect of heat treatment of human milk on absorption of nitrogen, fat, sodium, calcium and phosphorus by preterm infants. Arch Dis Child 1978; 53:555–63.
209. Alemi B, Hamosh M, Scanlon JW, et al. Fat digestion in very low birth weight infants: Effect of addition of human milk to low birth weight formula. Pediatrics 1981;68:484–9.
210. Hamosh M. Lingual and breast milk lipases. Adv Pediatr 1982;29:33–67.
211. Hernell O, Blackberg L, Lindberg T. Human milk enzymes with emphasis on the lipases. In: Lebenthal E, editor. Textbook of gastroenterology and nutrition in infancy. New York: Raven Press; 1989. p. 209–18.
212. Hamosh M. Enzymes in human milk: their role in nutrient digestion, gastrointestinal function and nutrition in infancy. In: Lebenthal E, editor. Textbook of gastroenterology and nutrition in infancy. 2nd ed. New York: Raven Press; 1989. p. 121–34.
213. Hamosh M. Enzymes in human milk. In: Jensen RG, editor. Handbook of milk composition. San Diego: Academic Press; 1995. p. 388–427.
214. Marfan AB. Allaitment naturel et allaitment artificiel. Presse Med 1901;9:13–9.
215. Lombardo D, Fanuel J, Guy O. Studies on the substrate specificity of a carboxyl ester hydrolase from human pancreatic juice. I. Action on carboxyl esters, glycerides and phospholipids. Biochim Biophys Acta 1980;611:136–46.
216. Lombardo D, Guy O. Studies on the substrate specificity of a carboxyl ester hydrolase from human pancreatic juice. II. Action on cholesterol esters and lipid soluble vitamin esters. Biochim Biophys Acta 1980;611:147–55.
217. Blackberg L, Angquist K-A, Hernell O. Bile salt stimulated lipase in human milk: evidence for its synthesis in the lactating mammary gland. FEBS Lett 1987;217:37–42.
218. Freed LM, York CM, Hamosh M, et al. Bile salt stimulated lipase: the enzyme is present in non primate milk. In: Hamosh M, Goldman AS, editors. Human lactation. Vol II: Maternal environmental factors. New York: Plenum Press; 1986. p. 595–602.
219. Rene K, Zambaux J, Wong H, et al. cDNA cloning of carboxyl-ester lipase from human pancreas reveals a unique proline-rich repeat unit. J Lipid Res 1991;32:267–76.
220. Han JH, Stratowa C, Rutter WJ. Isolation of full-length putative rat lysophospholipase cDNA using improved methods for mRNA isolation and cDNA cloning. Biochemistry 1987; 26:1617–25.
221. Kissel JA, Fontaine RN, Turck C, et al. Molecular cloning and expression of cDNA for rat pancreatic cholesterol esterase. Biochim Biophys Acta 1989;1006:227–36.
222. Kyger EM, Wiegand RC, Lange LG, Cloning of the bovine pancreatic cholesterol esterase/phospholipase. Biochem Biophys Res Commun 1989;164:1302–9.
223. Colwell NS, Aleman-Gomez JA, Kumar BV. Molecular cloning and expression of rabbit pancreatic cholesterol esterase. Biochim Biophys Acta 1993;1172:175–80.
224. Gjellesvik DR, Lorens JB, Male R. Pancreatic carboxylester lipase from Atlantic salmon (Salmo salar) cDNA sequence and computer-assisted modelling of tertiary structure. Eur J Biochem 1994;226:603–12.
225. Lidmer AS, Kannius M, Lundberg L, et al. Molecular cloning and characterization of the mouse carboxyl ester lipase gene and evidence of expression in the lactating mammary gland. Genomics 1995;29:115–22.
226. Mackay K, Lown RM. Characterization of the mouse pancreatic-mammary gland cholesterol esterase-encoding cDNA and gene. Gene 1995;165:255–9.
227. Sbarra V, Bruneau N, Mas E, et al. Molecular cloning of the bile salt dependent lipase of ferret lactating mammary gland: an overview of functional residues. Biochim Biophys Acta 1998;1393:80–9.
228. Hamosh M. Physiological role of milk lipases. In: Lebenthal E, editor. Textbook of gastroenterology and nutrition in infancy. New York: Raven Press; 1981. p. 473–82.
229. Hamosh M, Hamosh P. Lipoprotein lipase. Its physiological and clinical significance. Mol Aspects Med 1983;6: 199–289.

230. Mehta NR, Jones JB, Hamosh M. Lipases in human milk: ontogeny and physiologic significance. J Pediatr Gastroenterol Nutr 1982;1:317–26.
231. Freed LM, Berkow SE, Hamosh P, et al. Lipases in human milk: effect of gestational age and length of lactation on enzyme activity. J Am Coll Nutr 1989;8:143–50.
232. Freudenberg E. Die Frauenmilch-lipase. Basel, Switzerland: Karger; 1953.
233. Freudenberg E. A lipase in the milk of the gorilla. Experientia 1966;22:317.
234. Blackberg L, Hernell O, Olivecrona T, et al. The bile salt stimulated lipase in human milk is a newcomer derived from a non-milk protein. FEBS Lett 1980;112:51–4.
235. Pamblanco M, Ten A, Conin J. Bile salt stimulated lipase activity in human colostrum from mothers of infants of different gestational age and birth weight. Acta Paediatr Scand 1987;76:328–31.
236. Hamosh M. Enzymes in human milk. In: Howell RR, Morris FH, Pickering LK, editors. Human milk in infant nutrition and health. Springfield, IL: Charles C Thomas; 1986. p. 66–97.
237. Freed LM, Neville MC, Hamosh M. Lipase activities in human milk during weaning [abstract]. Pediatr Res 1989;25:290A.
238. Dewit O, Dibba B, Prentice A. Breast-milk amylase activity in English and Gambian mothers: effects of prolonged lactation, maternal parity, and individual variations. Pediatr Res 1990;28:502–6.
239. Baba T, Downs D, Jackson KW, et al. Structure of human milk bile salt activated lipase. Biochemistry 1991;30:500–12.
240. Swan JS, Hoffman MM, Lord MK, Poechman JL. Two forms of human milk bile salt-stimulated lipase. Biochem J 1992;283:119–22.
241. Hall B, Muller DPR. Studies on bile salt stimulated lipolytic activity in human milk. II. Demonstration of two groups of milk with different activities. Pediatr Res 1983;17:716–20.
242. Erlanson-Albertsson C, Sternby B, Johannsson V. The interaction between human pancreatic carboxylester hydrolase (bile salt stimulated lipase of human milk) and lactoferrin. Biochim Biophys Acta 1985;839:282–7.
243. Freed LM, York CM, Hamosh P, et al. Bile salt stimulated lipase of human milk: characteristics of the enzyme in the milk of mothers of premature and full-term infants. J Pediatr Gastroenterol Nutr 1987;6:598–604.
244. Freed LM, Neville MC, Hamosh P, Hamosh M. Diurnal and within-feed variations in lipase activity and triglyceride content of human milk. J Pediatr Gastroenterol Nutr 1986;5:938–42.
245. Berkow S, Freed LM, Hamosh M, et al. Lipase and lipids in human milk: effects of freeze thawing and storage. Pediatr Res 1984;18:1257–63.
246. Hamosh M, Henderson TR, Ellis LA, et al. Digestive enzymes in human milk: stability at suboptimal storage temperatures. J Pediatr Gastroenterol Nutr 1997;24:38–43.
247. Hernell O, Olivecrona T. Human milk lipases. II. Bile salt stimulated lipase. Biochim Biophys Acta; 1974;369:234–44.
248. Wang CS, Hartsuck JA, Downs D. Kinetics of acylglycerol sequential hydrolysis by human milk bile salt activated lipase and effect of taurocholate as fatty acid acceptor. Biochemistry 1988;27:4834–40.
249. Hernell O, Blackberg L. Digestion of human milk lipids: physiological significance of sn-2 monoacylglycerol hydrolysis by bile salt-stimulated lipase. Pediatr Res 1982;16:882–5.
250. Morgan RGH, Borgstrom B. The mechanism of fat absorption in the bile fistula rat. Q J Exp Physiol 1969;54:228–43.
251. Signer E, Murphy GM, Edkins S, Andersson CM. Role of bile salts in fat malabsorption of premature infants. Arch Dis Child 1974;49:174–80.
252. Fredrikzon B, Hernell O, Blackberg L, Olivecrona T. Bile salt stimulated lipase in human milk: evidence of activity in vivo and of a role in the digestion of milk retinol esters. Pediatr Res 1978;12:1048–52.
253. Connor J, Butler PA, Yaghi BM. The effect of bile salt stimulated lipase on the interconversion of retinylpalmitate and retinol. N Z Med J 1988;101:583–4.
254. Hall B, Muller DPR. Studies on the bile salt stimulated lipolytic activity in human milk using whole milk as a source of both substrate and enzyme. I. Nutritional implications. Pediatr Res 1982;16:251–5.
255. Hernell O, Blackberg L, Chen O. Does the bile salt stimulated lipase of human milk have a role in the use of the milk long-chain polyunsaturated fatty acids? J Pediatr Gastroenterol Nutr 1993;16:426–31.
256. Hernell O, Gebre-Medhin M, Olivecrona T. Breast milk composition in Ethiopian and Swedish mothers. IV. Milk lipase. Am J Clin Nutr 1977;30:508–11.
257. Ginder J, Nwankwo MU, Omene JA, et al. Breast milk composition and bile salt stimulated lipase in well nourished and undernourished Nigerian mothers. Eur J Pediatr 1987;146:184–6.
258. Dupuy P, Sauniere JF, Vis HL, et al. Change in bile salt dependent lipase in human breast milk during extended lactation. Lipids 1991;26:134–8.
259. Kabara JJ. Lipids as host resistance factors of human milk. Nutr Rev 1980;38:65-73.
260. Gillin FD, Reiner DS, Wang CS. Human milk kills parasitic intestinal protozoa. Science 1983;221:1290–2.
261. Gillin FD, Reiner DS, Gault MJ. Cholate-dependent killing of *Giardia lamblia* by human milk. Infect Immun 1985;47:619–22.
262. Canas-Rodriguez A, Smith HW. The identification of the antimicrobial factors of the stomach contents of suckling rabbits. Biochem J 1966;100:78–82.
263. Hamosh M. Free fatty acids and monoglycerides: antiinfective agents produced during the digestion of milk fat by the newborn. Adv Exp Med Biol 1991;310:151–8.
264. Bechamp A. Sur la zymase du lait de femme. C R Acad Sci III 1883;96:1508–10.
265. Jones JB, Mehta NR, Hamosh M. α-amylase in preterm human milk. J Pediatr Gastroenterol Nutr 1982;1:43–8.
266. Fridhandler L, Berk JE, Montgomery KA, Wand D. Column chromatographic studies of isoamylase in human serum, urine, and milk. Clin Chem 1974;20:547–55.
267. Hegardt P, Lindbert T, Borjesson J, Skude G. Amylase in human milk from mothers of preterm and term infants. J Pediatr Gastroenterol Nutr 1984;3:563–6.
268. Henderson TR, Fay TN, Hamosh M. Effect of pasteurization on long chain polyunsaturated fatty acid levels and enzyme activity in human milk. J Pediatr 1998;132:876–8.
269. Heitlinger LA, Lee PC, Dillon WP, Lebenthal E. Mammary amylase: a possible alternate pathway of carbohydrate digestion in infancy. Pediatr Res 1983;17:15–8.
270. Hanafy MM, El-Khateeb S, Guirgis FJ, El-Lozy M. Diastase in human milk. Alexandria Med J 1971;17:299–305.
271. Mellersh A, Clark A, Hafiz S. Inhibition of *Neisseria gonorrhoeae* by normal human saliva. Br J Venereal Dis 1979;55:20–23.
272. Monti JC, Mermoud AF, Jolles P. Trypsin in human milk. Experientia 1986;42:39–41.
273. Borulf S, Lindberg T, Mansson M. Immunoreactive anionic trypsin and elastase activity in human milk. Acta Paediatr Scand 1987;76:11–5.
274. Lindberg T. Protease inhibitors in human milk. Pediatr Res 1979;13:969–72.

275. Udall JN, Dixon M, Newman AP, et al. Liver disease in antitrypsin deficiency: a retrospective analysis of the influence of early breast vs bottle-feeding. JAMA 1985;253:2679–82.
276. Ogra SS, Weintraub D, Ogra PL. Immunological aspects of human colostrum and milk. Fate and absorption of cellular and soluble components in the gastrointestinal tract of the newborn. J Immunol 1977;119:245–8.
277. Iyengar L, Selvaraj RJ. Intestinal absorption of immunoglobulins by newborn infants. Arch Dis Child 1972;47:411–4.
278. Udall JN, Pan K, Fritze L, et al. Development of gastrointestinal mucosal barrier. The effect of age on intestinal permeability to macromolecules. Pediatr Res 1981;15:241–4.
279. Florent C, L'Hirondel J, Desmazures C, et al. Intestinal clearance of α-1-antitrypsin: a sensitive method for the detection of protein losing enteropathy. Gastroenterology 1981;81:777–80.
280. Sveger T. Breast-feeding, antitrypsin deficiency and liver disease. JAMA 1985:254:3036–7.

CHAPTER 17

Ontogeny of the Intestinal Flora

Ingegerd Adlerberth, MB, PhD

Lars Åke Hanson, MD, PhD

Agnes. E. Wold, MD, PhD

When the fetus is expelled from the sterile womb into the world of microbes, bacteria start colonizing the skin, respiratory tract, and intestine. This is the beginning of the development of a complex ecosystem: the normal intestinal microflora. Groups of bacteria are established sequentially and the microflora is not fully developed until several years of age.[1,2]

The bacteria colonizing the neonate are acquired from the mother and various environmental sources.[3-5] The composition of the intestinal microflora may, therefore, be influenced by delivery mode, feeding mode, and the degree of environmental hygiene.[6-12]

Many bacteria that inhabit the intestine, especially aerobic or facultatively anaerobic bacteria, are potential pathogens, since they may spread to extra-intestinal sites. Certain features of the microflora of the newborn infant—for example, a high population level of aerobic and facultatively anaerobic bacteria—make the newborn infant vulnerable to a range of infections. On the other hand, the unique microbial flora of the neonate and young infant may be important for the maturation of the developing immune system.

This chapter describes the establishment of the intestinal microflora in the young infant. Factors affecting the colonization process are reviewed, and possible mechanisms whereby the intestinal microflora may influence infant health are discussed.

ORIGIN AND COLONIZATION OF BACTERIA

A number of studies have investigated the time of acquisition of the major bacterial groups inhabiting the intestine. The observed colonization rates and mean counts of different bacteria in the intestinal flora of neonates and infants vary considerably between studies, which reflects both methodologic differences and differences between the groups of infants studied. The results from 22 studies performed between 1971 and 1995 are summarized in Table 17–1.[1,6,7,10,13-32]

Aerobic and Facultatively Anaerobic Bacteria

The intestinal milieu is characterized by a positive oxidation-reduction potential during the first days of life.[33] This favors the metabolism and replication of bacteria capable of oxidative metabolism, that is, aerobes and facultative anaerobes. In contrast, strictly anaerobic bacteria require a negative oxidative-reduction potential to thrive.[6] They cannot, therefore, expand during the first days of life; and the intestinal microflora is then dominated by aerobic or facultative bacteria, such as *Escherichia coli* and other enterobacteria, enterococci, and staphylococci.[10,12,18,34] These bacteria multiply freely and often reach population levels of 10^{10} bacteria per g feces in the newborn infant, roughly 100 times more than the levels found in adults.[6,20]

Escherichia coli strains that colonize the neonate may derive from the mother's fecal flora, transferred during delivery. Bettelheim and coworkers found that about two-thirds of the neonates harbored at least one *E. coli* strain acquired from their mother's fecal flora.[3,4,35,36] Most other studies, however, report that less than one-third of newborn infants acquire maternal *E. coli* strains.[17,37-39] This has been ascribed to the use of enemas, washing the mother's perineal area with antiseptics, and other measures used to reduce fecal contamination of the baby during delivery. However, even during home deliveries in an urban slum in Pakistan, where aseptic techniques are not practiced, only 38% of the infants acquire *E. coli* strains from their mothers.[40] One can speculate that when mothers give birth lying on their back, exposure to maternal fecal flora is reduced; whereas a standing or kneeling delivery position, as practiced by certain indigenous populations, almost invariably leads to fecal contamination of the infant.[14]

Many neonates delivered in hospitals pick up *E. coli* strains from other infants at the ward, spread by the nurses' hands.[17,36] This type of transmission is greatly reduced when rooming-in is practiced; that is, when the mothers handle their babies themselves.[41] In the home, *E. coli* strains may be acquired from other members of the family.

Other enterobacterial species than *E. coli*, including *Klebsiella*, *Enterobacter*, and *Citrobacter*, are isolated from

TABLE 17–1
Major Groups of Intestinal Bacteria*

	Age of Individuals									
	1 Week		1 Month		6 Months		1–4 Years		Adult	
	%	Bacterial Counts†	%	Bacterial Counts	%	Bacterial Counts	%	Bacterial Counts	%	Bacterial Counts
Aerobic and facultatively anaerobic bacteria										
Enterobacteria										
Mean	92	8.7	96	8.8	100	8.6	100	7.9	99	7.5
Number of studies	7	8	9	10	2	2	2	2	3	7
Enterococci										
Mean	88	8.0	88	8.2	95	8.9	94	7.3	94	6.7
Number of studies	10	11	12	14	3	2	2	2	3	6
Staphylococci										
Mean	69	6.4	61	6.3	50	4.8	50	4	62	4.4
Number of studies	9	8	11	10	2	1	2	1	3	5
Anaerobic bacteria										
Bifidobacteria										
Mean	75	9.1	73	9.3	94	9.6	90	10.1	84	9.1
Number of studies	11	12	13	15	3	2	3	3	4	7
Bacteroides										
Mean	53	7.9	55	8.6	67	9.4	86	9.9	100	10.2
Number of studies	12	11	13	14	3	2	3	3	4	6
Clostridia										
Mean	54	6.5	56	7.3	52	7.1	86	6.3	95	6.8
Number of studies	10	11	12	14	3	2	2	2	3	5
Lactobacilli										
Mean	43	7.0	39	7.8	29	5.2	42	4	90	6.8
Number of studies	6	7	8	8	1	1	1	1	3	6
Eubacteria										
Mean	17	6.8	11	8.2	0	—	43	9.5	85	9.7
Number of studies	4	1	4	3	1	—	1	1	2	4
Gram+ cocci										
Mean	14	10.5	10	9.2	21	9.1	79	10.0	55	8.9
Number of studies	3	1	3	3	1	1	1	1	2	2
Veillonella										
Mean	35	6.3	47	7.3	97	9.2	93	7	60	6.0
Number of studies	5	4	6	6	2	1	1	1	3	3
Ratio anaerobic and aerobic bacteria										
Mean	1/1		10/1‡		100/1		100/1		500/1	
Number of studies	1		4		4		3		4	

Data summarized from references.[1,6,7,10,13–32]
*Frequency of isolation (% of individuals colonized) and mean† population levels (^{10}log) in culture-positive individuals of different ages.
‡The ratio is often higher in exclusively breastfed infants.[6,14]

20 to 60% of infants during their first weeks of life. The intestinal population levels of these bacteria are comparable to those reported for *E. coli*.[7,10,42] In contrast to *E. coli*, however, *Klebsiella, Enterobacter,* and *Citrobacter* are not found in the intestinal microflora of most adults.[24,43] The strains colonizing neonates are, therefore, rarely of maternal origin.[39,40,44,45] Instead, these enterobacteria are frequently spread between neonates in maternity wards and nurseries by the staff.[44,45] Furthermore, since *Klebsiella, Enterobacter,* and *Citrobacter* survive better than *E. coli* outside the human host,[46] they may also be acquired from nonhuman sources. For example, feeds administered to Pakistani newborn infants were commonly contaminated with *Klebsiella* and *Enterobacter* species, but never with *E. coli*.[40]

Enterococci (*Streptococcus faecalis* or *Streptococcus faecium*) are isolated from most neonates (see Table 17–1), and commonly reach population levels of 10^{10} CFU per g of feces.[6,21] They are found in the intestinal microflora of almost all adults, and they are likely transferred to the neonate by the same routes as *E. coli*, although this has not been specifically studied.

Staphylococci, e.g., *Staphylococcus epidermidis*, and less frequently *Staphylococcus aureus*, also establish in the intestine during the first days of life (see Table 17–1), and may reach population levels of 10^{10} bacteria per g feces.[10] Staphylococci are found in the intestine of approximately two-thirds of adult individuals, but their population level seldom exceeds 10^7 per g feces.[24] These bacteria are well-recognized as members of the skin microflora, which is probably the origin of many strains colonizing the infant. Transfer may occur during breastfeeding or during general caretaking.

Nonhemolytic streptococci are found equally early, but less frequently than enterobacteria, enterococci, or staphylococci.[21] Other groups of aerobic bacteria, for example,

Aeromonas, *Pseudomonas,* and *Acinetobacter*, may be transiently isolated from neonates during the first week of life,[34,40,47] but usually disappear with the establishment of bacteria better adapted to the intestinal milieu.[40,47]

Anaerobic Bacteria

When the aerobic and facultatively anaerobic bacteria expand, they consume oxygen and lower the redox-potential to negative values. This in turn enables anaerobic bacteria to start multiplying.[6,20] Anaerobic bacteria colonizing soon after include *Bacteroides*, bifidobacteria, and clostridia (see Table 17-1).[6,10,19,21,23,25,29] These bacteria are isolated from a majority of infants, and may reach populations of 10^{9-11} per g feces within a week after birth.[6,14,21]

Bacteroides

Bacteroides are strict anaerobes, which means they die rapidly in contact with environmental oxygen. They can, therefore, only with difficulty spread between neonates by the hands of the staff.[48] Although there are no studies directly investigating the transfer of *Bacteroides* from mother to infant, suggestive evidence indicates that this route of transfer is important. Thus, infants delivered by cesarean section, who do not come into contact with the maternal fecal flora at delivery, show a delayed colonization with *Bacteroides*. In this respect, *Bacteroides* seems more affected than other anaerobes.[10,42,48,49] Moreover, the *Bacteroides* species most common in the microflora of newborn infants are the same as those that dominate in adults: *Bacteroides vulgatus*, *B. thetaiotaomicron*, *B. fragilis,* and *B. distasonis*.[22,26]

Bifidobacterium

Bifidobacteria are aero-tolerant anaerobes. They may, thus, survive for some time outside the intestine, a capacity that facilitates their horizontal transfer. An indication of environmental spread is that the infants' intestinal carriage of bifidobacteria varies between different maternity wards.[7,18] Furthermore, the species and biotypes of bifidobacteria most common in infants, that is, *Bifidobacterium bifidum* type B, *B. infantis* spp. *infantis*, and *B. longum* spp. *longum* type B, rarely dominate in adult individuals. These instead most often carry *B. adolescentis*, *B. longum* spp. *longum* type A, and *B. bifidum* type A.[18] However, transfer of bifidobacteria from mother to infant also occurs. Colonization with bifidobacteria is delayed after cesarean section;[9,48] Tannock and coworkers isolated similar strains of bifidobacteria in mother and child in two cases out of five.[5]

Lactobacillus

Whether lactobacilli form part of the early intestinal microflora or not is controversial. Many recent studies suggest that lactobacilli are important early colonizers, being present at 10^{7-9} per g feces in 60 to 80% of infants at one month age.[28,31,49] This contrasts with several earlier studies that reported infrequent colonization with lactobacilli during the first year(s) of life.[1,6,14] The discrepancy may relate to differences in isolation and identification methods, or to a changed colonization pattern during the last decades.

The vagina has a stable *Lactobacillus* microflora.[50] Although vaginal bacteria are often ingested by the baby during delivery, as shown by their presence in gastric aspirates,[51,52] there is little evidence that these lactobacilli can establish in the infant's intestinal tract. In a small study involving five mother-infant pairs, lactobacilli present in the vagina of the mother did not in any case colonize the intestine of the baby.[5]

Lactobacilli colonizing the neonate may instead derive from the mother's oral or fecal flora. *Lactobacillus plantarum*, the dominating species in the intestinal flora of Swedish neonates,[9] is also the dominant species in the oral cavity, and colon of adults.[53] A delayed colonization with *L. plantarum* is observed after cesarean section,[9] indicating that bacteria of maternal origin normally colonize the neonate. However, as most lactobacilli are aero-tolerant, they are probably easily acquired also from other sources. Within one month, section-delivered infants carry lactobacilli at a rate similar to vaginally-delivered infants.[49]

Clostridium

Clostridia are important members of the early intestinal microflora. *Clostridium perfringens*, *C. paraputrificum*, *C. difficile,* and *C. tertium* are the most common species in neonates.[21,26] *Clostridium perfringens* and *C. paraputrificum* are common in adults as well,[24] but *C. difficile*, which is isolated from approximately one-third of healthy neonates,[54] is found in less than 4% of adults.[24,55] Similarly, *C. tertium* is found in 30% of infants,[26] but occurs in less than 10% of adults.[24]

Clostridia form spores and, thus, have a unique potential to survive outside the human host. The spores resist most disinfectants, and are frequently found in the hospital milieu.[56] Thus, *Clostridium perfringens* is usually the first anaerobe to colonize infants after cesarian section deliveries,[48] indicating rapid acquisition from the environment. Strains of *C. difficile* colonizing neonates are almost never acquired from the mother, but are frequently spread between neonates in maternity and neonatal wards.[57–59]

Other Anaerobes

Many other anaerobic bacteria form stable intestinal populations in adults, such as *Veillonella*, *Eubacterium*, *Peptostreptococcus*, *Peptococcus,* and *Ruminococcus*.[24] *Veillonella* are isolated from 10 to 50% of newborn infants (see Table 17-1).[18,21,26,31] Although two-thirds of all adults harbor *Veillonella*, this species reaches higher population levels in neonates and young infants (up to 10^9 per g feces) than in adults (10^{5-7} per g feces).[1,6,24]

Few studies have investigated the presence of eubacteria in neonates. In these studies, colonization rates vary between 0 and 40 % during the first weeks of life,[7,18,21] and less than 50 % are colonized at 9 to 12 months of age.[6,14,60] The anaerobic gram-positive cocci *Peptostreptococcus* and *Peptococcus* generally do not appear until solid foods are introduced,[6,26] but are present in a majority of infants 12 months old.[6,14,60] *Ruminococcus* are only occasionally isolated during the first year of life.[14,26]

The successive establishment of different anaerobic species proceeds over a period of several years.[1,2] During this process, some early anaerobes disappear or decline in numbers, especially *C. difficile* and *Veillonella*,[1,55,61] whereas others—for example, bifidobacteria and *Bacteroides*—remain in high numbers throughout life.

GLOBAL DIFFERENCES IN COLONIZATION PATTERNS

The degree of environmental bacterial exposure of the newborn infant varies markedly between rich and poor countries. In developing countries, the newborn infant is exposed to massive numbers of bacteria from various sources. In Western industrialized societies, on the other hand, strict hygienic hospital standards and general household cleanliness have strongly reduced the exposure to certain groups of bacteria. This difference is reflected in the pattern of intestinal colonization.

Enterobacteria

Infants born in poor areas in developing countries acquire intestinal bacteria very early. In indigenous Guatemalan infants, most of the meconium samples passed at four to seven hours after birth contain bacteria,[14] most commonly enterobacteria and streptococci. These bacteria reach high numbers during the first days of life, but already by the end of the first week a pronounced bifidobacterial dominance is established, and the facultatives are suppressed. The Guatemalan mothers investigated gave birth in a kneeling position, and maternal feces commonly contaminated the baby during delivery.[14] Thus, the early establishment of both facultative and anaerobic bacteria was presumably the result of a direct transfer of bacteria from mother to infant.

However, several studies demonstrate a very early acquisition of enterobacteria also in section-delivered neonates in developing countries,[11,34] reflecting a pronounced exposure to environmental bacteria. Whether delivered in the hospital or at home and regardless of delivery mode, Pakistani infants from poor areas are significantly earlier colonized than Swedish hospital-delivered infants.[11,40] Within three days after birth, all Pakistani infants harbored enterobacteria, many of them several different enterobacterial species simultaneously. In contrast, only 75% of Swedish neonates were colonized with enterobacteria at one week of age, and usually with only one species.[11] Late acquisition of enterobacteria has been observed also in other studies of Swedish infants.[7,12,62]

Among Pakistani infants, the isolation rate of enterobacteria other than *E. coli* is high during the first week, but declines already from the second week of life, when *E. coli* starts to dominate.[40] The replacement of, for example, *Klebsiella* and *Enterobacter* by *E. coli* thus occurs earlier than among Swedish infants, who commonly carry *Klebsiella* until several months of age.[62] This may, in turn, reflect an earlier establishment of anaerobic bacteria in the Pakistani infants.

During the first six months of life, different *E. coli* strains replace each other repeatedly in the intestinal flora of Pakistani infants.[40] This contrasts sharply with the stable pattern observed among infants in industrialized societies, in whom a single *E. coli* strain usually dominates the enterobacterial microflora for prolonged periods.[17,63]

Gram-Positive Bacteria

Colonization with enterococci and lactobacilli occurs earlier in Ethiopian than in Swedish neonates.[12] One-year-old infants in Sweden carry lactobacilli and eubacteria significantly less frequently than Estonian infants.[60]

Instead, in Western infants, intestinal colonization with skin bacteria like *S. epidermidis* and sporeformers like clostridia becomes more prominent, since they lack competition from other bacteria. Thus, early colonization with *S. epidermidis* is more common in Sweden than in Ethiopia.[12] Similarily, in French[64] and U.S. neonates,[65] *S. epidermidis* rather than *E. coli* or enterococci are the first bacteria to colonize the intestine. One-year-old Swedish children harbor more clostridia, and are more often colonized with *C. difficile* than Estonian infants.[60]

ANTIBIOTICS AND NEONATAL INTENSIVE CARE

Newborn infants cared for in neonatal intensive care units (NICU) acquire an intestinal flora that differs from that of healthy neonates in certain aspects. *Klebsiella* and *Enterobacter* are usually the dominant enterobacteria, whereas *E. coli* is less frequently isolated.[45,66,67] Colonization with anaerobes is reduced.[27,49,68,69]

Infants cared for in NICU are often prematurely born, delivered by cesarean section, and treated with antibiotics. Several antibiotics, including penicillin G, ampicillin, cephalosporins, and aminoglycosides markedly affect the intestinal microflora of newborn infants.[8,9] Most anaerobic bacteria are profoundly suppressed, and clostridia are often the only anaerobes that remain detectable.[8,9] The rate of carriage of *C. difficile* may be increased.[57] Also, the aerobic microflora is pertubed: *E. coli* decreases, whereas *Klebsiella*, *Enterobacter*, and *Pseudomonas* increase.[8,66] Antibiotic-resistant strains of enterobacteria appear in the intestinal microflora.[70–72] In most cases, the intestinal microflora returns to normal within a few weeks of treatment, but it may take months before *Bacteroides* counts are back to normal.[8,9]

When a substantial portion of infants cared for in a ward are treated with antibiotics, this also affects the intestinal colonization pattern of untreated infants.[72] As antibiotics suppress anaerobic bacteria in treated neonates, a reduced spread of anaerobic strains between infants could be expected. This could explain the generally low colonization rate with anaerobic bacteria in NICU.[27,49,69,73]

BREASTFEEDING AND INTESTINAL COLONIZATION

Breastfeeding clearly influences the intestinal microbial colonization pattern. A great number of studies have been performed since 1900[74] focusing on differences in the composition of the microflora between breastfed and bottlefed infants (Table 17–2).[6,7,10,18,19,23,25,26,28–32,68,75–83] Although the results vary between studies, the most pronounced and persistent difference found is that breastfed infants have much lower counts of clostridia and enterococci than bottlefed infants.[6,10] Instead, breastfed infants tend to have higher counts of staphylococci, especially during the first weeks of life.[7,10,23] It may be that staphylococci from the nipple are swallowed.[84]

In a number of studies performed before the 1980s, high bifidobacterial counts were regarded as the most characteristic feature of the intestinal flora of the breastfed infant.[19,75–77] Most recent studies, however, report similar counts of bifidobacteria in breastfed and bottlefed infants (see Table 17–2).[7,10,23,30–32] Some, but far from all, studies show more *Bacteroides* in bottlefed than in breastfed infants.[25,26,68,77] Nevertheless, it may be that more breastfed than bottlefed infants harbor a flora dominated by bifidobacteria, an effect of marginally-increased bifidobacterial counts in combination with lower levels of other bacterial groups.[10,29] The fecal pH of breastfed infants is lower than that of bottlefed infants due to the low buffering capacity of human milk. This was assumed to permit the proliferation of acid-tolerant bifidobacteria, whereas *E. coli* and other enterobacteria would be suppressed.[77] There is, however, no correlation between fecal pH and bifidobacterial counts.[10,23,75] Furthermore, there is no correlation between high bifidobacterial and low enterobacterial counts in the intestine of breastfed infants.[78]

Colonization with lactobacilli does not seem to be much influenced by the feeding mode, although there are some studies showing significantly higher numbers of lactobacilli in bottlefed than in breastfed infants.[26,31,81]

There is a tendency, in many studies, that breastfed infants have lower counts of enterobacteria than bottlefed infants (see Table 17–2), but the difference is usually marginal.[10,25] More important, the enterobacterial flora differs at the species and strain level between breast- and bottlefed infants. Breastfed infants have fewer enterobacteria other than *E. coli*: for example, *Klebsiella* or *Enterobacter*.[10,11,62,77,85] Breastfed infants also have a more stable enterobacterial flora than bottlefed infants, with fewer *E. coli* serotypes being present concomitantly,[85,86] and a lower turnover of *E. coli* strains with time.[86]

There are studies indicating that breastfeeding selectively promotes the growth of *E. coli* strains of low virulence in the

TABLE 17–2
Studies Comparing the Intestinal Microflora of Breastfed and Bottlefed Infants

		Breastfed Compared to Bottlefed						
Reference	Age of Infants*	Fewer Clostridia	Fewer Bacteroides	Fewer Enterococci	Fewer Enterobacteria	More Bifidobacteria	More Staphylococci	Fewer Lactobacilli
75†	1,2w	Yes	NT	NT	No	Yes	NT	NT
76†	1w	NT	NT	NT	No	Yes	NT	NT
77†	1–7w	Yes	Yes	Yes	Yes	Yes	NT	NT
19†	1–6w	Yes	No	Yes(4–6w)	No	Yes	NT	NT
68	<2, 2–4, >4d	NT	Yes (>4d)	NT	No	NT	NT	NT
78†	1w	NT	NT	NT	No	Yes	NT	NT
18		NT	NT	NT	Yes	No	NT	NT
6†	1w – 12m	Yes	No	Yes	Yes	No	No	No
23	2,4,6 w	Yes (2,4w)	No	Yes (4,6w)	No	No	Yes	NT
25†	1–6d, 1m	NT	Yes	Yes	Yes	Yes	No	No
79	1–5d, 3,6w	NT	NT	NT	No	No	NT	No
26	28–46d	Yes	Yes	Yes	Yes	No	NT	Yes
7	5d, 3,8w	No	No	No	No	No	Yes (5d,3w)	No
80	3–7d	Yes (7d)	Yes (7d)	No	Yes (7d)	Yes (7d)	NT	No
81	1–12w	Yes	No	Yes	Yes	No	NT	Yes
82†	1–6d	NT	No	NT	No	Yes	NT	NT
28	1,4w	NT	NT	No	No	No	No	No
10	4d–4w	Yes (2–4w)	No	Yes(2–4w)	Yes (4d, 4w)	No	Yes	NT
83	2,7,11,15w	No	Yes (2w)‡	Yes (2,7w)	Yes(2w)	Yes (2w)‡	Yes (2,7w)	No
29	1w, 1,3m	Yes (1w)	No	Yes (1m)	No	No	NT	NT
30	2,4w	Yes (2w)	No	Yes	Yes	No	Yes	No
31	1,2w, 1,2,3m	Yes (2w–3m)	No	Yes (2w–3m)	Yes (2m)§	No	No	Yes (2w)
32	1w, 1m	No	No	Yes	No	No	No	NT
Studies before 1980		3/3	2/3	2/2	2/7	5/6	NT	NT
Studies after 1980		9/12	4/14	11/13	9/16	4/16	5/10	3/11
All studies		12/15	6/17	13/15	11/23	9/22	5/10	3/11

Results refer to breastfed babies in comparison to infants receiving different formulas. In studies including tests for statistical significance, only statistically significant differences are considered in the table.
* Age of infants in days (d), weeks (w), or months (m).
† No tests for statistical significance were performed.
‡ = significantly different from infants fed a casein-based formula.
§ = significantly different from infants fed a whey-based formula.
NT = not tested.

intestine. *Escherichia coli* isolated from breastfed infants are, thus, more sensitive to the bactericidal effect of human serum,[87] and less frequently carry K1 than *E. coli* from bottlefed infants.[85] The K1 capsular antigen protects the bacteria from the action of complement and phagocytes, and is an important virulence factor in *E. coli* causing extra-intestinal infections.[88,89]

Breastfeeding also favors *E. coli* carrying type 1 fimbriae,[90] possibly because type 1 fimbriae bind to the mannose-containing carbohydrates on secretory IgA present in large amounts in human milk.[91] In contrast, *E. coli* expressing mannose-resistant adhesins are isolated less frequently from breastfed infants,[62,90] possibly due to the selective promotion of type 1-fimbriated strains. Type 1 fimbriae of *E. coli* have not been linked to pathogenicity, whereas mannose-resistant adhesins, including, for example, P fimbriae, are well-recognized virulence factors in extra-intestinal infections; for example, urinary tract infections and septicemia caused by *E. coli*.[92]

Factors in Breastmilk that Could Modulate the Intestinal Microflora

It is not known which of the many factors present in breastmilk could be responsible for the differences in the bacterial flora between breastfed and bottlefed infants. Factors of suggested, but not proven, ability to influence the intestinal microflora include secretory IgA, lactoferrin, lysozyme, complex oligosaccharides, and nucleotides.[30,90,93–97] However, attempts to add bovine lactoferrin or nucleotides to infant formulas have not changed the intestinal microflora of the infants studied toward a more breastfed pattern.[28–30,94] The low casein and phosphate content of human milk results in a poor buffering capacity. Acid metabolites are thus not neutralized, which creates a low pH in the intestine of the breastfed infant.[19] However, lowering the casein and phosphate content of infant formulas does not result in a low intestinal pH in infants receiving the formula.[83] One may safely conclude that the complexity of factors in human milk is tremendous, and meticulously-performed studies will be required to dissect potential effects of individual factors.

INFLUENCE OF INTESTINAL MICROFLORA ON INFANTS

Characteristics and Functions of the Intestinal Microflora

Biochemical Reactions

The development of the intestinal ecosystem can be followed by assessing biochemical reactions performed by the intestinal bacterial population. A large number of different bacteria produce different short-chain fatty acids, such as acetate, proprionate, and butyrate, which are the preferred substrate for colonic epithelial cells.[98] The variety of short-chain fatty acids increases as a more complex microflora is established.[2,99] Certain bacteria—for example, *Eubacterium lentum*—convert cholesterol excreted in the bile to coprostanol,[100] and others—for example, *C. ramosum*—transform bilirubin to urobilins.[101] Some anaerobes, such as certain strains of *Ruminococcus* and *Bifidobacterium*, degrade mucin and liberate monosaccharides, which in turn may be the substrate for other bacteria.[102,103] Yet other bacteria, such as *Bacteroides distasonis*, are capable of inactivating pancreatic trypsin in the intestinal lumen.[104]

By assessing various biochemical parameters in feces, one may obtain an indication of whether bacterial groups responsible for certain key metabolic reactions have established or not. In general, this proceeds in a sequential manner: production of short-chain fatty acids is one of the first functions to be established, followed by bilirubin conversion and mucin degradation. A coprostanol-producing flora is acquired during the second year of life, and the capacity of the microflora to inactivate trypsin continues to develop beyond that period.[105] In Swedish children, some biochemical functions characteristic of a complete microflora are not established yet at five years.[2,105]

Suppression of Aerobic and Facultatively Anaerobic Bacteria

When the anaerobic bacterial populations expand in the intestine, the facultative bacteria decline in numbers.[6,14] Within a few weeks or months, reduced counts of, for example, *Klebsiella*, *Enterobacter*, and staphylococci are observed.[1,10,21,30,31,40,45,62] Other facultative bacteria, such as *E. coli* and enterococci, retain quite high population levels in the presence of anaerobes,[42] demonstrating that facultative bacteria differ in their ability to withstand the competition from anaerobes.

The relatively simple anaerobic flora of infants is not capable of suppressing facultative bacteria as effectively as the complex adult anaerobic microflora, estimated to harbor several hundred different anaerobic species.[24,106] In animal studies, mice monoassociated with *E. coli* have been used as a model of the early neonatal intestinal flora. When *E. coli* is present as the only colonizing species, levels of 10^{10-11} bacteria per g feces are obtained. To bring the *E. coli* population down to the levels found in conventional animals, 95 different anaerobic strains isolated from conventional mice were required.[107,108] The same phenomenon is seen in human infants, in whom relatively high numbers of both facultative and anaerobic bacteria may be present during the first months,[6,20] or even years, of life.[1] In the study by Ellis-Pegler et al. the mean ratio of anaerobic over facultatively anaerobic and aerobic bacteria was 1.5:1 in infants before four months, 10:1 in four to 12-month-old infants, and 50:1 in children one to four years old, as compared to a ratio of 200:1 in adults.[1]

Colonization Resistance

The intestinal microflora confers colonization resistance: that is, an ecologic pressure against the establishment of new bacterial strains into the ecosystem.[108,109] Colonization resistance is mainly a function of the anaerobic microflora.[108,110,111] It seems that the greater the variety of anaerobic species, the greater the resistance conferred by the microflora to implantation of invading bacterial strains. Several mechanisms have been proposed. Competition for nutrients is regarded as the most important factor in regulating the sizes of intestinal bacterial populations and in the resistance toward the incursion of new strains.[108] If the concentration of nutrients is low, bacteria are unable to multiply at a rate exceeding the normal transit time of the intestinal contents, and they are eliminated from the intestine. Competition for binding sites may also be of importance: bacteria associating with the intestinal mucosa are thought to have the advantage, as they are less easily eliminated.[108] Furthermore, metabolites elaborated by anaerobic bacteria—for example, short-chain fatty acids and hydrogen sulphide—may suppress the growth of certain bacteria, and thus prevent their establishment in the intestinal microflora.[108,112]

The relatively simple anaerobic flora of infants is likely to provide less colonization resistance than the diversified anaerobic microflora of adults. This can be demonstrated by the relative ease with which infants, as compared with adults, can be experimentally colonized with a new strain of E. coli.[113–116]

Role of the Intestinal Microflora in Neonatal Infections

The young infant is at higher risk to develop certain infections than older children or adults. Thus, urinary tract infections and septicemia are especially common in the neonatal period,[42,117,118] and diarrheal disease is common throughout the first two years of life, especially in developing countries.[118] The increased risk for bacterial infections may in part relate to special features of the infants' intestinal microflora.

Urinary Tract Infection

Urinary tract infection is usually caused by E. coli from the intestine that first colonize the periurethral area and then ascend into the urinary tract.[117,119] The periurethral area is heavily colonized with E. coli in both boys and girls during the first weeks of life, but such colonization decreases with age.[120] Urinary tract infection strikes 0.8% of boys and 1% of girls during the first year of life, but this incidence declines sharply with age.[117]

Certain E. coli strains are more likely than others to cause urinary tract infection. These strains possess so-called virulence factors: for example, P fimbriae and certain O and K antigens.[89,92] The P fimbriae mediate adherence to the uroepithelium, and thus permit bacteria to stick to the mucosa and resist being flushed out by the urinary flow.[121,122] However, P fimbriae also adhere to human colonic epithelial cells[123,124] and promote large intestinal colonization, especially in the neonate.[40,125,126] It is, thus, possible that P fimbriae have evolved primarily as a colonization factor for the intestinal milieu. Intestinal carriage of P-fimbriated uropathogenic E. coli strains increases the risk to contract urinary tract infection.[127,128]

Klebsiella is the second-most-common cause of urinary tract infection in neonates,[129] but is rare in older children.[117] This probably relates to the uniquely high incidence of intestinal colonization with Klebsiella in early life.

Septicemia

The incidence of neonatal septicemia is one to four in 1000 live births in Western countries, and the mortality rate is at least 20%.[130–132] In developing countries, the reported incidence is much higher.[118,133] Thus, 1% of Pakistani neonates are thought to die from septicemia.[134] Intestinal bacteria such as E. coli, Klebsiella, and other enterobacteria, enterococci, and Pseudomonas cause 30% of the septicemia cases in developed countries,[135–137] and up to 80% of those in developing countries.[133,138,139] The majority of cases in industrialized societies are instead due to S. aureus, S. epidermidis, and group B streptococci.[135–137] As mentioned, staphylococci are common inhabitants of the intestinal microflora of newborn infants, especially in countries with high hygienic standards; and it is possible that the intestine acts as a site of entry for staphylococci in some cases of neonatal septicemia.[65] In developing countries, the early intestinal colonization with a variety of different enterobacterial strains is likely to increase the risk of encountering pathogenic ones, and this colonization pattern could thus be an important factor in the high incidence of neonatal septicemia.

Intestinal bacteria may reach the bloodstream by a direct translocation over the intestinal epithelial barrier. Those that escape phagocytosis and other innate immune mechanisms may spread further and cause septicemia.[140] Enterobacteria, staphylococci, and enterococci are able to translocate: that is, pass viably over the intestinal epithelium to the mesenteric lymph nodes, blood, and other organs.[141] In experimental animals, translocation occurs when these bacteria reach population levels above 10^{7-8} bacteria per g feces.[141,142] The high risk of septicemia during the first period of life may relate to the high levels of facultative bacteria in the intestinal microflora. Although translocation has not been formally proven in human infants, transient bacteremia occurs in a considerable proportion of healthy neonates at the time of intestinal colonization.[143] Most infants show no symptoms, and the bacteria are cleared spontaneously in a few days.

Treatment with antibiotics results in a suppression of anaerobic bacteria and, in turn, a pronounced expansion of the populations of enterobacteria other than E. coli, which may increase the risk for neonatal septicemia. In a Swedish study, 23 of the 27 infants who contracted sepsis from gram-negative bacteria other than E. coli had all received antibiotics prior to diagnosis. The four remaining infants struck by septicemia had been delivered by cesarean section, which is also likely to result in a deficient anaerobic flora.[144]

Necrotizing Enterocolitis

Necrotizing enterocolitis is a life-threatening intestinal disease that primarily affects premature neonates. The clinical manifestations include abdominal distention and rectal bleeding. In severe cases, the intestinal wall is perforated. The condition is thought to emerge as the result of ischemic injury to an immature gut, accelerated by a direct action of intestinal bacteria.[145] The reported clustering of cases has suggested certain bacteria to be causative, but the bacteria isolated from the intestines of affected infants are normal members of the neonatal gut flora: most commonly, *Klebsiella*, *E. coli*, and clostridia.[146]

Diarrhea

Infants are more susceptible than adults to diarrhea caused by bacterial pathogens. For instance, infections due to *Campylobacter*, *Salmonella*, and enteropathogenic *E. coli* peak during the first year of life.[147–149] The intestinal flora of neonates and young infants provides less resistance to colonization with enteric pathogens than that of adults. Thus, ingestion of as few as 40 *Salmonella* can cause infection in an infant, whereas the infectious dose in adults is about 10^6 bacteria.[150]

Diarrhea in itself induces disturbances in the intestinal microflora. For example, the numbers of anaerobic bacteria decrease transiently,[151] perhaps because the rapid motility increases the oxygen contents in the intestinal lumen.

In a developing country, diarrhea was the main cause of death during the first two years of life, and a majority of the deaths in diarrhea occurred among the chronic cases.[134] Chronic diarrhea, defined as diarrhea persisting for more than two weeks, develops in approximately 15% of the acute cases in developing countries.[152] Defined diarrheal pathogens are rarely identified, but the small intestine may be colonized by bacteria normally present only in the colon. This condition, termed bacterial overgrowth, is believed to contribute to the pathogenesis.[153–156] For example, the bacteria may cause injury to the small-intestinal epithelium, leading to disaccharidase deficiency, which results in osmotic diarrhea. Further, a number of bacterial metabolites, such as hydroxylated fatty acids, alcohols, and deconjugated bile acids, may increase intestinal secretion.[157]

Antibiotics are frequently given to infants with diarrhea in developing countries.[152] This habit is detrimental, since antibiotics suppress most anaerobes, and thus decrease the colonization resistance. Not only is the treatment ineffective; it may also render the infant more susceptible to new episodes of diarrheal disease, or to chronic diarrhea.

Clostridium difficile-Associated Disease

The frequent colonization of young infants with *C. difficile* in large numbers does not have any clear adverse effects on health.[54,57,158] In adults, *C. difficile* is an important pathogen that elaborates toxins that cause antibiotic-associated diarrhea and pseudomembranous colitis if the bacterium reaches too high numbers in the intestinal flora.[159] Young infants colonized with toxigenic *C. difficile* almost invariably remain asymptomatic.[56,57,160] The reason for this resistance to *C. difficile*-induced gastrointestinal disease is unknown, but it has been speculated that infants could have a lower density of receptors for *C. difficile* enterotoxin in their intestinal mucosa.[158]

An association between intestinal carriage of toxigenic bacteria—for example, *C. difficile*—and the sudden infant death syndrome has been proposed.[161] It is hypothesized that if toxins elaborated by these bacteria reach the circulation and achieve a critical concentration, it may evoke host responses resulting in sudden death of the infant.[162]

Protection of Breastfeeding against Infectious Diseases

Breastfeeding confers significant protection from urinary tract infection, septicemia, necrotizing enterocolitis, and diarrheal disease.[163,164] This protective effect could partly relate to special features of the intestinal microflora in the breastfed baby. Thus, a selection for less-virulent enterobacterial strains is likely to contribute to the protection conferred by breastfeeding against urinary tract infection, septicemia, and diarrheal disease.[163,165] A reduction of enterobacteria, especially in the small intestine,[166] could result in a decreased translocation rate and a reduced risk for septicemia, and possibly a reduced risk for necrotizing enterocolitis.

However, even when colonization with potentially pathogenic bacteria is not inhibited by breastfeeding, human milk may decrease their ability to cause disease. For example, fully breastfed infants may be colonized with diarrheal pathogens and still remain perfectly healthy.[14] A number of factors in human milk may contribute to this kind of protection. Secretory IgA may neutralize bacterial toxins and prevent the attachment of bacteria to the intestinal mucosa,[163,167] which could be important in the protection against gastroenteritis.[168–172] The coating of bacteria with secretory IgA decreases their ability to translocate over the intestinal epithelium.[173,174] Furthermore, breast milk contains a number of cytokines, hormones, growth factors, and immune cells that may influence the growth and function of the infant's lymphoid system and the development of intestinal barriers, and enhance antibacterial defences.[163,164,175]

Influence of the Intestinal Flora on the Immune System

The intestinal microflora is an important stimulus for the intestinal lymphoid tissue. Animals harboring a normal intestinal flora have 10 times more IgA-producing cells in the gut than germ-free animals.[176]

The buildup of IgA-producing cells in the mucosa and secretory IgA antibodies in exocrine secretions is probably the result of repeated stimulation by the steady stream of newly-colonizing bacteria. As mentioned, bacteria establishing in the intestine may translocate over the intestinal epithelium, which brings them in direct contact with the immune apparatus and triggers a specific immune response,[174,177] including secretory IgA antibodies specific for bacterial surface components.[178] The secretory IgA is exported to the intestinal lumen, where it coats the bacteria.[179] This coating does not prevent the bacteria from thriving in the intestine, but destroys their ability to translocate.[174] Therefore, it is likely that bacterial strains colonizing for extended periods only exert a limited influence on the immune system after the initial colonization phase. A rapid replacement of individual bacterial strains in the microflora is probably a more powerful stimulus.

Aerobic or facultative bacteria are more likely to elicit a specific immune response than anaerobic bacteria, possibly due to their pronounced ability to translocate.[177,180] However, circulating antibodies against anaerobic bacteria, such as *Bacteroides, Clostridium,* and *Bifidobacterium* species, have been detected in several studies,[180–182] and anaerobic bacteria in the intestinal lumen are coated with secretory IgA.[179]

Oral Tolerance and the Intestinal Microflora

Unlike intestinal bacteria food proteins are poor immunogens, and often induce a state of specific unresponsiveness, termed oral tolerance.[183,184] To uphold a state of tolerance to food proteins and other harmless antigens is an important task of the immune system; in the absence of such mechanisms, inflammatory and hypersensitivity reactions can occur.

It is evident from animal studies that the presence of a normal bacterial flora in the gut facilitates the induction of oral tolerance to food antigens.[185,186] The mechanisms behind these interactions are not defined, but it is possible that certain bacterial structures might have a prononunced influence on the way the immune system handles different antigens. Adjuvant activity of bacterial components is a well-known phenomenon and means that the presence of these components influences the antigen presentation (for example, a protein antigen) with which they are mixed, thus rendering it more immunogenic. In analogy, certain bacterial structures may influence antigen-presenting cells so that they handle food proteins in a tolerogenic, rather than an immunogenic, way. For example, the lipopolysaccharide (LPS) molecule in the outer membrane of *E. coli* and other enterobacteria seems to enhance tolerance induction: if LPS is administered together with food antigens, the tolerizing effect of feeding is increased.[187] Other bacterial components might have adverse effects. Thus, cholera toxin and the heat-labile toxin of enterotoxin-producing *E. coli* may break oral tolerance to food proteins.[188,189] An adjuvant role of certain bacterial DNA sequences has recently been proposed.[190,191] Such DNA sequences may promote cell-mediated immunity, but suppress, for example, IgE synthesis against coadministered antigens,[192] which in turn could have implications for the development of IgE-mediated hypersensitivity reactions.

It is possible that the early establishment of high population levels of certain bacteria in the neonatal intestine provides a physiologic stimulus for the developing immune system, which facilitates the induction and maintenance of tolerance to harmless antigens, such as food proteins and inhaled environmental antigens. By contrast, in Western societies too-limited exposure to indigenous bacteria such as enterobacteria, enterococci, and lactobacilli in the neonatal period could result in a deficient stimulation of the immune system, and that tolerance is not developed.[60,193] The incidence of atopic allergy is steadily increasing in Western European countries, and vastly supersedes the incidence in Eastern European countries and the Third World.[194–196] The high incidence of allergy in Western countries may relate to an inadequately-developed intestinal microflora in infants in these societies.

REFERENCES

1. Ellis-Pegler RB, Crabtree C, Lambert HP. The faecal flora of children in the United Kingdom. J Hyg Lond 1975;75:135–42.
2. Midtvedt A-C. The establishment and development of some metabolic activities associated with the intestinal microflora in healthy children [thesis]. Stockholm: Stockholm Univ.; 1994.
3. Bettelheim KA, Breadon A, Faiers MC, et al. The origin of O-serotypes of *Escherichia coli* in babies after normal delivery. J Hyg Lond 1974;72:67–70.
4. Bettelheim K, Teoh-Chan C, Chandler M, et al. Spread of *Escherichia coli* colonizing newborn babies and their mothers. J Hyg Lond 1974;73:383–7.
5. Tannock GW, Fuller R, Smith SL, Hall MA. Plasmid profiling of members of the family *Enterobacteriaceae*, lactobacilli, and bifidobacteria to study the transmission of bacteria from mother to infant. J Clin Microbiol 1990;28:1225–8.
6. Stark PL, Lee A. The microbial ecology of the large bowel of breast-fed and formula-fed infants during the first year of life. J Med Microbiol 1982;15:189–203.
7. Lundequist B, Nord CE, Winberg J. The composition of faecal microflora in breastfed and bottlefed infants from birth to 8 weeks. Acta Paediatr Scand 1985;74:54–8.
8. Bennet R, Eriksson M, Nord C-E, Zetterström R. Fecal bacterial microflora of newborn infants during intensive care management and treatment with five antibiotic regimens. Pediatr Infect Dis J 1986;5:533–9.
9. Bennet R, Nord C-E. Development of the faecal anaerobic microflora after caesarean section and treatment with antibiotics in newborn infants. Infection 1987;15:332–6.
10. Balmer SE, Wharton BA. Diet and faecal flora in the newborn: breastmilk and infant formula. Arch Dis Child 1989;64:1672–7.
11. Adlerberth I, Carlsson B, de Man P, et al. Intestinal colonization with *Enterobacteriaceae* in Pakistani and Swedish hospital delivered infants. Acta Paediatr Scand 1991;80:602–10.
12. Bennet R, Eriksson M, Tafari N, Nord C-E. Intestinal bacteria of newborn Ethiopian infants in relation to antibiotic treatment and colonization with potentially pathogenic Gram-negative bacteria. Scand J Infect Dis 1991;23:63–9.
13. Gorbach SL, Nahas L, Lerner PI, Weinstein L. Studies of intestinal microflora. I. Effects of diet, age, and periodic sampling on numbers of fecal microorganisms in man. Gastroenterology 1967;53:845–55.
14. Mata LJ, Urrutia JJ. Intestinal colonization of breastfed children in a rural area of low socio-economic level. Ann N Y Acad Sci 1971;176:93–109.
15. Maier BR, Flynn MA, Burton GC, et al. Effects of a high-beef diet on bowel flora: a preliminary report. Am J Clin Nutr 1974;27:1470–4.
16. Drasar BS. Some factors associated with geographical variations in the intestinal microflora. In: Skinner FA, Carr JG, editors. The normal microbial flora of man. New York: Academic Press; 1974. p. 187.
17. Gothefors L, Carlsson B, Ahlstedt S, et al. Influence of maternal gut flora and colostral and cord serum antibodies on presence of *Escherichia coli* in faeces of the newborn infant. Acta Paediatr Scand 1976;65:225–32.
18. Mitsuoka T, Kaneuchi C. Ecology of the bifidobacteria. Am J Clin Nutr 1977;30:1799–810.
19. Bullen CL, Tearle PV, Stewart MG. The effect of "humanised" milk and supplemented breastfeeding on the faecal flora of infants. J Med Microbiol 1977;10:403–13.
20. Hoogkamp-Korstanje JAA, Lindner JGEM, Marcelis JH, et al. Composition and ecology of the human intestinal flora. Antonie Van Leeuwenhoek 1979;45:335–40.

21. Rotimi VO, Duerden BI. The development of the bacterial flora in normal neonates. J Med Microbiol 1981;14:51–62.
22. Rotimi VO, Duerden BI. *Bacteroides* species in the normal neonatal faecal flora. J Hyg Lond 1981;87:299–304.
23. Simhon A, Douglas JR, Drasar BS, Soothill JF. Effect of feeding on infants' faecal flora. Arch Dis Child 1982;57:54–8.
24. Finegold SM, Sutter VL, Mathisen GE. Normal indigenous intestinal flora. In: Hentges DJ, editor. Human intestinal microflora in health and disease. London: Academic Press; 1983. p. 3.
25. Yoshioka H, Iseki K, Fujita J. Development and differences of intestinal flora in the neonatal period in breastfed and bottlefed infants. Pediatrics 1983;72:317–21.
26. Benno Y, Sawada K, Mitsuoka T. The intestinal microflora of infants: composition of the fecal flora in breastfed and bottlefed infants. Microbiol Immunol 1984;28:975–86.
27. Sakata H, Yoshioka H, Fujita K. Development of the intestinal flora in very low birth weight infants compared to normal fullterm newborns. Eur J Pediatr 1985;144:186–90.
28. Gil A, Corral E, Martínez A, Molina JA. Effects of the addition of nucleotides to an adapted milk formula on the microbial pattern of faeces in at term newborn infants. J Clin Nutr Gastroenterol 1986;1:127–32.
29. Roberts AK, Chierici R, Sawatzki G, et al. Supplementation of an adapted formula with bovine lactoferrin: 1. Effect on the infant faecal flora. Acta Paediatr Scand 1992;81:119–24.
30. Balmer SE, Hanvey LS, Wharton BA. Diet and faecal flora in the newborn: nucleotides. Arch Dis Child 1994;70:F137–40.
31. Kleessen B, Bunke H, Tovar K, et al. Influence of two infant formulas and human milk on the development of the faecal flora in newborn infants. Acta Paediatr Scand 1995;84:1347–56.
32. Langhendries JP, Detry J, Van-Hees J, et al. Effect of a fermented infant formula containing viable bifidobacteria on the fecal flora composition and pH of healthy fullterm infants. J Pediatr Gastroenterol Nutr 1995;21:177–81.
33. Grutte FK, Horn R, Haenel H. Ernahrung und biochemisch-mikrookologische vorgange in enddarm von sauglingen. Z Kinderheilkd 1965;93:28–39.
34. Rotimi VO, Olowe SA, Ahmed I. The development of bacterial flora in premature neonates. J Hyg Camb 1985;94:309–18.
35. Bettelheim K, Teoh-Chan C, Chandler M, et al. Further studies of *Escherichia coli* in babies after normal delivery. J Hyg Lond 1974;73:277–85.
36. Bettelheim KA, Lenox-King SMJ. The acquisition of *Escherichia coli* by newborn babies. Infection 1976;4:174–9.
37. Gareau FE, Macker DC, Boring JR, et al. The aquisition of fecal flora by infants from their mothers during delivery. J Pediatr 1959;54:313–8.
38. Murono K, Fujita K, Yoshikawa M, et al. Acquisition of nonmaternal *Enterobacteriaceae* by infants delivered in hospitals. J Pediatr 1993;122:120–5.
39. Fryklund B, Tullus K, Berglund B, Burman LG. Importance of the environment and the faecal flora of infants, nursing staff and parents as sources of Gram-negative bacteria colonizing newborns in three neonatal wards. Infection 1992;20:253–7.
40. Adlerberth I. Bacterial adherence and intestinal colonization in newborn infants [thesis]. Göteborg, Sweden: Göteborg University; 1996.
41. Bettelheim K, Peddie B, Chereshsky A. The ecology of *Escherichia coli* in a maternity ward in Christ Church, New Zealand. Zentralbl Bakteriol Mikrobiol Hyg B 1983;178:389–93.
42. Bennet R. The faecal microflora of newborn infants during intensive care management and its relationship to neonatal septicemia [thesis]. Stockholm: Stockholm University; 1987.
43. Tannock GV. Normal microflora. An introduction to microbes inhabiting the human body. London: Chapman & Hall; 1995.
44. Shinebaum R, Cooke EM, Brayson JC. Acquisition of *Klebsiella aerogenes* by neonates. J Med Microbiol 1979;12:201–5.
45. Fryklund B. Epidemiology of enterobacteria and risk factors for invasive Gram-negative bacterial infection in neonatal special-care units [thesis]. Stockholm: Stockholm Univ.; 1994.
46. Cooke EM. *Escherichia coli*: distribution in nature: epidemiology. In: Cooke EM, editor. *Escherichia coli* and man. Edinburgh: Churchill Livingstone; 1974. p. 13.
47. Pazzaglia G, Escalante J, Sack R, et al. Transient intestinal colonization with multiple phenotypes of *Aeromonas* species during the first week of life. J Clin Microbiol 1990;28:1842–6.
48. Neut C, Bezirtzoglou E, Romond C, et al. Bacterial colonization of the large intestine in newborns delivered by caesarean section. Zentralbl Bakteriol Mikrobiol Hyg A 1987;266:330–7.
49. Hall MA, Cole CB, Smith SL, et al. Factors influencing the presence of faecal lactobacilli on early infancy. Arch Dis Child 1990;65:185–8.
50. Masfar AN, Duerden BI, Kinghorn GR. Quantitative studies of vaginal bacteria. Genitourin Med 1986;62:256–63.
51. Carlsson J, Gothefors L. Transmission of *Lactobacillus jensenii* and *Lactobacillus acidophilus* from mother to child at the time of delivery. J Clin Microbiol 1975;1:124–8.
52. Brook I, Barett C, Brinkman C, et al. Aerobic and anaerobic bacterial flora of the maternal cervix and newborn gastric fluid and conjunctiva: a prospective study. Pediatrics 1979;63:451–5.
53. Ahrné S, Nobaek S, Jeppson B, et al. The normal *Lactobacillus* flora on healthy human oral and rectal mucosa. J Appl Bacteriol 1998;85:88–94.
54. Bolton RP, Tait SK, Dear PRF, Losowsky MS. Asymptomatic neonatal colonization by *Clostridium difficile*. Arch Dis Child 1984;59:466–72.
55. Rolfe RD. Asymptomatic intestinal colonization by *Clostridium difficile*. In: Rolfe RD, Finegold SM, editors. *Clostridium difficile*: its role in intestinal disease. New York: Academic Press; 1988. p. 201.
56. Wilson KH. The microecology of *Clostridium difficile*. Clin Infect Dis 1993;16 Suppl 4:S214–8.
57. el Mohandes AE, Keiser JF, Refat M, Jackson BJ. Prevalence and toxigenicity of *Clostridium difficile* isolates in fecal microflora of preterm infants in the intensive care nursery. Biol Neonate 1993;63:225–9.
58. Kato H, Kato N, Watanabe K, et al. Application of typing by pulsed-field gel electrophoresis to the study of *Clostridium difficile* in a neonatal intensive care unit. J Clin Microbiol 1994;32:2067–70.
59. Martirosian G, Kuipers S, Verbrugh H, et al. PCR ribotyping and arbitrary primed PCR for typing strains of *Clostridium difficile* from a Polish maternity hospital. J Clin Microbiol 1995;33:2016–21.
60. Sepp E, Julge K, Vasar M, et al. Intestinal microflora of Estonian and Swedish infants. Acta Paediatr Scand 1997;86:956–61.
61. Rolfe RD. Probiotics: prospects for use in *Clostridium difficile*-associated intestinal disease. In: Fuller R, Heidt PJ, Rusch V, Van der Waaij D, editors. Old Herborn University Seminar Monograph. Vol. 8. Herborn-Dill: Institute for Microbiology and Biochemistry, Germany; 1995. p. 47.
62. Tullus K. Fecal colonization with P-fimbriated *E. coli* between 0 and 18 months of age. Epidemiol Infect 1988;100:185–91.
63. Kühn I, Tullus K, Möllby R. Colonization and persistence of *Escherichia coli* phenotypes in the intestines of children aged 0 to 18 months. Infection 1986;14:7–12.

64. Borderon JC, Lionnet C, Rondeau C, et al. Aspects actuels de la flore fecale du noveau-ne sans antibiotheerapie les sept premiers jours: enterobacteries, enterocoques, staphylocoques. Pathol Biol (Paris) 1996;44: 416–22.
65. el Mohandes AE, Keiser JF, Johnson LA, et al. Aerobes isolated in fecal microflora of infants in the intensive care nursery: relationship to human milk use and systemic sepsis. Am J Infect Control 1993;21:231–4.
66. Goldmann DA, Leclair J, Macone A. Bacterial colonization of neonates admitted to an intensive care environment. J Pediatr 1978;93:288–93.
67. Tullus K, Berglund B, Fryklund B, et al. Epidemiology of fecal strains of the family *Enterobacteriaceae* in 22 neonatal wards and influence of antibiotic policy. J Clin Microbiol 1988;26:1166–70.
68. Long SS, Swenson RM. Development of anaerobic fecal flora in healthy newborn infants. J Pediatr 1977;91:298–301.
69. Stark PL, Lee A. The bacterial colonization of the large bowel of pre-term low birth weight neonates. J Hyg Camb 1982;89:59–67.
70. Borderon JC, Gold F, Laugier J. Enterobacteria of the neonate: normal colonization and antibiotic induced selection. Biol Neonate 1981;39:1–7.
71. Bourillon A, Brackman D, Boussougant Y, de Paillerets F. Cefotaxime effects on the intestinal flora of the newborn. Dev Pharmacol Ther 1984;7 Suppl 1:144–9.
72. Tullus K, Burman LG. Ecological impact of ampicillin and cefuroxime in neonatal units. Lancet 1989;Jun 24:1405–7.
73. Graham JM, Taylor J, Davies PA. Some aspects of bacterial colonization in III, low-birthweight and normal newborns. In: Stern L, editor. Intensive care of the newborn. New York: Masson Publishing; 1976. p. 59.
74. Tissier H. Recherches sur la flore intestinale des nourrissons (etat normal et pathologique). Paris Thèses, 1900:1–253.
75. Willis AT, Bullen CL, Williams K, et al. Breastmilk substitute: a bacteriological study. BMJ 1973;iv:67–72.
76. Hewitt JH, Rigby J. Effects of various milk feeds on numbers of *Escherichia coli* and *Bifidobacterium* in the stools of newborn infants. J Hyg Lond 1976;77:129–39.
77. Bullen CL, Tearle PV, Willis AT. Bifidobacteria in the intestinal tract of infants—an in vivo study. J Med Microbiol 1976; 9:325–33.
78. Dolby JM, Honour P, Valman HB. Bacteriostasis of *Escherichia coli* by milk. I. Colonization of breastfed infants by milk resistant organisms. J Hyg Lond 1977;78:85–94.
79. Rose SJ. Bacterial flora of breastfed infants. Pediatrics 1984;74:563–4.
80. Mevissen-Verhage EAE, Marcelis JH, Harmsen-van Amerongen WCM, et al. Effect of iron on neonatal gut flora during the first week of life. Eur J Clin Microbiol Infect Dis 1985; 4:14–8.
81. Mevissen-Verhage EAE, Marcelis JH, Harmsen-Van Amerongen WCM, et al. Effect of iron on neonatal gut flora during the first three months of life. Eur J Clin Microbiol Infect Dis 1985;4:273–8.
82. Moreau M-C, Thomasson M, Ducluzeau R, Raibaud P. Cinétique d'établissement de la microflore digestive chez le nouveau-né humain en fonction de la nature de lait. Reprod Nutr Dev 1986;26:745–53.
83. Balmer SE, Scott PH, Wharton BA. Diet and faecal flora in the newborn: casein and whey proteins. Arch Dis Child 1989; 64:1678–84.
84. Gothefors L. Studies of antimicrobial factors in human milk and bacterial colonization of the newborn [thesis]. Umeå, Sweden: Umeå University; 1975.
85. Ørskov F, Biering-Sørensen K. *Escherichia coli* serogroups in breastfed and bottlefed infants. Acta Pathol Microbiol Scand B 1975;83:25–30.
86. Mevissen-Verhage EAE, Marcelis JH, Guiné PAM, Verhoe J. Effect of iron on serotypes and haemagglutination patterns of *Escherichia coli* in bottle-fed infants. Eur J Clin Microbiol Infect Dis 1985;4:570–4.
87. Gothefors L, Olling S, Winberg J. Breastfeeding and biological properties of faecal *Escherichia coli* strains. Acta Paediatr Scand 1975;64:807–12.
88. Robbins JB, McCracken GH Jr, Gotschlish EC, et al. *Escherichia coli* K1 capsular polysaccharide associated with neonatal meningitis. N Engl J Med 1974;30:1216–20.
89. Ørskov I, Ørskov F. *Escherichia coli* in extra-intestinal infections. J Hyg Lond 1985;95:551–575.
90. Slaviková M, Lódinová-Zadníková R, Adlerberth I, et al. Increased mannose-specific adherence and colonizing ability of *Escherichia coli* O83 in breastfed infants. Adv Exp Med Biol 1995;371A:497–500.
91. Wold AE, Mestecky J, Tomana M, et al. Secretory immunglobulin A carries oligosaccharide receptors for *Escherichia coli* type 1 fimbrial lectin. Infect Immun 1990;58: 3073–7.
92. Johnson JR. Virulence factors in *Escherichia coli* urinary tract infection. Clin Microbiol Rev 1991;4:80–128.
93. Gyllenberg H, Carlberg G. The nutritional characteristics of the bifid bacteria (*Lactobacillus bifidus*) of infants. Acta Pathol Microbiol Scand 1958;44:287–92.
94. Balmer SE, Scott PH, Wharton BA. Diet and fecal flora in the newborn: lactoferrin. Arch Dis Child 1989;64:1685–90.
95. Kunz C, Rudloff S. Biological functions of oligosaccharides in human milk. Acta Paediatr Scand 1993;82:903–12.
96. Teraguchi S, Ozawa K, Yasuda S, et al. The bacteriostatic effects of orally administered bovine lactoferrin on intestinal *Enterobacteriaceae* of SPF mice fed bovine milk. Biosci Biotechnol Biochem 1994;58: 482–7.
97. Teraguchi S, Shin K, Ozawa K, et al. Bacteriostatic effect of orally administered bovine lactoferrin on proliferation of *Clostridium* species in the gut of mice fed bovine milk. Appl Environ Microbiol 1995;61:501–6.
98. Roediger WEW. Role of anaerobic bacteria in the metabolic welfare of the colonic mucosa in man. Gut 1980;21:793–8.
99. Midtvedt A-C, Carlstedt-Duke B, Norin KE, et al. Development of five metabolic activities associated with the intestinal microflora of healthy infants. J Pediatr Gastroenterol Nutr 1988;7:559–67.
100. Eyssen HJ, Parmentier GG, Compernolle FC, et al. Biohydrogenation of sterols by *Eubacterium* ATCC 21, 408 - *Nova* species. Eur J Biochem 1973;36: 411–21.
101. Midtvedt T, Gustavsson BE. Microbial conversion of bilirubin to urobilins in vitro and in vivo. Acta Pathol Microbiol Scand 1981;B89:57–60.
102. Hoskins LC, Agustines M, McKee WB, et al. Mucin degradation in human colonic ecosystems. Isolation and properties of fecal strains that degrade ABH blood group antigens and oligosaccharides from mucin glycoproteins. J Clin Invest 1985;75:944–53.
103. Hoskins LC. Mucin degradation in the human gastrointestinal tract and its significance to enteric microbial ecology. Eur J Gastroenterol Hepatol 1993;5:205–13.
104. Ramare F, Hautefort I, Verhe F, et al. Inactivation of tryptic activity by a human-derived strain of *Bacteroides distasonis*. Appl Environ Microbiol 1996;62:1434–6.
105. Norin KE, Gustavsson BE, Lindblad BS, Midtvedt T. The establishment of some microflora associated biochemical characteristics in feces from children during the first years of life. Acta Paediatr Scand 1985;74:207–12.
106. Moore WEC, Holdeman LV. Human fecal flora: the normal flora of 20 Japanese-Hawaiians. Appl Microbiol 1974;27: 961–79.

107. Freter R, Abrams GD. Function of various intestinal bacteria in converting germfree mice to the normal stage. Infect Immun 1972;6:119–26.
108. Freter R. Factors affecting the microecology of the gut. In: Fuller R, editor. Probiotics—the scientific basis. London: Chapman & Hall, 1992. p. 111.
109. Van der Waaij D. Bioregulation of the digestive tract microflora. Rev Sci Tech 1989;8:333–45.
110. Wells CL, Maddaus MA, Jechorek RP, Simmons RL. Role of intestinal anaerobic bacteria in colonization resistance. Eur J Microbiol Infect Dis 1988;7:107–13.
111. Vollaard EJ, Clasener HAL. Colonization resistance. Antimicrob Agents Chemother 1994;38:409–14.
112. Hentges DJ. Role of intestinal flora in host defence against infection. In: Hentges DJ, editor. Human intestinal microflora in health and disease. New York: Academic Press; 1983. p. 311.
113. Cooke EM, Hettiaratchy IGT, Buck AC. Fate of ingested *Escherichia coli* in normal persons. J Med Microbiol 1971;5:361–9.
114. Jodal U, Ahlstedt S, Hansson LÅ, et al. Intestinal stimulation of the serum antibody response against *Escherichia coli* O83 antigen in healthy adults. Int Arch Allergy Appl Immunol 1977;53:481–9.
115. Lodinová R, Juoja V, Wagner V. Serum immunoglobulins and coproantibody formation in infants after artificial intestinal colonization with *Escherichia coli* O83 and oral lysozyme administration. Pediatr Res 1973;7:659–69.
116. Lari AR, Gold F, Borderon JC, et al. Implantation and in vivo antagonistic effects of antibiotic-susceptible *Escherichia coli* strains administered to premature newborns. Biol Neonate 1990;58:73–8.
117. Winberg J, Andersen HJ, Bergström T, et al. Epidemiology of symptomatic urinary tract infection in childhood. Acta Paediatr Scand Suppl 1974;257:1–20.
118. Zaman S, Jalil F, Karlberg J, Hanson LÅ. Early child health in Lahore, Pakistan: VI. Morbidity. Acta Paediatr Scand Suppl 1993;390:63–78.
119. Grüneberg RN. Relationship of infecting urinary organisms to the faecal flora in patients with symptomatic urinary infections. Lancet 1969;ii:766–8.
120. Bollgren I, Winberg J. The periurethral aerobic bacterial flora in healthy boys and girls. Acta Paediatr Scand 1975;65:74–80.
121. Svanborg-Edén C, Lidin-Janson G, Lindberg U. Adhesiveness to urinary tract epithelial cells of fecal and urinary *Escherichia coli* isolates from patients with symptomatic urinary tract infections or asymptomatic bacteriuria of varying duration. J Urol 1979:185–8.
122. Leffler H, Svanborg-Edén C. Chemical identification of a glycosphingolipid receptor for *Escherichia coli* attaching to urinary epithelial cells and agglutinating human erythrocytes. FEMS Microbiol Lett 1980;8:127–34.
123. Wold AE, Thorssen M, Hull S, Svanborg-Edén C. Attachment of *Escherichia coli* via mannose- or Gal 1-4Gal containing receptors to human colonic epithelial cells. Infect Immun 1988;56:2531–7.
124. Adlerberth I, Hanson LÅ, Svanborg C, et al. Adhesins of *Escherichia coli* associated with extra-intestinal pathogenicity confer binding to colonic epithelial cells. Microb Pathog 1995;18:373–85.
125. Tullus K, Kühn I, Ørskov I, et al. The importance of P- and type 1-fimbriae for the persistence of *Escherichia coli* in the human gut. Epidemiol Infect 1992;108:415–21.
126. Wold AE, Caugant DA, Lidin-Janson G, et al. Resident colonic *Escherichia coli* strains frequently display uropathogenic characteristics. J Infect Dis 1992;165:46–52.
127. Tullus K, Hörlin K, Svenson SB, Källenius G. Epidemic outbreaks of acute pyelonephritis by nosocomial spread of P fimbriated *Escherichia coli* in children. J Infect Dis 1984;150:728–36.
128. Plos K, Jodal U, Marklund B-I, et al. Intestinal carriage of P-fimbriated *Escherichia coli* and susceptibility to urinary tract infection in young children. J Infect Dis 1995;171:625–31.
129. Bergström T, Larson H, Lincoln K, Winberg J. Studies of urinary tract infections in infancy and childhood. XII. Eighty consecutive patients with neonatal infection. J Pediatr 1972;80:858–66.
130. Wilson HD, Eichenwald HF. Sepsis neonatorum. Pediatr Clin North Am 1974;21:571–82.
131. Siegel JD, McCracken GH. Sepsis neonatorum. N Engl J Med 1981;304:642–7.
132. Eriksson M. Neonatal septicaemia. Acta Paediatr Scand 1983;72:1–8.
133. Dawodu AH, Alausa OK. Neonatal septicaemia in the tropics. Afr J Med Med Sci 1980;9:1–6.
134. Khan SR, Jalil F, Lindblad BS, Karlberg J. Early child health in Lahore, Pakistan: X. Mortality. Acta Paediatr Suppl 1993;390:109–17.
135. Freedman RM, Ingram DL, Gross I, et al. A half century of neonatal sepsis at Yale. 1928–1978. Am J Dis Child 1981;135:140–4.
136. Bennet R, Eriksson M, Zetterström R. Increasing incidence of neonatal septicemia: causative organism and predisposing risk factors. Acta Paediatr Scand 1981;70:207–10.
137. Bennet R, Eriksson M, Melen B, Zetterström R. Changes in the incidence and spectrum of neonatal septicemia during a fifteen-year period. Acta Paediatr Scand 1985;74:687–90.
138. Ohlsson A, Serenius F. Neonatal septicaemia in Riyadh, Saudi Arabia. Acta Paediatr Scand 1981;70:825–9.
139. Bhutta ZA, Naqvi SH, Muzaffar T, Farooqui BJ. Neonatal sepsis in Pakistan. Presentation and pathogens. Acta Paediatr Scand 1991;80:596–601.
140. Van Camp JM, Tomaselli V, Coran AG. Bacterial translocation in the neonate. Curr Opin Pediatr 1994;6:327–33.
141. Berg RD. Bacterial translocation from the gastrointestinal tract. Trends Microbiol 1995;3:149–54.
142. Herías MV, Midtvedt T, Hanson LÅ, Wold AE. Role of *Escherichia coli* P fimbriae in intestinal colonization in gnotobiotic rats. Infect Immun 1995;63:4781–9.
143. Albers WH, Tyler CW, Boxerbaum B. Asymptomatic bacteremia in the newborn infant. J Pediatr 1966;69:193–7.
144. Bennet R, Eriksson M, Zetterström R. Bacterial etiology of neonatal septicemia in relation to prior antibiotic treatment. Acta Paediatr Scand 1987;76:673–4.
145. Egan AE. Neonatal necrotizing enterocolitis. In: Lebenthal E, editor. Textbook of gastroenterology and nutrition in infancy. New York: Raven Press; 1981. p. 979.
146. Kosloske AM. Epidemiology of necrotizing enterocolitis. Acta Paediatr Suppl 1994;396:S2–7.
147. Cooperstock MS, Zedd AJ. Intestinal flora of infants. In: Hentges DJ, editor. Human intestinal microflora in health and disease. New York: Academic Press; 1983. p. 79.
148. Cohen ML. The epidemiology of diarrheal disease. Inf Dis Clin North Am 1988;2:557–70.
149. Schlager AT, Guerrant RL. Seven possible mechanisms for *Escherichia coli* diarrhea. Inf Dis Clin North Am 1988;2:607–24.
150. Lipson A. Infectious dose of *Salmonella*. Lancet 1976;i:969.
151. Fujita K, Kaku M, Yanagase Y, et al. Physicochemical characteristics and flora of diarrhoeal and recovery faeces in children with acute gastroenteritis in Kenya. Ann Trop Paediatr 1990;10:339–45.

152. Mahmud A, Jalil F, Karlberg J, Lindblad BS. Early child health in Lahore, Pakistan: VII. Diarrhoea. Acta Paediatr Suppl 1993;390:79–85.
153. Challacombe DN, Richardson JM, Rowe B, Anderson CM. Bacterial microflora of the upper gastrointestinal tract in infants with protracted diarrhea. Arch Dis Child 1974;49:270–7.
154. Gracey M. The intestinal microflora in malnutrition and protracted diarrhoea in infancy. In: Lebenthal E, editor. Chronic diarrhoea in children. New York: Raven Press; 1984. p. 223–6.
155. Healy MJ, Walshe K, Weir DG, et al. Effect of *Bacteroides melaninogenicus* culture supernatant and deconjugated bile salt on lipid absorption. Dig Dis Sci 1995;40:2456–9.
156. de Boissieu D, Chaussain M, Badoual J, et al. Small-bowel bacterial overgrowth in children with chronic diarrhea, abdominal pain, or both. J Pediatr 1996;128:203–7.
157. Kirsch M. Bacterial overgrowth. Am J Gastroenterol 1990;85:231–7.
158. Kotloff K, Wade JC, Morris JG. Lack of association between *Clostridium difficile* toxin and diarrhea in infants. Pediatr Infect Dis J 1988;7:662–3.
159. Kelly CP, Pothoulakis C, LaMont JT. *Clostridium difficile* colitis. N Engl J Med 1994;330:257–61.
160. Valenzuela Montero M, Lobos T, Valenzuela A, et al. Prevalence of *Clostridium difficile* among healthy Chilean infants: evaluation by commercial enzyme immuno assay versus standard cytotoxin assay. Clin Infect Dis 1995;20 Suppl 2:259–60.
161. Murrell WG, Stewart BJ, O'Neill C, et al. Enterotoxigenic bacteria in the sudden infant death syndrome. J Med Microbiol 1993;39:114–27.
162. Siarakas S, Damas E, Murrell WG. The effect of enteric bacterial toxins on the catecholamine levels of the rabbit. Pathology 1997;29:278–85.
163. Wold AE, Hanson LÅ. Defence factors in human milk. Curr Opin Gastroenterol 1994;10:652–8.
164. Hanson LÅ, Telemo E. Immunobiology and epidemiology of breast feeding in relation to prevention of infections from a global perspective. In: Bienenstock J, editor. Mucosal immunology. New York: Academic Press; 1998. [In press]
165. Giugliano LG, Meyer CJ, Arantes LC, et al. Mannose-resistant hemagglutination (MRHA) and haemo-lysin production of strains of *Escherichia coli* isolated from children with diarrhoea: effect of breastfeeding. J Trop Pediatr 1993;39:183–7.
166. Steinwender G, Schimpl G, Sixl B, et al. Effect of early nutritional deprivation and diet on translocation of bacteria from the gastrointestinal tract in the newborn rat. Pediatr Res 1995;39:415–20.
167. Fubara ES, Freter R. Protection against enteric bacterial infection by secretory IgA antibodies. J Immunol 1973;111:395–403.
168. Glass RI, Svennerholm A-M, Stoll BJ, et al. Protection against cholera in breast-fed children by antibodies in breastmilk. N Engl J Med 1983;308:1389–92.
169. Cruz JR, Gil L, Cano F, Caceres P, Pareja G. Breast-milk anti-*Escherichia coli* heatlabile toxin IgA antibodies protect against toxin-induced infantile diarrhea. Acta Paediatr Scand 1988;77:658–62.
170. Ruiz-Palacios GM, Calva J, Pickering LK. Protection of breastfed infants against *Campylobacter* diarrhoea by antibodies in human milk. J Pediatr 1990;116:707–13.
171. Hayani KC, Guerrero ML, Morrow AL, et al. Concentration of milk secretory immunoglobulin A against *Shigella* virulence plasmid-associated antigens as a predictor of symptom status in *Shigella*-infected breast-fed infants. J Pediatr 1992;121:852–6.
172. Walterspiel JN, Morrow AL, Guerrero ML, et al. Secretory anti-*Giardia lamblia* antibodies in human milk: protective effect against diarrhea. Pediatrics 1994;93:28–31.
173. Maxson RT, Jackson RJ, Smith SD. The protective role of enteral IgA supplementation in neonatal gut origin sepsis. J Pediatr Surg 1995;30:231–3.
174. Shroff KE, Meslin K, Cebra JJ. Commensal enteric bacteria engender a self-limiting humoral mucosal immune response while permanently colonizing the gut. Infect Immun 1995;63:3904–13.
175. Donovan SM, Odle J. Growth factors in milk as mediators of infant development. Annu Rev Nutr 1994;14:147–67.
176. Crabbé P, Bazin H, Eyssen H, Heremans J. The normal microbial flora as a major stimulus for proliferation of plasma cells synthesizing IgA in the intestine. Int Arch Allergy Appl Immunol 1968;34:362–75.
177. Hohmann A, Schmidt G, Rowley D. Intestinal and serum antibody responses in mice after oral immunization with *Salmonella*, *Escherichia coli* and *Salmonella-Escherichia coli* hybrid strains. Infect Immun 1979;25:27–33.
178. Wold AE, Dahlgren U, Hanson LÅ, et al. Difference between bacterial and food antigens in mucosal immunogenicity. Infect Immun 1989;57:2666–73.
179. van der Waaij L, Limburg P, Mesander G, van der Waaij D. In vivo IgA coating of anaerobic bacteria in human feces. Gut 1996;38:348–54.
180. Berg R. Host immune response to antigens of the indigenous intestinal flora. In: Hentges D, editor. Human intestinal microflora in health and disease. New York: Academic Press; 1983. p. 101.
181. Dastur F, Awatramani V, Dixit S, et al. Response to single dose of tetanus vaccine in subjects with naturally acquired tetanus antitoxin. Lancet 1981;ii:219–21.
182. Kimura K, McCartney AL, McConnell MA, Tannock GW. Analysis of fecal populations of bifidobacteria and lactobacilli and investigation of the immunological responses of their human host to the predominant strains. Appl Environ Microbiol 1997;63:3394–8.
183. Weiner HL, Friedman A, Miller A, et al. Oral tolerance: immunologic mechanisms and treatment of animal and human organ-specific autoimmune diseases by oral administration of autoantigens. Annu Rev Immunol 1994;12:809–37.
184. Telemo E, Karlsson M, Dahlman-Höglund A, Dahlgren U, Lundin S. Oral tolerance in experimental animals. Int Arch Allergy Immunol 1997;113:219–23.
185. Moreau MC, Corthier G. Effect of gastro-intestinal microflora on induction and maintenance of oral tolerance to ovalbumin in C3H/HeJ mice. Infect Immun 1988;56:2766–8.
186. Sudo N, Sawamura S, Tanaka K, et al. The requirement of intestinal bacterial flora for the development of an IgE production system fully susceptible to oral tolerance induction. J Immunol 1997;159:1739–45.
187. Kim JH, Ohsawa M. Oral tolerance to ovalbumin in mice as a model for detecting modulators of the immunologic tolerance to a specific antigen. Biol Pharm Bull 1995;18:854–8.
188. Elson CO, Ealding W. Cholera toxin feeding did not induce oral tolerance in mice and abrogated oral tolerance to an unrelated protein antigen. J Immunol 1984;133:2892–7.
189. Gaborieau-Routhiau V, Moreau M-C. Gut flora allows recovery of oral tolerance to ovalbumin in mice after transient break down mediated by cholera toxin or *Escherichia coli* heatlabile enterotoxin. Pediatr Res 1996;39:625–9.
190. Klinman DM, Ae-Kyung Y, Beaucage SL, et al. CpG motifs present in bacterial DNA rapidly induce lymphocytes to secrete interleukin 6, interleukin 12 and interferon-γ. Proc Natl Acad Sci U S A 1996;93:2879–83.
191. Pisetsky D. DNA and the immune system. Ann Intern Med 1997;126:169–71.

192. Roman M, Martin-Orozco E, Goodman JS, et al. Immunostimulatory DNA sequences function as T helper-1-promoting adjuvants. Nat Med 1997;3:849–54.
193. Wold AE, Adlerberth I, Herías V. Bacterial regulation of immunity. In: Old Herborn University Seminar Monograph. Vol. 11. Herborn-Dill: Institute for Microbiology and Biochemistry; 1998. [In press]
194. Strachan DP. Hay fever, hygiene and household size. BMJ 1989;289:1259–60.
195. von Mutius E, Martinez FD, Fritzsch C, et al. Prevalence of asthma and atopy in two areas of West and East Germany. Am J Respir Crit Care Med 1994;149:358–64.
196. Björkstén B. Risk factors in early childhood for the development of atopic diseases. Allergy 1994;49:400–7.

CHAPTER 18

Genetic Models of Gastrointestinal Development

Alan N. Mayer, MD, PhD

W. Allan Walker, MD

Much of our current understanding of gut development derives from descriptive embryologic studies of chick, frog, and mouse performed in the late nineteenth to mid-twentieth centuries.[1] The classic works created a gross- and microanatomic framework of intestinal morphogenesis, highlighting the regional specialization seen along the anterioposterior (AP), dorsoventral (DV), and crypt-villus (CV) axes. During the 1960s, 70s, and 80s, transplantation studies addressed more mechanistic questions, such as when precursor cells become committed to intestinal fate, how the mesenchyme contributes to enterocyte differentiation, and from where the intestine derives positional information. These studies revealed the intestine to be a complex, dynamic tissue fashioned by a combination of autonomous and inductive influences, the latter provided by the surrounding mesenchyme. Attempts to further dissect these processes on the molecular level have met with limited success, mostly because induction is a transient phenomenon that occurs across small distances. It involves minute quantities of short-lived proteins that often remain physically associated with the cell surface or extracellular matrix. Biochemically isolating and identifying the mediators of induction involves massive quantities of starting materials and multistep purification schemes punctuated by tedious biologic assays.

Molecular genetic technology has changed the approach to animal development by allowing disruption, isolation, and manipulation of the genes that direct morphogenesis. Two landmark papers that arguably ushered in the era of modern development biology were that by Sidney Brenner, in which he described the use of the nematode *Caenorhabditis elegans* as a genetic model for development,[2] and that by Nusslein-Volhard and Wieschaus, in which they reported the comprehensive screening and classification of *Drosophila* mutants with defects in body patterning.[3] The common feature of these works is the demonstration of mutagenesis and large-scale screening as a feasible approach to identifying genes controlling animal development. The genetic approach has specific advantages compared to biochemistry, in that no assumptions are made regarding the structure, localization, or function of a gene product; rather, the only source of bias is in which phenotypes are considered interesting to the investigator. A good example is provided below in the isolation of the MOM genes in *C. elegans*. In that case three gene products that likely participate in the same signaling pathway—a secreted molecule, a receptor, and a transcription factor—were identified on the basis of a similar phenotype. Thanks to recombinant deoxyribonucleic acid (DNA) technology mapping, cloning, and expressing the genes identified in this manner will allow for their detailed biochemical characterization.

The field of gastrointestinal (GI) development now stands to benefit from the experimental framework erected by advances in molecular technology. Two of the model systems that have provided the bulk of raw material for progress in this area are *Drosophila* and *C. elegans*. Accordingly, this chapter will primarily review GI development in these systems, with an emphasis on the molecular pathways that guide formation of the endoderm and the gut tube. When relevant, vertebrate counterparts to the worm or fly genes will be mentioned, with the caveat that structural differences between the organs often preclude direct functional correlation. The zebrafish, a relatively new model, seeks to bridge these differences by offering the novel advantages of a classic genetic system applied to the study of a vertebrate.[4] Because vertebrates share many homologous organs,[5] genetic and morphologic data from the zebrafish can be extrapolated more readily to mammalian systems than from invertebrates such as *Drosophila*. The zebrafish is still in its infancy as an experimental system, but work thus far suggests a promising future.

CAENORHABDITIS ELEGANS

General Features

Caenorhabditis elegans is a simple, free-living worm about 1 mm in length. It is a member of the phylum *Nematoda*, and has the body plan of two concentric tubes separated by a space, the pseudocelom. The inner tube is the intestine, and the outer tube contains the cuticle, musculature, and

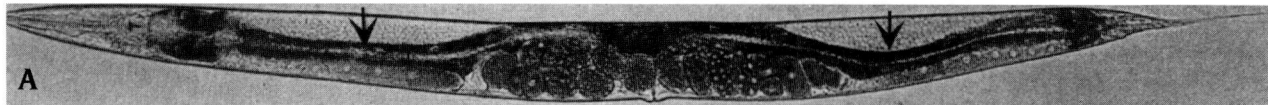
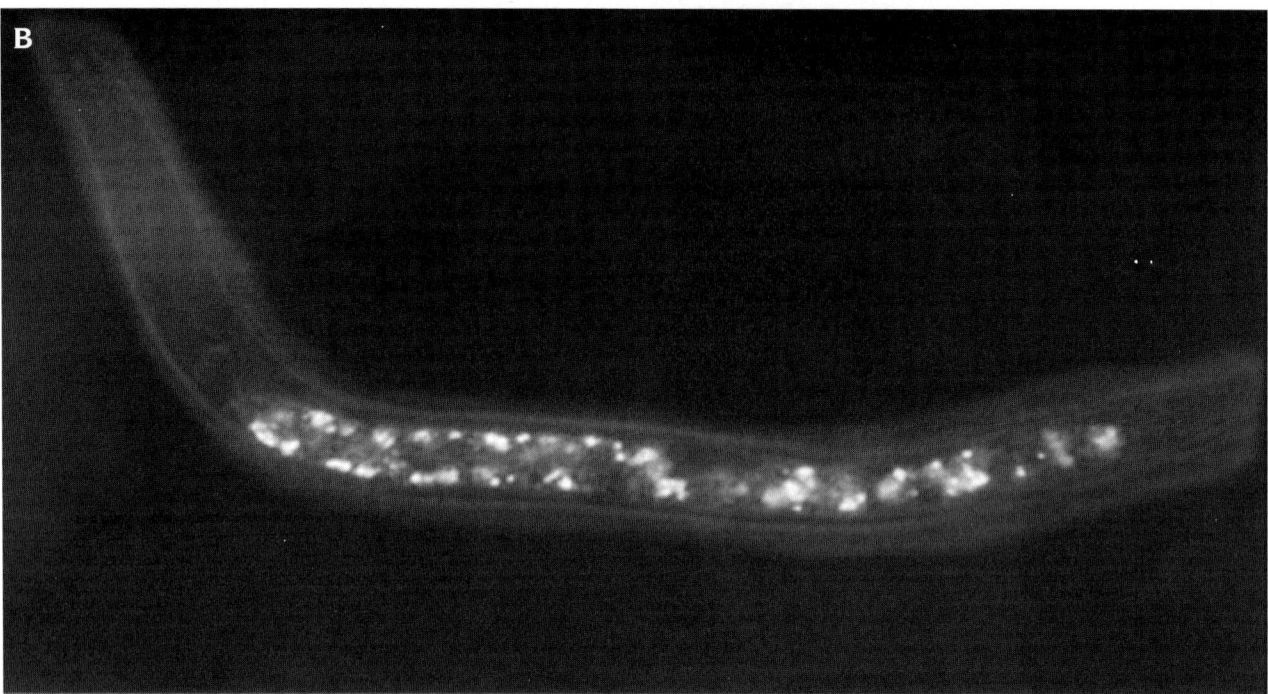

FIGURE 18–1. A, Photomicrograph of adult hermaphrodite worm; arrows point to gut tube. (Reproduced with permission from Wood WB, editor. The nematode *Caenorhabditis elegans*. 1st ed. Cold Spring Harbor (NY): Cold Spring Harbor Press; 1988.) B, Nomarski photomicrograph showing birefringent rhabditin granules exclusively located in the intestinal cells. (Courtesy of C. Rocheleau.)

neurons (Figure 18–1A). It was introduced to the field of developmental biology as a model organism in 1974 with the publication of the classic paper by Sidney Brenner[2] describing the first experimental use of *C. elegans* as a model genetic system.

The *C. elegans* genome contains an estimated 14,000 genes within 1×10^8 bases of DNA. The genome has been mapped to six linkage groups, which correspond to six haploid chromosomes. These include five autosomes and a sex chromosome (X). Both the hermaphrodites and males are diploid for the autosomes, but the hermaphrodite is diploid for the sex chromosome (XX) and the male is haploid (XO). Males arise spontaneously by nondisjunction of the X chromosome at a frequency of about 1:500.

The animals can be maintained on agar plates or in liquid culture medium, with *Escherichia coli* as a food source. The life cycle is three days under optimal conditions. Mutagenesis can be induced easily by either radiation or chemical mutagens such as EMS (ethylmethanesulfonate), and heterozygote hermaphrodites can be identfied by the homozygous phenotype in one-quarter of the progeny. Genetic crosses can be carried out by mating hermaphrodites with males. One notable technique for generating de facto null mutants is ribonucleic acid (RNA) interference.[6] Injection of either sense or antisense RNA into the hermaphrodite gonads will inhibit expression of the RNA-encoded gene in the progeny, resulting in maternal-effect null mutants for any gene of interest. The mechanism for this phenomenon is unknown.

Gastrointestinal Tract Development

The adult worm comprises only 959 cells, all of which have been assigned to a cell lineage by direct observation of the living animal using Nomarski optics and by earlier work using fixed sections.[7] The *C. elegans* intestine is made up of a ring of four cells anteriorly, followed posteriorly by a chain of eight pairs of cells, all of which surround a central lumen that connects to the anus near the tail (see Figure 18–1A). These cells are polarized epithelium, bearing microvilli on the apical surface and directly contacting the hypodermis and associated musculature at the basal surface. A unique property of intestinal cells that facilitates their study is the presence of rhabditin granules. These granules, products of tryptophan catabolism, develop only in the gut and are the only birefringent structures in the embryo (Figure 18–1B).[8] Fate mapping studies have shown that all 20 intestinal cells are derived from a single progenitor, known as the E blastomere of the eight-cell stage embryo.[7] The intestine is the only somatic tissue of *C. elegans* derived from a single founder cell. This feature

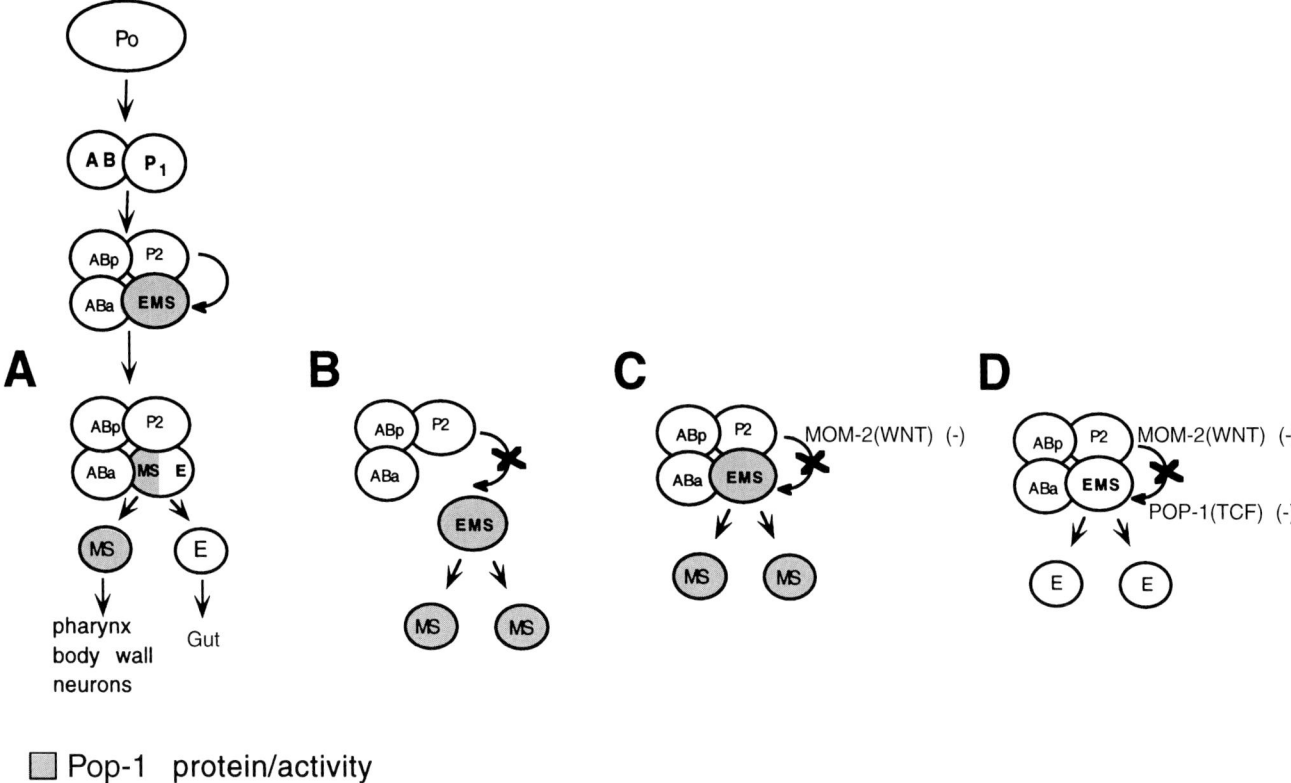

FIGURE 18–2. Molecular signals between the P2 and EMS blastomeres in the C. *elegans* embryo. A, Wild type, no manipulations. The MOM-2 protein produced by P2 interacts with EMS and localizes the POP-1 protein to the incipient MS pole of EMS. B, Physical separation of EMS from P2 resulting in disruption of P2-EMS signaling and consequent lack of POP-1 localization; MS cell forms in place of E-cell.[10] C, Genetic disruption of signaling. The MOM-2 mutant phenotype mimics physical separation of P2 and EMS. D, MOM-2::POP-1 double mutant results in endoderm formation in both progeny of EMS. (Adapted from Han M. Gut reaction to Wnt signaling in worms. Cell 1997;90:581–4.)

provides an opportunity to identify both the sources and mediators of endoderm induction in the early embryo.

Sources of Endoderm Induction

The finding that the E blastomere gives rise exclusively to the intestine offers an opportunity to address the long-held question of how cells becomes specified to an endodermal fate. Is the information inherited via asymmetric cell divisions, or does a neighboring cell induce its differentiation by some signal? In early embryogenesis during the second round of division, the P1 blastomere gives rise to an unpolarized cell EMS and a polarized cell P2, whereas AB divides to yield ABa and ABp, which have equal developmental potential (Figure 18–2A). EMS then divides into E and MS. E proceeds to differentiate into intestinal cells, and the MS lineage gives rise to mesodermal structures, such as pharyngeal and body wall muscle, gonads, and neurons.[7]

Given this information, a series of embryologic studies by Goldstein[9–11] addressed the question of how the E lineage acquires the potential to form intestine. Using newly developed blastomere culture techniques, it was demonstrated that direct contact between P2 and EMS in the four-cell stage was necessary for gut to differentiate from the E lineage of EMS. In the absence of P2, EMS gives rise to two MS cells (Figure 18–2B). This inductive effect was found to be position-dependent, in that isolating P2 and placing it on the presumptive MS side of EMS induced the reversal of E and MS identities, and gut accordingly developed from the progeny of what would have been MS. P2 was unable to induce gut development in ABa or ABp, indicating that the signal originating in P2 requires some competence factor (e.g., receptor) expressed by EMS for interpretation. In addition, when EMS was sandwiched between two P2 cells, only one of the progeny (either side) gave rise to endoderm, indicating that this signal inhibits the opposite side from responding. The mechanism by which P2 induces E formation seems to be via cell polarization and cytoskeletal reorganization, because agents which inhibit microtubule or microfilament polymerization also prevented endoderm induction in the four-cell but not the eight-cell stage embryo.[11]

Molecular Mediators of Endoderm Induction

The findings described set the stage for identifying the molecules that mediate the P2-EMS signal. Exploiting the power of genetics, screens were set up to identify mutants with altered pharyngeal development, a tissue with an easily visualized phenotype that derives from the EMS blastomere. This approach yielded mutants with abnormal intestine formation as well, such as SKN1, which lacks both pharyngeal and intestinal cells.[12] This mutation affects solely the fate of the EMS cell, leading it to produce only hypodermal and bodywall musculature, tissues it does not normally produce. In addition, a later role for SKN1 in maintaining intestinal cell differentiation is suggested by the phenotype of heterozygotes with a combined severe SKN1 allele and a chromosomal deficiency that deletes the SKN1 gene. These worms develop into larvae, but have defects in their intestinal cells that worsen with age. By the late larval stage the intestinal cells become severely atrophied, and the animals die.[12] Sequence analysis of the SKN1 gene was found to encode a putative transcription factor with sequence similarity to the basic region of the basic-leucine-zipper family of transcription factors. Its expression pattern in the wild-type worm shows an unequal distribution between AB and P1, with AB containing low amounts of SKN1 protein and P1 having higher amounts.[13] SKN1 is found in equal amounts in P2 and EMS, and in daughters E and MS. Thus, SKN1 is necessary, but not sufficient to specify the endoderm; later polarization and/or signaling events must specify the differential fates of E and MS.

Candidate genes for E and MS specification were sought by further screening for pharyngeal mutants. This effort identified POP-1, whose phenotype is the absence of pharyngeal cells and an excess of intestinal cells.[14] In the POP-1 mutant, the EMS blastomere gives rise to two daughter E cells, in effect converting the MS cell to an E-cell fate. The requirement for POP-1(+) activity in MS formation was further tested by constructing double mutants between the POP-1 mutant strain and mutant strains that produce ectopic MS-like cells in various locations.[15,16] The hypothesis was that if POP-1 confers a cell-autonomous signal essential for specifying the MS fate, then the development of ectopic MS-like blastomeres should be affected by POP-1 mutations independent of their position in the embryo. The result was that in the double mutants POP-1:PAR-1, POP-1:PIE-1, and POP-1:MEX-1, cells that would otherwise adopt MS-like fates at ectopic sites adopted E-like fates. These data support an essential role for the wild-type POP-1(+) gene in specifying MS- versus E-cell fate, either as an inducer of mesoderm or as an inhibitor of endoderm formation. The latter alternative was supported by the finding that signaling from P2 results in polarization of the EMS blastomere, with immunoreactive POP-1 protein being localized to the incipient E pole of EMS.[14]

Sequence analysis of the POP-1 gene revealed an open reading frame encoding a 487 amino acid protein with a high degree of homology to the transcription factors T-cell factor (TCF)-1 and lymphoid enhancer-binding factor (LEF)-1.[14] These proteins all contain domains known as the high-mobility group (HMG) box, which has been shown to bind DNA and promote transcriptional activation. Most significantly, the TCF-1/LEF-1 proteins have been implicated as targets of the WG-WNT signaling pathway,[17,18] which controls a host of cell-differentiation and pattern-formation processes from Drosophila to humans.[19] Thus the regulation of POP-1 activity in endoderm induction was suggested to be governed by a WNT-like signal.

To isolate mutants with defects specifically in P2-EMS signaling, genetic screens were focused on worms with abnormally high amounts of mesoderm and defective intestinal development, which is the opposite of the POP-1 phenotype. The rationale for this approach was that genetic defects in the P2-EMS interaction would lead to gutless worms with *mo*re *m*esoderm (MOM) phenotypes, just as physically disrupting the P2-EMS interaction resulted in two MS daughter cells and more mesoderm at the expense of endoderm.[9,10] Two groups independently isolated 29 mutants corresponding to 5 complementation groups. Three of the MOM genes were cloned, and shown to encode proteins homologous to components of the WNT-signaling pathway.[20,21]

Gene sequencing revealed that MOM-2 encodes a WNT-like molecule, MOM-5 encodes a Frizzled (FZ)-like receptor, and MOM-1 encodes a protein similar to Porcupine, which is required for WNT processing in Drosophila. Using cultured chimeric embryos, Thorpe et al.,[20] demonstrated that MOM-1(PORC), -2(WNT), and -3(uncloned) were required in the P2 (signaling) blastomere, whereas MOM-4(uncloned) was required in the EMS (target) blastomere. The penetrance of the MOM-5 allele precluded testing in this manner, but its homology to the Drosophila FZ gene family, previously shown to encode a WG receptor,[22] makes it likely to function in the target cell. Disrupting other downstream components of the WNT pathway had similar effects on endoderm formation. Using the RNA interference technique,[6] the β-catenin/armadillo homolog WRM-1 and the APC homolog APR-1 were also shown to be required for endoderm induction, further establishing a role for the WNT pathway in P2-EMS signaling.[21]

The target of this pathway is presumed to be POP-1(TCF). In all previous work on the WNT pathway (i.e., in Drosophila) TCF mutants have a phenotype similar to that of upstream factors WNT, ARM, and APC.[23] However, in P2-EMS signaling, the POP-1 mutant phenotype is opposite that of the upstream mutants, suggesting that WNT signaling inhibits POP-1 activity. Interestingly, immunoreactive POP-1 protein in EMS is localized away from the P2 signal toward the side that becomes the MS cell. Thus, the subcellular localization of POP-1 seems to mediate the differential cell fates of the EMS progeny because physically or genetically disrupting P2-EMS signaling results in elevated immunoreactive POP-1 protein in the presumptive E blastomere, converting it to an MS cell. Furthermore, in MOM::POP-1 double mutants, endoderm formation is restored, suggesting that once POP-1 is inactivated, the E cell proceeds to form gut in a cell-autonomous manner. It is unclear if POP-1 acts directly as a repressor of endoderm-specific genes, or if it activates transcription of downstream repressors. Future studies will ultimately reveal how TCF-POP-1 leads to inhibition of endoderm formation by the MS cells by identifying the molecular targets of WNT signaling.

DROSOPHILA MELANOGASTER

General Features and Background

(For an accessible introduction to fly genetics, see Greenspan, 1997.[24])

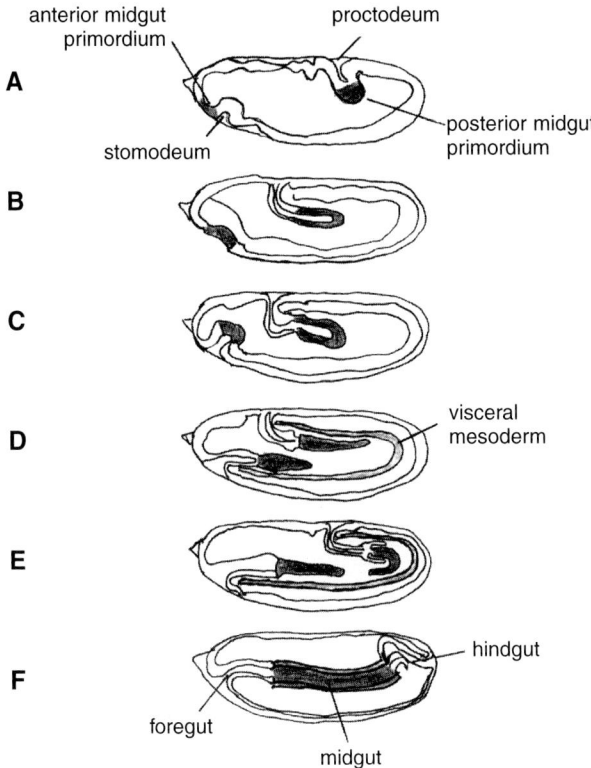

FIGURE 18-3. Diagram of intestinal morphogenesis. A, Stage 8: the posterior midgut primordium invaginates into the embryo and proceeds to lengthen as the germband extends anteriorly. B, Stage 9: the anterior midgut primordium becomes associated with the invaginating stomodeum. C, Stage 10: midgut primordia lose epithelial polarity. D, Stage 11: extended germband; endodermal mesenchyme migrating over palisades of visceral mesoderm. E, Stage 12: germband shortening; lobes of endoderm move toward each other, eventually meeting at 50% egg length. F, Stage 13: midgut cells reform as polarized epithelium lining a contiguous gut tube. (Adapted from Lawrence PA. The making of a fly. London: Blackwell Scientific Publications; 1992.)

Drosophila has played a central role in developmental genetics because it offers distinct advantages as an experimental system, some of which are intrinsic and some a product of the cumulative ingenuity of fly workers over the past century. In addition to the requisite features of any robust genetic system (rapid generation time, external development, easily scored phenotypes, inexpensive to maintain), features unique to *Drosophila* include the absence of recombination in males and the use of balancer chromosomes to control recombination in females, thus allowing the construction of complex genotypes. P element-mediated transposition enables the introduction of exogenous genetic material into the germline,[25] and has proven its usefulness in different ways. Insertional mutagenesis via P element transposition allows rapid identification of a disrupted gene by cloning the DNA adjacent to the P element. The technique of enhancer trapping,[26] in which transposition of a marker (i.e., lacZ) is followed by screening for strains with expression patterns limited to a tissue of interest, provides both a useful experimental tool and a marker for cloning a tissue-specific enhancer element. Given these tools, a wide variety of biologic phenomena have been explored using *Drosophila* genetics, including the development of the digestive tract.

While *Drosophila* became a model organism for the study of genetics in the late nineteenth century, not until the twentieth century was serious attention paid to its embryonic development. With the advent of molecular genetics in the 1970s, mutagenesis and screening became the prelude to mapping and cloning, resulting in a deluge of molecular information that needed an embryologic framework. During the 1980s, *Drosophila* embryology experienced a renaissance out of this necessity, and the expression patterns of any cloned gene naturally became part of its characterization. Body patterning was the first embryologic phenomenon to benefit from the capacity to "see" a gene expressed in time and space. Organ development, however, received less attention, perhaps due to the fact that many patterning defects were embryonic-lethal and consequently pre-empted organogenesis. The global defects seen in the body-patterning mutants led many workers to believe that mutating genes important for the control of organ formation would result in uninterpretable phenotypes. Nevertheless, in the last 10 years great strides have been made in organ development in *Drosophila*, and GI tract development, in particular, has proven an exemplary model for mesenchymal-epithelial interactions.

Anatomy and Histology of Larval Gastrointestinal Tract

The *Drosophila* larval intestinal tract consists of three sections: the foregut, midgut, and hindgut.[27] Of these sections only the midgut epithelium is derived from endoderm, with the foregut and hindgut forming from ectoderm. The foregut connects to the anterior midgut at the proventriculus, a three-layered, folded structure made of an internal layer of distal esophagus and a double layer of anterior midgut folded back on itself to form the gastric valve. The midgut has three distinct subdivisions (anterior, middle, and posterior) that are populated by different cells types. The anterior midgut bears four gastric cecae, which are diverticula emerging just distal to the proventriculus. The middle midgut is distinguished by further subdivisions along the AP axis that are populated by differentiated cell types: "copper cells," "large flat cells," and "iron cells." Of these, the specification of copper cells has been studied in the most depth and will be discussed in detail below. The malpighian tubules arise from the hindgut that connects to the rectum.

Overview of Gut Development in the Embryo

(Figures 18-3 for a general review of *Drosophila* development see Lawrence.[28])

Drosophila embryos are staged by specific anatomic features that are reproducible and readily identifiable.[29] In stages 1 to 5, the fertilized egg contains a syncytium of nuclei that divide and migrate to the periphery, culminating in the cellularization of the blastoderm. During this time, the initially homogeneous blastoderm becomes specified to various cells fates as the body plan of the embryo is laid out. Gastrulation occurs during stages 6 to 7, during which cells along the ventral midline form a furrow and dive into the embryo. Movement of cells on the ventral surface also takes place along the A-P axis, termed germband extension, during which cells of the ventral midline are pushed around the posterior end and advance along the dorsal aspect in the anterior direction (stages 7 to 11). At stage 6, the future anterior and posterior midgut anlagen begin their journey from the anterior and posterior poles inward, joining midway during stage 12 as the germband retracts (see Figure 18–3). By stage 13, germband retraction is complete, and the midgut epithelium becomes invested with an outer sheath of visceral mesoderm. In subsequent stages, the midgut epithelium differentiates by anatomic region into distinct cell subtypes.

Gut Morphogenesis

Early Events

The anlagen of the foregut, midgut, and hindgut reside in the unsegmented poles of the blastoderm embryo. Specification of the poles is accomplished by maternal-effect genes expressed during oogenesis, including both the terminal and anterior groups.[30] The latter is exemplified by bicoid, which determines anterior versus posterior identity. The terminal-group gene products form a signal cascade that results in activation of the terminal-gap genes tailless (TLL) and huckebein (HKB). Tailless mutants have severe hindgut defects that correspond to its pattern of expression, except in the most terminal region.[31] Tailless is a member of the nuclear steroid receptor superfamily.[31] A mammalian homolog of TLL was cloned, but there was no expression seen in endoderm derivatives in the mouse.[32] Huckebein mutants lack the entire midgut, but develop a stomodeum, proctodeum, and malpighian tubules.[33] One gene product thought to mediate activation of TLL and HKB is the *Drosophila* homolog of the vertebrate protein HNF4, a steroid-receptor transcription factor expressed specifically in liver, kidney, and intestine of the mouse.[34] The *Drosophila* homolog HNF4(D) is detected initially in the syncytial blastoderm terminalia, and then later in the early midgut endoderm. A *Drosophila* chromosomal deletion that includes HNF4(D) disrupts the formation of the midgut primordia and other gut-related structures.[35] The phenotype of the mouse HNF4 knockout was lethality prior to gastrulation, and thus its role in gut development could not be assessed.[34] HNF4(D) may act through TLL and HKB to specify the gut anlagen, but it may activate other genes, and its expression in later structures suggests an additional role in organogenesis.

Recent work on hindgut development[36] has implicated caudal, a homeodomain transcription factor, as essential for invagination of the hindgut primordium, acting through target genes folded gastrulation (FOG), forkhead (FKH), and wingless (WG). In their discussion, Wu and Lengyel point out the strikingly conserved expression patterns of these genes between fly and vetebrates. This led to the proposal that the blastopore equivalent of chordates and the amnio-proctodeal invagination of insects are homologous domains, both representing centers of specification for internal organ formation via conserved molecular pathways.

Specification of the Endoderm

The specification of the gut anlagen takes place in the stage 5 blastoderm embryo just prior to cellularization, when transcripts of the FKH gene are first detected in two domains at both poles of the embryo.[37] The genes TLL and HKB are required for FKH gene activation, and FKH is required for foregut and hindgut formation.[37] In the FKH mutant, these structures undergo a transformation in which the esophagus and proventriculus are replaced by components of the head skeleton; posteriorly, the malpighian tubules and the hindgut are also replaced by head structures. These changes signify a homeotic role for the FKH gene, since nonsegmented ectoderm is altered to produce terminal structures that normally arise from segmented regions.[38] The midgut endoderm also requires FKH for normal development, but homeotic transformation does not take place. Instead, the midgut degenerates shortly after invagination of the primordia. One theory to account for the difference relative to foregut and hindgut is that cells of the midgut may lack the necessary capacity to differentiate into alternative structures, either for lack of cellular components or interpretable external signals.

The FKH gene encodes a nuclear protein with a DNA-binding domain of about 110 amino acids that forms a "winged helix" structure on x-ray crystallographic analysis.[39] Winged helix proteins have been isolated from a variety of organisms, from yeast to human, and in all cases tested the proteins are sequence-specific DNA-binding proteins that serve as tissue-specific transcriptional activators. In fact, the first vertebrate FKH homologs were identified independently as a family of liver-enriched transcription factors.[40] The central role of FKH in gut development in *Drosophila* prompted investigation of the HNF3 proteins in the formation of endoderm and derivative structures in the mouse.[41] Study of expression patterns in mouse embryos revealed that the HNF3α, β, and γ genes are expressed sequentially during early development.[42] HNF3β expression is initiated 6.5 days postcoitus (dpc) in the node at the anterior end of the primitive streak, which later on gives rise to the notochord and gut endoderm. HNF3α expression is first detected at 10 dpc in midline endodermal cells in the invaginating foregut, and then in the notochord, gut endoderm, and ventral neural tube, along with HNF3β. HNF3γ then appears upon hindgut development. Later in embryogenesis, the HNF3 proteins are expressed predominantly in endoderm-derived tissues (intestine, liver, and lung), suggesting that the temporospatial expression pattern early on influences the axial patterning of the gut. Mice homozygous for an HNF3β deletion show multiple developmental anomalies, and die at 9.5 dpc with defects in the foregut and notochord, but molecular and histologic analyses indicate that some definitive endoderm tissue is present.[43] These findings are difficult to interpret due to the pleiotropic effects and early lethality of the null mutant, but they show that HNF3β is not required for initial formation of the intestine. Other FKH homologs remain to be tested.

Invagination, Outgrowth, and Fusion of the Midgut

The formation of the hollow gut tube is guided by a combination of cell-autonomous and inductive determinants, underscoring the complexity of intestinal development. Invagination of the gut primordia is tightly coordinated with gastrulation, as the embryo internalizes the precursor cells that are subsequently guided to form the internal organs. A common feature of the invagination process is the apical constriction of a subset of blastoderm cells, followed by cell movements to the interior of the embryo. This is seen in ventral furrow, stomodeum, proctodeum, and midgut primordia formation. After the anterior and posterior endoderm anlagen invaginate at the poles of the blastoderm embryo, these cells lose their polarity and become mesenchymal, forming two bilobed masses attached to the stomodeum (foregut primordium) and proctodeum (hindgut primordium), respectively (Figure 18–4). Germband lengthening is accompanied by expansion of the midgut primordia, followed by meeting and fusion of the two ends as they are brought together during germband shortening.[44]

On a cellular level, dramatic changes take place in the appearance and organization of the midgut primordia as the gut tube is fashioned. During germband shortening, the intestinal precursor cells migrate over the visceral mesoderm and undergo a transformation to a columnar epithelial phenotype with apicobasal polarity (Figure 18–5A).[45] By observation of the formation of the midgut in mutant embryos with defects in different aspects of visceral mesoderm development these events have been demonstrated to require direct contact between the endoderm and visceral mesoderm.[45] For example, in twist (twi) mutants, the mesoderm and its derivatives do not develop; the endoderm in these embryos invaginates during gastrulation but remains as solid clusters of mesenchymal cells. In tinman mutants, the visceral mesoderm is specifically defective, with only small islands of immunohistochemically-detectable tissue; only the endoderm cells in direct contact with these islands were able to form polarized epithelium. In addition, contact between epithelial cells was shown to be important for columnar morphology. These data support the argument that direct contact is necessary for epithelialization of the midgut primordia. Vertebrate model systems of intestinal development have produced similar findings, in which the formation and maintenance of a polarized epithelium is dependent on cell-substratum and cell-cell interactions.[46]

Independent of the inductive effects of the visceral mesoderm, specification of epithelial fate also requires the activity of two sets of genes, known as the neurogenic and proneural groups. The neurogenic group includes Notch, Delta, neuralized, and Enhancer of split. The Notch pathway controls many different cell fates by regulating cell responses to tissue-specific differentiation or proliferation signals.[47] By an unclear mechanism, activation of the receptor encoded by Notch impedes otherwise effective differentiation signals. In both Notch and Delta (a Notch ligand), mutant cells of the anterior midgut fail to invaginate and remain as a cluster of mesenchymal cells near the anterior pole.[48] Similar abnormalities are found in neuralized and Enhancer of split mutants, which shift the cell-type distribution of the midgut primordia. The principal midgut epithelial cells (PMEC) are specifically lost, whereas the adult midgut precursor (AMP) cells increase in number.[49] The loss of Notch activity may lead to uncontrolled specification of AMP cells in response to a local inducer, and consequently deplete the pool of cells that gives rise to the PMEC; this is analogous to the abnormal proliferation of neuroblasts from neurogenic ectodermal cells accompanied by a decrement in hypodermal (skin) cells seen in Notch mutants.[50] Despite direct contact of the AMP cells with the visceral mesoderm, epithelium fails to form in these mutants, thus accounting for the gutless phenotype. Genes homologous to Notch and Delta have been found in vertebrates, but there is no direct evidence yet for their participation in intestinal development. A possible role for the Notch pathway in liver development is suggested by the recent finding that Alagille syndrome (intrahepatic bile duct paucity) is caused by mutations in the Jagged1 gene,[51,52] which encodes a Notch receptor ligand. The significance of this, in molecular and embryologic terms, has yet to be determined.

Regional Specification of the Midgut

After the midgut primordia fuse and form a hollow epithelium-lined tube, regional differentiation along the AP axis of the midgut further specifies subtypes of cells, resulting in three midgut domains (anterior, middle, and posterior) distinguished by their cell morphologies (Figure 18–5B). Considering the endoderm's intrinsic lack of segmentation, this ordered configuration of cell types implies that the undifferentiated precursors receive positional information from a nearby source, namely the visceral mesoderm (VM). The differentiation of one cell type, the cuprophilic (or copper) cell, has been studied in detail to reveal a complex regulatory network within the VM that transduces positional information to the subjacent endoderm, resulting in spatially restricted cell-type differentiation. As outlined below, the mediators of this program were identified by harnessing the power of Drosophila genetics to yield our first detailed glimpse of the molecules that guide intestinal cell-subtype differentiation.

The VM inherits positional information conferred by segmentation genes whose expression is localized along the body axis during early embryogenesis.[53] The five primary homeotic genes that are expressed in domains along the AP axis in the thoracic and abdominal ectoderm are found expressed in the visceral mesoderm in the same linear AP configuration, although with different parasegment boundaries.[54] One of these genes, ultrabithorax (UBX), is expressed in a precisely demarcated domain (parasegment 7) owing to genetic interactions with neighboring homeotic genes antenapoedia (ANTP) anteriorly, abdominal-A (ABD-A) posteriorly, and the pair rule genes fushi tarazu (FTZ) and even skipped (EVE).[55] Ultrabithorax activates a signal cascade mediated by WG and decapentaplegic (DPP), extracellular proteins which act synergistically to induce the localized expression of labial (LAB), a homeotic gene required for copper cell differentiation.[56] Expression of UBX is maintained by positive feedback from DPP and WG, resulting in a "parautocrine" loop that continuously reassesses position along the AP axis.

Wingless was originally described as one of the segment polarity mutants in Drosophila.[3] Subsequently, the mouse

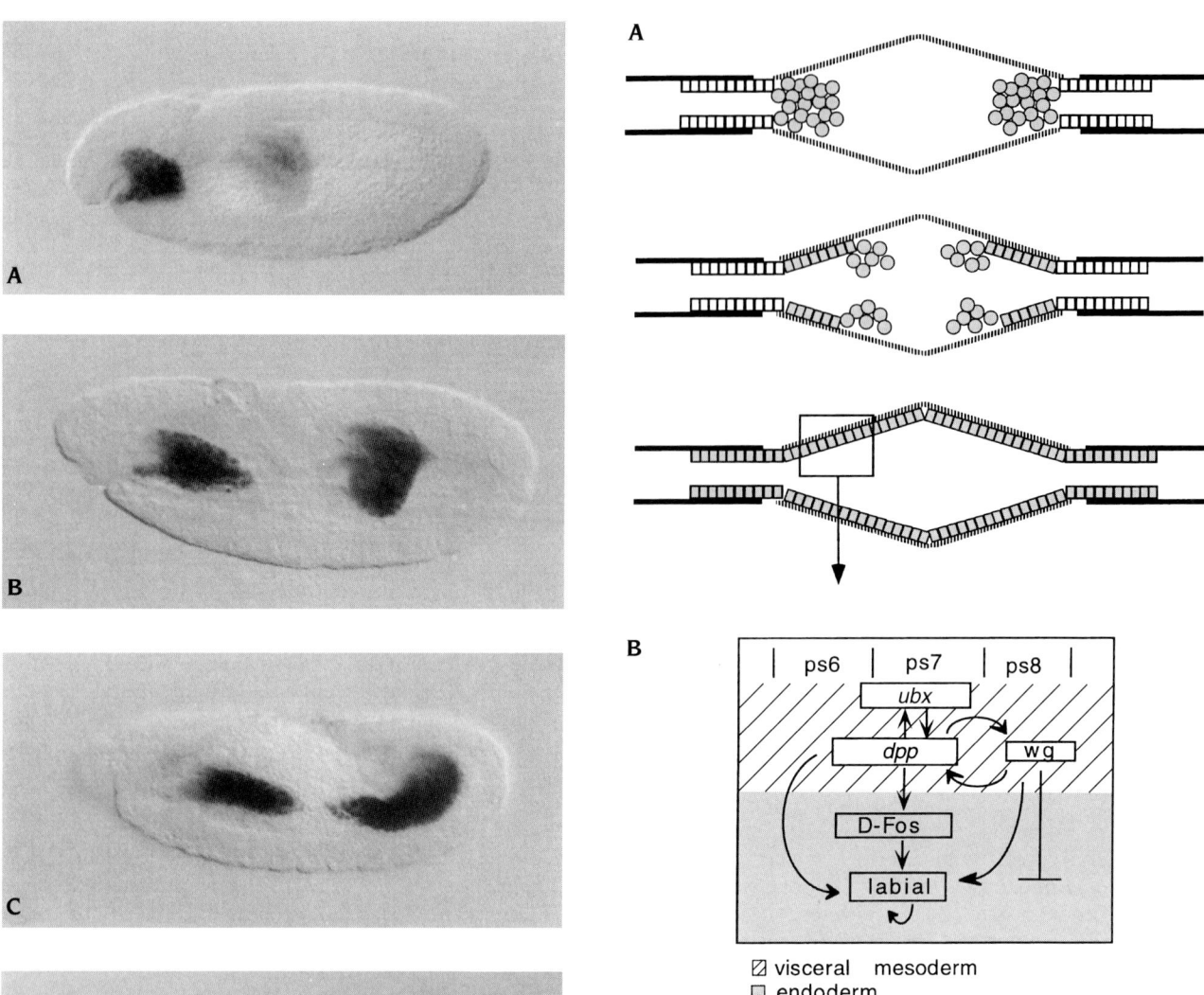

FIGURE 18-4. Embryos genetically engineered to carry enhancer trap elements expressed in the midgut, stained with antibody to β-galactosidase to highlight midgut embryogenesis. Anterior is to the left. In this line, the anterior midgut primordium stains before the posterior. A and B, Stage 11: the anterior and posterior midgut primordia consist of masses of cells attached to the developing foregut and hindgut, respectively. Note how germband extension has brought the proctodeal invagination to the dorsal side of the embryo. C and D, Stage 12: germband shortening accompanies the movement of the posterior midgut primordium toward the interior of the embryo, where it meets with the anterior midgut primordium to form a contiguous gut tube. (Reproduced with permission from Skaer H. The alimentary canal. In: Bate M, Martinez-Arias A, editors. The development of *Drosophila melanogaster*. Cold Spring Harbor: Cold Spring Harbor Press; 1993. p. 941–1012.)

FIGURE 18-5. Midgut formation and regional specification. A, Schematic diagram of midgut epithelial morphogenesis. *Circles*, unpolarized endodermal mesenchymal cells; *shaded squares*, polarized principal midgut epithelial cells; *open boxes*, foregut and hindgut epithelium; *broken line*, visceral mesoderm. The three drawings, corresponding roughly to stages depicted in A, C, and D from Figure 18-4, illustrate how the intestinal precursor cells begin as masses of unpolarized mesenchyme that migrate over the visceral mesoderm. After contact with the latter, they are transformed to an organized epithelium lining the midgut. Genetic experiments (see text) demonstrated that this direct interaction is necessary for epithelial cell formation. (Adapted from Tepass and Hartenstein.[45]) B, Genetic interactions in the specification of the middle midgut epithelium. The genetic signaling network between the outer gut layer (visceral mesoderm, *lightly shaded*) and epithelium (inner endoderm, *dark shading*) is shown by *arrows* (activation) and a *bar* (inhibition). *White boxes* represent the expression domains of a given gene. Note that UBX expression is maintained by a self-stimulating loop that sustains expression of labial. No signaling from visceral mesoderm to endoderm has yet been identified. (Adapted from Bienz.[60])

proto-oncogene int-1 was found to be identical to WG.[57] Over the last several years, an extended family of WNT (wingless-int) genes has been found to encode extracellular signaling molecules that guide tissue patterning and differentiation from worm to human via a conserved signal transduction pathway.[19] In the midgut, DPP in VM ps7 stimulates WG expression in the posteriorly adjacent VM ps8. The target of the WG signal is the transcription factor TCF/LEF-1/pangolin.[17,18,58] Activation of TCF is accomplished by a WNT-dependent stabilization of the Armadillo protein, which binds to TCF, forming a complex that accumulates in the nucleus. The ARM-TCF complex binds to the WG-response element of target genes (i.e., UBX and labial), stimulating their transcription. Interestingly, the WG signal in the midgut has a dual effect, inhibiting labial expression in the endoderm directly subjacent to ps8, but stimulating it anteriorly. By genetic manipulation of WG expression, Hoppler and Bienz[59] have shown that WG acts at two distinct threshold concentrations to control labial expression in the midgut epithelium. At high concentrations of WG (in the endoderm directly subjacent to VM ps8), labial expression is repressed, and large flat cells rather than copper cells develop. At the intermediate WG levels found anteriorly, labial expression is stimulated and copper cells are induced. The result is a sharp posterior demarcation of the copper cell domain at the ps7-8 border, and a graded anterior border through ps6. While the molecular basis for this has yet to be elucidated, the findings suggest participation of additional WG target genes that mediate a distinct response to higher WG levels. The widespread use of the wingless pathway in many tissue-patterning processes suggests the existence of tissue-specific factors that interpret incoming signals by interacting with the core elements of this pathway. One question that remains is whether the inhibitory effects of WG are mediated by TCF or a different nuclear target. The latter is suggested by the finding that separate WG target sites within the labial control regions respond to WG stimulation or repression.[60]

Another signaling molecule secreted under the control of UBX is DPP, a member of the transforming growth factor (TGF)-β family. Transforming growth factor-β homologs control body patterning, growth, and differentiation in many contexts.[61,62] In the midgut, DPP is expressed in the VM ps7, where it activates UBX within the same parasegment and WG in the VM ps8, thus forming part of the autoregulatory loop that maintains copper cell differentiation.[63] Decapentaplegic also activates D-FOS (a transcription factor related to AP-1)[64] and labial in the subjacent endoderm,[65] both of which are required for copper cell differentiation. Decapentaplegic signaling is mediated through a DNA sequence known as a cAMP-responsive element (CRE) in the upstream flanking regions of its target genes.[66] It is not known exactly how DPP signals through this site, but a likely mediator includes the Mothers against DPP (MAD) proteins, part of a conserved group of cytoplasmic proteins that are translocated into the nucleus in response to DPP signaling.[62]

One notable feature of the copper cell-induction model is the absence of reciprocal endoderm-to-mesoderm signaling. This stands in contrast to vertebrate systems in which bidirectional signaling has been demonstrated using transplantation[67] and, more recently, molecular techniques (see Chapter 6). In one case, avian gizzard endoderm was incidentally found to induce fibroblasts from fetal rat lung and skin to differentiate into visceral smooth muscle.[68] Fourteen years later, ectopic expression of the Sonic hedgehog gene in the incipient pancreatic endoderm of transgenic mice induced the formation of functional heterotopic intestinal smooth muscle in place of pancreatic mesenchyme.[69] This finding (and others discussed in detail by Roberts in Chapter 1) raises the question of whether the endoderm is capable of signaling to the VM in Drosophila. The Drosophila hedgehog gene may be a candidate for this messenger, since two of the known targets of the hedgehog signaling pathway are WG and DPP, both of which play key roles in endoderm induction, as discussed. Thus, among the many questions remaining as to how the Drosophila midgut is patterned, that of endoderm-to-mesoderm signaling remains conspicuously open to investigation.

DANIO RERIO (ZEBRAFISH)

General Features and Background

Despite the many technical advantages of Drosophila and C. elegans, one problem inherent in studying organ development in invertebrate models is the lack of homologous vertebrate structures, which points out the need for a vertebrate model system that would be amenable to genetic manipulation. Speaking to this issue, the zebrafish has emerged in recent years as a model for vertebrate development. Because the embryos are transparent and development takes place outside the female, all stages of development, from fertilization to organ formation, can be studied over the course of 5 days.[4,70,71] Saturation mutagenesis and large-scale genetic screens are feasible owing to the short generation time (3 months), the large number of eggs laid by females (50 to 100 per week), external fertilization and gestation, and low per capita maintenance costs.[72,73] Functional analysis of developmental mutants is enabled by the accessibility of the living embryo to examination and manipulation. Consequently, cell-lineage tracing, in situ labeling, and single-cell transplantation techniques are well established.[74] The development of a high-resolution genetic map is under way to facilitate positional cloning of genes that underlie interesting mutant phenotypes.[75]

Gastrointestinal Tract Development

The zebrafish digestive tract contains many features found in humans, including: a gut lined by epithelium organized into villi, derivative organs, such as liver, gallbladder, and pancreas; and AP regionalization.[76] The epithelium contains goblet cells and endocrine cells in addition to absorptive cells, but no Paneth's cells or crypts. The mucosa is surrounded by an inner circular layer and outer longtitudinal layer of smooth muscle that, regulated by enteric nerves, provide peristaltic movements to the gut tube. There is no stomach, for the pharynx is connected to the intestine via a short segment lined with stratified squamous epithelium, representing the esophagus.

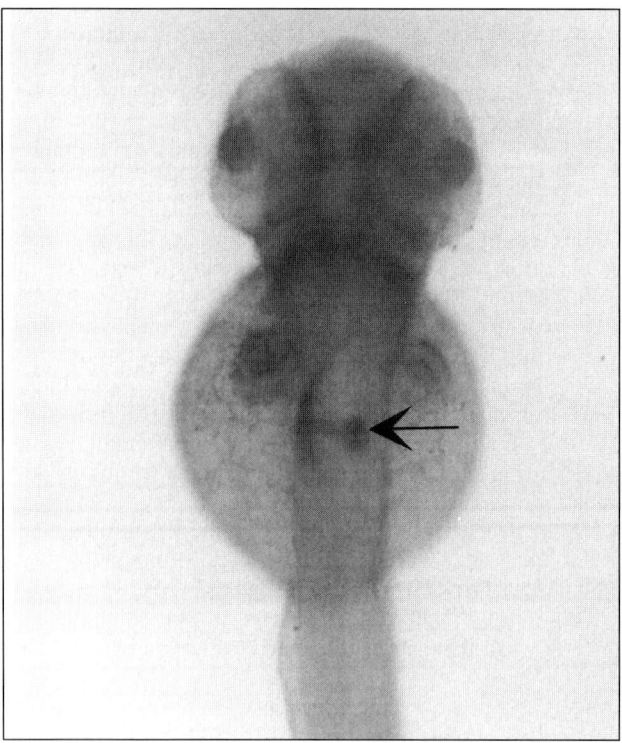

FIGURE 18–6. Dorsal view of a wild-type zebrafish embryo at 48 hpf, stained by in situ hybridization with a nucleic acid probe complementary to the zebrafish PDX gene. The arrow indicates the pancreatic primordium budding from the intestine. (Courtesy of J.-N. Chen and M. Fishman, Massachusetts General Hospital, MA.)

The development of the digestive organs can be monitored in living embryos using a dissecting microscope, although it is relatively obscured by overlying structures compared to other organs (i.e., the heart). The intestine becomes visible by 3 days postfertilization (dpf), and by 4 dpf peristalsis is evident. Histologically, the intestine can be identifed at 24 hours postfertilization (hpf) as unpolarized, radially aligned cells, and the liver becomes evident 12 hours later. The depth of the digestive tract structures has prompted the development of organ-specific markers to help visualize early events by in situ staining. Examples include GATA5 (liver, exocrine pancreas, intestinal epithelium), insulin (pancreatic islets), carboxypeptidase A (exocrine pancreas), and PDX (early intestine and pancreatic bud). Staining for PDX mRNA, for example, enables visualization of the developing foregut and pancreas in a 48 hpf embryo (Figure 18–6). Altered staining patterns may indicate defects in diverse processes, from gut-tube patterning to induction of pancreas and liver.

The power of the zebrafish as a genetic system for studying development is illustrated by the results of two large genetic screens recently completed by groups at Massachusetts General Hospital in Boston[77] and at the Max Planck Institute in Tubingen, Germany,[78] which yielded several hundred mutants in body patterning and organ formation. In the Boston screen, about 500 genomes were screened for defects in digestive organ development, and seven intestinal mutants were isolated.[76] The prevailing phenotype of these mutants is normal development until 4 dpf, at which time the epithelium is noted to become thin, lacking normal folds, with only scattered microvilli and no evident polarization. Degeneration of the epithelium occurs by 4 to 5 dpf. In the foregut mutants, exocrine pancreas development fails as well. In the Tubingen screen, two intestinal mutants were isolated with phenotypes consisting of thinned mucosa lacking normal folds and absent peristalsis.[79]

The identity of the mutated genes responsible for these defects are currently being sought by positional cloning. Since this approach remains quite time consuming, another method of mutagenesis using random viral insertion is currently under development.[80] This strategy involves developing a vector capable of inserting its genome into the germline of developing fish, thereby disrupting the target gene. In analogy to P-mediated mutagenesis in *Drosophila*, the advantage of this approach is the ease with which disrupted genes are cloned, since the agent that disrupts the gene acts as a marker as well. At present, the efficiency of this method is still orders of magnitude lower than EMS, making its application to a narrow screen prohibitive in terms of the number of fish that would have to be processed.

Because organogenesis occurs relatively late in the development of the embryo, and thus depends on multiple earlier events, a genetic approach might not have yielded useful results, since perturbation of important pathways could produce nonspecific, pleiotropic effects. The results of these large screens support the contrary notion that discrete organ defects can be induced by single intragenic mutations. It is now feasible to perform more detailed screens for defects in digestive organ development using whole-mount in situ staining with tissue-specific RNA or antibody probes as described above. Preliminary results from such dedicated organogenesis screens have identified additional mutants with defects in gut, liver, and pancreas formation, including laterality defects that affect heart situs, reminiscent of situs inversus and heterotaxy syndromes seen in humans (J.-N. Chen and M. C. Fishman, personal communication).

Beside providing structural information, the transparency of the zebrafish embryo and its external development allows monitoring of dynamic processes such as intestinal motility and may form the basis for genetic screens in the future. This approach may provide molecular insight into the function of the enteric nervous system, and ultimately lead to new treatments for common motility disorders such as gastroesophageal reflux. Another function that can be monitored in the live embryo is bile excretion. Embryos that appear jaundiced or lack intraluminal bile may have defects in bile synthesis or transport or in biliary tract formation. Such mutants may offer hope in identifying the underlying etiology of biliary atresia, and may provide specific targets for treating cholestasis.

CONCLUSION

The complexity of the GI tract lies in its composite nature, for many different primordial tissues contribute to its mature structure. As such, the central theme of this chapter has been intercellular communication. To specify, shape, and differentiate the endoderm, surrounding tissues must sense and transmit appropriately timed and placed signals. Classic studies of organ development have demonstrated that induction of endoderm is mediated by diffusible substances, and molecular genetic studies are beginning to reveal their identities. For example, by demonstrating the direct involvement of the WNT pathway in P2-EMS signaling, the work in *C. elegans* offers the first detailed genetic dissection of endoderm induction in a pregastrulation embryo. Although homologous signaling molecules are conserved in humans, it will be considerably more difficult to sort out exactly how WNT signaling affects endoderm development in the mammalian context, since 13 WNT homologs have been identified in vertebrates.[81] Thus, simpler models such as *C. elegans* will always have a role in human biology. Of note, the P2-EMS interaction described in *C. elegans* is the first in which a WNT signal has been shown to inhibit its target POP-1-TCF, raising the critical question of where this may be relevant in more complex organisms.

Direct contact with the visceral mesoderm has been shown to be required for maintenance of a polarized epithelium in vertebrates, and this was confirmed to be the case in *Drosophila* by genetically interfering with visceral mesoderm formation. Extension of such studies may help identify exactly which molecules interact with endodermal precursors to induce their polarization, and which molecules are needed for maintenance of epithelial-epithelial contact. This information may be useful in devising treatments for illnesses that feature compromised integrity of the intestinal mucosa, such as necrotizing enterocolitis, an often fatal condition that primarily affects premature infants.

Investigation of the AP regionalization of the intestinal epithelium in *Drosophila* using copper cell differentiation as a model system has revealed a molecular control network that translates positional information from a segmented tissue VM to an unsegmented one (endoderm). The molecules that populate this network include the homeobox protein UBX, WNT, and DPP, all of which have vertebrate homologs. Whether or not these proteins act in a similar capacity in vertebrate intestinal differentiation remains to be tested. What seems clear is that morphogenetic events rely on a finite number of signaling molecules that act in a context-dependent fashion. Accordingly, a WNT signal can induce cells to differentiate along many different paths; which one is chosen depends on previous developmental decisions and other signals from surrounding tissues. Genetic models will be crucial to understanding which combinations of signals leads to particular developmental fates. In the future, the zebrafish may serve as the vertebrate model to fulfill this need, but many technological advances will be necessary before its full potential as an experimental system, on par with *Drosophila* or *C. elegans*, can be realized.

REFERENCES

1. Gilbert SF, Raunio AM, editors. Embryology: constructing the organism. Sunderland, (MA): Sinauer; 1997.
2. Brenner S. The genetics of *Caenorhabditis elegans*. Genetics 1974;77:71–94.
3. Nusslein-Volhard C, Wieschaus E. Mutations affecting segment number and polarity in *Drosophila*. Nature 1980;287:791–801.
4. Driever W, Fishman MC. The zebrafish: heritable disorders in transparent embryos. J Clin Invest 1996;97:1788–94.
5. Wake MH, editor. Hyman's comparative vertebrate anatomy. 3rd ed. Chicago: University of Chicago; 1979.
6. Guo, S, Kemphues KJ. *Par-1*, a gene required for establishing polarity in *C. elegans* embryos, encodes a putative Ser/Thr kinase that is asymmetrically distributed. Cell 1995;81:611–20.
7. Sulston JE, Schierenberg E, White JG, Thomson JN. The embryonic cell lineage of the nematode *Caenorhabditis elegans*. Dev Biol 1983;100:64–119.
8. Babu P, Siddiqui S. Genetic mosaics of *Caenorhabditis elegans*: a tissue-specific fluorescent mutant. Science 1980; 210:330–2.
9. Goldstein B. Induction of gut in *Caenorhabditis elegans* embryos. Nature 1992;357:255–7.
10. Goldstein B. Establishment of gut fate in the E lineage of *C. elegans*: the roles of lineage-dependent mechanisms and cell interactions. Development 1993;118:1267–77.
11. Goldstein B. An analysis of the response to gut induction in the *C. elegans* embryo. Development 1995;121:1227–36.
12. Bowerman B, Eaton BA, Priess JR. Skn-1, a maternally expressed gene required to specify the fate of ventral blastomeres in the early *C. elegans* embryo. Cell 1992;68:1061–75.
13. Bowerman B, Draper BW, Mello CC, Priess JR. The maternal gene skn-1 encodes a protein that is distributed unequally in early *C. elegans* embryos. Cell 1993;74:443–52.
14. Lin R, Thompson S, Priess JR. Pop-1 encodes an HMG box protein required for the specification of a mesoderm precursor in early *C. elegans* embryos. Cell 1995;83:599–609.
15. Kemphues KJ, Priess JR, Morton DJ, Cheng N. Identification of genes required for cytoplasmic localization in early *C. elegans* embryos. Cell 1988;52:311–20.
16. Mello CC, Draper BW, Krause M, et al. The pie-1 and mex-1 genes and maternal control of blastomere identity in early *C. elegans* embryos. Cell 1992;70:163–76.
17. Riese J, Yu X, Munnerlyn A, et al. LEF-1, a nuclear factor coordinating signaling inputs from wingless and decapentaplegic. Cell 1997;88:777–87.
18. Van de Wetering M, Cavallo R, Dooijes D, et al. Armadillo coactivates transcription driven by the *Drosophila* segment polarity gene dTCF. Cell 1997;88:789–99.
19. Miller JM, Moon RT. Signal transduction through beta catenin and specification of cell fate during embryogenesis. Genes Dev 1996;10:2527–39.
20. Thorpe CJ, Schlesinger A, Carter JC, Bowerman B. Wnt signaling polarizes an early *C. elegans* blastomere to distinguish endoderm from mesoderm. Cell 1997;90:695–705.
21. Rocheleau CE, Downs WD, Lin R, et al. Wnt signaling and an APC-related gene specify endoderm in early *C. elegans* embryos [see comments]. Cell 1997;90:707–16.
22. Bhanot P, Brink M, Samos CH, et al. A new member of the frizzled family from *Drosophila* functions as a Wingless receptor. Nature 1996;382:225–30.
23. Nusse R. A versatile transcriptional effector of Wingless signaling. Cell 1997;89:321–3.
24. Greenspan RJ. Fly pushing. Cold Spring Harbor (NY): Cold Spring Harbor Press; 1997.
25. Spradling AC, Rubin GM. Transposition of cloned P elements into *Drosophila* germ line chromosomes. Science 1982;218: 341–7.
26. O'Kane C, Gehring WJ. Detection in situ of genomic regulatory elements in *Drosophila*. Proc Natl Acad Sci U S A 1987; 84:9123–7.
27. Skaer H. The alimentary canal. In: Bate M, Martinez-Arias A, editors. The development of *Drosophila melanogaster*. Cold Spring Harbor: Cold Spring Harbor Press; 1993. p. 941–1012.
28. Lawrence PA. The making of a fly. London: Blackwell Scientific Publications; 1992.

29. Campos-Ortega JA, Hartenstein V. The embryonic development of *Drosophila melanogaster*. Berlin: Springer-Verlag; 1985.
30. St. Johnston R, Nusslein-Volhard C. The origin of pattern and polarity in the *Drosophila* embryo. Cell 1992;68:201–19.
31. Pignoni F, Baldarelli RM, Steingrimsson E, et al. The *Drosophila* gene tailless is expressed at the embryonic termini and is a member of the steroid receptor superfamily. Cell 1990;62:151–63.
32. Monaghan AP, Grau E, Bock D, Schutz D. The mouse homolog of the orphan nuclear receptor tailless is expressed in the developing forebrain. Development 1995;121:839–53.
33. Weigel D, Jurgens G, Klingler M, Jackle H. Two gap genes mediate terminal pattern information in *Drosophila*. Science 1990;248:495–8.
34. Chen WS, Manova K, Weinstein DC, et al. Disruption of the HNF-4 gene, expressed in visceral endoderm, leads to cell death in embryonic ectoderm and impaired gastrulation of mouse embryos. Genes Dev 1994;8:2466–77.
35. Zhong W, Sladek FM, Darnell JE. The expression pattern of a *Drosophila* homolog to the mouse transcription factor HNF-4 suggests a determinative role in gut formation. EMBO J 1993;12:537–44.
36. Wu LH, Lengyel JA. Role of caudal in hindgut specification and gastrulation suggests homology between *Drosophila* amnioproctodeal invagination and vertebrate blastopore. Development 1998. [In press]
37. Weigel D, Bellen HJ, Jurgens G, Jackle H. Primordium specific requirement of the homeotic gene fork head in the developing gut of the *Drosophila* embryo. Roux's Arch Dev Biol 1989;198:201–10.
38. Jurgens G, Weigel D. Terminal versus segmental development in the *Drosophila* embryo: the role of the homeotic gene fork head. Roux's Arch Dev Biol 1988;197:345–54.
39. Clark KL, Halay ED, Lai E, Burley SK. Co-crystal structure of the HNF-3/fork head DNA recognition motif resembles histone H5. Nature 1993;364:412–20.
40. Lai E, Prezioso VR, Tao WF, et al. Hepatocyte nuclear factor 3 alpha belongs to a gene family in mammals that is homologous to the *Drosophila* homeotic gene fork head. Genes Dev 1991;4:1427–36.
41. McMahon AP. Mouse development: winged helix in axial patterning. Curr Biol 1994;4:903–6.
42. Monaghan AP, Kaestner KH, Grau E, Schutz G. Postimplantation expression patterns indicate a role for the mouse forkhead/HNF-3 alpha, beta and gamma genes in determination of the definitive endoderm, chordamesoderm and neuroectoderm. Development 1993;119:567–78.
43. Ang SL, Rossant J. HNF-3 beta is essential for node and notochord formation in mouse development. Cell 1994;78:561–74.
44. Poulson DF. Histogenesis, organogenesis and differentiation in the embryo of *Drosophila melanogaster*. In: Demerec M, editor. Biology of *Drosophila*. New York: Hafner Publishing Company; 1950. p. 275–367.
45. Tepass U, Hartenstein V. Epithelium formation in *Drosophila* midgut depends on the interaction of endoderm and mesoderm. Development 1994;120:579–90.
46. Louvard D, Kedinger M, Hauri HP. The differentiating intestinal epithelial cell: establishment and maintenance of functions through interactions between cellular structures. Annu Rev Cell Biol 1992;8:157–95.
47. Artavanis-Tsakonas S, Matsuno K, Fortini M. Notch signaling. Science 1995;268:225–32.
48. Hartenstein AY, Rugendorff A, Tepass U, Hartenstein V. The function of the neurogenic genes during epithelial development in the *Drosophila* embryo. Development 1992;116:1203–20.
49. Tepass U, Hartenstein V. Neurogenic and proneural genes control cell fate specification in the *Drosophila* endoderm. Development 1995;121:393–405.
50. Lehman R, Jimenez F, Dietrich U, Campos-Ortega JA. On the phenotype and development of mutants of early neurogenesis in *Drosophila melanogaster*. Roux's Arch Dev Biol 1983;192:62–74.
51. Li L, Krantz ID, Deng Y, et al. Alagille syndrome is caused by mutations in human Jagged1, which encodes a ligand for Notch1. Nat Genet 1997;16:243–51.
52. Oda T, Elkahloun AG, Metzler PS, et al. Mutations in the human Jagged1 gene are resposible for Alagille syndrome. Nat Genet 1997;16:235–42.
53. Lawrence PA, Morata G. Homeobox genes: their function in *Drosophila* segmentation and pattern formation. Cell 1994;78:181–9.
54. Tremml G, Bienz M. Homeotic gene expression in the visceral mesoderm of *Drosophila* embryos. EMBO J 1989;8:2677–85.
55. Bienz M. Homeotic genes and positional signalling in the *Drosophila* viscera. Trends Genet 1994;10:22–6.
56. Hoppler S, Bienz M. Specification of a single cell type by a *Drosophila* homeotic gene. Cell 1994;76:689–702.
57. Rijeswijk F, Schuermann M, Wagenaar E, et al. The *Drosophila* homolog of the mouse mammary oncogene int-1 is identical to the segment polarity gene wingless. Cell 1987;50:649–57.
58. Brunner E, Peter O, Schweizer L, Basler K. Pangolin encodes a Lef-1 homologue that acts downstream of Armadillo to transduce the Wingless signal in *Drosophila*. Nature 1997;385:829–33.
59. Hoppler S, Bienz M. Two different thresholds of wingless signalling with distinct developmental consequences in the *Drosophila* midgut. EMBO J 1995;14:5016–26.
60. Bienz M. Induction of the endoderm in *Drosophila*. Semin Cell Dev Biol 1996;7:113–9.
61. Massague J, Attisano L, Wrana JL. The TGF-beta family and its composite receptors. Trends Cell Biol 1994;4:172–8.
62. Massague J. TGF-beta signaling: receptors, transducers, and Mad proteins. Cell 1996;85:947–50.
63. Bienz M. Endoderm induction in *Drosophila*: the nuclear targets of the inducing signals. Curr Opin Genet Dev 1997;7:683–8.
64. Riese J, Tremml G, Bienz M. D-Fos, a target gene of Decapentaplegic signalling with a critical role during *Drosophila* endoderm induction. Development 1997;124:3353–61.
65. Tremml G, Bienz M. Induction of labial expression in the *Drosophila* endoderm: response elements for dpp signalling and for autoregulation. Development 1992;116:447–56.
66. Eresh S, Riese J, Jackson DB, et al. A CREB-binding site as a target for decapentaplegic signalling during *Drosophila* endoderm induction. EMBO J 1997;16:2014–22.
67. Haffen K, Kedinger M, Simon-Assman P. Mesenchyme-dependent differentiation of epithelial gut progenitor cells in the gut. J Pediatr Gastroenterol Nutr 1987;6:14–23.
68. Haffen K, Lacroix B, Kedinger M, Simon-Assmann PM. Inductive properties of fibroblastic cell cultures derived from rat intestinal mucosa on epithelia differentiation. Differentiation 1983;23:226–33.
69. Apelqvist A, Ahlgren U, Edlund H. Sonic Hedgehog directs specialized mesoderm differentiation in the intestine and pancreas. Curr Biol 1997;7:801–4.
70. Solnica-Krezel L, Stemple DL, Driever W. Transparent things: cell fates and cell movements during early embryo-genesis of zebrafish. Bioessays 1995;17:931–9.
71. Kimmel CB, Ballard WW, Kimmel SR, et al. Stages of embryonic development of the zebrafish. Dev Dyn 1995;203:253–310.

72. Mullins MC, Hammerschmidt M, Haffter P, Nusslein-Volhard C. Large-scale mutagenesis in the zebrafish: in search of genes controlling development in a vertebrate. Curr Biol 1994;4:189–202.
73. Solnica-Krezel L, Schier AF, Driever W. Efficient recovery of ENU-induced mutations from the zebrafish germline. Genetics 1994;136:1401–20.
74. Westerfield M, editor. The zebrafish book. 3rd ed. Eugene: The University of Oregon Press; 1995.
75. Knapik EW, Goodman, A, Atkinson OS, et al. A reference cross DNA panel for zebrafish (*Danio rerio*) anchored with simple sequence length polymorphisms. Development 1996;123:451–60.
76. Pack M, Solnica-Krezel L, Malicki J, et al. Mutations affecting development of zebrafish digestive organs. Development 1996;123:321–8.
77. Driever W, Solnica-Krezel L, Schier AF, et al. A genetic screen affecting embryogenesis in the zebrafish. Development 1996;123:37–46.
78. Haffter P, Granato M, Brand M, et al. The identification of genes with unique and essential functions in the development of the zebrafish, *Danio rerio*. Development 1996;123:1–36.
79. Chen J-N, Haffter P, Odenthal J, et al. Mutations affecting the cardiovascular system and other internal organs in zebrafish. Development 1996;123:293–302.
80. Gaiano N, Amsterdam A, Kawakami K, et al. Insertional mutagenesis and rapid cloning of essential genes in zebrafish. Nature 1996;382:829–32.
81. Moon RT, Brown JD, Torres M. WNTs modulate cell fate and behavior during vertebrate development. Trends Genet. 1997;13:157–62.

CHAPTER 19

Ectopic Transplantation Techniques for Evaluating Gastrointestinal Development

Tor C. Savidge, PhD

Many insights into gastrointestinal development can be gained by studying the regeneration and differentiation of ectopic grafts in suitable recipient animal hosts. This chapter will relate work on ectopic transplantation of fetal and neonatal tissues as an experimental tool to further our knowledge of molecular factors that regulate mammalian gastrointestinal development. The potential applications of grafting techniques to clinical practice will also be considered. Our focus will be primarily on developmental studies of the small intestine.

MORPHOLOGIC AND FUNCTIONAL DEVELOPMENT OF THE SMALL INTESTINE

Gastrointestinal ontogenesis is associated with proliferation and cytodifferentiation of several characteristic epithelial cell lineages that emerge in a specific spatial and chronological fashion.[1-4] In the mouse, a poorly developed stratified intestinal endoderm persists until embryonic (E) day 16, after which time it rapidly differentiates, starting initially in proximal regions.[5] Primitive villi lined with a columnar epithelium are evident by E18, although crypts of Lieberkühn remain poorly developed until after birth. Mouse C57BL/6J lac(B6):SWR aggregation chimeras, showing *Dolichos biflorus* agglutinin (DBA) lectin-binding polymorphism specified by DLB-1 alleles, have proved useful tools for developmental studies of small-intestinal crypt clonality and epithelial migration on villi.[6-8] Use of the DBA lectin to identify N-acetyl-D-galactosaminyl oligosaccharide residues on epithelial cells in tissue sections and in tissue whole mounts has demonstrated that the intervillous epithelium or immature "crypts" observed in late fetal and early neonatal life harbor a mixed genotype of epithelial stem cells that results in polyclonal glands. However, as the crypts mature during the first 3 weeks of postnatal life, a "purification" process occurs by means of stem-cell selection, leading to monoclonality.[8,9] Colonic crypts are also monoclonal, as indicated using the X-chromosome-linked lineage-marker enzyme glucose-6-phosphatase dehydrogenase.[10-12] Although adult human intestinal crypts demonstrate a similar monoclonality, it is unknown whether this is achieved through a similar purification step.[12,13] Further crypt maturation is associated with an increased cell population and production rate, resulting from the establishment of a complex stem-cell hierarchy.[14-16] Crypt fission is also active during the postnatal period, increasing the number of glands feeding each villus.[2] As several adjacent crypts supply epithelial cells onto individual villi, the latter structures tend to be polyclonal, the degree of which is region-specific.[6-13]

Studies using conventional, chimeric, and transgenic mice all indicate that a single pluripotent stem cell is anchored near the crypt base that ultimately restores the epithelial population by generating daughter cells that undergo division, lineage allocation, and cytodifferentiation during bipolar migration.[5,14,15] In the small intestine, 4 major epithelial cell lineages are evident, with absorptive enterocytes, peptide-producing enteroendocrine cells, and mucus-producing goblet cells undergoing cytodifferentiation during upward migration to the villus apical-cell extrusion zone.[1] This orderly process of migration, decycling, cytodifferentiation, and exfoliation is completed within 4 days and is segregated as vertical coherent bands on villi that originate from individual monoclonal crypts. Paneth cells, which produce small antimicrobial peptides[17] such as α-defensins and lysozyme, migrate downwards towards the crypt base, where they remain for approximately 3 weeks, partly in order to prevent translocation of luminal bacteria across the epithelial barrier.

The gastrointestinal tract in rodents displays two major phases of functional development.[4,18] The first phase occurs late in gestation and is limited to morphologic maturation, with gene expression focusing largely on producing proteins that are required for the digestion and absorption of milk components during the suckling period: e.g., lactase-phlorizin hydrolase, sodium-dependent glucose cotransporter (SGLT1), intestinal and liver fatty acid-binding proteins (I-FABP and L-FABP), and apolipoproteins (APOA-1, APOA-IV and

APOB). The second maturation phase occurs with the onset of weaning during the third postnatal week. At this time, the small intestine dramatically increases the gene expression of proteins required for digestion and absorption of carbohydrate in solid food: e.g., sucrase-isomaltase, trehalase, maltase-glucoamylase, and the fructose transporter GLUT5. Coincident with the acquisition of mature digestive and absorptive functions, protein required during the suckling period, e.g., lactase, is markedly reduced due to altered gene expression, protein translation, and turnover.[4,5,18] This period is also associated with profound immunologic changes that are both antigen-independent due to mucosal imprinting (e.g., of vascular addressins), and antigen-dependent due to an increased exposure of the gastrointestinal mucosa to luminal food and bacterial antigens.[19] Altered mucosal immune reactions are also capable of selectively regulating the gene expression of epithelial brushborder hydrolases, in particular lactase.[20]

Human gastrointestinal development differs drastically from that in rodents in that structural and functional maturation is precocious, occurring largely in utero in the absence of the luminal stimulation of postnatal life.[4,21–23] The small intestine is recognized as a simple tube by 4 weeks of gestation, with primative villi and crypts appearing by 8 and 10 weeks, respectively. Active glucose transport and peptidases are present by 10 weeks, whereas active transport of amino acids, alkaline phosphatase, and disaccharidase activity is detectable 2 weeks later. At this time, intestinal muscle layers and enteroendocrine cells appear, although Paneth cells are not evident until 24 weeks of gestation. After 38 weeks maturity is achieved. The procacious maturation of the human gastrointestinal tract is probably due to intrinsic timing mechanisms of the intestinal mucosa and high surges of glucocorticoids that have the ability to elicit procacious maturation in a number of experimental animal models.[4,18,24,25] It has been proposed, therefore, that an independent molecular pathway of glucocorticoid-induced gut maturation may have evolved to impart a selective advantage to offspring, allowing an early switch to solid food should this be required.[4,18]

USE OF ECTOPIC TRANSPLANTATION TO STUDY THE INFLUENCE OF LUMINAL AND CIRCULATORY SIGNALS ON GASTROINTESTINAL DEVELOPMENT

Signals derived from luminal contents have been implicated as regulators of epithelial cell proliferation and cytodifferentiation, especially following regional adaptation to segmental resection.[26–28] A number of ectopic transplantation studies have used gastrointestinal isografts and xenografts to examine the role of luminal contents in regulating gastrointestinal development.[29–50] By transplanting fetal tissues into adult hosts, this provides an attractive alternative method to investigate physiologic and genetic determinants that regulate gastrointestinal development in vivo in the absence of specific ontogenic signals from either the lumen or the circulation. Systemic hormones associated with pregnancy and luminal contents present in amniotic fluid, bile salts, and pancreatic secretions, as well as enteric bacteria and food antigens encountered in early postnatal life, all constitute potential regulatory factors.[51,52]

Early pioneering work established the feasibility of ectopic grafting of gastrointestinal tissues into adult recipient hosts.[29–36] Tissue growth was achieved following transplantation under the kidney capsule, into the subcutaneous fascia parallel to the paravertebral line, anterior chest wall, or the anterior chamber of the eye. These studies demonstrated that free, syngeneic intestine rapidly vascularizes and grows into a morphologically distinct tissue that retains an ability to produce brushborder enzymes[34,37–40] (e.g., lactase, sucrase and maltase), to absorb nutrients[35] (e.g., glucose, glycine and oleic acid), and to undergo peristalsis.[35] In a landmark study, Ferguson et al.[34] transplanted E19 fetal jejunal isografts under the kidney capsule of adult CBA mice and demonstrated that the developmental changes in brushborder lactase and sucrase activity that normally occur in the intestinal epithelium during the third postnatal week were also apparent in the isografts. This led to the concept that one or more timing mechanisms are intrinsic to the intestinal mucosa, thereby providing a spatial and temporal "memory" enabling appropriate tissue development in the absence of luminal signals and systemic hormones encountered during late gestation and the early postnatal period.

More recent experiments have used murine fetal gastrointestinal isografts of a younger gestational (E15 to 16) age to ascertain whether appropriate spatiotemporal patterns of tissue development are present prior to endodermal cytodifferentiation.[44–47] Fetal small intestine harvested at this stage of gestation possesses a stratified, undifferentiated endoderm lacking characteristic epithelial proteins, such as brushborder hydrolases and I-FABP/L-FABP. Subcutaneous implantation of E15 to 16 isografts into young adult male CBy/B6 nude recipients resulted in rapid vascularization and mucosal growth. In a fashion similar to older-gestational-age tissues, an appropriate morphologic pattern of epithelial cytodifferentiation was demonstrated both along the cephalocaudal (i.e., proximal-to-distal) and crypt-villus axes when tissue isografts were harvested 4 to 6 weeks after transplantation. Marked differences in villus height and crypt depth were apparent along the duodenal-to-ileal axis. Region-specific differences in epithelial proliferation and cytodifferentiation programs for each of the four principal cell lineages were also evident, indicating that the intrinsic timing occurred prior to endodermal cytodifferentiation and was not dependent on luminal or circulatory signals. Appropriate organotypic development was also evident after implanting fetal stomach[47] and colonic isografts.

Similar findings have been reported for human fetal intestine grown as xenografts in immunodeficient hosts,[42,43,48–50] although in these studies tissues were implanted after initial endodermal cytodifferentiation (Figure 19–1). In contrast to murine isografts, human and porcine[54] xenografts grown in *scid* mice were shown to initially undergo an extensive period of tissue degeneration. This was followed by angiogenesis and epithelialization, initially restricted to focal areas of necrosis but later spreading out to seal a luminal cavity. At this early stage of xenograft regeneration, the epithelium was pseudostratified

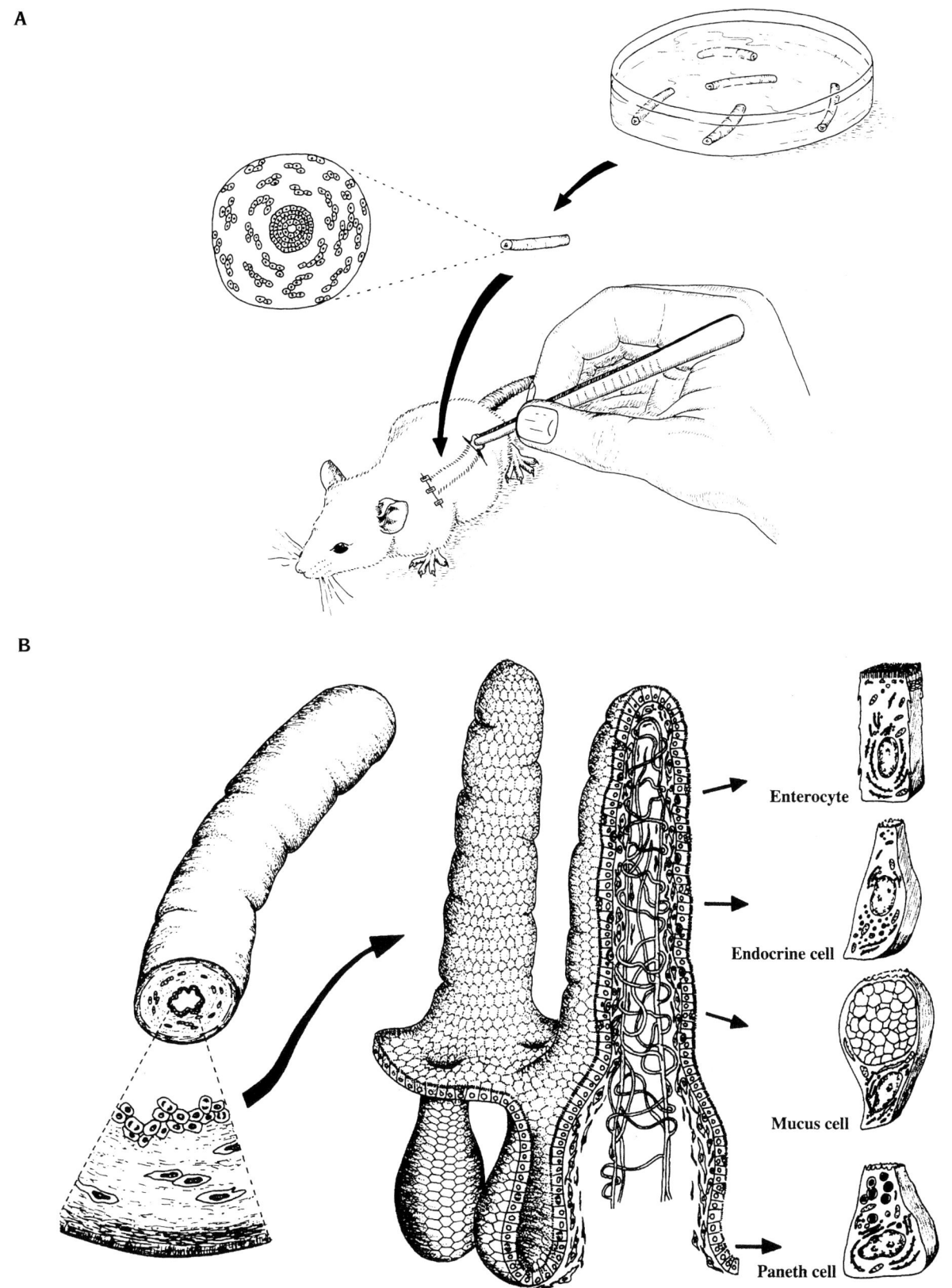

FIGURE 19–1. Schematic illustration of A, subcutaneous transplantation of a human fetal intestinal xenograft into a C.B-17 *scid* mouse recipient; B, mucosal development and epithelial cytodifferentiation following ectopic xenotransplantation of human fetal small intestine. (Reproduced with permission from Savidge TC, Shmakov AN, Walker-Smith JA, Phillips AD. Intestinal proliferation and infection in childhood. In: Halter F, Winton D, Wright NA, editors. The gut as a model in cell and molecular biology. London: Kluwer Academic; 1997. p. 111–20.)

and closely resembled the rapidly proliferating epithelial tissue of human fetal intestine prior to cytodifferentiation. With time (10 weeks after transplantation), xenografts developed a mucosal architecture that was entirely dependent on the region of fetal intestine chosen for engraftment.[48] Typically, villi were tall and ridgelike in proximal small-intestinal xenografts, and were significantly shorter in distal sites approaching the ileocecal junction. Genetic determination of host and donor cell types using in situ hybridization with species-specific DNA probes demonstrated an exclusively human origin for the epithelium and muscle layers. Although the submucosa and lamina propria were comprised of a chimeric mixture of cells, murine cells rarely contacted the epithelium, which interacted primarily with human-derived myofibroblasts and human intraepithelial lymphocytes. These studies proposed that a "selection" process may operate to maintain species-specific heterotypic cell interactions with the epithelium in these grafts, which may in turn be instrumental in regulating epithelial cytodifferentiation.[48,49]

TEMPORAL AND SPATIAL DISTRIBUTION OF EPITHELIAL CELL PROLIFERATION AND LINEAGE DEVELOPMENT IN ECTOPIC INTESTINAL GRAFTS

Crypt Cell Proliferation

Ectopically transplanted fetal stomach and small and large bowel all form well-developed crypts that show appropriate patterns of epithelial cell division.[43,47–50] Cell proliferation studies have demonstrated many similarities in MIB-1 monoclonal antibody immunoreactivity towards the cell-cycle dependent antigen Ki-67, as well as other cell-cycle markers, including proliferating cell nuclear antigen (PCNA), bromodeoxyuridine, [^{3}H]-thymidine and propidium iodide staining in human xenograft and pediatric small bowel. These investigations demonstrated that epithelial cell proliferation is not only restricted to xenograft crypts in a conventional fashion, but that it shows normal spatial distributions of G_1SG_2M, G_1G_2M, S- and M-phase cells. Detailed analysis of the DNA-synthesizing population demonstrated that the S-phase consistently represented 50% of the growth fraction, indicating cell-cycle homogeneity throughout the crypt proliferation compartment.[50] In addition, xenograft crypts demonstrated clear evidence of synchronous proliferative behavior, which is a typical feature of normal epithelial cell division in vivo.

These findings reflect common kinetic parameters in xenografted human fetal and pediatric small bowel: i.e., growth fractions, cell-cycle durations, epithelial cell migration rates, and the number of transit divisions before cells decycle and exit the crypts. Hence, there are basic regulatory mechanisms in ectopically transplanted fetal intestine that are sufficient to initiate and maintain the spatial arrangement of cellular proliferation. Luminal factors do not, therefore, appear to play an essential role in generating and maintaining an appropriate spatiotemporal regulation of crypt cell proliferation. Rather, these factors may play a "fine-tuning" role, as subtle differences were noted in the pattern of proliferation in xenograft and pediatric bowel, such as smaller crypts and lower proliferation indices in the former. The absence of conventional luminal stimuli in xenografted tissues, especially a bacterial flora, is the most likely explanation for these differences.[49,50] This is indicated by recording elevated crypt epithelial-cell proliferation rates following inoculation of bacteria into the lumen of human intestinal xenografts.[55–58]

Absorptive Cells

In small intestinal grafts, absorptive cells represent the major epithelial cell lineage. These appear highly differentiated, with well-developed apical tight junctions, glycocalyx, and brushborder microvillus membrane (Figure 19–2). As described above for duodenal isografts, human small intestinal xenografts also develop significant cephalocaudal and crypt-villus gradients in brushborder enzyme activity.[48] Appropriate spatiotemporal epithelial glycosylation patterns have also been demonstrated in isografts using a panel of lectins to examine defined carbohydrate specificities in the respective cell lineages.[46] This panel, which included the lectins CTB (*cholera toxin β-subunit*; αNeu5AC/α-Neu5Gc), DBA (*Dolichos biflorus* agglutinin; N-acetyl-D-galactosaminyl), HPA (*Helix pomatia*; N-acetyl-D-galactosaminyl), PNA (*Arachis hypogaea*; α/β-D-galactosyl), Jacalin (*Artrocarpus integrifolia*; α/β-D-galactosyl), TKA (*Trichosantes kirilowii*; α/β-D-galactosyl), and UEAI (*Ulex europaeus* I; α-L-Fucosyl), demonstrated that the cell lineage and region-specific patterns of lectin labeling were identical in isograft and intact intestine from 6-week-old FVB-N mice. Using a 20-member lectin panel, our laboratory has compared epithelial glycosylation patterns in human fetal, xenograft, and pediatric small bowel. Although xenograft epithelial cells showed many similarities with pediatric intestine, distinct fetal-specific glycosylation patterns were still apparent even 12 months after transplantation (unpublished observations). Luminal and circulatory signals may, therefore, be required for appropriate regulation of epithelial glycosylation during human gastrointestinal development.

Goblet and Paneth Cells

Mucus-producing goblet cells are readily identified using periodic acid-Schiff or alcian blue staining of intestinal ectopic grafts, with an appropriate region-specific increase in numbers in distal small-intestinal and colonic tissues. Goblet cells in these tissues possess large numbers of homogenous mucus granules located between the basally-situated crescent-shaped nucleus and the apical brushborder. The most apically-positioned granules are occasionally seen to discharge into the luminal environment (Figure 19–3A), especially after infection of the xenograft lumen with enteric pathogens, e.g., *Salmonella typhi* (unpublished observations). Although the abundant goblet-cell population in human intestinal xenografts appears histochemically and ultrastructurally mature, similarities are apparent when

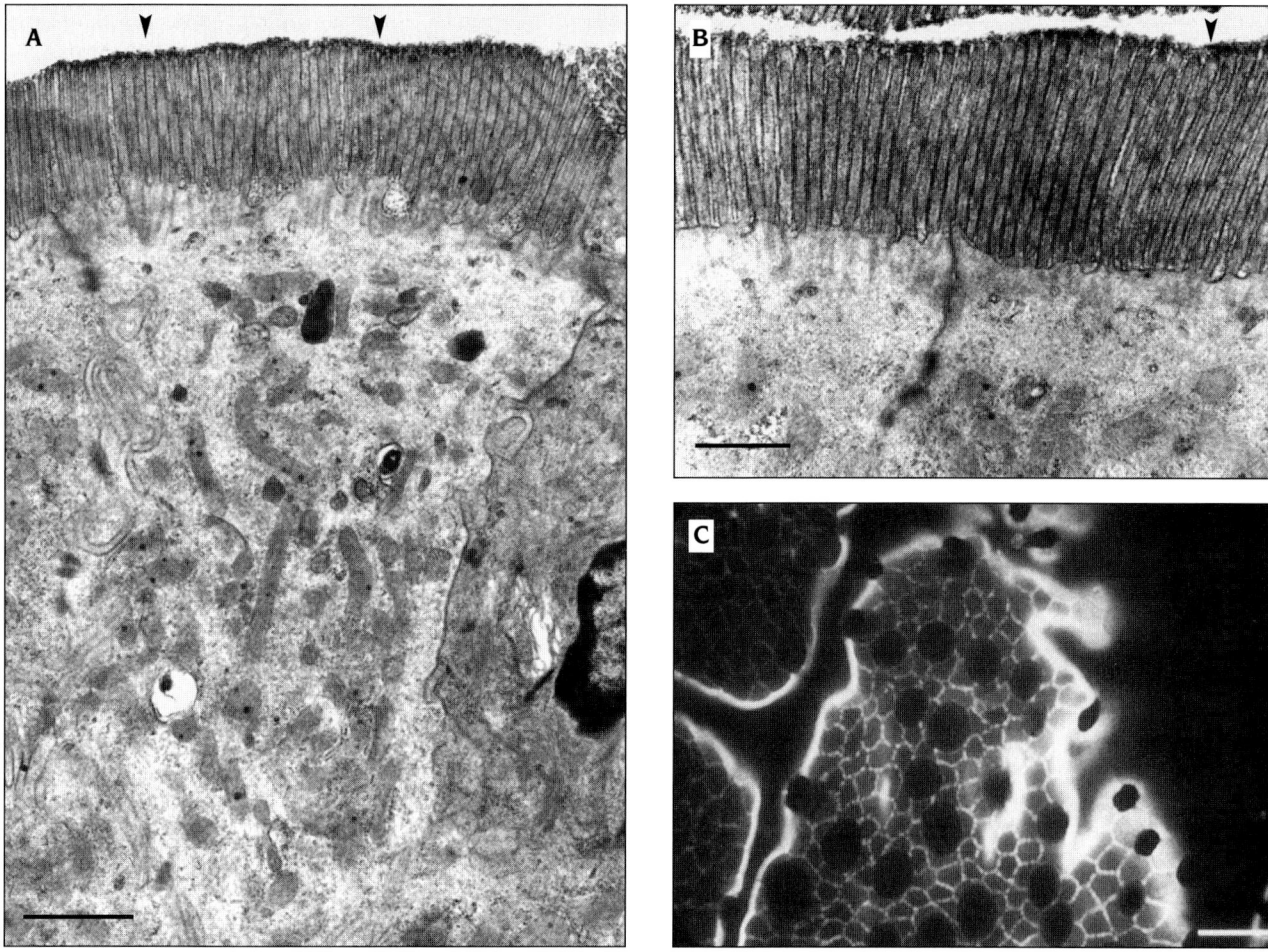

FIGURE 19–2. Epithelial cell polarity in human small intestinal xenografts. A and B show the well-developed brushborder membrane, with tight junctions and glycocalyx that form during xenograft regeneration. C, A confocal micrograph showing intense actin staining in the brushborder of a xenograft small intestinal villus. This is absent in the goblet-cell population. Scale bars represent 2.5, 1, and 20 µm in A, B and C, respectively.

comparing mucin gene expression, in particular MUC2 and MUC3, with human fetal bowel.[59] Luminal and circulatory signals may, therefore, be required for appropriate regulation of epithelial mucin gene expression during human gastrointestinal development.

Paneth cells express a number of antimicrobial peptides: e.g., lysozyme, a feature which aids in their identification.[44,45] Clear region-specific differences in Paneth cell numbers are also maintained in ectopic grafts where cells are abundant in small intestinal crypts but are rarely recorded in large bowel. Ultrastructurally, characteristic homogenous and electron-dense secretory granules are situated in the supranuclear region (Figure 19–3B), and show evidence of discharge into the crypt lumen following luminal infection of human intestinal xenografts with enteric pathogens. Although Paneth cells are normally collectively located at the base of intestinal xenograft crypts, we have observed occasional evidence of dysplasia and de novo differentiation of Paneth cells in "invading crypts" of human small- and large-intestinal xenografts, respectively.[50]

Enteroendocrine Cells

Enteroendocrine cells are readily identified at the light microscopic level in ectopic grafts, where antibodies are used to specific neuroendocrine components: e.g., antichromogranin, which stains the entire cell lineage in human intestine.[48] Chromogranin-positive enteroendocrine cells represent a minority cell type in intact and ectopic intestine, constituting approximately 1% of the total epithelial cell population (Figure 19–3C). In human intestinal xenografts enteroendocrine cells are found in numbers comparable to those with pediatric bowel, and often cluster throughout the crypt-villus axis. In contrast to goblet and Paneth cells, enteroendocrine cells are more numerous in human fetal and regenerating xenograft intestine, suggesting a putative role for their peptide products in gastrointestinal ontogenesis, where rapid growth is a necessity.[48]

Elegant multilabel immunohistochemical studies have defined the spatiotemporal development of specific functional subclasses of enteroendocrine cells in murine intestinal isografts.[44,45] A complex interrelationship exists between the expression of neuroendocrine products that is established early following initial cytodifferentation of fetal endoderm, and that depends on the location of enteroendocrine cells along cephalocaudal and crypt-villus axes. Rubin et al.[44,45] investigated the relative expression of eight distinct subclasses of enteroendocrine cells (serotonin, Peptide YY, cholecystokinin, gastrin, glucagon-like peptide 1, neurotensin, glucose-dependent insulinotropic peptide, and secretin-immunoreactive cells) in proximal-to-distal isograft segments, comparing these to differentiation pathways evident in intact bowel. Appropriate spatiotemporal coexpression of neuropeptides in all subclasses of enteroendocrine cells was accurately mimicked in isograft intestine, indicating that these complex differentiation pathways are not luminally or systemically regulated

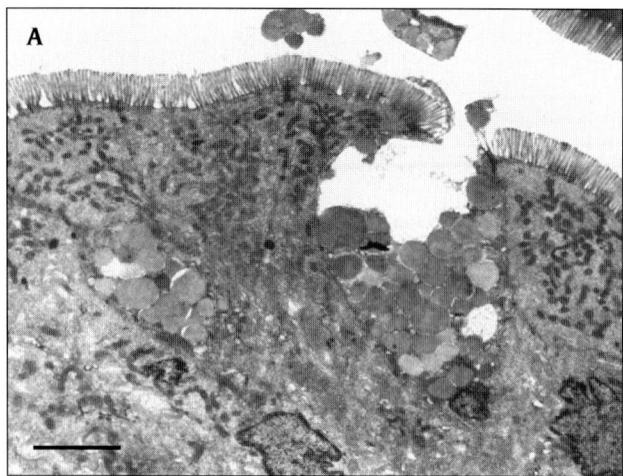
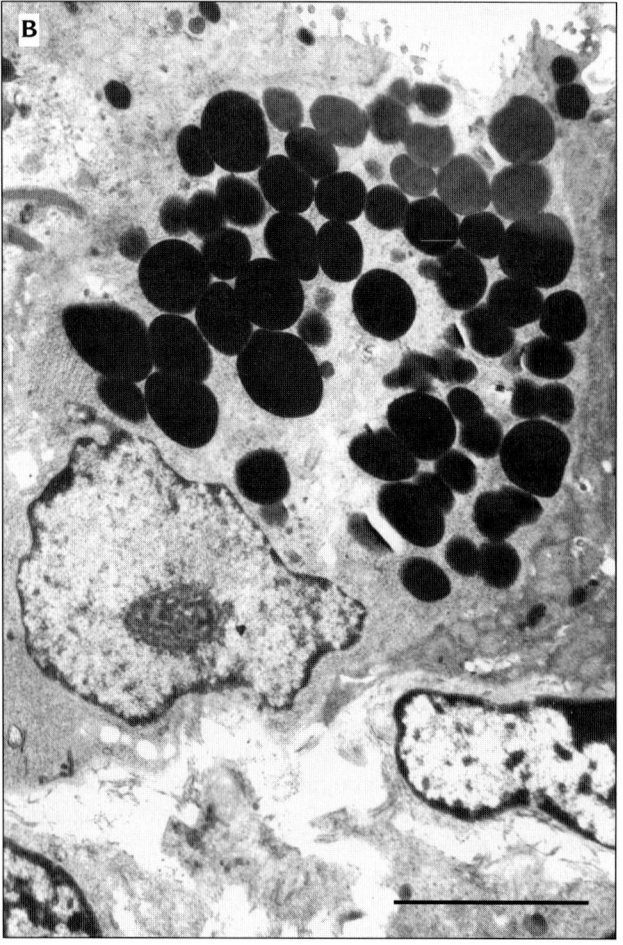
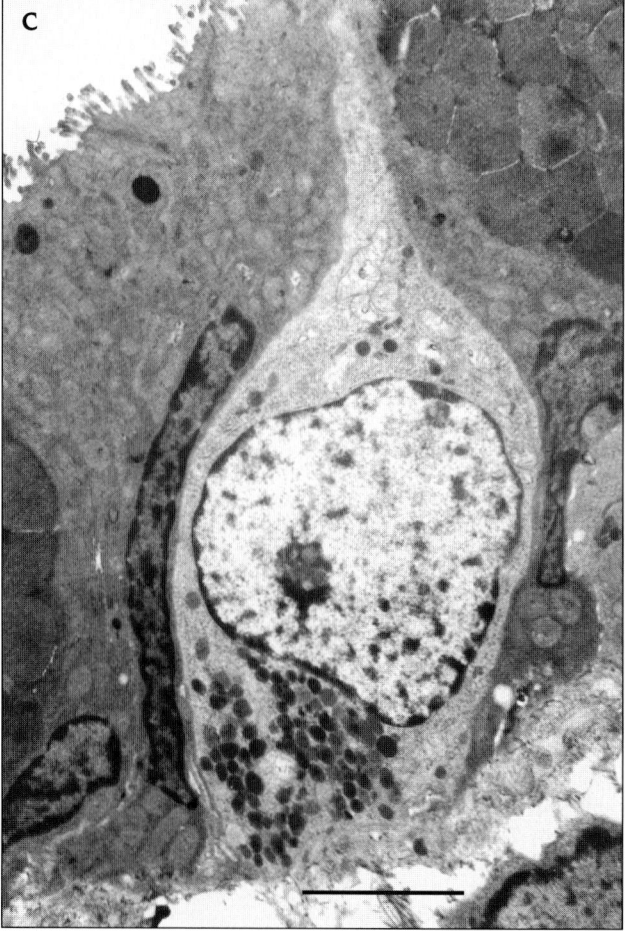

FIGURE 19–3. Electron micrographs showing a human small intestinal xenograft. A, goblet cell discharging mucus granules, B, Paneth cell, and C, enteroendocrine cell. Scale bars represent 5 μm in A, B, and C.

during gastrointestinal development. Typically, serotonin-expressing enteroendocrine cells remained the most abundant subclass, and were distributed uniformly throughout all the different types of intestinal isografts. In contrast, a proximal-to-distal decline in numbers was maintained for CCK- and GIP-immunoreactive cells, whereas for PYY-expressing cells a reverse pattern was preserved. Appropriate cytodifferentiation pathways were also apparent along the crypt-villus axis in isografts as judged by enteroendocrine cells coexpressing serotonin-substance P in crypts and serotonin-secretin on villi.

MOLECULAR REGULATION OF INTESTINAL EPITHELIAL CELL CYTODIFFERENTIATION IN ECTOPIC GRAFTS

Studies using heterotopic embryonic recombinants, aggregation chimeras, mutant and transgenic mice have greatly advanced our knowledge of cis- and transacting factors that regulate gastrointestinal development, and have been facilitated by ectopic transplantation approaches.[5] The fact that appropriate spatiotemporal epithelial regulation is evident along the crypt-villus and cephalocaudal axes in ectopically-transplanted gastrointestinal tissues can be explained by assuming that this information is contained within the crypt epithelial stem-cell population. This information may either be intrinsic to stem cells or derived from extracellular non-luminal signals.

Distinct cephalocaudal expression of gastrointestinal-specific homeobox genes,[60,61] such as CDX1 and CDX2, undoubtedly represents one potential source of positional information to ectopically-transplanted epithelial stem cells. CIS-acting elements, such as the 5'-nontranscribed domains of rat FABPL and FABPI genes, are also able to provide appropriate spatiotemporal regulation of Human Growth Hormone Reporter-gene expression in transgenic murine isografts.[44,55] This is demonstrated as isograft and intact gastrointestinal tissues show a similar expression of FABPL and FABPI confined to epithelial cells on the villus, with highest levels detected in the duodenum and jejunum. Characteristic differences in the expression of FABPL and FABPI are also maintained in ileal and colonic isografts. In ileal isografts FABPL is expressed in coherent bands of enterocytes extending along the whole villus, whereas FABPI is expressed more uniformly. In colonic isografts there is no evidence of FABPL expression, whereas FABPI is transcribed in differentiated colonocytes.

Developing mesodermal components in the gastrointestinal tract also constitute a potential source of positional information available to epithelial stem cells, directing appropriate spatiotemporal control over cytodifferentiation. Elegant transplantation models, involving heterospecific and heterotopic embryonic endodermal-mesenchymal recombinants, have established the importance of epithelial-mesenchymal crosstalk during gastrointestinal development.[62-70] These studies demonstrated that the tissue-specific morphologic and functional development of the gastrointestinal tract clearly involves instructive information contained within the endoderm itself, but is also supported by complex contact-dependent permissive information provided by the underlying mesenchyme. Potential transacting molecular factors that mediate this developmental crosstalk include differential expression of extracellular matrix components and fibroblast-derived growth factors. These mechanisms are described in detail in Chapter 6.

The intrinsic developmental programming of the intestinal mucosa is, therefore, regulated by local signals contained within the endoderm itself and the juxtaposed mesenchyme. In addition, isograft studies have demonstrated that the morphologic and functional maturation of ectopic grafts is dependent on endogenous (and exogenous) systemic hormones and growth factors.[34,37,71-73] Ferguson et al.[34] demonstrated that exogenous addition of cortisone to hosts bearing jejunal isografts resulted in a precocious induction of brushborder disaccharidases. These findings are similar to those described in intact neonatal animals. Small-intestinal isografts transplanted under the kidney capsule of hypophysectomized or diabetic adult rats demonstrate a significant reduction in their ability to develop, a feature reversed by exogenous addition of growth hormone and insulin, respectively.[71] These studies have indicated that both growth hormone and insulin are necessary for normal growth of ectopically-transplanted fetal intestine, although mucosal growth is not stimulated further in intact hosts, as is evident in transgenic isografts expressing the Human Growth Hormone Reporter gene.[44,45] Similar experiments have been extended to subcutaneous human intestinal xenografts in *scid* mice. Our laboratory has demonstrated that exogenous recombinant epidermal growth factor and keratinocyte growth factor are able to stimulate epithelial cell proliferation and mucosal growth of human ectopic grafts, whereas human growth hormone has a minimal effect (unpublished observations). In rodent isografts, infusion of antisera against epidermal growth factor into ectopic sites harboring fetal rat intestine significantly inhibited the growth of jejunal tissues, although ileal tissues remained unaffected.[72] Infusion of antisera to basic fibroblast growth factor also significantly inhibited mucosal growth and differentiation of rat intestinal isografts.[73] These studies therefore indicate that, although gastrointestinal development may be endodermally "hardwired" with positional and temporal information, this may be superseded to a marked degree by endogenous or exogenous hormones and growth factors.

Isograft studies have also suggested that luminal signals are required to initiate the expression of certain genes in epithelial cells, as has been demonstrated in neonatal animals.[4,18] For example, luminal signals do appear to influence Human Growth Hormone Reporter-gene expression in enteroendocrine cells of FABPL/hGH transgenic jejunal isografts, as the total number of reporter-gene immunoreactive enteroendocrine cells is lower than in intact gut.[44,45] Although normal enteroendocrine subpopulations are present in jejunal isografts, only a heterogenous population within these subgroups are able to express the transgene. Intestinal isografts prepared from transgenic animals may, therefore, represent good tools to study transacting luminal factors that control reporter-gene expression within defined epithelial populations, as these may differ markedly; i.e., for enterocytes and enteroendocrine cells.

USE OF ECTOPIC GRAFTS TO DEMONSTRATE MUCOSAL IMPRINTING OF INNATE INTESTINAL IMMUNITY

Rodent fetal intestine does not contain intraepithelial lymphocytes, plasma cells, or organized gut-associated lymphoid tissue, such as Peyer patches, at the time of epithelial cytodifferentiation. Although common-leukocyte antigen immunoreactive cells are detectable in developing (E15) small intestinal tissues, T (TcRαβ) and B cells only appear in substantial numbers postnatally. This feature differs drastically from the precocious development of immune function in human fetal intestine. Ectopic grafting approaches have been used to study developmental patterns of intestinal immunity in the absence of luminal antigens.[33,54,74–77] Ferguson and Parrot[33] demonstrated that murine small intestine transplanted under the kidney capsule of syngeneic adult hosts not only developed a conventional mucosal immune system with numerous diffuse lamina propria and intraepithelial lymphocytes, but these also formed primary Peyer patch-lymphoid follicles. These findings were later confirmed using rat small-intestinal isografts transplanted subcutaneously into adult syngeneic hosts. In this case, Peyer patches first appeared in isografts 1 to 2 weeks after transplantation, and reached a maximal size after 4 to 6 weeks.[74] IgA- and IgG-secreting plasma cells were are also present in isografts, as demonstrated by immunohistochemistry and immunoelectrophoresis. Development of plasma cells is an antigen-dependent process, as indicated by the succinct absence of such cells in fetal intestine. Cholera toxin immunization via the isograft intestine promotes this response further, as it generates specific antibody-producing cells in both ectopic isografts and in the recipient's own intestine.[75]

Importantly, the sequence of immunological development observed in these isografts mimicked the natural postnatal development of the intestinal tract, even though these cells are abundant in adult hosts. More recent studies have suggested this spatiotemporal acquisition of mucosal immune cells is predominantly due to selective migration of host immune cells into the isografts, and is stimulated further by immunization with cholera toxin.[76] Likely mechanisms regulating this selective lymphocyte migration in isografts are the developmental expression of tissue-specific tropic factors and of mucosal vascular addressins, especially mucosal-addressin cell-adhesion molecule 1 (MAdCAM-1), which is a ligand for the strongly gut-trophic lymphocyte integrin $\alpha^4\beta^7$. The developmental expression of MAdCAM-1 is therefore not dependent on luminal or systemic signals, because it is abundantly expressed in isografts, where it mediates lymphocyte entry.

We have demonstrated similar findings in fetal porcine (55 to 65 day gestational age) proximal and ileocecal small-intestinal xenografts in *scid* mice.[54] Only the ileocecal fetal tissues form substantial Peyer patch tissue during normal gestation, and therefore we used this feature to compare Peyer patch development and xenogeneic lymphocyte trafficking in the two different xenograft types. Although Peyer patch morphologic features were not fully recapitulated in ileocecal xenografts, invading murine blood vessels within these grafts displayed high endothelial venule (HEV)-like characteristics and expressed MAdCAM-1. These features were not observed in proximal intestinal grafts. In addition, ileocecal vessels supported xenogeneic trafficking of CD45 allotypic porcine peripheral blood lymphocytes, which was blocked using specific antibodies to MAdCAM-1 (MECA-367 and MECA-89), but not to the peripheral lymph-node vascular addressin PNAD (MECA-79). We have previously shown in mature human intestinal xenografts that the vasculature is chimeric in origin,[58,59] possessing murine endothelial cells that are supported by vimentin-positive human pericytes. This was also observed in porcine xenografts where the new host endothelium develops functional vascular addressins that are specific to the intestinal mucosa. As subcutaneous blood vessels in *scid* mice normally lack these vascular addressins, one may propose that instructive information is supplied to the invading endothelium by the intestinal-derived mesenchyme, possibly via the chimeric pericytes, in order for these to express tissue-specific lymphocyte-homing receptors. These findings may be of relevance to discordant bowel transplantation in humans, as xenogeneic gastrointestinal tissues would not only develop a human microvasculature, but would express appropriate and functional vascular addressins.

POTENTIAL CLINICAL APPLICATIONS OF ECTOPIC TRANSPLANTATION MODELS

The use of transgenic or genetically modified intestinal isografts or xenografts has a number of potential clinical applications. This type of model may represent a useful tool in evaluating the role of luminal signals in regulating oncogene expression or tumor progression in ectopic grafts harboring specific genetic mutations. For example, mice heterozygous for a mutant allele of APC (MIN) develop adenomas throughout the gastrointestinal tract. Recent work has shown that genetic modifier loci, such as MOM1, which encodes the secretory phospholipase Pla2g2a, influence tumor multiplicity and size in MIN mice. Both small- and large-intestinal isografts derived from a MIN genetic background develop tumors ectopically.[51] MIN1 and MOM1 therefore act in a tissue-autonomous fashion, as no tumors were detected in the gastrointestinal tract of the transplant recipient, which would have been expected if either had a systemic effect on tumor development. Unlike small-intestinal isografts, the frequency of tumor formation in colonic isografts is lower than that in intact tissue in MIN mice. Therefore, the MIN phenotype is not autonomous in the large bowel, and the development of colonic tumors appears to be dependent on luminal signals. Microenvironmental factors such as digestive secretions, dietary components, or intestinal flora may, therefore, represent critical factors in contributing to the development of MIN-induced colonic tumors.

Studies of abnormal human gastrointestinal development, such as the pathogenesis of colorectal carcinoma and its metastases, can also be rendered experimentally possible through ectopic xenotransplantation of normal and diseased tissues.[78–80] For example, comparing patterns of xenograft regeneration in biopsy specimens from a colon adenocarcinoma to metastases from the same patient has provided insights into potential metastatic mechanisms. Both tissue types express equivalent levels of cytokeratin, neuron-specific enolase and carcinoembryonic antigen, although significantly higher levels of β-galactosidase-specific receptors were identified in the latter, indicating a potential metastatic role for this differential pattern of membrane glycosylation.[79] On a similar note, the developmental susceptibility of human intestine to different types of metastases has also been investigated using ectopic grafts.[81]

Ectopic grafting models are also being developed to examine the feasibility of small-intestinal neomucosal growth in colonic sites.[82–91] This would have a potential application to a number of clinical disorders, including short bowel syndrome, familial adenomatous polyposis, and ulcerative colitis. Recent work has demonstrated an ability for enzymatically-isolated rat postnatal epithelial-cell aggregates, harboring functional stem cells, to be grafted subcutaneously or into mucosal-depleted colonic muscle of adult recipients.[82–87] The enzymatic disaggregation method used to prepare epithelial cell aggregates maintains the stem cells within a suitable niche embraced by pericryptal myofibroblasts, which remain attached during the isolation procedure. This heterotypic cell-to-cell contact is an essential prerequisite for appropriate small-intestinal neomucosal growth, supported by a permissive role of the underlying colonic muscle layer. This is demonstrated as transplanted cell aggregates successfully regenerate a small-intestinal neomucosa displaying crypts and villi lined with an epithelium possessing all major small-intestinal-cell lineages and showing a degree of function: i.e., nutrient transport and brushborder enzyme activity. In addition, ectopic neomucosa demonstrates a proliferative response to exogenous epidermal growth factor,[88–91] which represents one possible therapeutic approach for stimulating neomucosal growth in humans, as has been suggested from its use in necrotizing enterocolitis.[92] In addition, studies are currently in progress that aim to engineer artificial tubular intestinal tissues by seeding epithelial cells onto polymeric delivery vehicles, such as poly D,L-lactic-co-glycolic acid.[93]

Developmental genetic defects in gastrointestinal function—e.g., sucrase-isomaltase deficiency and cystic fibrosis—may in the future be remedied through novel drug treatment[94] or by gene-targeting to gastrointestinal epithelial stem cells.[95–99] In the latter case, an understanding of physiological mechanisms that govern the maintenance of normal crypt architecture in human gastrointestinal tissues is important in devising strategies for the development of less transient forms of gene therapy. However, identification of the stem-cell component in the intestinal crypt is difficult, as the majority of markers for the proliferative compartment label predominantly the substem-cell component. The time taken to populate the whole crypt with cells derived from mutated stem cell(s) varies among tissues and species. In the mouse small intestine and colon, it is estimated that this time is approximately 6 and 1.5 months, respectively, whereas in the human colon it may be as long as two years. Whether this finding can be explained on the basis of different numbers of cells within the stem cell niche or on differing stem cell intermitotic intervals of different species or tissues is not yet clear. It is, therefore, likely that the development of ectopic grafting models using human gastrointestinal tissues will be important when studying the kinetics of the expression of transgenes introduced into the gut mucosa.

CONCLUSION

Investigating mechanisms that regulate mucosal development are important, since a number of human gastrointestinal diseases are associated with defective mucosal maturation. This chapter has focused largely on providing an overview of the ability of undifferentiated fetal endoderm to develop normally as ectopic grafts in the absence of conventional luminal and systemic signals present during fetal and postnatal life. This finding is particularly notable in murine intestinal isografts, where an intrinsic mucosal memory not only accurately recapitulates appropriate spatiotemporal development of epithelial cytodifferentiation, but also of mesenchymal, vascular, and immune cells within the ectopic grafts. Human fetal intestine also grows into well-developed xenografts, although additional luminal and/or systemic signals appear to be required to regulate appropriate epithelial cytodifferentiation pathways.

Ectopic transplantation of fetal intestinal tissues has demonstrated that this tissue possesses an intrinsic developmental program that is present prior to endodermal cytodifferentiation. These complex events are likely to be orchestrated, in part, by local transacting factors produced by neighbouring epithelial, mesenchymal, neuronal, and immune cells; by luminal stimuli present in gastrointestinal secretions; by direct cellular crosstalk between the heterotypic-cellular associations that form during intestinal crypt-villus formation; and by genetic information encoded within the functional epithelial stem-cell population that repopulates the intestinal grafts. These transplantation techniques represent a potentially exciting new approach to study novel clinical regimes aimed at treating gastrointestinal developmental disorders: for example, adopting epithelial stem-cell transplantation or gene targeting.

The author thanks Drs. Alan Phillips, Adrienne Morey, Anthony Whyte, and Geoff Morgan for their valuable advice and assistance in producing the figures.

REFERENCES

1. Cheng H, Leblond CP. Origin, differentiation and renewal of the four main epithelial cell types in the mouse small intestine. V. Unitarian theory of the origin of the four epithelial cell types. Am J Anat 1974;141:537–62.
2. Klein RM, McKenzie JC. The role of cell renewal in the ontogeny of the intestine. I. Cell proliferation patterns in adult, fetal, and neonatal intestine. J Pediatr Gastroenterol Nutr 1983;2:10–43.
3. Louvard D, Kedinger M, Hauri HP. The differentiating intestinal epithelial cell: establishment and maintenance of functions through interactions between cellular structures. Annu Rev Cell Biol 1992;8:157–95.
4. Henning DJ, Rubin DC, Shulman RJ. Ontogeny of the intestinal mucosa. In: Johnson LR, editor. Physiology of the gastrointestinal tract. 3rd ed. New York: Raven Press; 1994. p. 34–46.

5. Gordon JI, Hermiston ML. Differentiation and self-renewal in the mouse gastrointestinal epithelium. Curr Opin Cell Biol 1994;6:795–803.
6. Schmidt GH, Wilkinson MM, Ponder BAJ. Cell migration pathway in the intestinal epithelium: an in situ marker system using mouse aggregation chimeras. Cell 1985;40:425–9.
7. Winton DJ, Bluont MA, Ponder BAJ. A clonal marker induced by mutation in mouse intestinal epithelium. Nature 1988;333:463–6.
8. Winton DJ. Intestinal stem cells and clonality. In: Halter F, Winton D, Wright NA, editors. The gut as a model in cell and molecular biology. London: Kluwer Academic; 1997. p. 3–13.
9. Schmidt GH, Winton DJ, Ponder BAJ. Development of the pattern of cell renewal in the crypt-villus unit of chimaeric mouse small intestine. Development 1988;103:785–90.
10. Griffiths DRF, Davies SJ, Williams D, et al. Demonstration of somatic mutation and crypt clonality by X-linked enzyme histochemistry. Nature 1988;333:461–3.
11. Williams ED, Lowes AP, Williams D, Williams GT. A stem cell niche theory of intestinal crypt maintenance based on a study of somatic mutation in colonic mucosa. Am J Pathol 1992;141:773–6.
12. Williams ED. The stem cell niche hypothesis, mutation and neoplasia. In: Halter F, Winton D, Wright NA, editors. The gut as a model in cell and molecular biology. London: Kluwer Academic; 1997. p. 14–9.
13. Cambell F, Fuller CE, Williams GT, Williams ED. Human colonic stem cell mutation frequency with and without irradiation. J Pathol 1994;174:175–82.
14. Potten CS, Loeffler M. Stem cells: attributes, spirals, pitfalls and uncertainties. Lessons for and from the crypt. Development 1990;110:1101–20.
15. Winton DJ, Ponder BAJ. Stem cell organisation in mouse small intestine. Proc R Soc London Biol Sci 1990;241:13–8.
16. Jankowski JA, Wright NA. Epithelial stem cells in gastrointestinal morphogenesis, adaptation and carcinogenesis. Semin Cell Biol 1992;3:445–56.
17. Quellette AJ, Darmoul D, Selsted ME. Paneth cells, host defence and the crypt microenvironment. In: Halter F, Winton D, Wright NA, editors. The gut as a model in cell and molecular biology. London: Kluwer Academic; 1997. p. 82–8.
18. Henning SJ. Gastrointestinal development: an overview. In: Halter F, Winton D, Wright NA, editors. The gut as a model in cell and molecular biology. London: Kluwer Academic; 1997. p. 49–60.
19. Sanderson IR, Walker WA. Uptake and transport of macromolecules by the intestine: possible role in clinical disorders (an update). Gastroenterology 1993;104:633–9.
20. Savidge TC, Smith MW, Mayel-Afshar MS, et al. Selective regulation of epithelial gene expression in rabbit Peyer's patch tissue. Eur J Physiol 1994;428:391–9.
21. Dahlqvist A, Lindberg T. Development of the intestinal disaccharidase and alkaline phosphatase activities in the human fetus. Clin Sci (Colch) 1966;30:517–28.
22. Grand RJ, Watkins JB, Torti FM. Development of the human gastrointestinal tract: a review. Gastroenterology 1976;70:790–810.
23. Moxey PC, Trier JS. Specialised cell types in the human small intestine. Anat Rec 1978;191:269–86.
24. Nanthakumar NN, Henning SJ. Ontogeny of sucrase-isomaltase gene expression in rat intestine: responsiveness to glucocortocoids. Am J Physiol 1993;264:G306–11.
25. Shulman RJ, Schanler RJ, Heitkemper MA. Antenatal glucocorticoids decrease intestinal permeability in low birth weight infants. Pediatr Res 1994;35:255A.
26. Altmann G, Leblond CP. Factors influencing villus size in the small intestine of adult rats as revealed by transposition of intestinal segments. Am J Anat 1970;127:15–36.
27. Dowling RH. Small bowel adaptation and its regulation. Scand J Gastroenterol 1982;17:53–74.
28. Rubin DC, Levin MS. Regulation of epithelial cell proliferation and differentiation in small bowel adaptation after resection and during ontogeny. In: Halter F, Winton D, Wright NA, editors. The gut as a model in cell and molecular biology. London: Kluwer Academic; 1997. p. 217–36.
29. Greene HSN. The heterologous transplantation of embryonic mammalian tissues. Cancer Res 1943;3:809–15.
30. Toolan HW. Growth of embryonic gut and stomach in the exterior chest wall of adult cortisone-treated homologous hosts. Cancer Res 1957;17:707–14.
31. Phillips B, Grazet JC. Growth of human foetal tissues in mice treated with antilymphocyte serum. Nature 1969;222:1292–4.
32. Zinzar SN, Leitina BI, Tumyan BG, Svet-Moldavsky GJ. Very large organ-like structures formed by syngeneic foetal alimentary tract transplanted as a whole or in parts. Rev Europ Etudes Clin Et Biol 1971;XVI:455–8.
33. Ferguson A, Parrot DMV. Growth and development of "antigen-free" grafts of fetal mouse intestine. J Pathol 1972;106:95–102.
34. Ferguson A, Gerskowitch VP, Russel RI. Pre- and post-weaning disaccharidase patterns in isografts of fetal mouse intestine. Gastroenterology 1973;64:292–7.
35. Leapman SB, Deutsch AA, Grand RJ, Folkman J. Transplantation of fetal intestine: survival and function in a subcutaneous location in adult animals. Ann Surg 1974;179:109–14.
36. Povlsen CO, Skakkebaek NE, Rygaard J, Jensen G. Heterotransplantation of human foetal organs to the mouse mutant *nude*. Nature 1974;248:247–9.
37. Kendall K, Jumawan J, Koldovsky O, Krulich L. Effect of the host hormonal status on development of sucrase and acid β-galactosidase in isografts of rat small intestine. J Endocrinol 1977;74:145–6.
38. Kendall K, Jumawan J, Koldovsky O. Development of jejunoileal differences of activity of lactase, sucrase and acid β-galactosidase in isografts in fetal rat intestine. Biol Neonate 1979;36:206–14.
39. Jolma VM, Kendall K, Koldovsky O. Differences in the development of jejunum and ileum as observed in fetal rat intestinal isografts; possible implications related to the villus size gradient. Am J Anat 1980;158:211–5.
40. Montgomery RK, Sybicki MA, Grand RJ. Autonomous biochemical and morphological differentiation in fetal rat intestine transplanted at 17 and 20 days of gestation. Dev Biol 1981;87:76–84.
41. Schwartz MZ, Flye MW, Storozuk RB. Growth and function of transplanted fetal rat intestine: effect of cyclosporine. Surgery 1985;97:481–6.
42. Friedberg JS, Ryan DP, Driscoll SG, Folkman J. Human small bowel transplants into athymic mice and rats. Surg Forum 1985;36:375–8.
43. Winter HS, Hendren RB, Fox CH, et al. Human intestine matures as nude mouse xenografts. Gastroenterology 1991;100:89–98.
44. Rubin DC, Roth KA, Birkenmeier EH, Gordon JI. Epithelial cell differentiation in normal and transgenic mouse intestinal isografts. J Cell Biol 1991;113:1183–92.
45. Rubin DC, Swietlicki E, Roth KA, Gordon JI. Use of fetal intestinal isografts from normal and transgenic mice to study the programming of positional information along the duodenal-to-colonic axis. J Biol Chem 1992;267:15122–33.
46. Falk P, Roth KA, Gordon JI. Lectins are sensitive tools for defining the differentiation programs of mouse gut epithelial cell lineages. Am J Physiol 1994;266:G987–1003.
47. Rubin DC, Swietlicki E, Gordon JI. Use of isografts to study

proliferation and differentiation programs of mouse stomach epithelia. Am J Physiol 1994;267:G27–39.
48. Savidge TC, Morey AL, Ferguson DJP, et al. Human intestinal development in a severe-combined immunodeficient xenograft model. Differentiation 1995;58:361–71.
49. Shmakov AN, Morey AL, Ferguson DJP, et al. Conventional pattern of human intestinal proliferation in a severe-combined immunodeficient xenograft model. Differentiation 1995;59: 321–30.
50. Shmakov AN, Savidge TC. Cellular proliferation in the crypt epithelium of human small intestinal xenografts. Epith Cell Biol 1995;4:104–12.
51. Gould KA, Dove WF. Action of Min and Mom1 on neoplasia in ectopic intestinal grafts. Cell Growth Differ 1996;7:1361–8.
52. Mulvihill SJ, Stone MM, Debas HT, Fonkalsrud EW. The role of amniotic fluid in fetal nutrition. J Ped Surg 1985; 20:668–72.
53. Adrian TE, Soltesz G, MacKenzie LZ, et al. Gastrointestinal and pancreatic hormones in the human fetus and mother at 18–21 weeks of gestation. Biol Neonate 1995;67:47–53.
54. Whyte A, Locke D, Savidge T, License ST. Pig lymphocytes utilise mouse MADCAM-1 to enter fetal gut xenografts in *scid* mice. Cell Immunol 1997;25:38–44.
55. Savidge TC, Shmakov AN, Walker-Smith JA, Phillips AD. Intestinal proliferation and infection in childhood. In: Halter F, Winton D, Wright NA, editors. The gut as a model in cell and molecular biology. London: Kluwer Academic; 1997. p. 111–20.
56. Huang GTJ, Eckmann L, Savidge TC, Kagnoff MF. Infection of human intestinal epithelial cells with invasive bacteria upregulates apical intercellular adhesion molecule-1 (ICAM-1) expression and neutrophil adhesion. J Clin Invest 1996; 98:572–83.
57. Eckmann L, Stenson WF, Savidge TC, et al. Role of intestinal epithelial cells in the host secretory response to infection with invasive bacteria: bacterial entry induces epithelial prostaglandin H synthase-2 expression, and prostaglandin E2 and F2α production. J Clin Invest 1997;100:296–309.
58. Thulin JD, Kuhlenschmidt MS, Gelberg HB. Development, characterization and utilisation of an intestinal xenograft model for infectious disease research. Lab Invest 1991;65: 719–31.
59. Buisine MP, Devisme L, Savidge TC, et al. Mucin gene expression in human embryonic and foetal intestine. Gut 1998;43: 519–24.
60. Shaw-Smith CJ, Walters JR. Regional expression of intestinal genes for nutrient absorption. Gut 1997;40:5–8.
61. Traber PG. Mechanisms of sucrase-isomaltase gene transcription: implications for intestinal development. In: Halter F, Winton D, Wright NA, editors. The gut as a model in cell and molecular biology. London: Kluwer Academic; 1997. p. 253–65.
62. Le Dourain N, Bussonnet C, Chaumont F. Etude des capacites de differenciation et du role morphogene de l'endoderme pharyngien chez l'embryon d'oiseau. Ann Embryol Morpholog 1968;1:29–39.
63. Grumpel-Pinot M, Yasugi S, Mizuno T. Differentiation d'epitheliums endodermiques associes au mesoderme splanchnique. C R Acad Sci Hebd Seances Acad Sci D 1978;286: 117–21.
64. Kedinger M, Simon PM, Grenier JF, Haffen K. Role of epithelial-mesenchymal interactions in the ontogenesis of intestinal brush-border enzymes. Dev Biol 1981;86:339–47.
65. Lacroix B, Kedinger M, Simon-Assmann PM, Haffen K. Effects of human fetal gastroenteric mesenchymal cells on some developmental aspects of animal gut endoderm. Differentiation 1984;28:129–35.
66. Haffen K, Kedinger M, Simon-Assmann P. Cell contact dependent regulation of enterocyte differentiation. In: Lebenthal E, editor. Human gastrointestinal development. New York: Raven Press; 1989. p. 89–97.
67. del Bouno R, Fleming KA, Morey AL, et al. A nude mouse xenograft model of fetal intestine development and differentiation. Development 1992;114:67–73.
68. Yasugi S. Role of epithelial-mesenchymal interactions in differentiation of epithelium of vertebrate digestive organs. Dev Growth Differ 1993;35:1–9.
69. Duluc I, Freund J, Leberqueier C, Kedinger M. Fetal endoderm primarily holds the temporal and positional information required for mammalian intestinal development. J Cell Biol 1994;126:211–21.
70. Fritsch C, Simon-Assmann P, Kedinger M, Evans GS. Cytokines modulate fibroblast phenotype and epithelial-stroma interactions in rat intestine. Gastroenterology 1997; 112:826–38.
71. Cooke PS, Yonemura CU, Russell SM, Nicoll CS. Growth and differentiation of fetal rat intestine transplants: dependence on insulin and growth hormone. Biol Neonate 1986;49:211–8.
72. Alarid ET, Chen P, Schaudies RP, Nicoll CS. Differential effects of an antiserum to epidermal growth factor on the development of transplanted rat embryos and fetal structures in vivo. Growth Factors 1993;8:235–43.
73. Liu LM, Russel SM, Nicoll CS. Analysis of the role of basic fibroblast growth factor in growth and differentiation of transplanted fetal rat paws and intestines. Endocrinology 1990; 126:1764–70.
74. Kantak AG, Goldblum RM, Schwartz MZ, et al. Fetal intestinal transplants in syngeneic rats: a developmental model of intestinal immunity. J Immunol 1987;138:3191–6.
75. Mosley RL, Klein JR. Peripheral engraftment of fetal intestine into athymic mice sponsors T cell development: direct evidence for thymopoietic function of murine small intestine. J Exp Med 1992;176:1365–73.
76. Okuyama S, Rubin D, Woodley M, Peters MG. Regional expression of murine intestinal immune cells in normal and isografted intestine. Cell Immunol 1995;163:198–205.
77. Okuyama S, Rubin D, Streeter PR, Peters M. Murine isograft studies of gut immunity: recirculation and homing of mononuclear cells. Gastroenterology 1997;112:1241–9.
78. Verstijnen CPHJ, Kate JT, Arends JW, et al. Xenografting of normal colonic mucosa in athymic mice. J Pathol 1988;155: 77–85.
79. Vehmeyer K, Kunze E, Ciesiolka T, et al. Xenografts from a human colon carcinoma and its metastases: establishment, characterisation and differences in the pattern of carbohydrate-binding proteins. Anticancer Res 1989;9:277–84.
80. Joshi SS, Jackson JD, Sharp JD. Comparison of the growth and metastasis of four human intestinal tumor cell line xenografts. Tumour Biol 1989;10:117–25.
81. Shtivelman E, Namikawa R. Species-specific metastasis of human tumor cells in the severe combined immunodeficiency mouse engrafted with human tissue. Proc Natl Acad Sci U S A 1995;92:4661–5.
82. Tait IS, Evans GS, Flint N, Campbell FC. Colonic mucosal replacement by syngeneic small intestinal stem cell transplantation. Am J Surg 1994;167:67–71.
83. Campbell FC, Tait IS, Flint N, Evans GS. Transplantation of cultured small bowel enterocytes. Gut 1993;34:1153–5.
84. Tait IS, Evans GS, Kedinger M, et al. Progressive morphogenesis in vivo after transplantation of cultures small bowel epithelium. Cell Transplant 1994;3:33–40.
85. Tait IS, Flint N, Campbell FC, Evans GS. Generation of neomucosa *in vivo* by transplantation of dissociated rat postnatal small intestinal epithelium. Differentiation 1994;56:91–100.

86. Tait IS, Penny JI, Campbell FC. Does neomucosa induced by small bowel stem cell transplantation have adequate function? Am J Surg 1995;169:120–6.
87. Patel HRH, Tait IS, Evans GS, Campbell FC. Influence of cell interactions in a novel model of postnatal mucosal regeneration. Gut 1996;38:679–86.
88. Thompson JS, Sharp JG, Saxena SK, McCullagh KG. Stimulation of neomucosal growth by systemic urogastrone. J Surg Res 1987;42:402–10.
89. Thompson JS, Saxena SK, Sharp JG. Effect of urogastrone on intestinal regeneration is dose-dependent. Cell Tissue Kinet 1988;21:183–91.
90. Thompson JS, Saxena SK, Greaton C, et al. The effect of the route of delivery of urogastrone on intestinal regeneration. Surgery 1989;106:45–51.
91. Saxena SK. Thompson JS. Sharp JG. Role of epidermal growth factor in intestinal regeneration. Surgery 1992;111:318–25.
92. Sullivan PB, Brueton MJ, Tabara ZB, et al. Epidermal growth factor in necrotising enteritis. Lancet 1991;338:53–4.
93. Mooney DJ, Organ G, Vavanti JP, Langer R. Design and fabrication of biodegradable polymer devices to engineer tubular tissues. Cell Transplant 1994;3:203–10.
94. Savidge TC, Shmakova A. Human gastrointestinal drug delivery; an experimental chimeric approach. J Drug Target 1995;3:71–4.
95. Engelhardt JF, Yankaskas JR, Wilson JM. In vivo retroviral gene transfer into human bronchial epithelial of xenografts. J Clin Invest 1992;90:2598–607.
96. Hyde SC, Gill DR, Higgins CF, et al. Correction of the ion transport defect in cystic fibrosis transgenic mice by gene therapy. Nature 1993;362:250–4.
97. Henning SJ. Gene transfer into the intestinal epithelium. Adv Drug Del Rev 1995;17:341–7.
98. Jacomino M, Lau C, James SZ, et al. Gene transfer into fetal rat intestine. Hum Gene Ther 1996;7:1757–62.
99. Slorach EM, Dorin JR. Towards gene correction for cystic fibrosis in intestinal stem cells. In: Halter F, Winton D, Wright NA, editors. The gut as a model in cell and molecular biology. London: Kluwer Academic; 1997. p. 34–46.

Index

Absorptive capacities, 134
Absorptive cells, 310
  terminal web of, 58
Acetylation, 104
Achalasia, 216
Acinetobacter, 281
Actin, 26, 57
Actin core filaments, 58–59
Actin cytoskeleton, 72
Actin filaments, 57
Activation domains, 19
Activator domain, 14
Activators, 16
Activins, 46
ADA expression, 23–24
Adapters, 14
Addressins, 184
Adenosine deaminase
  modular regulation of, *15*
Adenosine monophosphate, 253
Adenylate cyclase, 71
Adjuvant activity, 287
Adrenalectomy, 38, 45
Adrenergic agonists, 263
Adrenocorticotropic hormone (ACTH), 37
Aerobes, 279–281
  bacterial counts, *280*
  ratio, 284
  suppression of, 284
Aeromonas, 281
Aganglionosis, 202–203, 206
Aging, 105–106
Agonists, 74
Albumin, serum
  in breast milk, 227, *228, 233*, 234
  in colostrum, *228*
  function, *232*
Alcoholism, 263
Aldohexose transport, 131
Alkaline phosphatase, 40, 249
  EGF and, 45
Allergies, 78, 287
Alport's syndrome, 89
Amino acids
  absorption of, 45
  uptake, *140*
Amino acid transport, 125, *126*, 132
  abnormalities, 139–140
  initial, *130*
  intake of, 134
  molecular mechanism, 135
Aminopeptidase N (APN), 22
Amniotic fluid, 43, 48
  amylase in, 261
  nutrients in, 246
  swallowing, 134, 245
Amphiregulin, 44
α-Amylase, 227
  antibacterial effect of, 270
  in colostrum, *228*
  function, *232*, 235
  in human milk, *228*, 235, 270
  milk amylase, 270
  structure, 265
Amylase activity
  development of, *267*
  pancreatic, 247, 264–265
  salivary, 247, 261
Anaerobes, 281–282
  bacterial counts, *280*
  facultative, 279–281, 284
Anal sphincter muscle, 5
Anaphylactic shock, 189
Anergy, 188–189
Anion exchange activity, 40
Anterior intestinal portal, 2
Anterior-posterior axis, 3–8, 10
  gene regulation, 20–22

Anterior-posterior regions, *3*
Antibacterial peptides, 20
Antibiotics, 285, 286
  and neonatal intensive care, 282
Antibody switching, 180–183
α1-Antichymotrypsin, *252*
Antigen uptake, 75
Anti-inflammatory factors, *252*
Antimicrobial peptides, 152–153
  function, 153
  structure, 153
Antimicrobial proteins, 147
  in human milk, *252*
Antioxidants, *252*
α₁-Antitrypsin, 235
  in colostrum, *228*
  function, *232*
  in human milk, *228*, 235, 270
Anus, 1
Apical membrane, 72, 129
Apolipoprotein, 23, 250
Apolipoprotein genes, 24, 250
Apolipoprotein regulatory factor (ARP), 21
Appendix, 2
ASBT, 136, 137
Ascorbate, *252*
Aspartic proteinases, 261
Autoimmune conditions, 189
Axial tissues, 5

B Cells
  in adult lamina propria, 167
  in fetal lamina propria, 165, 172
  IgA, 167
  TGF and, 48
B Lymphocytes, 175–190
  antibody diversity, 178–180
  antigen dependence, 181
  cytokines and, 185–186
  differentiation, 185–186
  migration, 175
  origins, 177
  precursors, 178
  subsets, 180
  surface antigen expression, *180*
Bacteria, intestinal, *280*
Bacterial fermentation, 255
Bacterial populations, 134
Bacteroides, 281, 282, 283, 284
  bacterial counts, *280*
  breastfed vs bottlefed, *283*
Barrett's esophagus, 150
Basal transcription factors, 14
Basement membrane, 84, 88–97, *86*
  crosstalk with CDX, 96–97
  formation, *87*
  homeobox genes and, 94–97
  molecules, 92–94
  muscular, 89
  subepithelial, 89
Basolateral membrane, 72, 131
Basolateral transporters, 132
Belt desmosome, 58
Betacellulin, 44
Betaglucosidase, 247
Betaglycan, 46
bHLH factors, 25–26
Bifidobacteria, 255, 281, 283, 284
  bacterial counts, *280*
  breastfed vs bottlefed, *283*
Bile acids
  conjugation, 50
  excretion, 250
Bile acid transport, 126, 131–132, 136
  abnormalities, 140
  rates, 136
Bile ducts, 8
Bile salts, 38, 249

  absorption of, 38
Bile salt-dependent lipase
  in human milk, 268–269
Bile salt-stimulated lipase (BSSL), 227, 235, 249
  in colostrum, *228*, 235
  function, *232*
  in human milk, *228*, 235
Bile salt transport, 38–39
  glucocorticoids and, 38
Biochemical maturation, 247–250
BMP expression, 7, 30
Bone morphogenetic proteins (BMP), 46
Breast milk, 78, 227–240
  serum albumin in, 227, 234
  antichymotryptic activity of, 270
  anti-inflammatory factors in, *252*
  antimicrobial agents in, *252*
  antitryptic activity of, 270
  digestive enzymes in, 268–270
  EGF in, 44
  fortifiers, 238
  function, 227, 240
  IgG in, 75, 76, 234
  immunoglobulins in, 234
  malnutrition and, 230, 269
  maternal infection, 231
  nitrogen in, 229–231
  oral contraceptives and, 231
  preterm milk, 230
  protection against infection, 286
  proteins in, *228*
  protein gene expression, 228
  proteolytic activity, 270
  role of, 250–253
  TGF in, 44, 48
  total protein in, 229–237
  volume, 229, 230
  whey-casein ratio, 229, 231
  whey proteins, *233*
Breastfed vs bottlefed infants, 238–240
  intestinal flora, 255, 283, 284
Bronchus-associated lymphoid tissues (BALT), 175, 183
Brunner's glands
  absence of, 29
Brushborder cytoskeleton, 58–59
Brushborder enzymes
  development of, 103–119
  regulation of, 40
Brushborder enzyme activity, 249
  EGF and, 45
Brushborder formation, 57–59
Brushborder lactase, 115
Brushborder membrane
  transport system, 125, 135
Bursa, 177

E-Cadherin, 167
Caenorhabditis elegans, 47, 293–296
  endoderm induction, 295–296
  GI tract development, 294–295
Calbindin-D9k gene, 23, 112
Calcium
  absorption of, 45, 59
  transport, 45
Caldesmon, 59
Calmodulin, 59
Caloric deficit, 231
Campylobacter, 286
Carbohydrate intolerance, 139
Carbohydrate malabsorption, 137–139
Carbonic anhydrase 1 (CA1), 23, 83, 112
Carboxypeptidases, 265
Carnivores, 134
β-Carotene, *252*
Cascades, 14
Casein, 227
  changes during lactation, 231–232

in colostrum, *228*, 229
   developmental pattern, *228*
   functions, *232*
   in human milk, *228*, 231–232
Casein mRNA, 228
CAT reporter transgene, 26
Cathepsin E, 261
Caudal intestinal portal (CIP), *7*
   formation, 2
Caudal-related homeodomain factor (CDX), 22, 95–97, 113
   binding sites, 23
   in colon cancers, 95
   expression, 27, 95–96
   function, 112–113
   overexpression, 95
   regulation, 95–96
Caveolae, 71
Caveolin, 71
Caveolin-coated vesicles, 71
CDX genes, 112
CDX proteins, 117
Ceca, 5
   formation, *7*
Cecropins, 153
Celiac disease, 189
Cell growth, inhibition of, 46
Chloramphenicol acetyl transferase (CAT), *24*
   expression, 26
Cholecystokinin, 214, 221
Cholesterol, 71
Cholic:chenodeoxycholic ratio, 249–250
Cholinergic agonists, 263
Chromatin, 16–17
Chymosin, 261
Chymotrypsin, 265
   development of, *267*
Chymotrypsinogen, 265
Circadian rhythm, 134
Cis-regulatory modules, 15
   definition, 15
Cis-regulatory sequences, 13–14
   organization, 14
Cis-regulatory systems
   modularity in, 15
Citrobacter, 279–280
Clathrin, 71–72, 74
Clathrin-coated pits/vesicles, 71–72, 73, 75
Cloaca, *3*, 5
   formation, *7*
Clostridia, 281, 282
   bacterial counts, *280*
   breastfed vs bottlefed, *283*
   colitis, 286
   sudden infant death syndrome, 286
Coactivators, 14
Cobalamin
   in human milk, 236
Colipase, 266, *268*
Colitis, 91, 94
Collagens, 84, *86*, *87*, 89–92
   expression, 90
Colon, 21
   adenocarcinomas, 108
   adenomas, 108
   development, 108–109
   disorders, 223
   immunity and, *149*
   lactase-phlorizin expression, 116–117
   motility, 222–223
   sucrose-isomaltase expression, 108–109
Colon endoderm, 88
Colonization resistance, 284–285
Colostrum, 229–230
   serum albumin in, 234
   α-amylase activity in, 235
   antiproteases in, 270
   α_1-antitrypsin, 235
   BSSL, 249
   EGF in, 237
   IGF-I in, 237, 251
   IGFBP in, 237
   immunoglobulins in, 234, 252–253
   intestinal growth and, 133
   lysozyme in, 235
   peroxidase activity in, 235–236
   proteins in, 229
   vitamin b_{12}-binding, 236
   whey proteins in, *227*, 229
Compartment for uncoupling of receptor and ligand (CURL), 72

Complement 3 (C3), *252*
Congenital megacolon, 202–204, 206
   See also Hirschsprung's disease
Connective tissue, differentiation of, 40
Coprostanol, 284
Core rootlets, 58
Corticosterone, EGF and, 45
Corticosterone surge, 136
Cortisol, *252*
Covalent modification, 16
Cranial-caudal axis, 1
Cripto, 44
Crohn's disease, 150, 190, 255
Crosstalk, 96–97, *253*
Crypt, 19–21
   formation, 64
Crypt cells
   production rate, 45
   proliferation, 310
   structure, 57, 67
   TGF and, 48
Crypt labeling index, 43
Crypt-to-villus axis, 1, 2, 3, 248
   gene regulation, 20–22
   transport systems, 132
Crypt-villus conjunction, 83
Cryptdin gene promoter, 155
Cryptdins, 154–156
   in goblet cells, 157
   immunoreactivity, 156
Crypts, 83, 307–308
   fission, 307
   maturation, 307
Crypts of Lieberkühn, 57, 150, 307
Crytdins, 84
Cyclosporin, 39–40
Cystic fibrosis, 127
   abdominal distress, 139
   defensin in, 153
   gastric lipase/dietary fat, 249
Cystinuria, 139
Cytochalasin D, 72
Cytodifferentiation, 1–5, 88
   regulators of, 308
Cytodifferentiation and proliferation, 307
   molecular regulation, 313
Cytokeratin, 57–67
   distribution, 62–63
   expression, *63*, 64–66
   function, 66
   structure/composition, 59–63
   See also Keratin
Cytokeratin filaments, 66
Cytokeratin gene expression
   regulation of, 61–62
Cytokines, 255
   B lymphocyte differentiation, 185–186
   major functions, *166*
   T cells and, *166*, *182*
Cytoprotection, 250, *252*
Cytoskeleton, 58–59
   proteins, 65

Danio rerio. *See* Zebrafish
Decorin, 90
Defensins, *149*, 150–159
   chromosome mapping, 157–158
   enteric, 157
   killing mechanism, 154
   in Paneth cells, 154
   structure, 153–154
Defensin-encoding mRNAs, 156
Defensin genes, 155–159
   antimicrobial activity of, 158–159
   expression, 155–157
   hematopoietic, 157–158
   myeloid, 157
   structure, 155–156
Defensin precursors, 155
Dendritic cells, 48, 177
   dome, 169
Deoxyribonucleic acid (DNA)
   binding, 16
   inhibition of, 29
   intramodular 16
Dephosphorylation, 16
Desmin
   phosphorylation of, 61
Desmosomes, 57
Developmental time axis
   gene regulation, 20

Dexamethasone, 38
   with T4, 39
Dextrocardia, 9
Diabetes, 28, 189
Diarrhea, 138–139, 286
Dietary shifts
   during gestation, 133
   perinatal period, 133
   suckling stage, 133–134
Diffuse esophageal leiomyomatosis, 89
Digestion
   development, 237–238
Digestive enzymes, 20
   hormonal regulation, 268
   in human milk, 268–270
   secretion, 261–270
Dimerization, 18
Disaccharidases, 247
   deficiency, 286
DNA-binding domains, 17–19
Domain formation, 17
Dorsal-ventral axis, 1, 8–9
Dorsal-ventral patterning, 8–9
Drosphila melanogaster, 47, 296–301, 303
   copper cell, 299, 301
   gut development, 297–298
   gut morphogenesis, 298
   hindgut, 298
   larval GI, 297
   midgut, 299, *300*
   morphogenesis, *297*
   "parautocrine" loop, 299
   specification of endoderm, 298
   ultrabithorax, 299
   winged helix proteins, 298
Duodenal atresia, incidence, 9
Duodenum, 21, 22
   contractile activity, 220
   pressure, 220
   transport systems, 132
Dynamins, 73–74
   expression, 73
   role, 73
Dysmotility, 140

E Blastomere, 294–296
EGF gene, 44
EGF receptor, 44, 251, 264
   distribution, 45
Elastase 1, 265
Electrolytes
   absorption of, 45
Embryogenesis, 2
EMS Blastomere, 295
"End-product" genes, 19
Endocytic compartments, 76–78
Endocytic pathways, 72–73
   regulation of, 73
Endocytosis, 71–78
   acute regulation, 74
   apical, *75*
   definition, 71
   in polarized cells, 72
Endoderm, 3
   differentiation, 4–5
   regionalization, 29
Endosomes, 75
   apical recycling, *72*, 73, 76
   basolateral, *72*
   early, *72*, 74
   late, *72*, 73, 74
   sorting, *72*, 74, 75
Endothelin, 205–206
   defect, 213
Endothelin receptor, 205, 206, 213
Endotubin, *72*, 76
Enhancers, 14, 17
   definition, 14
   intestinal-specific, 23–25
Enhancer binding protein (EBP), 28–29
Enhancer trapping, 297, *300*
Entactin, 84, 89
Enteral nutrition, 245
Enteric ganglia, 197
   precursors to, 201
Enteric nervous system, 197–207, 212–213
   abnormalities, 202–203
   as "gut brain," 211
   maturation, 212
   molecular markers, *199*
   precursors, 202

progenitors, 207
    signaling pathway, 205
Enteric neuroblasts, 198
Enterobacteria, 279–280, 283
    global differences, 282
    breastfed vs bottlefed, *283*
Enterococci, 280
    bacterial counts, *280*
    breastfed vs bottlefed, *283*
Enterocyte maturation, 59
Enterocytes, 20, 58, 307
    absorptive, 149
Enteroendocrine cells, 20, 213–214, 307, *312*
    coexpression of neuropeptides, 312
    distribution of, 311–313
    gene regulation in, 25
    keratin in, 66
    peptides, 214
    serotonin expression, 313
Enteroglucagon, 214
Enterokinase, 265
Enterokinase activity, 249
Enteropeptidase, 265
    activity, 265
    deficiency, 265
    role, 265
Enzyme synthesis/secretion, 263–264
Epidermal growth factor (EGF), 44–46, 250–251
    action of, 250
    biologic effect, 45
    in colostrum, *228*
    distribution, 44
    function, *232, 252*
    in human milk, *228*, 237, *252*
    lipase activity and, 264
    role, 250, 264, 268
    structure, 44
Epidermolysis bullosa, 89, 93
Epimorphin, 97
Epiregulin, 44
Epithelial cells, 313
    antimicrobial peptides in, 152
    development, 57–67
    differentiation, 93, 96, 308, *309*
    in fetal gut, 171
    lineage determination, 148, 310
    proliferation, 42, 48, 96
    proximodistal markers, *85*
    regulators of, 308, 313
    TGF as inhibitor of, 47
    turnover, 171
    types, 84
Epithelial growth, 97
Epithelial-mesenchymal complementarity, 91–92
Epithelial-mesenchymal interactions, 3–5, 86–88, 97
Epithelial-to-mesenchymal transition, 47
Escherichia coli, 279–280, 284
    global differences, 282
    urinary tract infection, 285
    virulence factors, 285
Esophageal body
    disorders of, 215
    motility in, 215
Esophagitis, 215
Esophagus, 214–215
Esterase gene, 30
Eubacteria, *280*
Eubacterium lentum, 284
Eukaryotic cells, 71
    transcription in, 13
Eukaryotic gene regulation, 14–19
Exopeptidases, 265
Extracellular matrix, 39, 213
    cytokines, 178
    induction of, 48
    make-up of, 88–89
    TGF and, 47
Ezrin, 59

Facilitators, 17
Fasting, 43
Fat
    absorption of, 250
    dietary, increasing, 249
    digestion of, 262–263
    milk, 269
Fatty acid binding proteins (FABP), 21–22, 83
    expression, 40
    patterns, 40
    regulation, 40

Fecal analysis, 237–238, 284
Fecal contamination, 279
Feed tolerance/intolerance, 221, 222, 223
Feedback loops, 14
Fermentation, 138
Fibronectin, 91, *252*
Fibulins, 90
Filament formation, 61
Fimbrin, 58–59
First feed, 213–214
Fodrin, 58–59
Folate-binding protein, 236–237
    in colostrum, *228*
    function, *232*
    in human milk, *228*, 236–237
Foregut
    differentiation, *7*
    formation, 2–9
    patterning, 6
    ventralization, 8–9
Fork head, 29–30
Fructose absorption rates, 136
Fructose-glucose-galactose malabsorption, 138
Fructose malabsorption, 138–139
Fructose transport, 124, 131, *136*
    luminal fructose and, 141
Fusion proteins, 17

Galactose absorption, 124
Galactosyltransferase, 233
Ganglioblasts, 198
Gastric acid output, 237
Gastric electrical slow-wave, 217
Gastric emptying, 217–218
Gastric lipase, 263–264
Gastric lipase activity, 262–264
Gastric motility, disorders of, 218
Gastric motor activity, 217
Gastric pH, 237
Gastrin, 214, 221, 248
    pH, 248
Gastritis, 150
Gastroenteritis, 139
Gastroesophageal reflux, 215, 216
GATA, 30
    function, 9
    LPH promoter and, 117
    proteins, 112
Gene expression, 19–27
    regulation of, 103–105
Gene regulation, 15
General transcription factors (GTF), 14
    TFII, 14
Genomic regulatory systems, 13–14
Gliadin, 189
Glial cells, 197, 198
β-Globin locus, 17
Glomerulonephritis, 89
Glucagon, 25, 112
Glucoamylase, 247
Glucoamylase activity, EGF and, 46
Glucocorticoids, 37–39, 92
    biochemistry, 37
    biology, 38
    in dietary regulation, 136
    lactase and, 38
    structure, 37
Glucocorticoid receptors, 37–38
Glucocorticoid response element, 265
Glucocosteroid-binding globulin, 38
Glucose absorption, 45, 124
    transcellular, 131
Glucose-galactose malabsorption, 138
Glucose transport, *128*, 129–131
    brushborder membrane, 130
    fetal, 248
    initial, *130*
    prenatal, 130
Glucose transporters (GLUT), 124–125, 135–139
    expression, 136
    mechanisms, 136
GLUT mRNA, 135, *136*
    expression, *137*
Glutamine, 133, 253
Glutamine synthetase activity, 249
Gluten-induced enteropathy, 139
Gluten-sensitive enteropathy, 189
Glycine transport, 45
Glycocalyx, 58
Glycosylation, 61, 64
Goblet cells, 20, 83, *312*

categories, 151
distribution of, 310–311
gene regulation in, 25
in inflammation, 149
keratin in, 66
mucus granules, 310
Golgi apparatus, 42
Goodpasture's syndrome, 89
Gram-positive bacteria, 282
Gram-positive cocci
    bacterial counts, *280*
"Ground state," 8–9
Growth factors, 20, 313
    in human milk, 237
GTPase, 73, 74
Guanylin, 23
Guanylyl cyclase, 23
Gut, 1
    characteristics, 83–85
    development, 84–85
Gut closure, 254
Gut endoderm, 1, 4

Haptocorrin
    in colostrum, *228*
    function, *232*
    in human milk, *228*, 236
Hartnup disease, 139
Heart, 9
Helix-loop-helix factors, 18, 29
Hemidesmosomes, *91*
Hensen's node, *7*, 9
Heparan sulfate proteoglycan. See Perlecan
Heparin-binding EGF, 44
Hepatic development, 7
Hepatic fibrosis, 48
Hepatic growth factor-scatter factor, 97
Hepatic nuclear factor (HNF), 21–22, 28, 111–112
    absence of, 28
    binding sites, 23–24
    expression, 7
    family, 29–30
    gene family, 27–28
    LPH gene and, 117
Heregulin, 44
Hindbrain, 5
Hindgut
    differentiation, *7*, 29
    formation, 2–7
Hirschsprung's disease, 94, 202–204, 206, 213, 223
    SOX and, 206
L-Histidine transport, 134
Histone, 149
Hollow visceral myopathy, 222
Homeobox (HOX) genes, 10, 30, 94–98, 113
    detection, 6
    enteric nervous system, 213
    expression, 5–7, 94–95
    function, 5–7, 94
    overexpression, 213
Host defense-effectors, 255
HOX protein, 111
Human growth hormone (hGH) mRNA, 155, 313
Human milk fortifiers, 238
    preterm formula, 238
Humoral controls
    development of, 213–214
Hydrolases
    brushborder, 103
    digestive, 83
Hypolactasia, 116

IgA
    in colostrum, *228*, 234
    in human milk, *228*, 234, *252*
    induction, 181
    mucosal, 175
    polymeric, 252
    responses, 182, 187
    role of, 177
    subclasses, 177
    uptake, 72
IgA deficiency, 189
IgA secretion, 167, 176–177, 286
    in colostrum, 229, 234
IgA synthesis, 176–177
    TGF and, 48
IgA transport, 75, 147
IgD, 180–182
IgE, 181–183

IGF receptor genes, 41–42
IGF RNA transcripts, 42
IGF-binding proteins (IGFBP), 40–42, 251
    actions, 42
    in colostrum, *228*, 237
    function, *232*
    in human milk, *228*, 237
IGFBP mRNA, 43
IgG
    in altered B lymphocyte function, 189–190
    in colostrum, *228*
    in endosomes, 75
    in human milk, *228*, 234
    transport, 75
IgM, 180–183
    in altered B lymphocyte function, 190
    in colostrum, *228*
    in human milk, *228*, 234
IgM transport, 75
Ileum, 22
    transport systems, 132
Immune homeostasis, 48
Immune system of gut (GALT), 165, 183, 188
Immune system
    intestinal flora and, 286
    TGF and, 48
Immunity, innate, 147–159, 314
    acquired, 147
    enteric, 147
    mucosal imprinting, 314
    peptide mediators, *149*
Immunity, mucosal, 75
Immunity, passive, 75, 78
Immunization, 187
Immunosuppressive drugs, 99
Inductive tissues, 176–177
Inflammation, 48
Inflammatory bowel disease, 94, 190
Innervation, 198
Insulin, 40–44
Insulin genes
    regulation, 29
Insulin-like growth factors (IGF), 40–44, 237
    biology, 42–43
    in colostrum, *228*, 237
    deficiency, 44
    distribution, 42
    elimination of function, 43–44
    function, *232*
    gene, 41
    in human milk, *228*, 237, 251–252
    mitogenic activities, 42
    proliferative effect of, 43
    as survival factor, 43
Integrins, 84, *89*, 90, 93
Integrin signaling, 97
Intercellular communication, 293–303
Interferon, 165, 171
    production, 172, 181
Interleukin (IL), 171
    production, 172, 181
    roles of various, 185–186, 255
Intermediate filaments (IF), 57–58
    cellular organization, 62
    classes, 59
Interstitial matrix, 88
Intervillus epithelium, 20
Intestinal bacteria, 279–287
    biochemical reactions, 284
    breastfeeding and, 282–284
    colonization resistance, 284–285
    competition, 285
    influence on infants, 284–287
    major groups, *280*
    modulation, 284
    neonatal infections, 285–286
    suppression, 284
    translocation, 285, 286
Intestinal barrier, 75–76
Intestinal cells of Cajal, 213, 217
Intestinal epithelium, 43, 103
    cell lineages, 148–149
    cellular specialization, 65
    gene regulation, 21–25
    markers, 65
    in mucosal immunity, 148
    organization, 19–20
    renewal process, 147
Intestinal flora, 255, 279–287
Intestinal growth, 246

Intestinal lumen, 245–256
    role, 245
Intestinal mass, increase in, 130
Intestinal pseudo-obstruction, 222, *223*
Intestinal surface, 127
Intestinal trefoil factor (ITF), 25
Intracellular signaling
    alterations due to, 94
    TGF mediated, 47
Intraluminal nutrients, 246
Iodothyronine deiodinase, 39
Irritable bowel syndrome, 138
Isoactin, 26
Isomaltase activity
    fetal, 247

Jejunum, 21, 22
    transport systems, 132
Junctional complex, 58, 124
Junction types, 58
Juvenile polyposis coli, 47

Kallikrein, 265
Keratin, 59
    cellular distribution, *64*
    classification, 60
    expression, 59–60, 64–66
    post-translational modification, 61
    regulation of, 65–66
Keratin intermediate filaments, 60–61
Keratin mRNA, 65
Keratin tonofilaments, 57
Keratinocyte growth factor, 97
Kinase activation, 47, 75
    inhibition, 47
    cyclin-dependent, 47
Klebsiella, 279–280, 283
    global differences, 282
    septicemia, 285
    urinary tract infection, 285
"Knockout," 43
Krüppel gene, 15
Krüppel-like factor, 29

α-Lactalbumin
    in colostrum, *228*, 229
    function, *232*
    in human milk, *228*, 231, 232–233
Lactase
    detection, *84*
    development, 83
    fetal, 247
    glucocorticoid and, 38
    regulation, 247
Lactase activity
    changes in, 38
    EGF and, 45–46
Lactase-phlorizin hydrolase (LPH), 23, 104, *106*, 112
    expression, 115–117
    fetal, 247
    precursor, 118
    promoter, 117
    regulation, 115–119
    structure, 118
    synthesis, 117
Lactation, 228–229
    exercise during, 231
    feedback inhibition of, 229
    protein intake during, 231
Lactobacilli, 255, 281, 283
    bacterial counts, *280*
    breastfed vs bottlefed, *283*
Lactoferrin, 233–234, 252
    in colostrum, *228*, 229, 234, 252
    excretion, *238*
    in feces, 237–238
    function, *232*, 233, 252
    in human milk, *228*, 231, 233–234, 251, *252*
    intake, *238*
    in low-birth-weight infants, 238
    structure, 233
Lactogenesis, 228
Lactoperoxidase, 236
    in colostrum, *228*, 236
    function, *232*
    in human milk, *228*, 236
Lactose malabsorption, 247
Lamina propria, 83, 165
    fetal, 165
Laminins, 84, *86*, *87*, 89

deficiency, 94
expression, 90
Hirschsprung's disease, 94
role of, 92–94
Large intestine, 5
    formation, 7
Left-right asymmetry, 9
Left-right axis, 9
Leucine uptake, 132
Leucine zipper factors, 18, 28
Limb bud, 5
Lipase, 249–250
    carboxylester, 266
    development, 265–266
    development of, *267*, *268*
    fat digestion, 266
    gastric, 263
    lingual, 263, 264
    pancreatic, 264, 266–269
    pregastric, 263
Lipase activity, 249, 251, 264
    lower, 266
Lipids, *252*
Lipid binding protein, 83
Lipolytic enzymes, 249
Liver, 8
Locus control region, 16
    definition, 17
Looping, 9
Low-birth-weight infants, 238
Low-density lipoprotein uptake, 72
Lower esophageal sphincter, 215–216
    disorders of, 216
    neural mechanisms, 215
    pressure, 215
LPH cDNA, 115
LPH mRNA, 115–118, 247–248
    processing, 118
    translation, 118
LPH promoter, 117
LPH protein expression, 116
Lumican, 5
Luminal and circulatory signals, 308–310, 311, 313
    nonluminal, 313
Luminal molecules, 255–256
Lung, 8
Lymphocytes, 147
    homing, *184*
    memory, 184
    recruitment of, 185
Lymphocytes, intraepithelial, 167, *168*,
    development, 172
    in immune system, 176
Lymphocytes, lamina propria, 165–167
Lymphoid tissue, 165–169
Lysosomal compartments, 77
Lysosomes, 73, 76–78
    giant, 77–78
Lysozyme, 150, 152, 157, 253
    in colostrum, *228*
    in human milk, *228*, 234–235, *252*, 253
    lactoferrin and, 234–235
    role, 253
Lysozyme mRNA, 151

M Cells, 75, 169, 245, 254
Macromolecular transport, 254–255
Macrophages, 168–169
Macrophage chemotactic protein-1 (MCP-1), 255
Macula adherens, 58
Magainin, 153
Malabsorption, 137–139
Malformations, 9–10
Malnutrition, 246, 269
Malrotation, 9, 222
Maltase activity, 253
    EGF and, 45
    fetal, 247, 253
Mammary gland function, 227
Mannose-6-phosphate receptor, 42, 46, 73
MASH, 206–207
Maternal infection, 231
Maternal nutrition, 230–231
Matrilysin, 157
Matrix-attachment regions (MAR), 17, 23
Maturational factors, *252*
Meconium, in utero passage, 223
Megacystis-microcolon–intestinal hypoperistalsis, 222
Membrane proteins, 73

Mesenchymal cells, 84
    properties, 88
Mesoderm, 3, 9
Messenger RNA, 13
Metalloprotease, 93
Metalloproteinase gene, 40
Metallothionein, 43
MHC class I & II, 169
    expression, 170–172, 255–256
Microbial colonization pattern, 282–284
Microvilli, 57
    apical, 103
    organization, 59
    structure, 59
Microvillus core, 58
Microvillus membrane, 59
Midceca, 5
Midgut
    differentiation, 7
    formation, 2–7
Milk fat globules, 263
Milk protein gene expression, 227–229
Milk volume, 229–230
Mitogen-activated-extracellular-related kinase (MEK-1), 97
Mitosis, 61
Modularity, 14–19
    complexity, 15–16
    definition, 14
Modules, 14–19
    architecture, 16
    cis-regularity, 17
    insulator, 17
    specialized, 17
    types, 17
Monosaccharides, transcellular absorption, 125
Monosaccharide transport, 248
Morphogenesis, 84
Motilin, 214
Motor activity, 211–223
    normal, 211–212
    structure, 212
    timetable, 211
Mouth, 1
Mucins, 252
Mucin genes, 83
Mucopolysaccharide barrier, 149
Mucosa-associated lymphoid tissues (MALT), 175, 183
Mucosal addressin cell adhesion molecule (MAdCAM), 166, 184–185, 314
Mucosal development, 309
Mucosal immune system, 175–190
    oral tolerance, 188–189, 287
Mucosal mass, 127
Mucosal memory, 315
Mucus, 20
Mucus cells, 83
Mucus gel layer, 254
Müllerian inhibiting substance, 46
Muscle-specific gene regulation, 25–27
Muscular dystrophy, 89
Muscularis, 25, 43
Muscularis mucosae, 25–26
Muscularis propria, 25–26
Mutagenesis, 294
Myeloperoxidase, 236
    in colostrum, 228, 236
    function, 232
    in human milk, 228
Myosin, 57
Myosins, 59

Na^+-K^+ATPase expression, 40
Necrotizing enterocolitis, 139, 222, 254, 285–286, 315
    defensin mRNA expression in, 157
Neonatal infections, 285–286
Neural crest, 197–202, 203, 212
    differentiation, 201–202
    migration, 198–201
Neural tube, 5
Neuregulin, 30, 97
Neurofilaments
    phosphorylation of, 61
Neurons, 197
    subclasses, 201
Neuropathic pseudo-obstruction, 218
Neuropeptides, 20
Neurotensin, 214
Neurotensin-neuromedin N, 25

Nidogen, 84, 86, 87, 89–92
Nitric oxide, 214
NKX, 8, 30
Nonerythroid spectin, 59
Nonprotein nitrogen in colostrum, 230
Nonsplanchnic mesoderm, 4
Notochord, 9
Nuclear lamins
    phosphorylation of, 61
Nucleotides, 253
Nutrient transport, 123–141
    affinity constants, 128
    birth and suckling, 129
    categorized, 131
    derangements, 137–140
    development, 128–137
    during gestation, 134
    measuring, 126–127
    molecular mechanisms, 134–137
    postnatal onset, 136–137
    prenatal development, 129
    prenatal onset, 134–136
    regulatory mechanisms, 127–128
    systems, 124–126, 132–133, 134–137
    uptake capacity, 128
    weaning, 129–130

Oligosaccharides, 252, 253
Omnivores, 134
Opsinins, 252
Oral contraceptives, 231
Oral tolerance, 188–189, 287
Oxytocin, 229

P1 Blastomere, 295
Pancreas
    atrophy of, 48
    organogenesis, 8
Pancreatic enzymes, 249
    secretory, 264–268
Pancreatic lipase-related proteins, 266, 268
Paneth cells, 20, 21, 84, 245, 307, 311, 312
    antimicrobial proteins/peptides in, 150
    cryptdin genes in, 155
    defence function, 148–150
    defensins in, 154–158
    deficiency, 151–152
    differentiation, 147, 150–151
    exocytic secretion by, 150
    gene regulation in, 25
    granules, 150
    intracellular Ca^{++} flux, 150
    keratin in, 66
    markers of, 150–151
    maturation, 152
    role, 255
Paracellular permeability, 59, 127
Parkinson's disease, 204
PDX, 8–9, 29
    expression, 8, 29, 94
    role, 94–95
Pepsinogen, 5, 83, 261
    development of, 248–249
    secretion, 262
    stimulants of, 262
Pepsinogen promoter, 88
Pepsins, 261–262
Pepsin activity, 237
Pepsin secretion, 237
Peptidases, 249
Peptidoglycans, 253
Peptides, 152–153
    antibiotics, 148, 149
    function, 153
    neurotransmitters, 214
    in phagocytes, 153
    phylogeny, 153
    structure, 153
Peptide transport, 135
Peptide YY, 214, 221
Peptococcus, 281
Peptostreptococcus, 281
Peripheral nervous system, 197–199
    sympathoadrenal, 199
    sympathoenteric, 199
Peristalsis, 197, 215
Perlecan, 86, 87, 90
    deposition, 92
    in inflammatory bowel disease, 94
Peroxidases
    in human milk, 235–236

Peyer's patches, 75, 165–169, 182–189
    in B cells, 168
    blasts, 165
    development, 167–169
    immune responses in, 176
    in T cells, 168
Phenylalanine hydroxylase (PAH), 28
Phospholipase, 150–151, 152
Phospholipid kinases, 76
Phosphorylation, 16, 104
    keratins, 61, 64
Plasma cells, 177
    precursors, 186
Plasma membrane lipids, 127
Plasmin, 46
Pleurocidin, 153
Polarization, 1, 7
Polyadenylation, 180
Polyoma enhancer motifs, 62
Polysaccharidases, 247
Postprandial motor response, 221–222
    activity modulators, 214
Pre-B lymphocytes, 178
Pre-propeptides, 155
Preinitiation complex, 14
Proglucagon gene
    expression, 25
Prolactase, 116
Prolactin, 228–229
Proline transport, 125
Promoter elements, 14, 104
Proptides, 155
Prostaglandins, 252
    role of, 250
Proteases, 265–266
Protease E, 265
Protein digestibility, 237–238
    in formula, 239
    in human milk, 238
Protein digestion, 262
Protein function, 103–105
Protein intake in infants, 238–240
    higher intake and morbidity, 238
Protein kinase, 76–75
Protein kinase C, 97
Protein requirements, 238–240
Proteoglycans, 84
Proteolytic activity, 248
Protofibrils, 60
Protofilaments, 60
Proximodistal cytodifferentiation, 87–88
Pseudomonas, 281, 282
    septicemia, 285
Pulmonary hemorrhage, 89
Pyloric atresia, 93

Rabs, 74
    expression, 74
    function, 74
Ras activation, 97
Rectum, 5
Recycling receptors, 75
Regionalization, 95
Regulatory networks, 14
Rennin, 261
Repressors, 16
RET receptor, 203, 204
c-RET, 199, 203–205
    downregulation, 207
    expression, 200, 203, 205
    mutations, 203–204
c-RET mRNA, 203
Retinoic acid, 62, 92
Retinoids, 62
Rhabditin granules, 294
Ribonucleic acid (RNA) polymerase, 13–14
Ribosomal RNA, 13
RNA synthesis
    differential splicing, 104, 180
    initiation of, 104
mRNA
    steady-state, 249
    transport of, 104
y^+ mRNA, 135
Ruminococcus, 282, 284

Salmonella, 286
Scaffold-associated regions (SAR), 17
β-Scaffold factors, 19
Secretagogues, 264
Secretin, 25

Secretory component, 75
Septicemia, 285
Serine-threonine kinase receptors, 47
Serum albumin
  in breast milk, 227, *228*, *233*, 234
  in colostrum, *228*
  function, *232*
SGLT mRNA, 135
SGLT protein, 135
Short bowel syndrome, 315
  acquired, 139
  congenital, 140
Short-chain fatty acids (SCFA), 138
Signaling molecule, 5, *295*
Signaling pathway, 296, 303
Silencers, 14
  definition, 14
Sjögren's syndrome, 189
Skin blistering, 89
Skin-blistering disease, 61
Smads, 47
Small intestine
  bacterial load, 147
  defensin gene expression in, *156*
  development, 106–107
  disorders, 222
  fasting motor activity, 220–221
  formation, *7*
  innate immunity in, 147–159
  lactase-phlorizin expression, 115–116
  LPH mRNA expression, 115–116
  maturation, 106
  motility, 218–222
  sucrase-isomaltase in, 106–107
Small-intestinal endoderm, 88
Smooth muscle, 25–27
  development, 213
  differentiation, 2–3
  disorders, 222
  electrical slow wave, 213
  formation, 7–9, 201
  origin, 1
Smooth muscle myosin, 26
Sodium
  electrochemical gradient, 127
Sodium transport, 45
Solvent drag, 127
Somatostatin, 214
Somatostatin genes
  regulation, 29
Somite, 5
Somitic mesoderm, 4
Sonic hedgehog, 5–9, 40, 96, 301
  as activator of HOXD, 5
  activators of, 7
  and BMP expression, 7
  misexpression, 7
SOX, *18*, 206–207
Sp1, 22
Spectrin, 57
Sphincter formation, 25
Splanchnic mesenchyme, 1, 84
  differentiation, 2
Splanchnic mesoderm, 1–3
Splicosomes, 104
Spot desmosome, 58–59, 66
Staphylococcus, 280, 282, 283
  bacterial counts, *280*
  breastfed vs bottlefed, *283*
  septicemia, 285
Starch digestion, 247
Starch supplements, 270
Stem cells, 57, 177–178, 307
  fetal, 181
  lymphoid, 178
Stomach, 216–218
  contractile activity, 217
  fasting motor activity, 217, 221
Streptococcus, 280
  septicemia, 285
Stromelysin, 40
Sucking, 214
  nutritive/non-nutritive, 214
Suckling
  response to, 130
Suckling-to-weaning transition, 136
Sucrase, 5
  detection, *84*
  development, 83
  expression, 93

Sucrase activity
  changes in, 38
  EGF and, 45–46
  fetal, 247
Sucrase gene, 88
Sucrase mRNA induction, 38
Sucrase-isomaltase, 104–115
  activity, 38, 104–105
  expression of, 105–109
  regulation of, 105–115
Sucrase-isomaltase footprint, 111
Sucrase-isomaltase gene, 22, 137
  regulation of, *114*
Sucrase-isomaltase mRNA, 105, 113
  transcriptional initiation, 113
Sucrose-isomaltase
  synthesis, 109
Sudden infant death syndrome, 286
Sugar transport, 124, 131
  mechanisms of, 134–135
  regulation, 135
Swallowing, 214
Systemic hormones, 308
Systemic lupus erythematosus, 189

T Cell apoptosis, 39–40
T Cells
  activation antigens, 166
  composition of, 165
  development of, 172
  in fetal intestine, 171–172
  in fetal lamina propria, 165–167
  markers, *166*
  "natural," 167
T-Cell receptors, 167, 169–172
  lineages, 169
  repertoire, 169–170
  variability, 169
T-Cell receptor enhancer, *16*
T Helper cells
  classification, 181
T Lymphocytes, 165–172, 175–179
  IgA regulation, 176
  migration, 175
  stimulation, 189
  switch, 182
TATA binding protein, 14
  associated factors, 14
Taurine transport, 132
Taurocholate transport, 38
Telokin expression, 26
Temporal "memory," 308
Tenascin, 91, 94
Terminal deoxynucleotidal transferase (Tdt), 180–181
Terminal web, 57–59
  assembly, 57–58
  ultrastructure, 58
TGF binding protein, 46
TGF gene, 44, 46
TGF receptors, 46–47
TGF signaling, 47
Thrombospondin, 46
Thymic precursors, 48
Thyroid hormones, 39–40
  biochemistry, 39
  intestinal development and, 39–40
  receptors, 40
  structure, 39
Thyroid hormone receptors, 39
Thyroid stimulating hormone (TSH), 39, 40
Thyroid, 8
Thyroxine (T4), 39
Timing mechanisms, 308
α-Tocopherol, *252*
Tonofilaments, 57
Trachea, ventralization of, 8
Tracheo-esophageal fistula, 8
Transcobalamin II
  in human milk, 236
Transcortin, 37
Transcription factors, 13–19
  bound to promoter elements, 14
  classification, 17–19
  gene regulation and, 27–31
  subregions, *18*
  TRANS-FAC database, 18
Transcription initiation, 13–14
Transcriptional initiation, 104–105
Transcriptional regulation, 118–119

Transcriptomes, 104
Transepithelial transport, 75
Transferrin
  transcytosis, 76
  uptake, 72
Transferrin mRNA, 229
Transforming growth factor (TGF), 30, 44–48
  biologic actions, 47–48
  biologic effect, 45
  deficiency, 48
  distribution, 44
  immune system and, 48
  overexpression, 48
  wound healing, 48
Transgenes, 26
Transport gradient, 132
Trefoil factor (mTFF), 149
Trefoil factors family, 83
Trehalase activity
  EGF and, 45–46
  fetal, 247
Triglycerides, 249
  hydrolysis of, 249, 263
  as source of energy, 263
Triiodothyronine (T3), 39
  hydrocortisone with, 62
Tropomyosin, 57, 59
Truncated proteins, 17
Trypsin, 265
  development of, *267*
  inactivation, 284
Trypsin-catalyzed proteolysis, 266
Trypsinogen
  activation, 265
  development, 265
Tryptophan, 239–240
TSH receptor, 40
Tufting enteropathy, 94
Tumor suppressor genes, 47
Turnover number, 127–128
Tyrosine hydroxylase, 201
Tyrosine kinase, 42, 44, 213
Tyrosine kinase receptors, 40, 84, 213

Ulcerative colitis, 150, 190
Urinary tract infection, 285

Vaccination, 186–188
Vagus nerve, 212
Vasoactive intestinal peptide, 214
Veillonella, 281
  bacterial counts, *280*
Villin, 57–59
Villus, 20, 21
  formation, 64
Villus cells,
  structure, 57, 66
Vimentin
  phosphorylation of, 61
Virulence factors, 284, 285
Vitamin B_{12}
  absorption, 236
  in human milk, 236
Vitamin B_{12} binding capacity
  of colostrum, *228*, 236
  of human milk, *228*, 236
Vitamins
  uptake, 72
Vitellogenin gene, 30
Volatile fatty acids, 255

Weaning, 308
  delayed, 246
  glucose transport, 131
  premature, 246
Whey proteins, 227–233
WNT, 5, 30
Wortmannin, 76

Xenopus, 39–40

Zebrafish, 301–303
  GI tract development, 301–302
  organ-specific markers, 302
Zinc fingers, 18, 30
Zinc finger-type nuclear receptor class, 21
Zonula adherens, 58
Zonula occludens, 58
Zymogen granules, 265, 268